Neuro-Ophthalmology
A Practical Text

Neuro-Ophthalmology
A Practical Text

Nancy M. Newman, MD
San Francisco, California

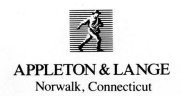

APPLETON & LANGE
Norwalk, Connecticut

92 93 94 95 96 / 10 9 8 7 6 5 4 3 2 1

Prentice Hall International (UK) Limited, *London*
Prentice Hall of Australia Pty. Limited, *Sydney*
Prentice Hall Canada, Inc., *Toronto*
Prentice Hall Hispanoamericana, S.A., *Mexico*
Prentice Hall of India Private Limited, *New Delhi*
Prentice Hall of Japan, Inc., *Tokyo*
Simon & Schuster Asia Pte. Ltd., *Singapore*
Editora Prentice Hall do Brasil Ltda., *Rio de Janeiro*
Prentice Hall, *Englewood Cliffs, New Jersey*

Library of Congress Cataloging-in-Publication Data
Newman, Nancy M., 1941–
    Neuro-ophthalmology : a practical text / Nancy M. Newman.
        p.   cm.
    Includes bibliographical references.
    ISBN 0-8385-6698-7
    1. Neuroophthalmology.   I. Title.
    [DNLM: 1. Eye—innervation.   2. Eye Diseases.   3. Nervous System
    Diseases—complications.   WW 101 N554n]
    RE725.N496   1991
    617.7—dc 20
    DNLM/DLC   91-22414
    for Library of Congress   CIP

Production Assistant: Sasha Kintzler
Designer: Michael J. Kelly

PRINTED IN THE UNITED STATES OF AMERICA

ISBN 0-8385-6698-7

9 780838 566985

90000

CONTENTS

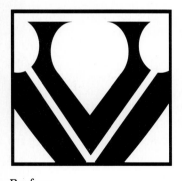

PREFACE

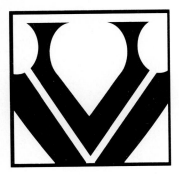

The visual sense *is* of paramount importance for most people; nearly a third of all afferent sensory input is visual. If the neural processes concerned with the control of eye movements are included, close to eighty percent of the brain is occupied with vision and related functions.

This book attempts to explore neuro-ophthalmology in a reasonably complete manner. It is a pragmatic clinical guide to neuro-ophthalmic disorders presented with a framework of basic scientific information. No attempt has been made to be exhaustive. The book is liberally laced with decision trees, tables, and bibliographic references so that, given a patient's complaint, symptoms, or findings, the reader may quickly move to the differential diagnosis, office and laboratory evaluation, and then treatment of the patient.

This work is intended to provide the basis for the highest quality care of the patient with a neuro-ophthalmic problem and/or medical problem that presents in a neuro-ophthalmic context. The bibliography for each chapter has been chosen to complement the text with references to more inclusive works (which will provide more complete bibliographic references), recent, especially pertinent or substantive citations, and a few particularly thoughtful or provocative titles. For details, please consult these works (to which the author is indebted also).

Even a single-authored volume is really dependent on the help and support of many "significant others," and for their contributions and unfailing support I gratefully thank: my parents, family, and friends; my mentors—Arthur Jampolsky, who pointed out the fascination of neuro-ophthalmology to a premed student at a time when barely a half dozen people considered themselves neuro-ophthalmologists, and Bernard Becker, Andy Gay, and the incomparable William F. Hoyt—all of whom provided sterling examples and intellectual challenge; my many colleagues for their comments and suggestions that helped to make this book better than it otherwise might have been*; my residents and staff, especially ophthalmic technicians, Alita Soon, Mary Wu, and Kathy Jones, and ophthalmic photographers Mary Federico and Michael Coppinger, who helped me continue to learn from my patients; my patients and their doctors who referred them to me; my editors; and, very specially, my secretary, Frank Collier, without whom this book would never have been finished.

---

* Again, especially William F. Hoyt, Dick Mills, Dick Sogg, Neil Miller, and Stephen Geiser; also, Bob Nelson, David Rodgers, John Heckenlively, Jim Corbett, David Zee, Mort Goldberg, Creig Hoyt, Klara Landau, Wayne Cornblauth, and Dick Weleber.

Section I
The Visual Afferent System

CHAPTER 1

THE VISUAL AFFERENT PATHWAYS
ANATOMIC CONSIDERATIONS

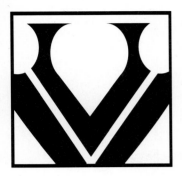

The eye is the paramount sense organ of the body, detecting the first threat of danger, the first stirring of the quarry, a veritable window on the world, open to information from afar, discerning the tiniest motes dancing in a sunbeam, discriminating the transient hues of a fleeting rainbow. Safe in their deep bony orbits, reposing on a cushion of fat, protected by the curtaining eyelids and moistened by glistening tears, the eyeballs move in conjunction, each with six slender muscles directing the intent gaze upon the object of suspicion or curiosity.

Lockhart

The eye develops as an outpouching of the brain (Fig. 1–1). Its pathology and physiology are like those of the central nervous system; it is one of the primary sense organs and the retina is its primary sensory element. The other ocular structures are the supportive and nutritive elements necessary for maintenance and function of the retina. The sclera is a structural and protective coating; the pigment epithelium, vascular choroid, and blood vessels are nutritive; the cornea, lens, and their accessory structures are the optics; and the aqueous and vitreous provide protective support, flux of nutrients, and optical access.

THE VISUAL PROCESS

The visual process begins as light rays enter the eye through the cornea; pass through the aqueous, lens, and vitreous; and strike the retina. The optical system, primarily the lens and cornea, acts to focus the image as does the lens of a camera. The focused image is reversed on the retina, both right to left and up to down (Fig. 1–2). If the eye is too long for its focusing power, the images form anterior to the retina and the patient is nearsighted (myopic); if too short, the image is focused behind the retina and the patient is farsighted (hyperopic). If the cornea is not perfectly spherical, light is refracted differently in various meridians, causing astigmatism.

THE RETINA

Classically, the retina is said to have 10 layers (Fig. 1–3). From innermost to outermost, they are the (1) internal limiting membrane, (2) nerve fiber layer, (3) ganglion cell layer, (4) inner plexiform layer, (5) inner nuclear layer, (6) outer plexiform layer, (7) outer nuclear layer, (8) external limiting membrane, (9) receptor elements (rods and cones), and (10) retinal pigment epithelium.

The three nuclear layers (3, 5, and 7) contain cell bodies, whereas most synapses occur in the plexiform layers (4 and 6). The retinal pigment epithelium is critical in the catabolic metabolism of the

Figure 1–1. The eye forms as an outpouching of the central nervous system. (The formation of the optic vesicle and cup in a 4-mm human embryo.) (*From Miller N, ed.* Walsh and Hoyt's Clinical Neuro-ophthalmology. *4th ed. Baltimore: Williams & Wilkins, 1982; 1; with permission.*)

3

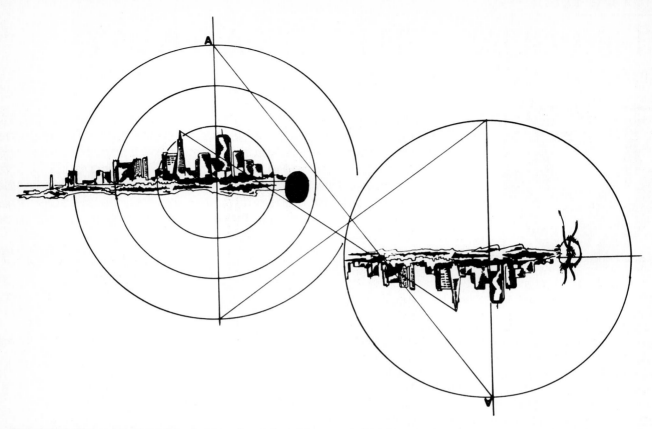

Figure 1–2. Diagrammatic portrayal of how the optics of the eye project the scene viewed onto the retina (reversed and upside-down).

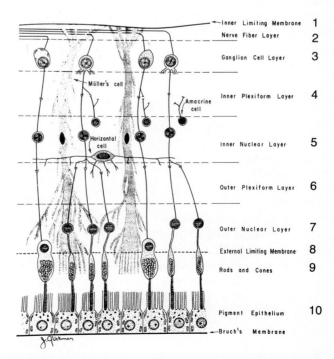

Figure 1–3. Layers of the retina. Diagram of neurons and glia within the retina based on a drawing by T. Kuwabara. (*Adapted from Cogan D. Neurology of the Visual System. Springfield, IL: Thomas, 1967, with permission.*)

photoreceptors; it ingests and disposes of their shed outer segments and facilitates their continued renewal. Uniquely, the glial Müller cells traverse the entire retina from the internal limiting membrane to the external limiting membrane. They provide the architectural skeleton and physiologic support of the neural cells.

The **receptors** (rods and cones) absorb much of the incident light that transverses the retina. The subsequent bleaching and isomerization of the receptor visual pigments, rhodopsin (rods) and iodopsin (cones), is the first step in the transduction of light energy into the electric energy of neural excitation. The receptor mechanism is exquisitely sensitive, responding to only a few quanta of light. As sensory organs, the rods and cones are analogous to the peripheral sensory endings (eg, pacinian corpuscles) of the other sensory pathways.

The *cones*, color- and light-sensitive receptors, are located primarily in the central retina, outnumbering rods in the macula and exclusively occupying the fovea. They are small and tightly organized, providing for a high order of visual discrimination. Because they are small in size and contain minimal

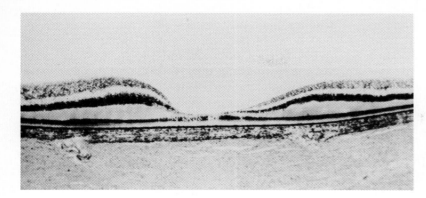

Figure 1–4. Cross section at the posterior pole of the eye including the macular and paramacular regions of the retina. Noteworthy is the attenuation of all the retinal layers, except the photoreceptors, in the center of the macula. (*From Cogan D. Ophthalmic Manifestations of Systemic Vascular Disease. Vol 2 in: Smith LH, ed.* Major Problems in Internal Medicine. *Philadelphia: Saunders, 1974, with permission.*)

visual pigment, however, they have a high threshold to stimulation. *Rods* are more important in peripheral vision and in low illumination. Because rods have a large amount of visual pigment relative to cones and many intracellular connections, they are more sensitive. Thus, the cones yield high visual acuity under photopic (well lit) conditions; the rods are more sensitive in scotopic (dimly lit) conditions, but discriminate poorly.

Many types of retinal cells, for example the A2 cell, which received input from both rods and cones, are being newly investigated and characterized. Their functional organization and roles are incompletely understood.

The **ganglion cells** form a layer with maximal thickness and density (8 to 10 layers) in the parafoveal macula, but are absent from the fovea itself (Fig. 1–4). This facilitates acute vision as the light rays traverse fewer retinal layers. With increased distance from the fovea, ganglion cell density decreases and dendritic field size increases.

Morphologically, the *ganglion cells fall into three categories.* The largest group (80%) are cells with small bodies that usually give rise to one dendrite (but occasionally yield two or three). These cells project to the dorsal layers, the parvocellular layers, of the lateral geniculate body (layers 1 to 4). These ganglion cells respond linearly to appropriate stimulation and show high resolution and color sensitivity. They have been termed P-beta or B cells in primates (somewhat analogous to X cells in cats), and are thought to participate in tasks requiring fine discrimination.

Another group of small-bodied ganglion cells is the group called P-gamma, C, or W cells, which constitutes 10% of the ganglion cells and which projects to the superior colliculus (SC) with a collateral projection to the lateral geniculate body. These cells have slow conduction velocities and sluggish responses.

TABLE 1–1. MAJOR SUBDIVISIONS AND CONNECTIONS OF THE PRIMATE GENICULOCORTICAL VISUAL SYSTEM

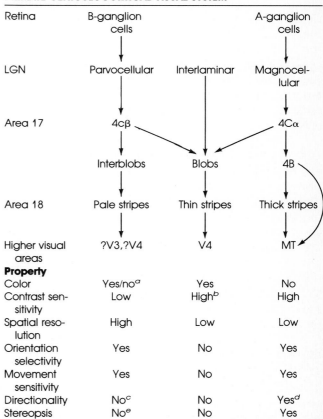

Retina	B-ganglion cells		A-ganglion cells
LGN	Parvocellular	Interlaminar	Magnocellular
Area 17	4cβ		4Cα
	Interblobs	Blobs	4B
Area 18	Pale stripes	Thin stripes	Thick stripes
Higher visual areas	?V3,?V4	V4	MT
Property			
Color	Yes/no[a]	Yes	No
Contrast sensitivity	Low	High[b]	High
Spatial resolution	High	Low	Low
Orientation selectivity	Yes	No	Yes
Movement sensitivity	Yes	No	Yes
Directionality	No[c]	No	Yes[d]
Stereopsis	No[e]	No	Yes

[a] Cells beyond 4Cβ do respond to color-contrast borders but are not overtly color-coded.
[b] By deoxyglucose.
[c] At least it is not prominent.
[d] Rare in thick stripes in area 18 but very common in layer 4B of area 17 and in MT.
[e] In anesthetized animals, we have seen only a few stereotuned cells in upper layer area 17. In attentive animals, cells coded for stereoscopic depth have been reported both above and below layer 4C of area 17, but are especially concentrated in layer 4B. We do not understand these differences in results, but one possibility is that the stereo mechanisms are built up in 18, and the stereotuning in 17 is the result of a back projection that is suppressed by anesthesia.
From Livingstone M, Hubel D. J. Neurosci. 1987;7:3420, with permission.

The third group of ganglion cells, also forming about 10% of the total population, is the group called M or A cells in primates (roughly analogous to Y cells in cats). These cells have large cell bodies and project to the magnocellular layers of the lateral geniculate body (layers 5 and 6); some also project to the superior colliculus. These cells give fast, short-lasting, nonlinear, broad-based, achromatic responses. They are very sensitive to low contrast and flicker; they have low acuity in contrast to P-beta (B, X) cells and are thought to encode movement.

Each ganglion cell type seems to have its own pattern of projection via parallel visual channels, each relaying information about different aspects of vision (see Table 1–1).

The **retinal nerve fiber layer** consists of ganglion cell axons that course radially toward the optic disc (Fig. 1–5). These are the tertiary neurons of the visual pathway. Bundles of axons pass toward the optic nerve within tunnels formed by the processes of the Müller cells and astrocytes (Fig. 1–6). As the retinal nerve fiber layer and optic disc, the anterior visual pathway is visible to the examiner as is no other part of the central nervous system (CNS).

Axonal Transport. Within neurons, retrograde and anterograde axoplasmic flow transports materials to and from the cell bodies. As all cellular proteins are produced in the cell body, this bidirectional traffic furnishes nutrition and building blocks to the far-flung cell processes, the axons and dendrites. Transmitter substances, viruses, cell organelles, and poisons are also transported by axonal flow. In fact, the access of some viruses and toxins (herpes, polio, tetanus) to the CNS is by retrograde axoplasmic flow. Some substances are even transported transsynaptically. When disease or mechanical factors slow axoplasmic flow, the dammed-up axoplasm causes neuronal swelling on either side of the damaged area. In the retina, these swollen cells show microscopically as cytoid bodies. Larger areas of axoplasmic stasis appear ophthalmoscopically as cotton-wool spots, confluent retinal whitening, and papilledema.

The Fovea and Macula

The fovea and macula are specialized retinal areas aligned with the optic axis of the eye; they subserve the finest visual acuity of any part of the eye. The discriminating capacity of the fovea determines the best possible visual acuity. The retina is thinnest at the fovea, where no blood vessels or ganglion cells overlie the photoreceptors (Figs. 1–7 and 1–4).

THE OPTIC DISC AND OPTIC NERVE

The fibers of the ganglion cells exit the globe at the optic disc (optic papilla, optic nerve head) to form the optic nerve. The optic nerve consists of four parts: (1) the ocular portion (1.5 mm), which transverses the sclera; (2) the orbital portion (40

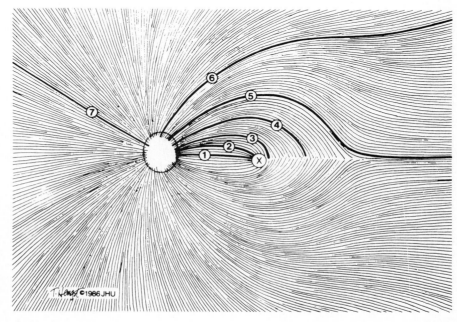

Figure 1–5. Schematic drawing of the pattern of nerve fibers in the retina. The **X** indicates the location of the fovea. Representative fiber pathways are highlighted with bold lines. 1. Nasal macular fiber originating near the horizontal meridian. 2. Nasal macular fiber originating a short distance above the horizontal meridian. 3. Perpendicular fiber. 4. Oblique fiber. 5. Fiber originating in the peripheral retina temporal to the fovea near the horizontal meridian (temporal raphé). 6. Fiber originating in the peripheral retina temporal to the fovea away from the horizontal meridian. 7. Fiber originating nasal to the optic disc. (*From Miller N, Pollock SC. The retinal nerve fiber layer. In: Beck R, ed. Int Ophthalmol Clin. 1986;26:207, with permission.*)

mm), which leads to (3) the canalicular portion, which passes through the optic canal; and (4) the intracranial portion, which joins its counterpart from the opposite side to form the optic chiasm. Within the orbit, the optic nerve is not tethered. Thus, because its length exceeds the distance from the optic canal to the eyeball, it has a sinuous course that allows for considerable excursion as the globe moves.

Because the eye is an embryologic outpouching of the forebrain, in reality the **optic nerve** is an externalized white-matter tract of the CNS. As it exits the globe, it becomes myelinated and is invested with vaginal sheaths, which through the optic canal are continuous with the meninges of the CNS (Fig. 1–8). The optic nerve sheaths similarly are composed of pia, arachnoid, and dura. The dura is continuous with the periorbita in the orbital apex. At the globe, it splays out to insert onto the sclera surrounding the optic nerve. The pia invests the optic nerve itself. Characteristic mesodermal septa of pia carry an intricate supply of blood vessels into the tissues of the optic nerve. The arachnoid ends at the sclera. It contains the cerebrospinal fluid, which is in continuity with that of the CNS. This relationship is important in the effects of intracranial pressure on the optic nerve head.

The nerve itself contains two tissue compartments: the **neuroectodermal compartment,** with the nerve tissue proper, neurons, and neuroglia; and the **mesodermal compartment,** with the supporting and nourishing tissues—the blood vessels, fibroblasts,

and meningothelial cells. These form orderly layers in which the neural elements are completely embedded in a glial cover; the glia in turn contacts the mesodermal elements that surround and form the blood vessels (Fig. 1–9).

At the optic disc, nerve fibers make up 90% of the optic nerve tissue; more posteriorly, nerve fibers still form the largest contribution to the optic nerve, but they are joined by a larger proportion of astrocytes. At the level of the sclera, the nerve fibers run through the collagenous tissue sheets of the lamina cribrosa.

The **lamina cribrosa** is a specialized, sieve-like region of scleral trabeculae through which the nerve fibers exit the eye (Fig. 1–10). Although these scleral trabeculae are relatively inert, many relationships critical to the integrity of the nerve occur in this region:

1. The nerve leaves the eye and its intraocular pressure and becomes invested with myelin and vaginal sheaths.
2. As the fibers acquire myelin, the nerve doubles in size from 1.5 to 3 mm (occasionally the myelin continues through the lamina as myelinated nerve fibers in the retina—see page 100).
3. In the orbit, the nerve is subject to the combined influences of orbital pressure and intracranial pressure (transmitted through the optic nerve sheaths).

With increased intraocular pressure, the lamina becomes physically distorted and bowed backwards,

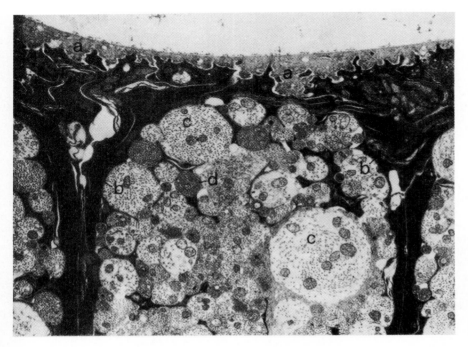

Figure 1–6. Nerve fiber layer of the retina. Two Müller cells (*top corners*) partly form the inner limiting membrane. Their radial fibers enclose bundles of nerves (×4000). (*From Hogan M, Alvarado J, Waddell J. Histology of the Human Eye: An Atlas and Textbook. Philadelphia: Saunders, 1971, with permission.*)

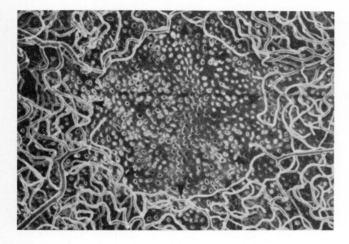

Figure 1–7. Retinal vascular organization in the fovea. Scanning electron micrograph shows the capillary-free zone of the fove-ola. (*From Miller N, ed. Walsh and Hoyt's Clinical Neuro-ophthalmology. 4th ed. Baltimore: Williams & Wilkins, 1982; 1; with permission.*)

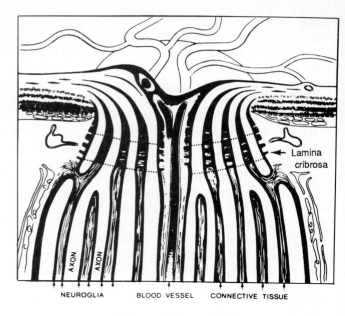

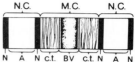

Figure 1–9. Layers of optic nerve. The intraorbital optic nerve is divided into two tissue compartments, neuroectodermal and mesodermal. In the neuroectodermal (*NC*) compartment, the axons (*A*) are surrounded by neuroglia (*N*). The neuroglial cells are in contact with the mesodermal compartment (*MC*) in which connective tissue (*cf*) surrounds the blood vessels (*BV*). (*From Newman NM. The Prechiasmal Visual Afferent Pathways. In: Clinical Neuro-ophthalmology: the Afferent Visual System. Karpe, J. and Burde, RM (eds.) Boston: Little, Brown, 1977, with permission.*)

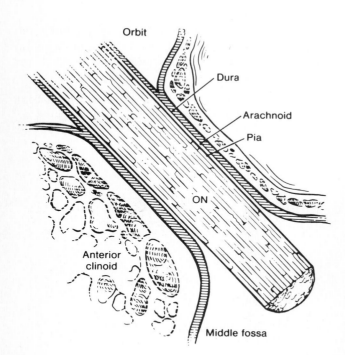

Figure 1–8. Schematic drawing of the optic nerve sheaths showing their relationship to the optic nerve (*ON*) and to the surrounding sphenoid bone. The dura is tightly adherent to the bone within the optic canal. Within the orbit it divides into two layers, one of which remains as the outer sheath of the optic nerve, and the other becomes the orbital periosteum (*periorbita*). Intracranially, the dura leaves the optic nerve to become the periosteum of the sphenoid bone. (*From Miller N, ed. Walsh and Hoyt's Clinical Neuro-ophthalmology. 4th ed. Baltimore: Williams & Wilkins, 1982; 1; with permission.*)

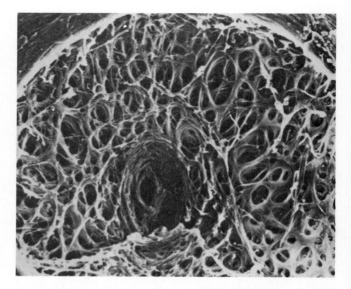

Figure 1–10. Scanning electron micrograph of the scleral laminar region viewed from the vitreous cavity. (*From Miller N, ed. Walsh and Hoyt's Clinical Neuro-ophthalmology. 4th ed. Baltimore: Williams & Wilkins, 1982; 1; with permission.*)

perhaps contributing to the nerve fiber damage in glaucoma (Fig. 1–11).

With many types of optic nerve insult, axoplasmic flow is blocked at the lamina cribrosa; the cellular organelles and axoplasm dam up, causing the clinical picture of disc swelling. It does not seem to make much difference whether the pathologic process is an increase in intracranial pressure, an increase in intraocular pressure, a decrease in intraocular pressure, or other insult to the optic nerve. Optic neuritis, optic neuropathies, optic nerve tumors, and vascular pathology all cause axoplasmic stasis at the lamina cribrosa. The ophthalmoscopic manifestation is a swollen disc.

The optic nerve fibers include predominantly visual fibers that project to the lateral geniculate body and pupillary fibers destined for the pretectal nuclei of the upper brain stem. About 10% of fibers are centrifugal fibers possibly involved in vascular regulation or modulation of neurologic function within the retina. In addition, some optic nerve fibers project to accessory visual pathways, which pass to the supraoptic nuclei, pulvinar nucleus, and superior colliculus. The functions of the centrifugal and accessory neurons are not well understood.

Thus, there are three main retinal ganglion cell outflows: those to the lateral geniculate body (mostly visual neurons), those to the pretectum (mostly pupillary neurons), and those to the superior colliculus and the accessory optic paths. In addition, there is a number of retinotopically organized but functionally distinct subcortical relays that form parallel and independent pathways from the retina to the visual cortex and the retinohypothalamic path to the supraoptic nuclei.

The **retinogeniculate path** (the VAP) is by far the largest projection. In addition, about 10% of ganglion cell axons (mostly the W type) conveys retinotopic information to the superior colliculus. Other input to the superior colliculus comes from the primary visual cortex. Outputs from the superior colliculus are to the pulvinar and to the tectospinal tract. These may function in adjusting eye and body positions in respect to the outer world. Projections to nuclei in the prectum (rostral brain stem) appear to deal with vestibulo-ocular and optokinetic reflexes. The **accessory optic tract** projects to the mesencephalon near the substantia nigra and pretectal area and appears to act to stabilize the retinal image.

Within the optic nerve, the ganglion cell fibers assume positions dependent on their origin in the retina. The nasal macular fibers pass directly to the disc as the papillomacular bundle and form a large part of the temporal portion of the optic nerve. In general, fibers from peripheral ganglion cells are peripheral in the optic disc and in the optic nerve,

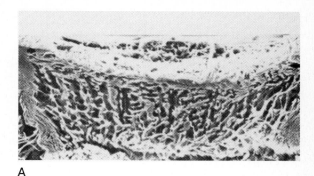

A

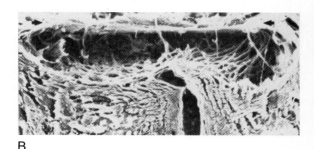

B

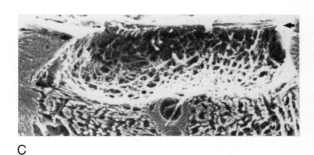

C

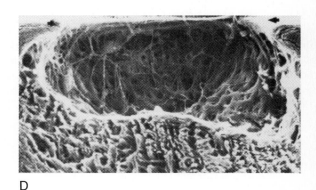

D

Figure 1–11. Bowed lamina cribrosa associated with optic nerve damage in human glaucoma. A series of lamina digests illustrates progressive posterolateral extension of floor of nerve head with increasing glaucoma damage. **A.** Normal adult. **B, C.** Moderately severe glaucoma. **D.** Blind glaucomatous eye. Note that the width of the scleral canal at the level of Bruch's membrane remains constant. ×80. (*From Quigley HA, Addicks EM, Green WR, Maumenee AE. Optic nerve damage in human glaucoma. Arch Ophthalmol 1981;99:635–649, with permission.*)

whereas fibers from more central ganglion cells exit into the central part of the nerve (Fig. 1–12), although recent studies in the cat show axons from adjacent ganglion cells can take divergent routes. Throughout the nervous system, superior visual fibers remain superior, and inferior fibers remain inferior; in the distal optic nerve, nasal fibers remain nasal and the temporal fibers remain temporal. As the nerve progresses toward the chiasm, the fibers from the papillomacular bundle move more centrally and in the posterior orbit occupy the central core of the optic nerve (Fig. 1–13).

Orbital Optic Nerve

In the orbit, the nerve lies within the muscle cone, cushioned in orbital fat, in turn protected by the bony walls of the orbit. It exits the orbit through the optic canal. Because the optic nerve may lose its bony protection and/or actually project into the ethmoid or sphenoid sinuses (Fig. 1–14), it is vulnerable to sinus infections, tumors, and trauma (especially basilar skull fractures and iatrogenic trauma in surgical procedures of the sinuses).

THE OPTIC CHIASM

The chiasmatic portion of the visual afferent path consists of the intracranial parts of the optic nerves, the optic chiasm, and the optic tracts. In the chiasm the neighboring fibers of each retina decussate or cross to the opposite side and become associated with the uncrossed temporal fibers from the opposite retina. The ratio of crossed to uncrossed fibers is 53:47. Thus, from the chiasm to the visual cortex the fibers of the visual path represent the ipsilateral halves of both retinas (but the contralateral visual fields!). The inferior ventral fibers move into the optic nerve of the opposite side, forming a "knee" known as Wilbrand's loop (Fig. 1–15; see also Chapter 2). The macular fibers decussate primarily in the

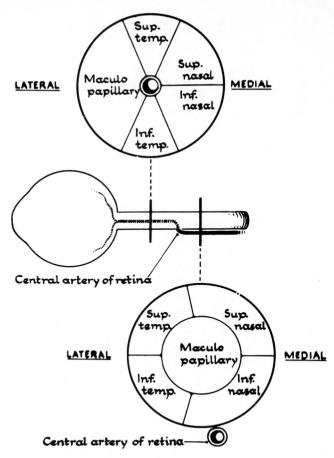

Figure 1–13. The arrangement of the nerve fibers in the optic nerve. (*From Reed H, Drance SM. The Essentials of Perimetry: Static and Kinetic. 2nd ed. London: Oxford, 1972, with permission.*)

posterior superior portion of the chiasm, and thus can be affected by dilation of the third ventricle, where the optic chiasm projects into the anterior ventricular floor between the chiasmatic and infundibular recesses (Fig. 1–16). Here, as in the subarachnoid space, it is bathed in CSF.

Anatomical Relationships

The chiasm is intimately related to many structures. It lies approximately 1 cm above the diaphragm sella, tilted at 45 degrees so that the anterior border is inferior to the posterior border (Fig. 1–17). The arterial circle of Willis is superior to the chiasm anteriorly and inferior to it posteriorly. Anteriorly the chiasm and the intracranial optic nerves receive their blood supply from the internal carotid arteries, anterior cerebral arteries, and anterior communicating artery, and even at times from more posterior portions of the circle of Willis.

The infundibular stalk passes posterior to the chiasm (Fig. 1–17) whereas the chiasm itself may

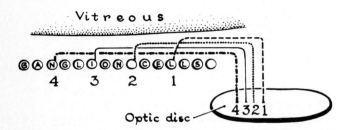

Figure 1–12. The relationship of the peripheral to the central nerve fibers in the retina and at the optic disc. (*From Reed H, Drance SM. The Essentials of Perimetry: Static and Kinetic. 2nd ed. London: Oxford, 1972, with permission.*)

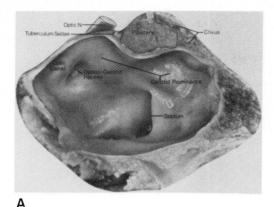

A

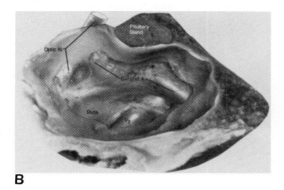

B

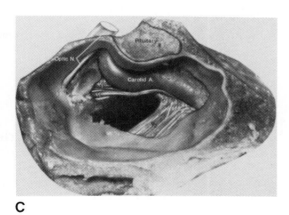

C

Figure 1–14. Stepwise dissection of the lateral wall of the right half of the sellar-type **sphenoid sinus** and adjacent structures. **A.** The sphenoid sinus and sellar area are divided in the midsagittal plane. The optic nerve is seen proximal to the optic canal. The opticocarotid recess separates the carotid prominence and the optic canal. The septum in the posterior part of the sinus is incomplete. **B.** The sinus mucosa and thin bone of the lateral sinus wall have been removed to expose the dura covering the carotid artery, the second trigeminal division (V2) just distal to the trigeminal ganglion, and the optic nerve. **C.** The dura has been opened to expose the carotid artery, optic nerve in the optic canal, second trigeminal division below the carotid artery, and abducens nerve (**VI**) between the first trigeminal division (V1) and the carotid artery. (*From Rhoton A Jr. Microsurgical anatomy of the sellar region. In: Wilkins R, Rengachary S, eds. Neurosurgery. New York: McGraw-Hill, 1985; 1; 811–821; with permission.*)

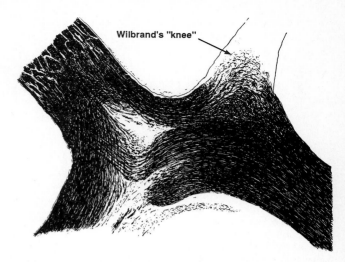

Figure 1–15. Wilbrand's "knee." (*From Polyak A. The Vertebrate Visual System. Chicago: University of Chicago Press, 1968, with permission.*)

vary somewhat in its position relative to the pituitary fossa. It may be prefixed, in normal position, or postfixed (Fig. 1–18). Therefore, the relative position of the chiasm in relation to tumors of the region accounts to some degree for the varied visual field defects associated with sellar and parasellar lesions. As mentioned above, the optic nerves may actually lie within the ethmoid or sphenoid sinuses as they approach the optic chiasm. The sphenoid sinus also has an important relationship with the carotid arteries, which frequently protrude into the sinus (Fig. 1–14).

THE OPTIC TRACT

The visual afferent fibers leave the posterior lateral aspect of the chiasm and form two diverging arms, the optic tracts, as they extend from the optic chiasm and proceed to the lateral geniculate body. Between the tracts lie the infundibulum and the cerebral peduncles (Fig. 1–19). Visual fibers from the corresponding portions of the two retinas are more closely associated here, prior to terminating on adjacent laminae in the lateral geniculate body. Thus, in the optic tracts, crossed and uncrossed visual fibers representing the entire hemifield of the opposite side are associated. Consequently, **all visual field defects resulting from lesions of the postchiasmal visual afferent pathways affect the opposite hemifield and cause homonymous hemianopias** (except for defects of the temporal crescent, page 44). The pupillary fibers leave the optic tracts before the lateral geniculate body and enter the superior brachium collicu-

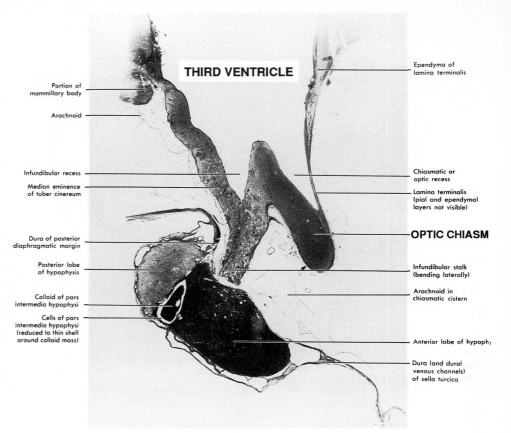

Figure 1-16. Exact midsagittal section through the chiasm and anterior part of the third ventricle (25 μm thickness). The infundibular stalk in this specimen deviates slightly laterally as it descends. It then angulates abruptly laterally (as seen on serial sections) before entering the posterior lobe. The distal part of the stalk is therefore here sectioned obliquely in a parasagittal plane and appears cut off from the hypophysis. (*From Rosenbaum AE, et al. Normal third ventrical. In: Newton TH, Potts DG, eds.* Radiology of the Skull and Brain. *St. Louis: Mosby, 1974; 4; with permission.*)

lus on their way to the posterior commissure and pretectal nuclei.

In the optic tracts, the orientation of the visual afferent pathways rotates nearly 90 degrees, such that the macular fibers that lie medially at the posterior aspect of the chiasm become more dorsal, the fibers from the inferior retinas come to lie laterally, and the superior fibers come to lie medially (Fig. 1–20).

THE LATERAL GENICULATE BODY

The first synapse of the retinal ganglion cell is in the lateral geniculate body (LGB). The lateral geniculate cell axons in turn project via the optic radiations to the visual cortex. The LGB is part of the thalamus, and its function as a neuronal relay station is similar to that of other thalamic nuclei, which relay somaesthetic impulses to the parietal cortex—for example, the medial geniculate bodies, which relay auditory information to the temporal lobe cortex. The optic tract fibers enter the anteroventral surface of the lateral geniculate body and the optic radiation fibers exit from its dorsolateral surface.

Each lateral geniculate body is triangular and striated in appearance, with six alternating gray and

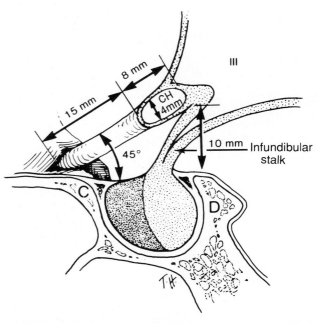

Figure 1–17. Infundibulum, chiasm. Relationships of the optic nerves and optic chiasm (CH) to the sellar structures and third ventricle (III). (C, anterior clinoid; D, dorsum sellae). (*From Miller N, ed.* Walsh and Hoyt's Clinical Neuro-ophthalmology. *4th ed. Baltimore: Williams & Wilkins, 1982; 1; with permission.*)

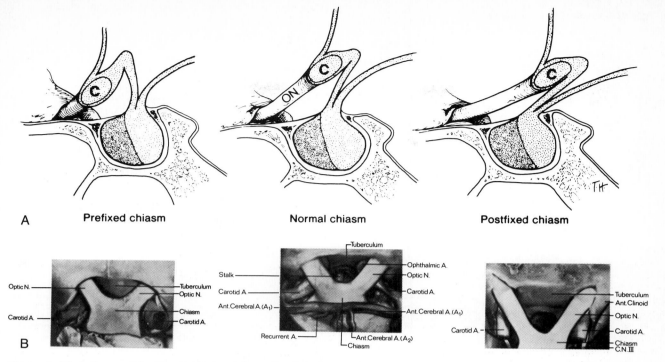

A Prefixed chiasm   Normal chiasm   Postfixed chiasm

B

Figure 1–18. A. Pre- and Postfixed chiasms. Schematic drawing of three sagittal sections of the optic chiasm and sellar region showing the positions of a prefixed chiasm above the tuberculum sellae (*left*), a normal chiasm above the diaphragma sellae (*center*), and a postfixed chiasm above the dorsum sellae (*right*). **B.** Superior view of the sellar region. *Left.* Prefixed chiasm. *Center.* Normal chiasm. The ophthalmic artery protrudes medial to the right optic nerve. The anterior cerebral arteries pass dorsal to the chiasm. The left recurrent artery arises from A₁ segment of the left anterior cerebral artery. The pituitary stalk lies between the optic nerves. *Right.* Postfixed chiasm. The diaphragma sellae and pituitary gland have been removed. Cranial nerve III lies ventral to the carotid artery. (*From Miller N, ed.* Walsh and Hoyt's Clinical Neuro-ophthalmology. *4th ed. Baltimore: Williams & Wilkins, 1982; 1; with permission.*)

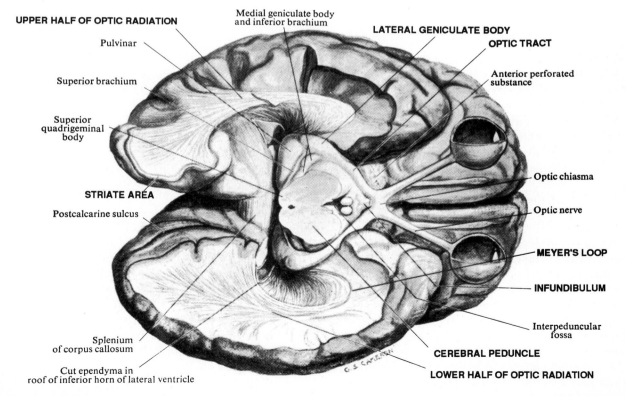

Figure 1–19. Cerebral hemisphere dissected from below showing the optic tracts surrounding the cerebral peduncles and infundibulum. On the right side (upper part of illustration) the dissection is carried further than on the left. (*From Lockhart RD, Hamilton GF, Fyfe FW.* Anatomy of the Human Body. *Philadelphia: Lippincott, 1959, with permission.*)

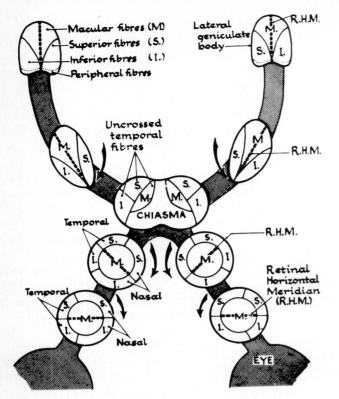

Figure 1–20. The rotation of the optic tracts. The nasal rotation of nerve fibers is shown very schematically. (*From Reed H, Drance SM. The Essentials of Perimetry: Static and Kinetic. London: Oxford, 1972, with permission.*)

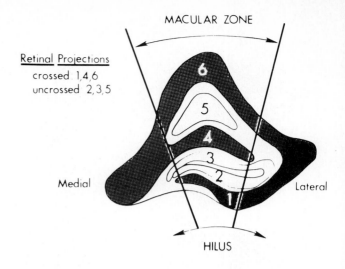

Figure 1–21. Coronal section of lateral geniculate nucleus. Note extensive macular representation. (*From Glaser J. Anatomy of the visual sensory system. In: Duane T, ed. Clinical Ophthalmology. Hagerstown, MD: Harper & Row, 1976; 2; with permission.*)

white layers. There are four dorsal layers of small cells (parvocellular layers) receiving axons of P-beta (B or X) retinal ganglion cells and two ventral layers of larger cells (magnocellular layers) receiving axons of P-alpha (A or Y) ganglion cells. Retinal fibers from the ipsilateral eye project to layers 2, 3, and 5; the contralateral eye projects to layers 1, 4, and 6. The apex of the lateral geniculate body carries the macular fibers, the lateral portion receives the inferior retinal fibers, and the medial portion the superior fibers (Fig. 1–21).

OPTIC RADIATION (GENICULO-CALCARINE TRACT)

The fibers of the last neuron of the primary visual afferent pathway emerge from the lateral geniculate body, traverse the internal capsule and head to the visual cortex, passing both above and below the posterior horn of the lateral ventricle. The fibers from the medial portion of the lateral geniculate body representing the upper retinas pass directly to the superior bank of the calcarine fissure on the medial aspect of the hemisphere. The fibers from the lateral

portion of the lateral geniculate body representing the inferior retinas course forward and outward in the roof of the descending horn of the lateral ventricle and loop around the anterior tip of the temporal horn (Meyer's loop); they are then directed posteriorly, as a thin curved sheet lateral to the posterior horn, to their termination in the inferior bank of the calcarine cortex (Fig. 1–19).

THE CALCARINE CORTEX

The occipital lobes form the posterior portions of the cerebral hemispheres. They are divided into three major segments: Brodmann areas 17, 18, and 19 (Fig. 1–22). The primary visual cortex is arrayed on the superior and inferior ridges of the calcarine cortex (striate cortex, V_1, area 17 of Brodmann). It extends medially in the intrahemispheric fissure to just beneath the corpus collosum. Laterally, the visual cortex extends approximately 1 to 2 cm onto the outer surface of the occipital lobe (Fig. 1–23). The total surface area included in the visual cortex varies from individual to individual. Yet consistently, nearly one half of the visual sensory cortex is devoted to the macular projections (Fig. 1–24).

The representation of the retina within the cortex is best visualized by imagining the posterior pole of the globe to overlie the ipsilateral cortex. The up-

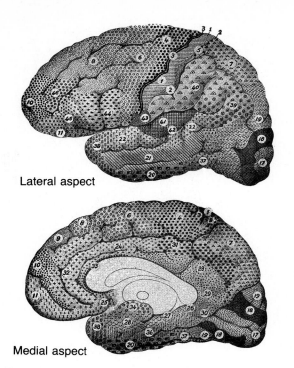

Figure 1–22. Primary visual cortex: 17. Striate area. 18. Parastriate area. 19. Peristriate area. (*From Duke-Elder A. System of Ophthalmology. London: H. Kimpton, 1961; 2; with permission.*)

Lateral aspect

Medial aspect

per retina corresponds to the upper bank of the calcarine cortex and the lower retina to the lower bank. The macula coincides with the posterior pole; the fovea is represented at the extreme tip of the occipital lobe and the peripheral nasal retina (represented by the uniocular temporal crescent of the visual field) represented by the medial anterior portion of the calcarine cortex within the intrahemispheric fissure, under the splenium of the corpus callosum (Fig. 1–25).

The **striate cortex** is divided into six laminae. The optic radiations terminate predominantly in layer IV. Axons from the parvocellular (dorsal) layers of the lateral geniculate body (where P-beta = x = B retinal ganglion cells project) arborize in sublayer IVc-beta and axons from the magnocellular (ventral) layers (where M = A = y retinal ganglion cells project) arborize in layer IVc-alpha.

On the basis of their receptive field properties, the cells of the visual cortex are classified into four groups by Hubel and Wiesel: circularly symmetric, simple, complex, and hypercomplex.

The **circularly symmetric cells** are similar in their properties to lateral geniculate and retinal cells. The **simple cells** respond to specific linear configu-

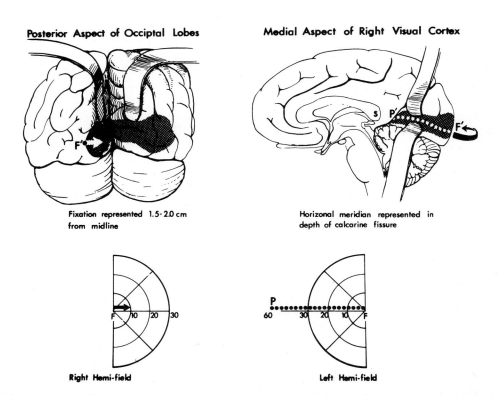

Posterior Aspect of Occipital Lobes

Fixation represented 1.5–2.0 cm from midline

Right Hemi-field

Medial Aspect of Right Visual Cortex

Horizonal meridian represented in depth of calcarine fissure

Left Hemi-field

Figure 1–23. Visual cortex. Location of visual cortex primarily in interhemispheral fissure. Lateral extension as illustrated is variable. Point F′ corresponds to central fixation point F in contralateral field. Peripheral field point P is represented in rostral portion of cortex, P′. (S, splenium of corpus callosum.) (*From Glaser J. Anatomy of the Visual Sensory System. In: Duane T, ed. Clinical Ophthalmology. Hagerstown, MD: Harper & Row, 1976; 2; with permission.*)

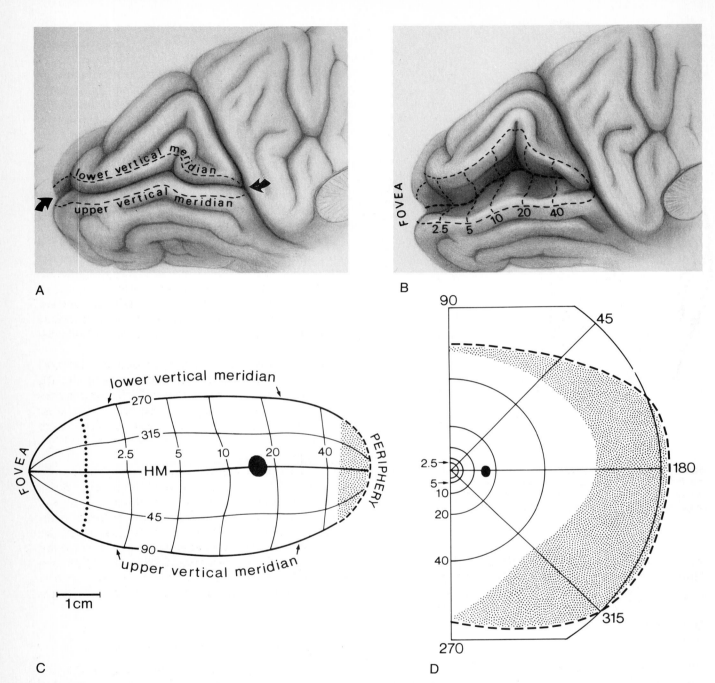

Figure 1–24. Schematic map of the representation of the visual field in human striate cortex. It is important to note that considerable variation occurs among individuals in the exact dimension and position of striate cortex. **A.** View of the left occipital lobe showing striate cortex, which is mostly hidden within the calcarine fissure (running between the arrows). The boundary (dashed line) between striate cortex (V1) and extrastriate cortex (V2) contains the representation of the vertical meridian. It is usually located along the exposed medial surface of the occipital lobe as shown, but variation occurs in specimens. **B.** View of the left occipital lobe with the calcarine fissure opened, exposing the striate cortex. Dashed lines indicate the coordinates of the visual field map. The representation of the horizontal meridian runs approximately along the base of the calcarine fissure. The vertical lines mark the isoeccentricity from 2.5° to 40°. Striate cortex wraps around the occipital pole to extend about 1 cm onto the lateral convexity, where the fovea is represented. **C.** The projection of the right visual hemifield (D) upon the left visual cortex, obtained by transposing the map illustrated in (B) onto a flat surface. Striate cortex is an ellipse about 80 mm by 40 mm, measuring roughly 2,500 mm² (40 mm × 20 mm × pi = 2,500 mm²). The row of dots indicates where striate cortex folds around the occipital pole: the small region between the dots and the foveal representation is situated on the exposed lateral convexity of the occipital lobe. The black oval marks the region of striate cortex corresponding to the visual field coordinates of the contralateral eye's blind spot. This region of cortex receives visual input only from the ipsilateral eye. HM indicates horizontal meridian. **(D).** Right visual hemifield showing the V4e isopter plotted with a Goldmann perimeter. The stippled region corresponds to the monocular temporal crescent which is mapped within the most anterior 8–10% of striate cortex (see stippled region of map C).

cells respond to binocular stimuli predominantly.

The visual cortical cells are arranged into interconnecting columns that, as the functional units of the visual cortex, bring together cells serving either orientation or dominance. Occupying approximately 1 cm of cortex, a complete set of columns is termed a **hypercolumn.** The hypercolumns brings common functions to adjacent points in the visual cortex. Spatial frequency and color selectivity also demonstrate a columnar organization. Together the hypercolumns form groups of cells that subserve visual stimuli from a specific retinal location with respect to pattern, color, brightness, movement, orientation, and depth perceptions. The magnocellular pathway appears to be involved with stereopsis, movement, and depth perception, and the parvocellular path with fine discrimination, form, and color (Table 1–1, page 5).

Although these mechanistic constructs (types of cells and separation of function) are helpful, they are only a step toward a fuller understanding of visual physiology. Many controversies exist about their details.

Beyond this hierarchically increasing integration of visual data, the visual cortex in layers II, III, and IV is also the first point at which homolateral points of both retinas project to the very same cells, forming the basis of binocular function. Fibers carry information from both eyes to the complex and hypercomplex cells.

In addition, terminals from each eye alternate in an organized pattern of stripes, the **ocular dominance columns.** The ocular dominance columns do not appear to be fully developed at birth. If an eye of a monkey or kitten is occluded, then the cells that correspond to that eye and its columns atrophy and their counterparts from the other eye hypertrophy. A similar phenomenon may be one mechanism in the development of amblyopia in humans (Chapter 15).

Parastriate and Peristriate Areas

The topographic parastriate cortex (area 18 of Brodmann) adjoins the visual cortex (area 17) and is also a six-layered granular cortex, but without the line of Gennari (Fig. 1–26). Area 18 is intimately connected to ipsilateral areas 17 and 19 and has prominent commissural connections with its contralateral counterpart via the splenium of the corpus callosum. In addition, it is well connected to the association areas, ipsilateral visuomotor cortex, and brain stem.

The peristriate cortex (area 19) extends anteriorly onto the lateral aspect of the parietal and temporal lobes and is connected predominantly with area 18, the pulvinar, and pretectum. It appears to be concerned with visual associations, integration of vi-

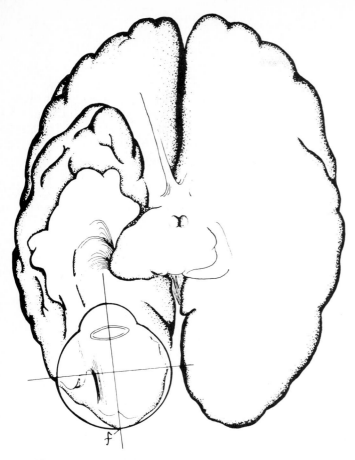

Figure 1–25. Representation of retina projected on visual cortex. The fovea is projected at the occipital pole. The nasal retina, which corresponds to the temporal crescent in the visual field, is projected anterior in the calcarine fissure.

rations, orientations, and directions of movement. Thus, for the first time in the visual afferent pathway, the visual cells respond to contours and patterns and show directional sensitivities, presumably by receiving and integrating input from the circularly symmetrical cells.

Complex cells also respond best to bars of specific orientation, direction, and speed. In contrast to circularly symmetric cells and simple cells, which are located predominantly in layer IV, complex cells are found in layers III and V. **Hypercomplex cells** require the same stimuli conditions as complex cells, but also demand that the stimulus must be of specific length; they appear to receive most of their input from complex cells.

Color vision is similarly served by color opponent cells in the visual cortex (using four classes of cells with the same functions as for uncolored information).

Thus, in area IV, cells react to monocular stimuli, whereas in layers II, III, V, and VI, individual

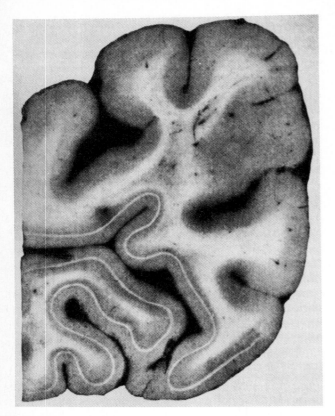

Figure 1–26. Line of Gennari. Coronal section of occipital lobe to show stria of Gennari in both walls of posterior calcarine fissure. (*From Woolf S.* Anatomy of the Eye and Orbit. *6th ed. Revised by EJ Last. London: Lewis, 1968, with permission.*)

sual information with other modalities, and visual memory.

Obviously, the primary visual cortex (area 17) is the hub for visual analysis. But it is only one site in an extensive network of cortical and subcortical structures that correlate visual input from the external world via connections to other sensory (eg, proprioception, hearing) and motor (eg, eye and head movement, limb movement) systems.

Other cells in the visual association areas integrate motion, form, color, depth, and directional information, but still respond only to selected features of the visual scene. They are organized in multiple functionally and physiologically distinct areas (V_2, V_3, and so forth) surrounding V_1. As we better define the functions and interrelationships, a more descriptive and physiologic map will replace the old topographic maps.

For now, how these bits of the mosaic become integrated into a whole vision, combined with percepts of the other senses, introduced into a conceptual framework, and combined with phylogenetic and individual experience, remains far from understood.

UNIFYING CONCEPTS

The exquisite sensitivity of the visual apparatus is remarkable, especially considering the peculiar inverse design of the eyeball. The light rays must transpierce not only the entire eye (cornea, anterior chamber, pupil, lens, and vitreous) but must also penetrate the full thickness of the retina before reaching the sensory elements, the rods and cones (Fig. 1–27). Thus, the optical quality of the ocular media and of the retina itself is critical to acute vision. Teleologically, the absence of retinal elements and blood vessels in the fovea is explained by the necessity of a clear path to the receptor elements.

The Retinal Nerve Fiber Layer and Temporal Raphé

The ganglion cell axons (the tertiary neurons of the visual system) converge on the optic disc where they exit the eye and form the optic nerves. (There are approximately 1.2×10^6 axons in each optic nerve.)

The axons of the nasal parafoveal cells proceed directly to the temporal border of the disc as the

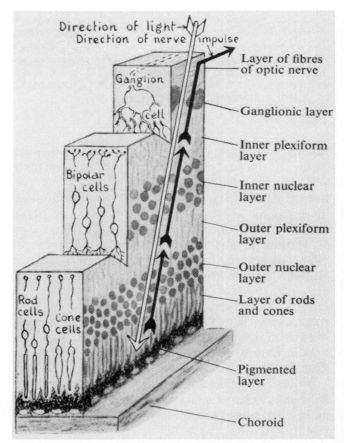

Figure 1–27. Light rays traversing the retinal layers. (*From Lockhart RD, Hamilton GF, Fyfe FW.* Anatomy of the Human Body. *Philadelphia: Lippincott, 1959, with permission.*)

papillomacular bundle. The axons from the portions of the ganglion cell layer that are nasal, superior, and inferior to the disc also proceed in a direct radial fashion. Fibers from the temporal retina must arc around the fibers of the papillomacular bundle. In the temporal periphery, the axons of the ganglion cells are divided by the retina into inferior and superior parts by the temporal raphé (Fig. 1–5). Throughout the retina, fibers from adjacent groups of ganglion cells travel together, initiating the retinotopic projection that continues to the visual cortex.

Topographic Anatomy of the Visual Afferent Pathways

Two major principles govern the organization of the visual afferent pathways and underly the analysis of visual fields. The first is **retinotopic projection,** the definite and stable arrangement of the retinal nerve fibers and their postsynaptic connections throughout the visual pathway from the retina to the visual cortex. Each point on the retina projects to a specific and predictable area in the primary visual cortex. This stable representation is one of the bases for the processing of visual information into meaningful visual perceptions. The second principle is the **hemidecussation of the visual pathways.** Each cerebral hemisphere is concerned with the environment of the opposite side. To accomplish this for the visual system, the nasal retinal fibers decussate in the optic chiasm, and the temporal retinal fibers project ipsilaterally. The division occurs at a vertical line through the fovea.

Visual processing occurs (1) in the retina, where information from many cellular interactions contributes to the receptive field of the individual ganglion cell; (2) at the lateral geniculate nucleus, where the ganglion cell axons and cells of the lateral geniculate body interact; (3) at the visual cortex, where each axon of the many lateral geniculate cells converges on as many as 5000 cortical cells; and (4) in the visual association areas, where visual, oculomotor, and other inputs are synthesized.

VASCULAR SUPPLY OF THE VISUAL AFFERENT PATHWAYS

The visual afferent pathways and the globe both have dual blood supplies. The blood supply to the visual afferent pathways comes from the internal carotid and vertebrobasilar (posterior cerebral artery) circulations; that of the globe, from the retinal (central retinal artery) and choroidal (posterior ciliary arteries) circulations, both originating from the internal carotid artery. The prechiasmal afferent visual pathways are supplied nearly exclusively by branches of the internal carotid artery. Thus, vascular disease in the internal carotid distribution gives rise to unilateral visual symptoms.

The chiasm takes its blood supply from many adjacent arteries, including the internal carotid, anterior cerebral, and anterior communicating arteries. The postchiasmal visual afferent pathways are supplied predominantly by branches of the basilar artery and the posterior cerebral artery and its calcarine branches. There are also contributions from the middle cerebral, posterior communicating, and anterior choroidal arteries (Fig. 1–28).

Blood Supply of the Orbit

The Ophthalmic Artery. The ophthalmic artery is the first major branch of the internal carotid artery (ICA) as it emerges from the cavernous sinus. After a brief course in the intracranial cavity, it lies inferior to the optic nerve within the optic canal, enters the orbit, and divides into three parts. The first part continues along the inferior lateral aspect of the optic nerve for approximately half the length of the nerve. Here the artery makes a sharp angle. The second portion usually passes over the optic nerve to the superomedial

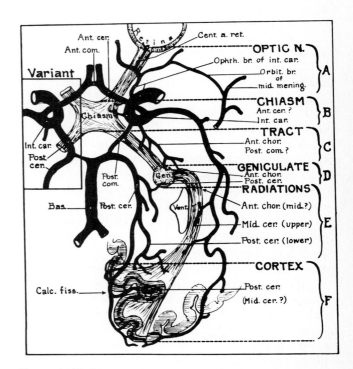

Figure 1–28. Blood supply of the anterior and posterior visual pathways. Note that each region of the visual pathway is supplied by multiple arteries. (*From Walsh FB, Smith GW. Ocular complications of carotid angiography: Ocular signs of thrombosis of internal carotid angiography.* J Neurosurg. *1952;9:517–537, with permission.*)

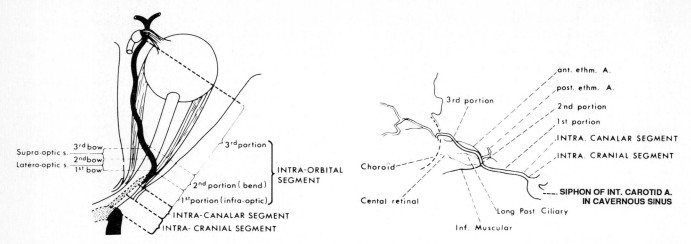

Figure 1–29. Diagram of the segments of the ophthalmic artery and its major branches. Axial (**left**) and lateral (**right**) views. (*From Vignaud J, Clay C, Aubin ML. Orbital arteriography. Radiol Clin North Am. 1972;10:39–61, with permission.*)

orbit; the third and most tortuous portion of the artery terminates as the dorsal nasal and supratrochlear branches (Fig. 1–29).

Almost all of the orbit is supplied by the ophthalmic artery with only minor contributions from other sources. The most important of these is the infraorbital branch of the maxillary artery from the external carotid artery (ECA), which often supplies some of the structures of the floor of the orbit in addition to the maxillary sinus.

Rarely, the ophthalmic artery arises via the meningeal artery as a branch of the ECA instead of the ICA. In this case it enters the orbit through a canal in the lateral portion of the sphenoid bone. But the central retinal artery still arises from the internal carotid artery; thus, in these cases the orbit is supplied by the ECA and the globe by the ICA.

Usually the central retinal artery is the first major branch of the ophthalmic artery, arising near its bend. The posterior ciliary arteries, muscular branches, and lacrimal artery arise next, followed by the posterior ethmoidal and supraorbital arteries, and then by more muscular branches and the anterior ethmoidal artery.

The ophthalmic artery has many anastomoses, especially with branches of the external carotid artery. These anastomoses are significant as alternate paths of emboli and as sources of collateral circulation. Orbital and intracranial arteriovenous malformations often involve these arteries, which are also important for interventional neuroradiology where catheterization or embolization of the cerebral and orbital circulations can sometimes have unintended effects if flow occurs via unusual routes. In most cases, the blood supply to the eye and orbit is sufficiently prolific that sudden occlusion of either the

internal carotid or the ophthalmic artery rarely causes permanent blindness.

On the other hand, significant and chronic stenosis can cause serious complications, primarily as a result of neovascularization. The "ischemic eyeball" gives rise to many signs, including neovascularization and venous statis (Chapter 8). Such cases signify severe generalized occlusive disease that involves the anastomosing circulations and prevents effective collateral flow to the eyeball.

Blood Supply of the Globe

The vascular supply of the eye is from ophthalmic artery branches via the choroidal and retinal circulations. The retinal and choroidal blood supplies are anatomically and physiologically quite different (Table 1–2). This dual blood supply of the globe

TABLE 1–2. CHARACTERISTICS OF RETINAL AND CHOROIDAL VASCULATURE

	Retina	Choroid
Source	Single artery and vein	Multiple vessels
Collaterals	Absent	Present
Pericytes	Present	Absent on inner surface Present on outer surface
Endothelium	Continuous	Fenestrated
A–VO$_2$ Difference	Maximal	Minimal
Autoregulation	Present	Absent
Rate of flow	Slow	Fast
Percentage of total blood flow	5%	95%

from the ciliary/choroidal and retinal vasculatures (Fig. 1–30) results in characteristic patterns of ocular vascular disease (see also Chapter 8). The choroidal system nourishes the outer retina and the central retinal artery system the inner retina.

The retinal vasculature has a discrete and relatively slow rate of flow that is not under neural regulation. Because of the slow flow and extremely high metabolism of the retina, there is maximum extraction of oxygen.

The quantity of blood flow through the choriocapillaris, on the other hand, is approximately 30 times that of the retina, a necessity to sustain the high metabolic rate of the rods and cones. The choroidal vasculature has fenestrated junctions and is under neural control. Because of the magnitude of the blood flow, the oxygen extraction is much less than that in the retina.

Analogous to the blood–brain barrier, there is a blood–retina barrier that has two components: (1) the continuous endothelium with tight junctions that lines the walls of the retinal vessels and (2) the retinal pigment epithelium that separates the retina from the fenestrated (leaky) vessels of the choriocapillaris.

Blood Supply of the Retina

The outer retinal layers are nourished by the posterior ciliary circulation by diffusion from the vascular choriocapillaris, which provides about 85% of the ocular blood flow. The retinal circulation per se supplies the inner retinal layers and originates from the central retinal artery, which generally branches into four arterioles, each serving a quadrant of the eye (Fig. 1–31). All are end arteries. As the areas supplied do not overlap, occlusion of one of these arterioles will produce a quadrantic visual field defect with its apex at the blind spot; occlusion of both upper or both lower branches will produce an altitudinal hemianopia. In approximately 5% of eyes, an artery at the temporal edge of the disc, a **cilioretinal artery,** originates from the choroidal circulation; on occasion, a

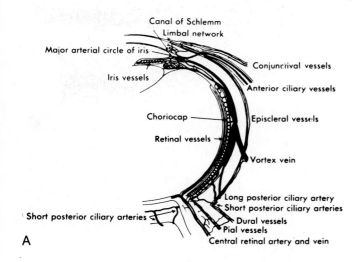

A

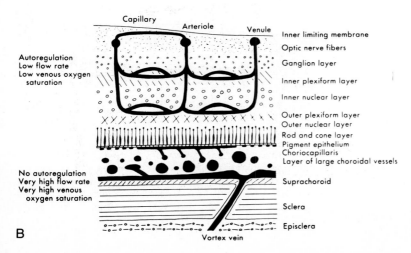

B

Figure 1–30. Dual blood supply of globe. **A.** Blood vessels of human eye. **B.** Retinal capillaries are distributed within inner layers of retina. Outer layer, 130 μm thick, has no blood vessels. It is nourished mainly from choroidal capillaries. (*From Alm A, Bill A. Ocular circulation. In: Moses R, ed. Adler's Physiology of the Eye: Clinical Application. 8th ed. St. Louis: Mosby, 1987, with permission.*)

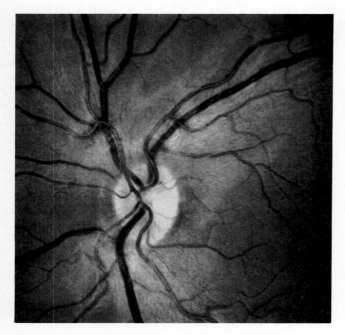

Figure 1–31. Branching of central retinal artery into four arterioles, each serving a quadrant of the eye.

cilioretinal artery may preserve vision in cases of central retinal arterial occlusion, or conversely, produce a central scotoma if it is occluded itself.

The veins of the retina carry blood back toward the optic nerve in nearly the same patterns as the arteries. When there are cilioretinal arteries, cilioretinal veins may be found.

In addition to its critical role in the nourishment of the retina, the retinal vascular tree is an important signpost of vascular disease, both systemic and retinal.

With gradual obstruction of venous circulation in the optic nerve, **optociliary shunt vessels** form. These are important clinical clues to pathology. In combination with decreased vision and optic atrophy, they form a triad nearly pathognomonic of optic nerve sheath meningioma. Optociliary shunt vessels also occur following venous occlusion and in glaucoma, although in the latter case, occult venous occlusion could be a causative factor.

Venous pulsations, present in 80% of normal eyes, may be lost as intracranial and intraocular pressure rise. However, because they are normally absent in 20% of individuals, their absence is significant only if their presence was previously noted.

Blood Supply of the Choroid

The **long posterior ciliary arteries** enter the choroid approximately 15–20 degrees lateral to the optic

nerve and run anteriorly in the suprachoroidal space to supply the ciliary body and iris.

The **short posterior ciliary arteries** perforate the sclera around the optic nerve and enter the choroid as separate nasal and temporal groups (Fig. 1–32). In the sclera the arteries run perpendicular to the choriocapillaris and divide by successive bifurcations. In contrast to the retinal vessels, the majority of these divisions takes place immediately upon entering the choroid. Thus, the outer layer of the choroid shows rows of arteries extending in radial bands from their entrance point (Fig. 1–33). Arteries destined for distal choroidal areas do not give branches to the proximal choriocapillaris.

In the posterior pole and equatorial areas, the terminal branches form lobules of choriocapillaris drained by choroidal veins into the vortex veins or the central retinal vein (Fig. 1–34). On fluorescein angiography, occlusion of the arteries creates a lobular disturbance of choroidal filling in the posterior pole (Fig. 1–35) and wedge-shaped defects peripherally (Fig. 1–36). Choroidal filling is always somewhat variable.

The submacular choriocapillaris receives an abundant arteriolar blood supply and thus is relatively protected from vascular occlusive disease.

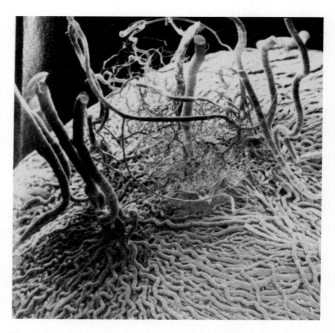

Figure 1–32. Choroidal vasculature. Low-power scanning electron micrograph in posterior view. Posterior ciliary arteries (short and long) and their choroidal branches are visualized lateral (temporal) and medial (nasal) to distal retrobulbar capillary plexus (× 15). (*From Risco J, Grimson B, Johnson P. Angioarchitecture of the ciliary artery circulation of the posterior pole. Arch Ophthalmol. 1981;99:864–868, with permission.*)

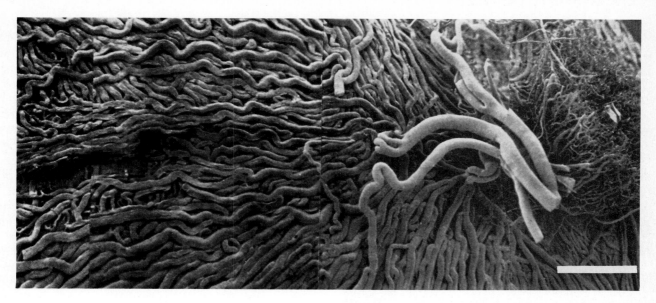

Figure 1–33. Choroidal vasculature. Papillomacular area of the choroid in scleral view. Arteries are located in the outer choroidal layer, and the veins occupy the middle choroidal layer in this area. The long posterior ciliary artery (LPCA) was removed from the specimen and its site is seen as horizontal groove (scale unit = 1mm). (*From Shimuzu K, Ujiie K.* Structure of the Ocular Vessels. *Tokyo: Igaku Shoin, 1978, with permission.*)

The choriocapillaris supplies the outer layers of the retina (the retinal pigment epithelium, rods and cones, and outer nuclear and plexiform layers), except in the fovea and extreme periphery, where it nourishes the whole thickness of the retina.

Blood Supply of the Optic Nerve

The intracranial and intracanalicular portions of the optic nerve derive their blood supply from the internal carotid, anterior cerebral, and ophthalmic arter-

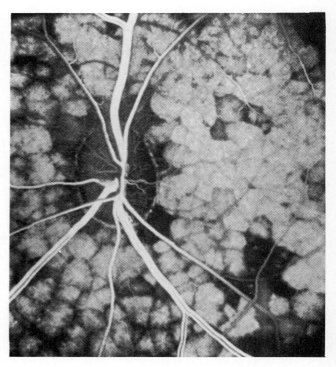

Figure 1–35. Choroidal vasculature. Choriocapillaris pattern in fluorescein fundus angiogram of monkey's eye, showing various units of choriocapillaris mosaic (each unit supplied by terminal choroidal arteriole). Note presence of some empty units among normally filled units. (*From Hayreh SS. Segmental nature of the choroidal vasculature. Br J Ophthalmol. 1975;59:631–648, with permission.*)

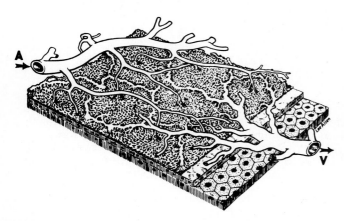

Figure 1–34. Choroidal vasculature. Three-dimensional schematic representation of choriocapillaris pattern. (A, choroidal arteriole; V, choroidal vein.) (*From Hayreh SS. The choriocapillaris. Arch Klin Exp Ophthalmol. 1974;192:165–179, with permission.*)

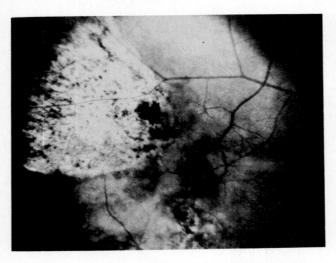

Figure 1–36. Choroidal vasculature. Triangular chorioretinal lesion in peripheral part of right eye of 68-year-old man with temoral arteritis, anterior ischemic optic neuropathy, and no perception of light. (*From Hayreh SS. Acute choroidal ischemia. Trans Ophthalmol Soc UK. 1980;100:409, with permission.*)

ies. The orbital optic nerve is supplied by the ophthalmic artery via the pial plexus, and the optic nerve head is nourished chiefly by the posterior ciliary branches of the ophthalmic artery.

At the globe, the prelaminar optic nerve head is supplied in sectoral fashion, almost entirely by branches of the short posterior ciliary arteries from the peripapillary choroid. These are relatively large choroidal vessels, **not** branches from the choriocapillaris. Although the central retinal artery branches from the ophthalmic artery and enters the optic nerve 10 mm from the globe, in this region it is only in transit; the retrobulbar optic nerve is supplied by the pial plexus. Only as the central retinal artery enters the interior of the eye does it begin to supply the ocular tissues; the surface nerve fiber layer of the disc is supplied by retinal arterioles that originate in the circumpapillary region (Fig. 1–37).

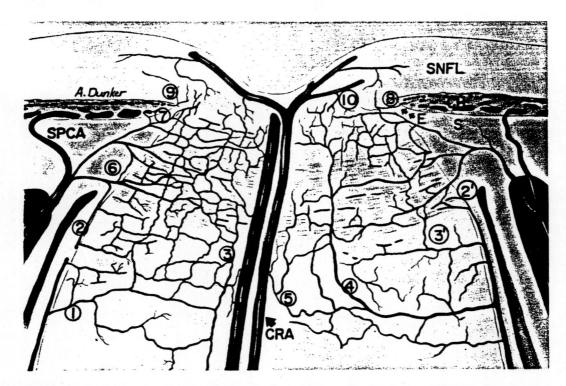

Figure 1–37. Vasculature of anterior optic nerve. Composite illustration to scale of various vascular arrangements. Venous vessels and superficial central retinal artery (CRA) plexus are not drawn in full. *Retrolamina.* 1. Pia mater as source of transverse and longitudinal vessels. 2, 2'. Recurrent short posterior ciliary artery (SPCA) to retrolamina, and pial vessels to lamina cribrosa. 3,3'. Pial-derived longitudinal arterioles course to and anastomose with laminar vasculature. 4. Occasionally realized large pial arteriole courses longitudinally through laminar tissue. 5. Intraneural branching of central retinal artery, with anastomosis to laminar and retrolaminar systems. *Lamina cribrosa.* 6. Transverse entry of scleral short posterior ciliary arteries that dominat laminar vasculature and mingle with longitudinal microcirculation. *Prelamina.* 7. Branch of short posterior ciliary artery courses through Elschnig tissue (E) at level of choroid (CH) and enters into nerve. 8. Occasional choroidal vessel to prelamina. (S, sclera.) *Superficial nerve fiber layer* (*SNFL*). 9. *Choriocapillaris "spur" capillary* anastomoses with other retinal and prelaminar vessels. 10. Both epipapillary and peripapillary branches of central retinal artery anastomose with prelaminar vessels. (*From Lieberman MF, Maumenee AE, and Green WR. Histologic studies of the vasculature of the anterior optic nerve. Am J Ophthalmol. 1976; 82:405–423.*)

Blood Supply of the Chiasm

The blood supply to the chiasm is provided by a host of arteries forming an arterial plexus that is derived from branches of the anterior cerebral, anterior communicating, internal carotid, meningeohypophyseal trunk, and posterior communicating arteries. The major blood supply to the chiasm itself is on its inferior aspect; disruption of this blood supply probably contributes to the production of the classic bitemporal hemianopia that occurs with lesions compressing the chiasm from below, especially pituitary tumors (Fig. 1–38).

Blood Supply of the Retrochiasmal Visual Afferent Pathways

Blood Supply of the Optic Tracts. The **optic tract** is supplied by the anterior choroidal artery and occasionally by direct branches from the internal carotid artery. The tract blood supply is very variable and has bridging anastomoses to the posterior communicating and posterior cerebral arteries.

Blood Supply of the Lateral Geniculate Body. These anastomoses, particularly those between the anterior and posterior choroidal arteries, also are abundant on the lateral surface of the **lateral geniculate body.** The numerous anastomoses explain why vascular lesions of the optic tract and lateral geniculate body are rarely identified.

The Blood Supply of the Optic Radiations. As described above, the optic radiations divide into two wings following their exit from the lateral geniculate body. The superior portion is supplied predominantly by penetrating branches of the middle cerebral artery; and the inferior portion, Meyer's loop, is supplied from the posterior cerebral artery.

The Blood Supply of the Visual Cortex. The most posterior parts of the visual afferent system, the visual cortices, are supplied predominantly by the vertebrobrasilar system through the posterior cerebral and calcarine arteries. The posterior cerebral artery (PCA) has been described by Hoyt, Newton, and Margolis as the artery of "seeing and looking." It is the predominant supply of the striate and peristriate cortex, although there are some anastomoses with branches of the middle cerebral artery, especially over the lateral surface of the occipital lobes. Accessory blood supplies from the parieto-occipital artery and the posterior temporal artery are present 50% of the time.

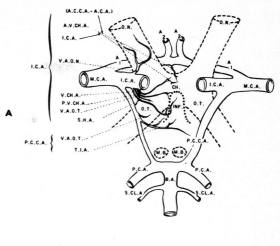

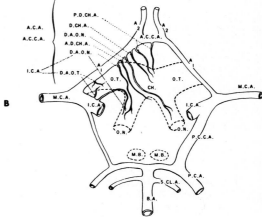

Figure 1–38. A. Diagram of the circle of Willis and ventral surface of the chiasm, infundibulum and adjacent optic nerves and optic tracts. **B.** Diagram of the circle of Willis and dorsal surface of the chiasm and adjacent optic nerves and optic tracts. A.C.A., Anterior cerebral artery (A₁, proximal); A.C.C.A., anterior communicating artery; I.C.A., internal carotid artery; P.D.CH.A., posterodorsal chiasmatic arteries; D.CH.A., dorsal chiasmatic arteries; D.A.O.N., dorsal arteries of optic nerve; A.D.CH.A., anterodorsal chiasmatic arteries; D.A.O.T., dorsal arteries of optic tract; A.V.CH.A., antero ventral chiasmatic arteries; V.CH.A., ventral chiasmatic arteries; V.A.O.T., ventral arteries of optic tract; TIA., tuberoinfundibular arteries; S.H.A., superior hypophysical arteries; V.A.O.N., ventral arteries of optic nerve. (*From Wollschlager G, Wollschlager PB. The circle of Willis. In: Newton TH, Potts DG, eds. Radiology of the Skull and Brain. St. Louis: Mosby, 1974; 3; with permission.*)

The PCA also supplies mesencephalic structures concerned with pupillary reflexes; gaze pathways (supranuclear, nuclear, and infranuclear); vestibulo-ocular reflexes; and facial, palpebral, and corneal reflexes. About 10% of the time, the posterior cerebral artery originates from the internal carotid, a so-called "fetal origin" of the PCA. This has obvious implications; in these cases symptoms usually attributed to the vertebrobasilar system can originate from occlusive or embolic disease in the carotid distribution.

BIBLIOGRAPHY

General

Hogan M, Alvarado G, Weddell J. *Histology of the Human Eye. An Atlas and Textbook.* Philadelphia: Saunders, 1971.

Miller N, ed. *Walsh and Hoyt's Clinical Neuro-ophthalmology.* 4th ed. Baltimore: Williams & Wilkins, 1982. (The "bible," a compendium of all neuro-ophthalmolgy. *The Source* for all the details. A good place to find pertinent references when you wish to explore further.)

Polyak S. *The Vertebrate Visual System.* Chicago: University of Chicago Press, 1968.

Vital-Durand F. Organization, development and early manipulations of primate's visual pathways. In: Jay B, ed. *Detection and Measurement of Visual Impairment in Pre-Verbal Children.* Boston: Dr. W. Junk, 1986.

Woolf S. *Anatomy of the Eye and Orbit.* 6th ed, revised by EJ Last. London: Lewis, 1968.

Axoplasmic Flow

Griffin JW, Wetson DF. Axonal transport in neurologic disease. *Ann Neurol.* 1988; 23:3–13.

Retinal Projections

Perry VH, Cowey A. Retinal ganglion cells that project to the superior colliculus and pretectum in the macaque monkey. *Neuroscience.* 1984; 12:1125–1137.

Perry VH, Oehler R, Cowey A. Retinal ganglion cells that project to the dorsal lateral geniculate nucleus in the macaque monkey. *Neuroscience.* 1984; 12:1101–1123.

Simpson JI. The accessory optic system. *Annu Rev Neurosci.* 1984; 7:13–41.

Stone J, Hoffman KP. Very slow conducting ganglion cells in the cat's retina: A major new functional type? *Brain Res.* 1972; 43:610–616.

Chiasm

Kupfer C, Chambler L, Downer JC. Quantitative histology of optic nerve, optic tract and lateral geniculate nucleus of man. *J Anat.* 1967; 101:395–401.

Visual Cortex

Hubel DH, Wiesel TN. Receptive fields, binocular interaction and functional architecture in the cat's visual cortex. *J Physiol.* 1962; 160:106–154.

Vascular Supply

Hayreh SS. The ophthalmic artery. In: Newton TH, Potts DG, eds. *Radiology of the Skull and Brain.* St. Louis: Mosby, 1974; 2:1333–1390.

Risco IM, Grimson Baird S, Johnson PT. Angioarchitecture of the ciliary artery circulation of the posterior pole. *Arch Ophthalmol.* 1981; 99:364–368.

Sagaties MJ et al. The structural basis of the inner blood–retinal barrier in the eye of *Macaca mulatta. Invest Ophthalmol Vis Sci.* 1987; 28:2000–2014.

Shimizu K, Ujiie K. *Structure of the Ocular Vessels.* Tokyo: Igaku Shoin, 1978.

CHAPTER 2

CLINICAL EVALUATION OF THE VISUAL AFFERENT PATHWAYS

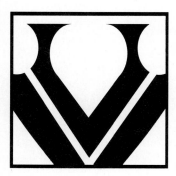

The previous chapter traced the light impulse from entry into the eye, to the stimulation of the rods and cones, and finally to the integration of the visual input in the parieto-occipital cortex. The following chapters will concentrate on the information necessary to localize problems, make diagnoses, and appropriately treat (or refer) the patient.

A wide spectrum of diseases affects the visual pathways. However, the multitude of disorders causes remarkably few visual signs and symptoms: loss of visual acuity, color perception, or field; afferent pupillary defects; alterations in the nerve fiber layer; swelling or atrophy of the optic discs; and abnormal visual sensations such as photopsias. For each disorder, the signs and symptoms are determined by the **anatomy** of the visual afferent pathways and the **character** of the causative lesion. Accompanying "neighborhood" signs also help to localize lesions—such as proptosis in orbital masses, seizures in temporal lobe lesions, and disconnection syndromes in parietal/occipital pathology.

Clinical evaluation begins with careful history-taking and proceeds to equally careful ophthalmologic and neuro-ophthalmologic examinations.

HISTORY

In neuro-ophthalmology, the history is of paramount importance. Taking a good history is **not** a rote rambling over routine questions. It is an adaptive process reacting to the patient's problem(s) and the information at hand; it is interactive; it is searching. A good history is complemented by close observation of the patient: Is there nervousness? "La belle indifference?" Exaggeration? The history should lead

to an hypothesis about the cause of the problem, an hypothesis to be sequentially refined as the evaluation proceeds.

For the patient with a presumed lesion of the visual afferent pathways, the history should differentiate between direct effects on the visual system, pathology that affects it from a distance, and symptoms that masquerade as visual afferent pathway problems (Fig. 2–1, next page).

First, determine the exact nature of the visual complaint. Is it loss of vision—acuity, color, field? Is it uniocular or binocular? Constant or variable?

At times, patients are unable to explain their visual problem precisely. In some cases, "blurred vision" may in fact be mild diplopia. Does the vision "blur" only in certain directions? In motility disorders, the amount of diplopia usually varies in different fields of gaze or at distance as opposed to near. The patient may recognize that vision blurs sometimes but at others becomes double as the images are separated further. Evanescent blur that blinks away may be due to problems of the tear film or cornea, or could be the obscurations associated with a swollen optic disc or optic disc anomalies.

Is the visual loss intermittent, transient or constant? How long has it been present? If intermittent, how long does it last?

Then, after determining the precise nature of the visual complaint, roughly localize the pathologic process. Is the visual problem monocular or binocular? Potential confusions include:

1. The patient with asymmetric bilateral visual loss. The visual loss in the better eye may be unnoticed in comparison with the more profound visual loss in the more affected eye.

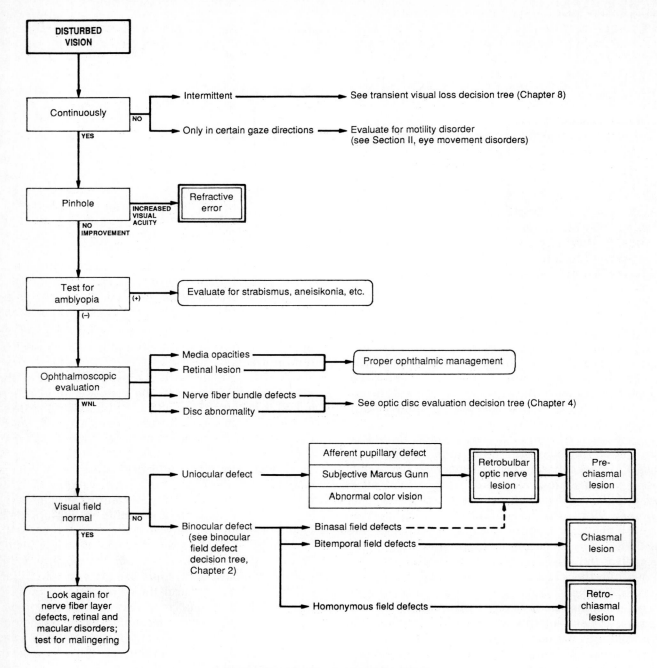

Figure 2–1. Decision tree. Disturbed vision.

2. The patient with a homonymous hemianopia who mistakenly attributes the visual loss to the eye on the side of the visual field defect. Even very bright patients who give an excellent history may do this; for example, a right homonymous hemianopia may be described as seeing poorly out of the right eye.

Is the visual problem more than a decrease in acuity? Are other changes in the quality of visual perception present—are colors faded, is there distortion or dimness, does the patient experience hallucinations? Does the problem go away if one eye is covered?

The tempo of the problem often gives a clue to the nature of the disease. Is it chronic? Did it have an abrupt onset, as in emboli? Is it acute or subacute, as in ischemic and demyelinating processes; or is it gradually progressive, as in compression of the visual pathways? Are the symptoms of constant severity? Are there associated symptoms? Do they point to the location of the lesion or a contributing systemic problem? Is the problem stable, improving, or progressively worse? Are there situations that either exacerbate or mitigate the symptoms? Are they related to posture, physical activity, or the ingestion of certain foods?

On the basis of your history, form an hypothesis: What is the most likely etiology of the patient's visual complaint? Refine that hypothesis with further questions about the patient's symptoms, and fit those facts into the context of the general medical history. What is the patient's age, sex, social history? Ask about alcohol and drugs, life-style, diet, stress. Is there a family history of visual loss? What is the past medical history? Are previous symptoms suggestive of a generalized illness that might now be affecting the visual pathways? Could use of medications or drugs be causing symptoms?

The history is not only the most important part of the patient evaluation, it should be the most extensive as well. However, history alone cannot always distinguish between ophthalmic and neurogenic visual loss.

Obtain as much information as you can contribute to the differential diagnosis, and then examine the patient. Careful examination usually detects changes in the media, macula, and retina or other ocular disease. But sometimes what at first seems to be a simple eye problem—"I need new glasses"—turns out to be a neurogenic decrease in visual acuity or even a refractive problem caused by neuro-ophthalmic trouble—for example, myopia, unilateral, as with Horner's syndrome or bilateral, as with a pretectal mass.

Avail yourself of all accessible records: previous medical evaluations, family and driver's license photos, and previous neuro-imaging studies. Review the originals yourself. It is astonishing how often a congenital Horner's syndrome, long-standing strabismus, or nystagmus will go unnoticed by patients and their families; how frequently casually ordered neuro-imaging, such as computed tomography (CT) or magnetic resonance imaging (MRI) scan will omit the orbit or sella turcica, which is the seat of the pathology.

While taking the history, observe the patient closely, not only for affect but also for the appropriateness of visual behavior in regard to the visual complaint. Look for abnormalities of the ocular adnexa, clues to guide the remainder of your exam. Close observation may reveal lid retraction (thyroid orbitopathy) or ptosis (Horner's syndrome or ophthalmoplegia); conjunctival telangiectasia (sickle-cell disease, ataxia telangiectasia, or Fabry's disease) or arterialization of the conjunctival veins (carotid-

cavernous fistula); or disorders of facial movement such as hemifacial spasm, blepharospasm, or myokymia (CPA tumor, intrinsic brain-stem glioma, or aberrant blood vessel).

Also, be aware of the "real" problem as perceived by the patient and the patient's family, and be sure to address it as well as your diagnosis.

General Principles

The prechiasmal visual afferent pathway (VAP) is the first portion of the tertiary visual neuron—that is, the retinal nerve fiber layer, optic disc, and optic nerve. What follows is a basic clinical approach to disorders that affect these structures. They present with *uniocular* loss of visual acuity, color vision, or visual field; afferent pupillary defects; and alterations in the retinal nerve fiber layer and optic discs, especially swelling or atrophy (Table 2–1).

Damage to the prechiasmal afferent visual pathways should be suspected when the patient complains of a *unilateral* visual disturbance (constant, progressive, or intermittent) or when an abnormal finding is unilatreal (eg, a swollen disc, optic atrophy, retinal nerve fiber layer defect, or afferent pupillary defect).

In contrast, disorders of the postchiasmal VAP cause signs and symptoms involving both eyes *homonymously*; chiasmal disorders typically cause bitemporal visual field defects but may also show evidence of optic nerve and optic tract dysfunction.

There are three tiers of examinations. The first evaluations should be done on *every* patient, either at bedside or in the office. The next group are those added to gain additional information or refine the differential diagnosis. The third group may be considered "laboratory" tests, where in general the patient needs to be sent off, whether it be just to the next room, down the block to the hospital, or across the state to a university center for the newest in neuro-imaging. Visual field testing, which can become quite elaborate and may mean referring your patient, is considered in the first section, because **you** must do at least some type of visual field evaluation on every patient.

TABLE 2–1. MANIFESTATIONS OF PRECHIASMAL VISUAL AFFERENT PATHWAY DISORDERS[a]

Decreased visual acuity
Decreased color vision
Decreased brightness sensation
Visual field defects
Afferent pupillary defect (Marcus Gunn pupil)
Alteration in retinal nerve fiber layer
Changes in the optic disc—especially swelling or atrophy

[a] All uniocular.

The **diagnostic evaluation** of patients with lesions of the prechiasmal afferent visual paths always should include:

1. Careful assessment of visual acuity.
2. Assessment of color vision.
3. Tests for afferent pupillary defects.
4. Comparison of brightness sensation between the two eyes (the "subjective Marcus Gunn test").
5. Testing of visual fields at least by confrontation and with red targets.
6. Ophthalmoscopic examination—looking for retinal nerve fiber layer damage, optic atrophy, a swollen disc or an abnormal optic disc (especially hypoplastic and "tilted" discs).

Purely ocular disorders that can mimic neurogenic visual loss must be ruled out. These include refractive errors, media changes, keratoconus, central serous retinopathy, cystoid macular edema, fundus flavimaculatus (Stargardt's disease), cancer-associated retinopathy (CAR syndrome), and solar retinopathy. Thus, do as much of a thorough general ophthalmologic evaluation as the circumstances of examination allow as well as neuro-ophthalmic exam.

An appropriate abbreviated neurologic exam tailored by the history and neuro-ocular findings will often add important information, as when increased deep tendon reflexes and papillitis point to multiple sclerosis (or other diffuse neurologic disease).

Much neuro-ophthalmic testing is either psychophysical or electrophysiologic. **Psychophysical tests** evaluate the patient's *subjective* response to a specific stimulus. Thus, the more carefully the stimulus and the testing conditions can be controlled, the more accurate the test. Theoretically, the response recorded is the threshold response, that which is seen 50% of the time and missed 50% of the time. In a psychophysics laboratory, the threshold is determined by gradually increasing a subthreshold stimulus until it is just perceived, and then decreasing a suprathreshold stimulus until it is not perceived (the "staircase" method). However, in the clinical setting, true staircase paradigms are infrequent. Visual acuity testing, visual field testing, contrast sensitivity, and dark adaptation are examples of psychophysical tests. The major disadvantage of psychophysical tests is that they call for a *subjective* response, and thus the cooperation and truthfulness of the patient.

In **electrophysiologic tests,** a specific stimulus is utilized and the electric response to the stimulus recorded and analyzed, sometimes by computer. The electrophysical response provides an *objective* measurement, and thereby has an advantage over the subjective psychophysical tests. However, some testing situations require patient cooperation, such as looking at and concentrating on the stimulus. Electrophysiologic tests include electroretinograms (ERG), pattern electroretinograms (PERG), and visual evoked potential (VEP) testing.

The effectiveness of any test depends on the test itself, the tester, and the testee. Thus, the potential impact of all test variables must be considered in interpreting the results.

Lesions of the prechiasmal pathway produce unilateral visual disturbances—such as uniocular decrease in visual acuity, uniocular diminution of color vision or brightness, and uniocular field loss (notably, nerve fiber bundle defects and central scotomas). When the macular outflow is affected, there is loss of visual acuity and color vision, an afferent pupillary defect (the Marcus Gunn pupil), a subjective brightness difference between the involved and uninvolved eyes, and a field defect involving the central portion of the visual field.

Subtle retinal nerve fiber layer damage can be the only evidence that there is anything amiss, especially in the early stages of disease (eg, in multiple sclerosis without overt optic neuritis, or in diseases such as glaucoma that tend to affect the peripheral or paracentral visual field more severely than central acuity). In these cases, visual field defects, pupillary defects, and decreases in visual acuity and color vision may also be subtle. Later, as destruction of ganglion cell axons progresses, obvious disc changes and dense field defects appear.

Lesions of the optic nerve eventually produce ophthalmoscopic evidence of their presence: nerve fiber bundle defects, optic atrophy, or disc swelling. However, after retrobulbar insult, visible findings may not appear for several weeks. In contrast, lesions of the retina or optic nerve head are almost always visible with the ophthalmoscope. The "asymptomatic" contralateral eye always should be checked *very* carefully. Bilateral abnormalities (signs or symptoms) imply chiasmal and retrochiasmal processes or bilateral ocular or optic nerve disease.

Unfortunately, the common visual function tests do not fully evaluate the physiologic properties of the 1.2 million axons in the optic nerve. It is possible for a patient to complain of subjective visual disturbance but have normal color vision by standard tests, no objective decrease in central visual acuity, and no obvious visual field abnormality. Nevertheless, the patient is acutely aware of a significant subjective deficiency in visual function; vision in the affected eye is "not as good, not as bright," and colors may appear faded. This is particularly true of patients who have recovered from an episode of retrobulbar neuritis. However, even this difficult group of patients often shows some abnormal findings on examination: an afferent pupillary defect (even with 20/15 vision) and/or retinal nerve fiber layer or optic disc atrophy. Electrophysiologic and/or psychophysical testing may be abnormal, especially contrast sensitivity tests.

BASIC CLINICAL EVALUATION OF THE VISUAL AFFERENT PATHWAYS

Start with an evaluation of the patient's general appearance and the external tissues of the eye and orbit (Table 2–2). Is there the smooth, pasty facies of pituitary deficiency? A scar from removal of skin cancer? Are abnormal blood vessels present, suggesting a dural arteriovenous malformation or hemoglobinopathy?

Visual acuity. The "best corrected" visual acuity **always** must be determined. That is, the very best vision possible with an accurate refraction on the date of examination—not without glasses and not as measured in somebody else's office, even if that last measurement was just made this morning. It is critical to obtain the best visual acuity you can, as a decrease in vision from 20/10 to 20/15 may be the only objective finding of an optic neuropathy. Test one eye at a time, because when tested binocularly, visual acuity is normally about one line better than the visual acuity of each eye separately (eg, visual acuity of 20/20 in each eye may be 20/15 when both eyes are used). A visual acuity less than 20/25 in either eye, or a drop in visual acuity, must be explained.

If you examine the patient in your office, this means the very best refraction that can be done. If you are in the emergency room or a hospital room, or you do not refract, then use the patient's most recent correction (glasses and/or contact lenses) and a pinhole. The pinhole, by allowing only the most central rays of light to enter the eye, minimizes the effect of refractive errors, yielding an acuity quite close to that of a correct refraction. However, because of dif-

fraction by the pupillary margin, the vision may be slightly less than best corrected visual acuity. Also remember that with a pinhole, a spurious decrease in visual acuity can appear if the patient has significant media opacities.

Visual acuity describes the optical resolution of the eye and is a measure of central (foveal, macular) vision (peripheral vision is tested by the visual field). Distance visual acuity is recorded as 20/X (see Table 2–3 for equivalents). The numerator indicates the theoretical testing distance (in practice, the distances are not always 20 feet, but the testing system is set up optically to simulate testing at 20 feet); and the denominator indicates the size of the smallest line of letters read by the patient. Thus, the standard designation of 20/20 indicates that the patient saw at 20 feet the line that a "normal" person is expected to see at 20 feet. When the notation is 20/100, the patient sees at 20 feet only those letters that a "normal" person would see at 100 feet. Most young, healthy people have 20/15 visual acuity and a few even test at 20/10; thus *20/20 may actually indicate visual loss.* Charts containing 20/20 as the most difficult line are therefore inappropriate for early detection of visual loss. When visual acuity is tested at near, it is usually registered as J1, J3, and so forth—the standard Jaeger notation (see Table 2–3 for Snellen equivalents). Most patients over the age of 45 (and some younger) will need a reading correction (a magnifying correction) to read clearly at near. Thus, when measuring a patient's near acuity in a hospital room, the inability to read small letters at near may represent only presbyopia (the decrease of accommodation that occurs with age) rather than a manifestation of neurogenic visual loss. When corrected, distance vision should always be the same as visual acuity at near, and so any discrepancy must be explained.

TABLE 2–2. THE BASIC EXAMINATION

External examination
Visual acuity
Color vision
Brightness comparison (subjective Marcus Gunn test)
Afferent pupillary defect (Marcus Gunn pupil)
Visual fields
Media: hand light or slit-lamp evaluation
Fundus: disc, vessels, nerve fiber layer
General ophthalmic examination: retinoscopy, etc

TABLE 2–3. EQUIVALENTS OF SNELLEN NOTATION

Snellen Notation	Decimal	Metric	Near Equivalent
20/10	2.0	6/3	—
20/15	1.3	6/4.3	—
20/20	1.0	6/6	J1 +
20/25	0.8	6/7.5	J1
20/30	0.6	6/9	J2
20/40	0.5	6/12	J3
20/50	0.4	6/15	J5
20/60	0.3	6/18	—
20/70	0.29	6/21	J7
20/80	0.25	6/24	—
20/100	0.2	6/30	J10
20/200	0.1	6/60	J16
20/400 (big "E")	0.05	6/120	—

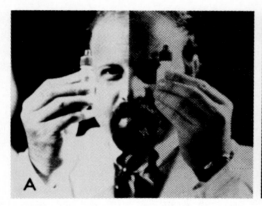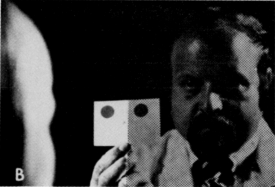

Figure 2–2. Color testing. Color comparison with objects presented to both sides of central fixation area. **A.** Mydriatic red bottle tops. **B.** Card with two large red patches. (*From Glaser J. In: Duane T, ed.* Clinical Ophthalmology. *Hagerstown, MD: Harper & Row, 1976; 2; with permission.*)

If the patient is unable to see any of the standard letters, vision is then recorded as count fingers (CF), [usually with a notation of distance following it, indicating the distance at which the patient was able to count the fingers—for example, 3 feet (CF 3') 1 foot (CF 1'), and so forth] hand motion (HM), light perception (LP), or no light perception (NLP—total blindness). Vision better than 20/400 necessitates macular vision. Total destruction of the macula, if the peripheral retina is normal, still allows visual acuity of at least count fingers. Thus, if the media are clear, hand-motion vision means both central and peripheral retinal disease or optic nerve disease. Visual acuity this low is not compatible with normal ambulation. So, note the consistency of the patient's visual performance with the visual acuity as tested.

A decrease in visual acuity nearly always indicates a prechiasmal or chiasmal lesion. Isolated postchiasmal pathology causes loss of visual acuity only if disease is bilateral and extensive. In fact, if even a very small percentage of macular fibers survives, visual acuity can be normal.

Color-vision testing. Color-vision testing should be a routine part of the neuro-ophthalmologic examination. For neuro-ophthalmic purposes, color testing is different than testing for hereditary dyschromotopsias. For neuro-ophthalmic evaluation, the color vision of one eye is compared with that of the other, whereas inherited anomalies of color vision are tested binocularly (if you refer your patient for color testing, eg, Farnsworth Munsell 100 Hue, you may need to specify separate testing of each eye). Grossly, a great deal of information can be obtained by noting the saturation of a colored target in one part of the field as compared to another (eg, nasal versus temporal, central versus paracentral). Testing with red targets on both sides of the vertical meridian seems to be especially sensitive for detecting bitemporal hemianopias (Fig. 2–2).

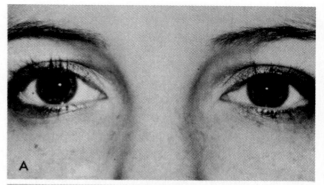

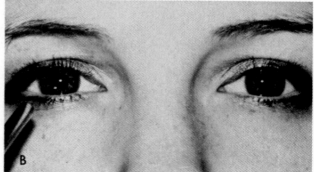

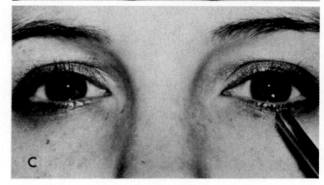

Figure 2–3. I. Testing for a relative afferent pupillary defect (normal). **A.** With diffuse illumination, pupils are of equal size. **B.** With light on right eye, both pupils constrict **C.** Pupils remain constricted when light is swung to left eye. (*From Beck RW, Smith CH. The neuro-ophthalmic exam.* Neurol Clin. *1983;1:807–830, with permission.*)

Color-vision testing evaluates central (macular) vision, predominantly cone function, which deteriorates early in optic nerve disease. Thus, color vision, especially red-green, deteriorates more in optic nerve disease than in a macular lesion with equal visual acuity loss; in contrast, patients with purely ocular disease often retain good color vision despite significant decrease in visual acuity.

Perhaps the fastest and easiest method for detecting a color-vision deficit is to have the patient compare colors as seen with each eye. This is quicker and frequently more rewarding than a formal test of color vision, because most color-vision test plates are designed for hereditary defects of color vision. In

the ophthalmologist's office, the test targets are frequently the tops of medication bottles, which come in a convenient selection of red, white, blue, and green. Pencils, neckties, or any colored object at hand and of convenient size can be used. It is useful as well to try two objects of the same color, but of different hue, to test color saturation. Compare the color sense between the two eyes to test for uniocular visual loss, between different parts of the visual field to check for a central scotoma or hemianopia, or against your own color sense, the "normal" reference (unless you happen to have a color deficiency). Recall that approximately 7% of men (and a smaller percentage of women) will have a red-green color

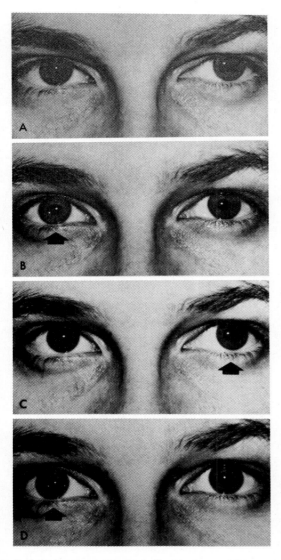

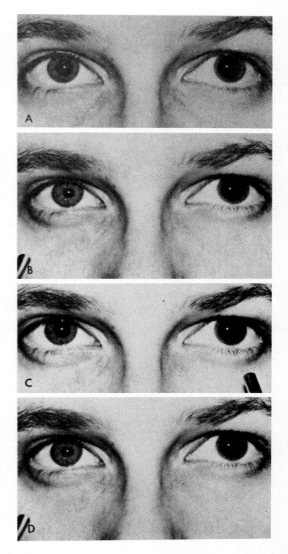

Figure 2–3. II. Marcus Gunn pupil. Testing for a relative afferent pupillary defect with a left optic neuropathy. (Arrows indicate eye on which bright line is directed.) **A.** With diffuse illumination, pupils are of equal size. **B.** With light on right eye, pupils constrict briskly. **C.** Pupils dilate slightly when light is swung to left eye. **D.** On swinging light back to right eye, both pupils constrict.

Figure 2–3. III. Testing for a relative afferent pupillary defect when one pupil is dilated. A left optic neuropathy is present. **A.** With diffuse illumination, left pupil is larger than right. **B.** With light on right eye, right pupil constricts but left does not. **C.** When light is swung to left eye, right pupil dilates slightly. **D.** It again constricts when light is swung back to right.

TABLE 2–4. EXTERNAL EXAM (SOME CLUES TO NEURO-OPHTHALMIC DISORDERS)

Lid retraction, stare—Thyroid orbitopathy
Ptosis—third-nerve palsy, Horner's syndrome
Hatchet face—Myotonic dystrophy
Moon face—Cushing's disease or syndrome
Temporal muscle atrophy or tortuosity of temporal vessels—
  Temporal arteritis
Blepharospasm or hemifacial spasm—Idiopathic vascular cross
  compression of VII nerve root
Myokymia—Brain-stem or cerebellopontine angle tumor
Abnormal conjunctival vessels—Dural carotid–cavernous fistula,
  Fabry's disease, sickle hemoglobinopathy
Café-au-lait spots—Neurofibromatosis (optic nerve and chias-
  mal gliomas, neurofibromas)

deficiency; very few people have other hereditary color deficiencies.

Ishihara color plates were designed to test hereditary red-green color loss and are not optimal for testing acquired neuro-ophthalmic visual defects. The **American Optical–Hardy-Rand-Ritler (AO-HRR) color plates,** although also primarily designed for testing familial color vision defects, work much better for neuro-ophthalmic disease because they measure the blue-yellow as well as the red-green axis. These are the test plates preferred by most neuro-ophthalmologists.

More formal color vision testing—such as the **D15, desaturated D15,** and **Farnsworth-Munsell 100 Hue tests,** as well as more complicated psychophysical tests of color vision such as anomaloscopes—are time consuming and do not add much additional information. However, they do provide an objective record that, like the charts from the AO-HRR plates, can be used on subsequent visits to evaluate progression or improvement. Occasionally, formal color testing is helpful in detecting a malingerer or hysteric by responses so poor in relation to the degree of visual loss as to be totally unbelievable.

Brightness sense (Subjective Marcus Gunn Testing). Just as the swinging flashlight test is used to observe pupillary function, it may be used to estimate the relative brightness sense of the two eyes. In this case, assuming that a light shining into the good eye is worth one dollar, the patient is asked to tell you the "value" of the light shining into the bad eye. Amazingly, even with very mild degrees of optic nerve dysfunction (especially in optic neuritis) the brightness value in the bad eye is significantly diminished. This decrement may be quantitated using crossed polaroids.

Afferent pupillary defect (Marcus Gunn pupil) Testing. Examine the patient for an afferent pupillary defect with the swinging flashlight test (Fig. 2–3). A positive afferent pupillary sign has been

called the most important pupillary abnormality in medicine and is all but pathognomonic of a defect in the prechiasmal afferent visual pathways. The afferent pupillary defect correlates with the decrease in sensitivity of the visual field; retinal or macular disease must be massive to cause an obvious afferent pupillary defect. Rarely, amblyopia is associated with an afferent pupillary defect, but so rarely that you should always suspect a primary optic nerve disorder before attributing a Marcus Gunn pupil to anisometropic or strabismic amblyopia.

Anisocoria (unequal pupils) is **not** caused by isolated lesions of the **visual afferent pathways.** *Anisocoria indicates a lesion of the efferent pupillary pathways* (see Chapter 16).

The **general ophthalmic exam** should detect ocular disease, such as keratoconus, which can present as a neuro-ophthalmologic problem; and subtle ocular signs of neuro-ophthalmic disorders (eg, the

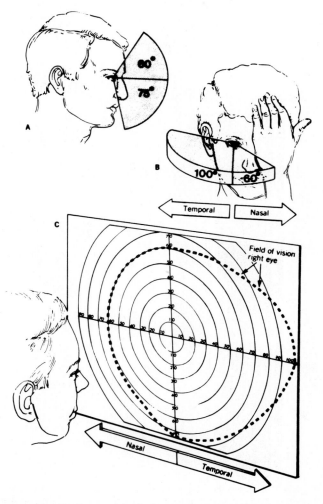

Figure 2–4. Extent of the visual field in degrees. (*From Anderson DR. Perimetry: With and Without Automation. 2nd ed. St. Louis: Mosby, 1987, with permission.*)

Kayser-Fleischer ring of Wilson's disease). It should assess the clarity of the media, especially their part in any decrease in visual acuity. (Media opacities may decrease visual acuity, contrast sensitivity, and the sensitivity of the visual field, but *almost never* cause an important visual field defect such as scotoma or nerve fiber bundle defect.) When not using a

slit-lamp to evaluate media opacities, a simple rule of thumb is: Your view into the fundus should equal the patient's view out. For example, if you estimate your view through a cataract is 20/40 while the patient sees only 20/200, you must rule out neurogenic visual loss—that is, explain the difference in visual acuity between 20/40 and 20/200. When the cause of

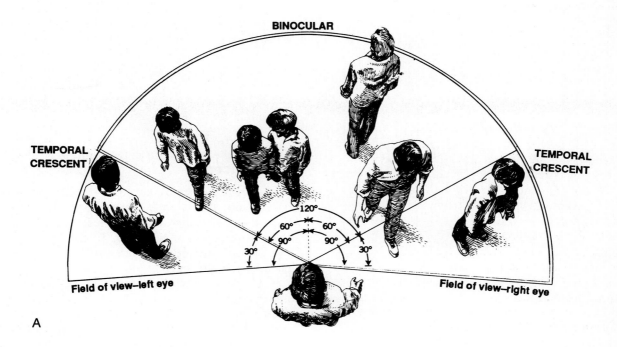

A

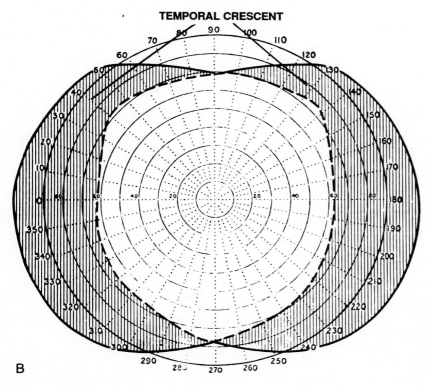

B

Figure 2–5. **A.** Binocular visual field. **B.** Binocular visual field showing the crescentic unpaired areas. (**A.** *from Traquair HM. An Introduction to Clinical Perimetry. 6th ed. St. Louis: Mosby, 1987, with permission.* **B.** *from Anderson, DR. Perimetry: With and Without Automation. 2nd ed. St. Louis: Mosby, 1987, with permission.*)

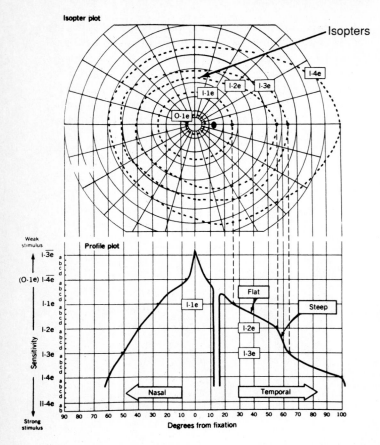

Figure 2–6. The blind spot, as seen on isopter and profile plots. (*From Anderson DR. Perimetry: With and Without Automation. 2nd ed. St. Louis: Mosby, 1987, with permission.*)

However, in a symptomatic patient, if all else appears normal, rule out subtle defects in color and brightness sense and contrast sensitivity. Then look again for subtle neuro-ophthalmic pathology—such as nerve fiber layer changes—and consider malingering.

Although it is rarely necessary to do a complete **neurologic exam** initially in addition to the neuro-ophthalmic evaluation, an estimate of mental status, gait, and station can be done simply. Observe how the patient navigates. The history should have included questions about motor function, sensation, and autonomic and sphincter function. Frequently, a quick check of reflexes or cerebellar function will point toward a generalized neurologic problem. Suspicion of diffuse neurologic disease necessitates a thorough neurologic evaluation.

The Visual Fields—Basic Definitions and Concepts

Visual field testing is a keystone of neuro-ophthalmic evaluation; it not only detects and defines visual field defects, it also localizes lesions and monitors their progression or recovery. To completely test the visual fields one must understand their anatomic basis and use appropriate methodology.

The visual field is that portion of space in which objects are visible at one time; it is the entire area seen when fixing steadily. The **uniocular visual field** is the visual field of one eye; it extends 60 degrees superiorly, 75 degrees inferiorly, 100 degrees temporally, and 60 degrees nasally (Fig. 2–4). The *binocular visual field* is the visual field seen simultaneously with both eyes, that is, the central area without the temporal crescents (Fig. 2–5).

The horizontal and vertical meridians divide the visual field into upper and lower, temporal and nasal halves by lines passing through fixation (the projection of the macula). At the optic disc, there is no retina and no receptive elements; therefore, the disc is a nonseeing area and corresponds to the blind spot

decreased visual acuity is obscure, evaluation of the ocular reflexes and surfaces by retinoscopy, keratometry, and slit-lamp exam becomes even more important. The external examination (Table 2–4) should note abnormalities such as facial myokymia (brainstem or cerebellar pontine angle tumor), ptosis (III nerve palsy, Horner's syndrome), lid retraction (thyroid orbitopathy), and proptosis (orbital tumor).

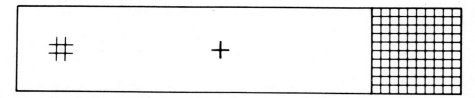

Figure 2–7. Blind spot. The completion phenomenon. Look at the cross in the figure with the right eye closed. Adjust the distance from the eye to the page until the left grid disappears (about 4 inches from your nose). This demonstrates the blind spot of the left eye. Now look at the cross with the left eye closed. No hole is seen in the right grid although the right eye has the same blind spot as the left. Higher visual processing "completes" the grid. (*Adapted from Gittinger JW Jr. Ophthalmology: A Clinical Introduction. Boston: Little, Brown, 1984, with permission.*)

FIELDS

RIGHT

Blind
spot

TEMP.

PATIENT

EXAMINER

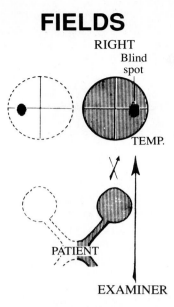

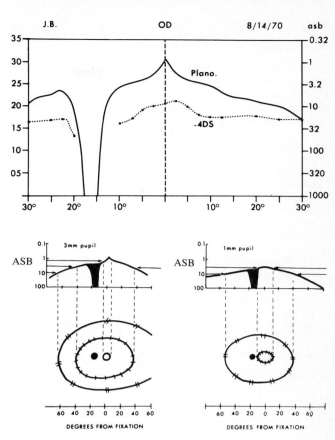

Figure 2—8. Projection of the visual field. Scheme to explain the custom of recording the visual field of the right eye on the right, and that of the left eye on the left. (*From Reed H, Drance SM. The Essentials of Perimetry: Static and Kinetic. London: Oxford, 1972, with permission.*)

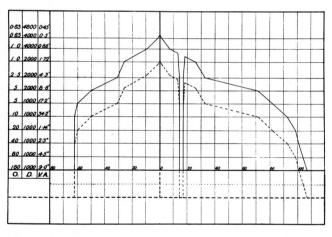

Figure 2—9. The field of vision regarded as a hill seen in section. The horizontal meridian is shown. The continuous horizontal base line indicates the extent of the field in degrees, the vertical lines, the visual acuity: O, the diameter of the test object in millimeters, D, its distance from the eye in millimeters, and V.A., the visual angle subtended at the nodal point. Beginning with an angle of 9 degrees, the visual angle is halved for each successive isopter; a modification is introduced by the substitution of 1/2000 and 1/4000 for the original figures of 2.5/4000 and 1.25/4000. The interrupted line shows the alteration produced by an imaginary uniform depression of the acuity over the whole as if its full width lay on the horizontal meridian instead of slightly below it. This chart is intended to illustrate a clinical rather than a mathematical conception of the composition of the visual field in terms of relative visual acuteness; it is at least approximately accurate. (*From Traquair HM. An Introduction to Clinical Perimetry. 6th ed. St. Louis: Mosby, 1949, with permission.*)

Figure 2—10. Effect of refraction and change in pupil size on field. **A.** Static profiles of horizontal meridian in a young adult showing the effect of a refractive change. The central portions of the visual field are particularly affected. **B.** Kinetic perimetry carried out with three targets and the corresponding static profile of the horizontal meridian show that when the pupil changed from 3 to 1 mm in diameter there was only a slight rise in differential threshold (evidenced by a lowering of the profile) yet the isopters showed a very marked change because of the very gradual slope of the areas tested. (*From Reed H, Drance SM. The Essentials of Perimetry: Static Kinetic. London: Oxford, 1972, with permission.*)

of the visual field (found about 15 degrees temporal to fixation and just below the horizontal meridian) (Fig. 2—6). Normally, you are not aware of your blind spot because the corresponding area of the other eye sees normally; even if you close one eye, neural processing tends to form a whole image. This explains why patients may be oblivious to good-sized visual field defects, especially if monocular. To demonstrate your blind spot and the phenomenon of completion, see Figure 2—7.

Representation of the Visual Field. Each eye is tested separately, generating two charts, one for the visual field of *each* eye. By convention the charts are drawn as if projected onto a plane in front of the patient. That is, the right visual field is projected to the right,

TABLE 2–5. GLOSSARY OF VISUAL FIELD TERMS

Types of Visual Field Defects

Hemianopia (hemianopsia) Defect of one half of the visual field, respecting either the horizontal or vertical meridian.
Macular sparing Hemianopic defect sparing at least 5 degrees centrally.
Macular splitting Hemianopic defect that does not spare central vision.
Quadrantanopia (quadrantopsia) Loss of one-fourth of the visual field, respecting either the horizontal or vertical meridian.
Scotoma An area of depressed function surrounded by areas of more normal function; usually perceived by patient as area gone from view.
    Arcuate Arcing around the fovea; a visual field defect representing damage to the nerve fiber layer, usually in the temporal arcades.
    Bjerrum Acruate nerve fiber bundle defect; visual field defect in line with blind spot (eg, at 15 degrees); typical of glaucoma.
    Central Involving fixation.
    Centrocecal Involving fixation and the blind spot.
    Congruous Homonymous defects very similar in each eye.
    Homonymous Affecting the same side of the visual field in both eyes.
    Incongruous Homonymous defects that are different in each eye.
    Paracentral In the central area, sparing fixation.
    Peripheral Outside 30 degrees.
    Positive Scotoma that appears as an obscuration between patient and object viewed, often colored, typical of central serous retinopathy.
    Ring Circle of depressed visual field, usually 20 to 40 degrees from center. Typical of retinitis pigmentosa (RP).
    Scintillating A positive scotoma associated with positive, usually bright, sometimes colored sensations typical of a migraine.
    Seidel Pathologic elongation of blind spot, comma-shaped visual field defect, an "early" Bjerrum scotoma.
    Total, complete No test target is visible.

Characteristics of Visual Field Defects

Contracted (constricted, absolute) Visual field with peripheral area in which no target is seen no matter how large or bright. ("Constricted" is commonly used to mean depressed; although common, this usage is wrong, according to Traquair and others.)
Depressed (relative) Area of visual field with partial loss of sensitivity (eg, in which smaller targets are not seen, but larger ones are). Some function is retained in depressed area but sensitivity is decreased.

Attributes of the Visual Field

Blind spot Physiologic nonseeing area (scotoma) of the visual field that occurs because there are no rods and cones in the optic disc; the representation of the optic disc in the visual field.
Central Within 30 degrees of fixation.
Isopter Line connecting points of equal sensitivity in the visual field like an isobar (weather map) or contour line (topographical map).
Peripheral Outside 30 degrees.

Types of Visual Field Testing

Automated Method of visual field testing in which a computer generates the patterns of stimulus presentation.
Kinetic Method of visual field testing with moving targets.
Profile plot Representation of visual field as a "hill" or "island" of vision used most often in static perimetry. Height of profile represents sensitivity of visual field at that point, equivalent to a cross section through "island of vision."
Static Method of visual field testing with nonmoving targets. Usually position and size of the targets are constant and intensity varies.

the same as your visual field is projected (Fig. 2–8). So any time you develop right/left confusion in the interpretation of visual fields, check the patient's field against your visual field.

The charts are a two-dimensional projection of the "island of vision" (originally called the "hill of vision" by Traquair). Kinetic visual fields are usually represented as topographical maps (Fig. 2–6A), but also can be shown as profile plots (Fig. 2–6B); static visual fields appear as cross sections of the islands (Fig. 2–9).

The height of the island in cross section represents the sensitivity of the retina. Normally, retinal sensitivity increases from the periphery to a maximum at the fovea. The 25- to 30-degree surrounding fixation (representing the fovea), known as the **central field,** is the area with the greatest sensitivity. It corresponds to the macular region of high spatial and color resolution where the cones dominate. In the area beyond this, the periphery, vision is 20/100 or less and is rod dominated; thus, the peripheral retina is more sensitive in the dark. With uncorrected refractive error, the island is flattened into a plateau (sensitivity decreases), as shown in Figure 2–10A. The larger isopters representing the relatively insensitive peripheral retinal areas are not affected by re-

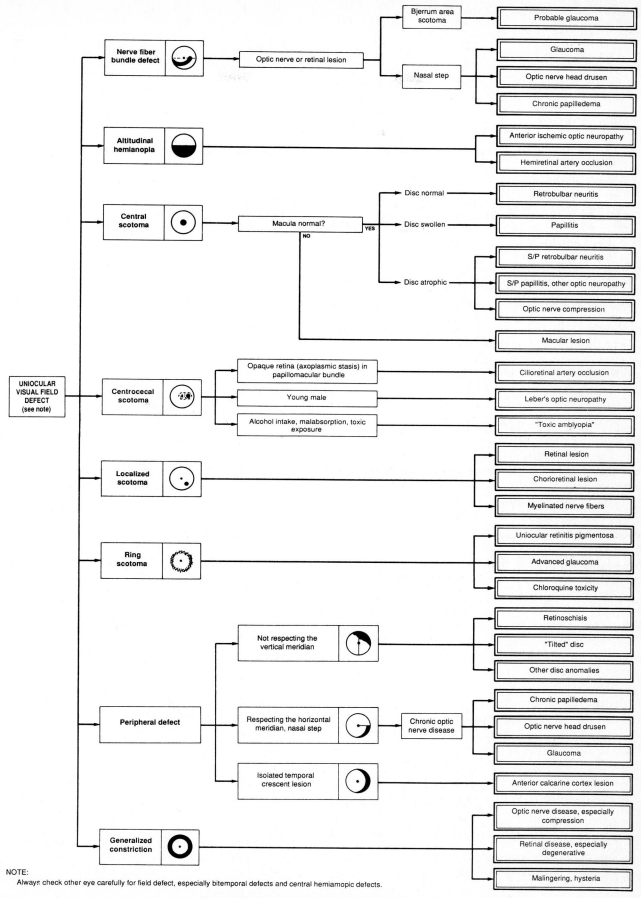

Figure 2–11. Uniocular Visual Field Defects.

NOTE:

Always check other eye carefully for field defect, especially bitemporal defects and central hemiamopic defects.

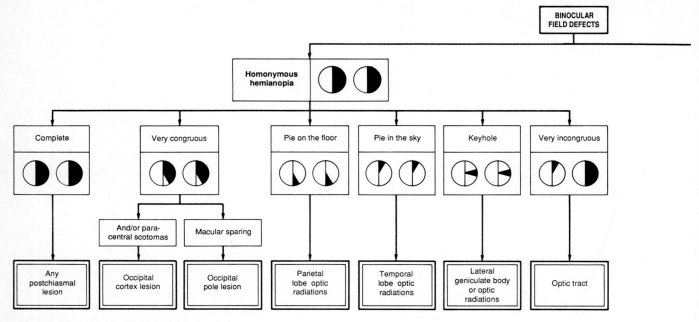

Figure 2–12. Binocular visual field defects.

fraction and are normal; the smaller isopters representing areas of retina where sensitivity is affected by refraction will shrink. Changes in pupil size and decreased clarity of the ocular media (eg, cataract) have similiar effects (Fig. 2–10B).

The Pathologic Field. Many terms are used to describe visual field defects (Table 2–5). The **contracted or constricted field** is a field reduced in size by an **absolute defect;** *no* target is ever visible in the lost visual field. The division between seeing and nonseeing areas is sharp; the isopters become bunched together because the edge of an absolute defect is the limit of visibility for all isopters (Fig. 2–13.) Contracted fields are rare. Additionally, prognosis for recovery is usually poor when the defect is total. These types of defects are frequently caused by structural or vascular abnormalities.

Depression is a reduction of the sensitivity of the field. This means that because small test targets will not be seen in the depressed area of the visual field, you must use larger test targets to quantify the defects; the isopters are compressed but still spread apart. The border between seeing and nonseeing differs for each isopter. The defect is **relative** (Fig. 2–14). Areas of depression usually indicate possibility for recovery and are typical of compressive lesions and the effect of media opacities.

Relative defects differ in size for different target objects and are equivalent to depressed areas of the visual field. **Absolute defects,** on the other

hand, are the same size for any target, no matter how large, and correspond to contracted parts of the visual field.

A **scotoma** is an area of depressed vision surrounded by an area of more normal vision. The blind spot, as mentioned above, is a scotoma normally present in each eye. The other terms used to describe scotomas (Table 2–5) are descriptive and usually refer to the area of the field involved and the appearance of scotoma (eg, central, centrocecal, paracentral, hemianopic, nerve fiber bundle).

Hemianopsia (hemianopia) means loss in half a field. Lesions in the chiasm or posterior to the chiasm cause hemianopic defects. **Homonymous** defects arise posterior to the chiasm. *A total homonymous hemianopia has no localizing value;* it only indicates a severe lesion posterior to the chiasm. The hemianopia is named according to its configuration. Hemianopia may be homonymous, bitemporal, altitudinal, and so forth.

Congruous defects are defects that are practically identical in the two eyes; **incongruous defects** are somewhat different in each eye. The degree of congruity in incomplete hemianopias is frequently useful in localization of a lesion. Incongruous defects usually are indicative of more anterior postchiasmal visual afferent path lesions (eg, tract or lateral geniculate body), whereas visual cortex lesions are exquisitely congruous by most methods of visual field testing. In automated perimetry, the expected

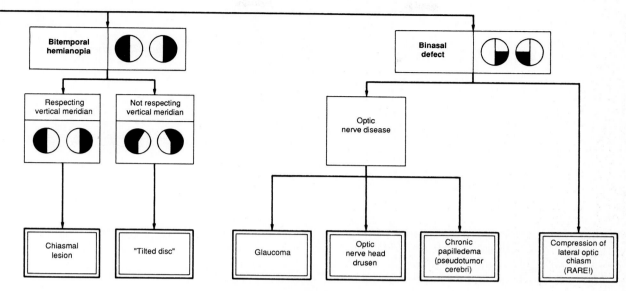

Figure 2-12. (cont.)

congruity sometimes is not found. Whether this is an artifact of extrapolation, an artifact of testing methods, or a revelation about the physiology of the visual field is yet to be determined.

Anatomic Basis of Visual Field Defects

Visual pathway disease often is localized by the pattern of visual field disturbance (Figs. 12–11 and 12–12). This useful property depends on retinotopic projection (page 19). That is, there is a definite and stable arrangement of nerve fibers from the retina to the cortex. The fibers from corresponding retinal points in the two eyes (points corresponding to the same spot in the visual field) are increasingly closely

aligned in the retrochiasmal visual pathways until in the visual cortex they project to the same elements.

Organization within the retina. The details of the retinal nerve fiber layer, its conformation and important relationships, were outlined in Chapter 1. Remember that most ganglion cell axons project to the disc in a linear fashion; the important exceptions are (1) the arcuate fibers, which must arc around the papillomacular bundle; and (2) the resultant horizontal *temporal raphe* (Fig. 2–15).

Lesions of the retinal nerve fiber layer cause visual field defects, scotomas, and nerve fiber bundle defects. The latter defects widen peripherally, point to the blind spot centrally, and respect the horizontal meridian (eg, nasal steps, altitudinal hemianopias).

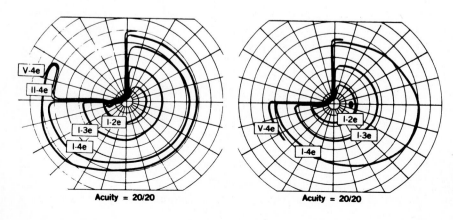

Figure 2–13. Contracted visual field. (*From Anderson DR.* Perimetry: With and Without Automation. *2nd ed. St. Louis: Mosby, 1984, with permission.*)

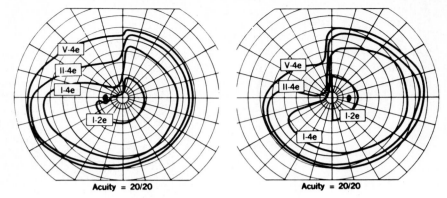

Figure 2–14. Depressed visual field. (*From Anderson DR.* Perimetry: With and Without Automation. *2nd ed. St. Louis: Mosby, 1984, with permission.*)

Other retinal lesions cause scotomas corresponding to their size and location. The ring scotoma is typical of retinitis pigmentosa.

Within the optic nerve, the macular fibers begin as the occupants of the temporal portion of the nerve where the papillomacular bundle reaches the optic disc. As the nerve approaches the chiasm, the macular fibers move toward its center.

Optic nerve lesions cause nerve fiber bundle defects (central and centrocecal scotomas, altitudinal hemianopias, nasal steps) and generalized depression of the visual field, with a tendency to affect the nasal field early and predominantly. Lesions at the junction of the optic nerve and chiasm affect Wilbrand's knee, causing the "junction scotoma" described by Traquair, a strictly unilateral paracentral hemianopic scotoma (Fig. 2–16). In fact, the junction scotoma described in many texts (Fig. 2–17) occurs somewhat later than the defect Traquair described. In any case, both field defects result from compres-

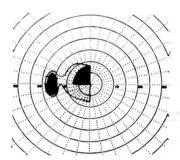

Figure 2–16. Junction scotoma. (*From Traquair HM.* An Introduction to Clinical Perimetry. *6th ed. St. Louis: Mosby, 1949, with permission.*)

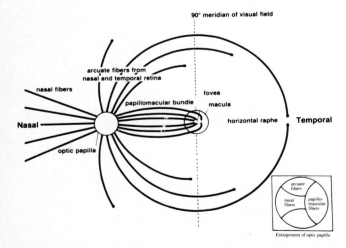

Figure 2–15. Organization of nerve fiber layer. Nerve fiber organization in the retina of the left eye. (*From Rosenberg M.* Neuroophthalmology. In: Wilkins R, Rengachary S, eds. Neurosurgery. *New York: McGraw-Hill, 1985, with permission.*)

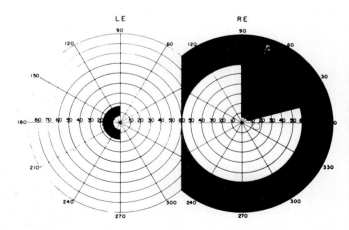

Figure 2–17. Junction scotoma. From a case of aneurysm of right anterior cerebral artery with compression of right optic nerve and anterior chiasm. (*From Harrington DO.* The Visual Fields: A Textbook and Atlas of Clinical Perimetry. *2nd ed. St. Louis: Mosby, 1964, with permission.*)

sion of the optic nerve, medially and inferiorly, just as it enters the chiasm.

Lesions of the ganglion cells and their axons in the prechiasmal visual afferent pathways cause uniocular visual field defects and uniocular decrease of visual acuity.

Sensory information from one half of the body is processed by the contralateral brain. This makes a crossing in the visual pathway, the optic chiasm, a necessity. Thus, nasal visual fibers must cross to join their counterparts, the temporal fibers from the other eye.

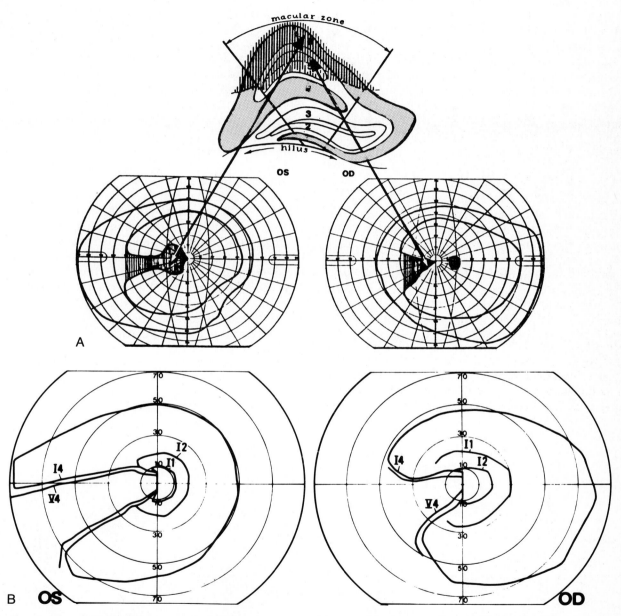

Figure 2–18. A. Lateral geniculate body visual field defect. Progressive geniculate hemianopia from astrocytoma involving the right lateral geniculate nucleus. Initial visual defects were relative and grossly incongruous. In the temporal field there was a "keyhole-shaped" defect, and in the nasal field a smaller wedge-shaped defect. The schematic diagram of the laminae in the right geniculate nucleus (at the top) indicates, in a midcoronal section, how a lesion at the dorsal crest of the lateral geniculate nucleus (LGN) produces greater involvement of lamina 6 and a larger visual defect in the paracentral temporal field of the contralateral eye. **B.** Tract visual field defects in a patient with sectorial optic atrophy felt to have a lateral choroidal artery syndrome. Note the relative congruity of the homonymous horizontal sectoranopia. (**A.** *from Hoyt WF. Geniculate hemianopsia: Incongruous visual defects from partial involvement of the lateral geniculate nucleus.* Proc Austral Assoc Neurol. *1975; 12:7–16, with permission.* **B.** *redrawn from Frisen L, Holmegaard L, Rosencrantz M.* J Neurol Neurosurg Psychiatr. *1978; 41:374–380. From Miller N, ed.* Walsh and Hoyt's Clinical Neuro-ophthalmology. *4th ed. Baltimore: Williams & Wilkins, 1982; 1; with permission.*)

The **classic chiasmal visual field defect** is the bitemporal hemianopia or bitemporal scotoma. As mentioned in Chapter 1, the actual position of the chiasm relative to the pituitary gland and to vascular structures in the parachiasmal area can be quite variable. Obviously, depending upon the exact position of the lesion, "chiasmal" visual field defects assume some of the character of optic nerve defects or optic tract defects in addition to the typical bitemporal configuration. Chiasmal lesions are often associated with decreased visual acuity.

Binasal defects not infrequently are mentioned in the literature and are generally attributed to pathology at the lateral aspects of the chiasm. In fact, this type of visual field defect is exceedingly rare in parachiasmal lesions. *Most binasal visual field defects are evidence of optic nerve disease.* Thus, given a binasal field defect, especially one with some tendency to adhere to the horizontal meridian rather than the vertical, look for optic nerve disease such as glaucoma, optic nerve head drusen, or chronic papilledema.

Postchiasmal lesions. Lesions of the postchiasmal afferent visual pathway cause **binocular, homonymous defects** and *very rarely* cause any decrease in visual acuity.

Lesions of the optic tract, when partial, are generally incongruous; those of the **lateral geniculate body,** because of its anatomy, can cause an unusual type of keyhole or sector defect (Fig. 2–18A). These lesions are exceedingly rare, perhaps because of the overlapping blood supply to the lateral geniculate body. Similar defects are seen in lesions of the anterior radiations (Fig. 2–18B).

In the **optic radiations,** the visual fibers spread out. The fibers from the lower portion of the path loop anteriorly and laterally around the temporal horn, forming **Meyer's loop** (Fig. 2–19). Temporal lobe lesions involving these lower fibers cause the classic "pie in the sky" visual field defect (Fig. 2–20). The superior fibers form the parietal radiations. Parietal lesions affect the superior fibers and cause defects denser below, giving a "pie on the floor" type of field defect (Fig. 2–21).

The optic pathways terminate in the **visual cortex.** Here, the lesions cause homonymous and congruous visual field defects as visual fibers from corresponding points on the retina associate more and more closely (Fig. 2–22). Small defects are generally paracentral in location; larger lesions cause homonymous hemianopias.

The anterior portion of the calcarine cortex contains the fibers from the temporal crescents. This area, near the splenium of the corpus callosum, is sometimes either affected in isolation or spared by visual cortex lesions (Fig. 2–23). Thus, visual field defects either involving or sparing this area should be thought of and searched for. *This is the only place in the retrochiasmal visual system that uniocular visual field defects can occur.*

Extensive bilateral cortical lesions can cause to-

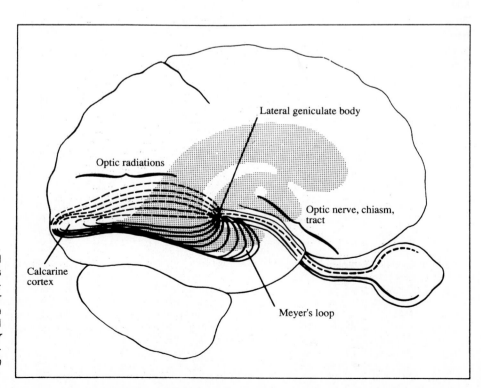

Figure 2–19. The optic radiations and Meyer's loop. Superior retinal projections remain superior (dashed lines), while inferior retinal projections remain inferior (solid lines). The inferior radiations arch around the temporal horn of the lateral ventricle (strippled area). (*From Gittinger JW Jr. Ophthalmology: A Clinical Introduction. Boston: Little, Brown, 1984, with permission.*)

Lateral geniculate body

Optic radiations

Optic nerve, chiasm, tract

Calcarine cortex

Meyer's loop

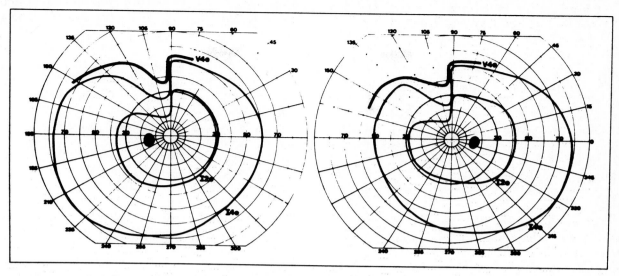

Figure 2–20. Left superior quadrantanopia, a "pie-in-the-sky" visual defect in temporal lobe lesions. (*From Gittinger JW Jr. Ophthalmology: A Clinical Introduction. Boston: Little, Brown, 1984, with permission.*)

tal loss of vision, but because the pupillary fibers leave the visual afferent pathway prior to the lateral geniculate body, in **cortical blindness** pupillary reactions are normal, an important point in differentiation of cortical from anterior visual pathway lesions.

There is much discussion of **macular sparing** in lesions of the visual cortex. Frequently, posterior lesions are associated with homonymous defects that seem to loop around central fixation, to "spare" the macula. However, visual fixation, especially in patients with diffuse or large neurologic lesions, is variable and can simulate macular sparing. Thus, if there appears to be macular sparing, be sure it is not due to poor fixation. The area of macula "spared" should be at least 3 degrees before macular sparing is even con-

sidered. Suggestions for the phenomenon include binocular representation of the macula, duplication of macular representation, overlapping blood supplies (middle cerebellar and posterior cerebellar arteries), and a host of others. Evidence from accurate microelectrode recording and retrograde labeling experiments demonstrates that the division of retinal fibers along a vertical line through the fovea is rarely perfect (Fig. 2–24); there are fibers from several degrees on either side of the vertical that reach the cortex on the "wrong" side but these cannot account for more than a few degrees of macular sparing. Meanwhile, true macular sparing (> 5 degrees; Fig. 2–25) usually means a visual cortex lesion, probably because of supplementary blood supplies.

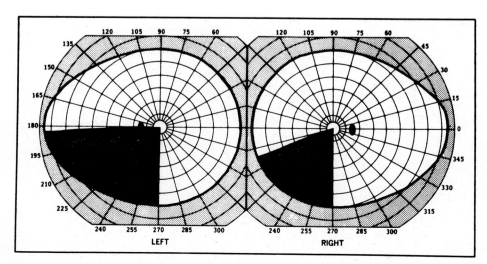

Figure 2–21. Parietal lobe lesions tend to affect the inferior quadrants of the contralateral visual field first. This is an example of a patient with a **right** parietal lobe lesion, a "pie-on-the-floor" visual field defect. (*From Bajandas F, Kline L. Neuro-ophthalmology Review Manual. 3rd ed. Thorofare, NJ: Slack, 1988, with permission.*)

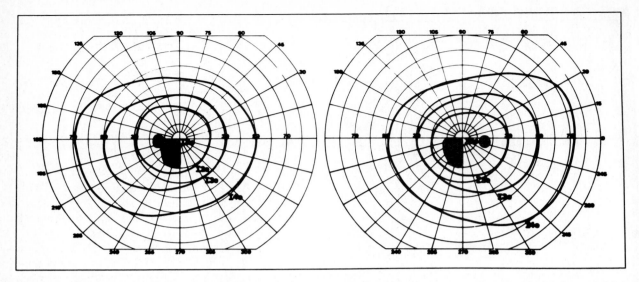

Figure 2–22. Homonymous paracentral scotomata from an occipital infarct. (*From Gittinger JW Jr. Ophthalmology: A Clinical Introduction. Boston: Little, Brown, 1984, with permission.*)

In contrast, **macular splitting** can occur in any hemianopic defect and has no localizing value.

Recent studies suggest that damage to one hemisphere should result in foveal splitting in the ipsilateral eye and foveal sparing in the contralateral eye. This is due to mingling of ipsilateral and contralateral projecting cells and their receptive fields on the nasal side of the foveal pit for 2 to 3 degrees. This finding needs confirmation in patients with hemisphere lesions.

Principles of Visual Field Testing

When you test the visual field, you test the patient's ability to see a target at a specific point. Thus, factors

that influence visibility of the target become important. These variables include the following.

1. *Target variables*—size, intensity, wavelength (brightness/color), and duration of presentation.
2. *Field variables*—background, room illumination, and color.
3. *Subject variables*—alertness, cooperation, steadiness of fixation, response time, refraction, clarity of the ocular media, and droopy lids. Pupillary size is an especially important patient variable (eg, pupil constriction as from glaucoma drops can cause an apparent depression of the visual field or enlargement

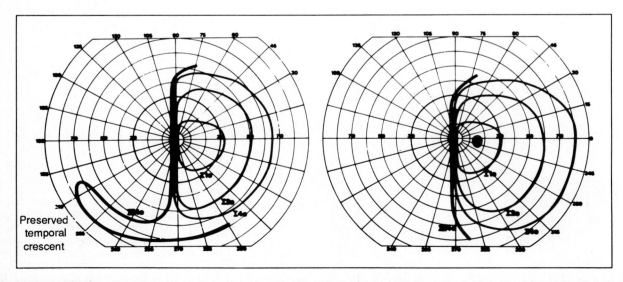

Preserved temporal crescent

Figure 2–23. Temporal crescent. In this left homonymous hemianopia there is a partially preserved temporal crescent of field in the left eye. (*From Gittinger JW Jr. Ophthalmology: A Clinical Introduction. Boston: Little, Brown, 1984, with permission.*)

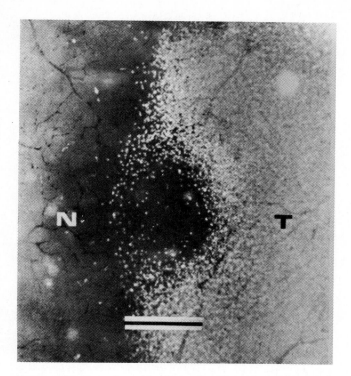

Figure 2–24. Projection of the fovea. Darkfield photomicrograph of flat-mounted fovea. Labeled cells on temporal side (T) that project to ipsilateral horseradish-peroxidase-injected lateral geniculate body appear white. Nasal retina (N) is predominantly unlabeled, with the exception of scattered labeled ganglion cells lying along the rim of the foveola. Fuzzy bright zones indicate adherent pigment epithelial cells below the plane of focus (×170). (*From Bunt A, Minckler D. Foveal Sparing: New anatomical evidence for bilateral representation of the central retina. Arch Ophthalmol. 1977; 95:1445–1447, with permission.*)

of a scotoma, just because less light gets into the eye. A cataract can have a similar effect; ptosis or dermatochalasis can simulate a superior field defect).

4. *Examiner variables*—rate of stimulation, repetition, and number of directions tested.
5. *Variables dependent on the testing method.*

Conceptual Basis of Visual Field Testing. There are two basic types of visual field testing, kinetic and static. To conceptualize the visual field and understand the differences between kinetic and static tests of the visual field, think of the field as an island of vision. In **kinetic visual field testing,** the stimulus is a moving target, usually moved from the periphery toward the center of the field. A mark is made at the point at which the target is first seen. For each stimulus an **isopter** defines the line connecting all of the points at which the stimulus is first detected (Fig. 2–26). This zone of isosensitivity is similar to a temperature isobar on a weather map or an altitude contour (isodine) on a topographical map. With the exception of the normal blind spot, the stimulus should be seen everywhere within its isopter and not seen anywhere outside it. Obviously, the position of the isopter is very sensitive to the speed of movement of the stimulus. **Kinetic visual field testing** is represented by tangent screen testing, arc perimetry, and Goldmann perimetry.

In contrast to kinetic field tests, **static perimetry** tests the height of the island of vision at many single

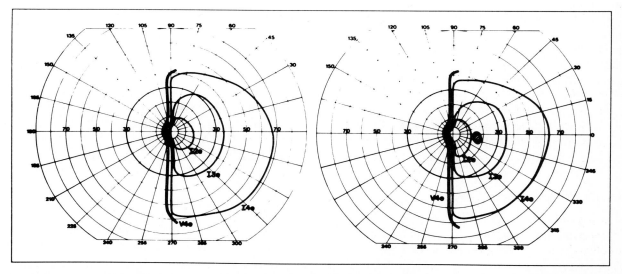

Figure 2–25. Left homonymous hemianopia with macular sparing. (*From Gittinger JW Jr. Ophthalmology: A Clinical Introduction. Boston: Little, Brown, 1984, with permission.*)

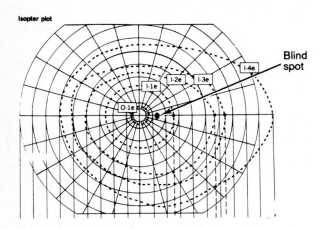

Figure 2–26. Isopter. (*From Anderson DR.* Perimetry: With and Without Automation. *2nd ed. St. Louis: Mosby, 1984, with permission.*)

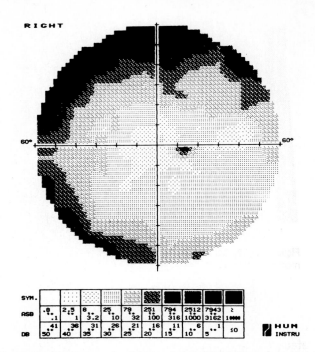

Figure 2–27. Gray scale. A normal visual field (Humphrey Field Analyzer). The visual field out to 60 degrees is represented on graytone printout. Note that on the nasal side the absolute edge of the field is reached (zero values for some points at the upper left). (*From Anderson DR.* Perimetry: With and Without Automation. *2nd ed. St. Louis: Mosby, 1984, with permission.*)

points on the island. In static perimetry, the stimulus is presented without movement. Thus, confrontation fields done by hands held steady in the visual field, as well as more sophisticated threshold and suprathreshold tests of the visual field, are types of static perimetry.

Suprathreshold perimetry is done with a target that exceeds the expected threshold. The stimulus is recorded as either seen or not seen.

Threshold perimetry theoretically determines the intensity at which the stimulus is detected 50% of the time. Although much more sensitive, this type of testing obviously depends on momentary fluctuations in both testing conditions and patient response. The threshold determinations can be recorded as a numeric value or shown as an interpolated gray scale (Fig. 2–27). In this case, the boundary between different densities of gray represents the boundary between areas of different sensitivity and corresponds roughly to an isopter on kinetic field charts. Static field testing yields a profile plot of sensitivity of the visual island. For both grids and profiles, some inaccuracies result from areas between tested spots which must be interpolated. Obviously, because there is space between the test spots, small defects may be missed.

Methods of Visual Field Testing

The patient history is a guide to where and how to test the visual field. Knowing where and how can be especially critical if the patient is a child, tired, or uncooperative. In those cases, test the field prior to doing any other examination and test areas of particular interest first. Use simple methods to get the information you need quickly. Always test the important things first. If you are concerned about a homonymous field defect, test alongside the vertical meridian; if you are concerned about a central scotoma, test the central portion first. If the patient is cooperative and not likely to fatigue quickly, test the better eye first, so that the patient knows what to expect from the testing procedure and what to look for in the stimulus.

Confrontation visual field testing. Screening visual fields should be done on every single patient; the easiest way to do this is by confrontation. In confrontation field testing the patient is confronted with a target (the other eye is covered) while he or she looks at your eye (*not* your nose, as the purpose is to compare the patient's visual field with your hopefully normal visual field). Be careful to present the target halfway between the patient and yourself, so that the target appears the same to both of you (Fig. 2–28).

Hold your hands on either side of the vertical meridian with one, two, three, five, or no fingers showing. Ask the patient to identify the number of fingers. Test all quadrants; also test homonymous quadrants with double simultaneous presentation. Ask the patient for any subjective difference between the clarity of the fingers presented in each quadrant.

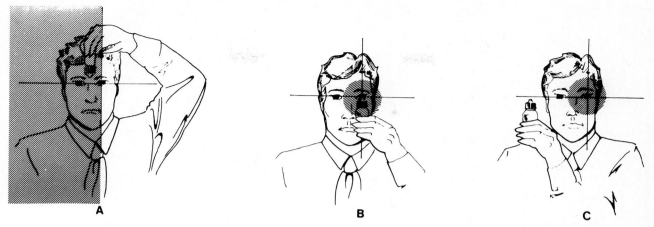

Figure 2–28. Color confrontation. **A.** Testing for a hemianopic defect. Compare color perception on both sides of the vertical meridian. **B. and C.** Testing for a central scotoma. Compare central (*B*) and peripheral (*C*) perception of color.

In this manner, you test for significant visual field defects in all quadrants, for hemianopias, and for parieto-occipital disease that causes difficulty in perceiving simultaneously presented targets (asimultagnosia). Presenting colored targets in the quadrants tests color fields.

It is frequently taught that fingers or small objects should be wiggled or moved from outside the visual field onto the visual field to test it. Although the visual fields **can** be tested in this manner, at times it can be very inaccurate because of the Riddoch phenomenon (the ability to see moving better than static targets in defective portions of the visual field). For this reason, stationary targets are preferable. Hand or finger waving can be useful in extremely depressed fields; occasionally, threatening gestures get a response in malingerers.

Advantages of confrontation field testing. The testing is rapid and simple. It is easily understood by the patient and needs little or no paraphernalia. It is often the only way to get important field information from a child or an uncooperative, demented, or obtunded patient.

As mentioned elsewhere, **color confrontation testing** can be very sensitive for detecting bitemporal hemianopias and in fact can give clearly abnormal answers when results by automated perimetry or Goldmann field testing are equivocal. Color confrontation fields should be done on every patient where a hemianopic defect is suspected. Color confrontation compares the color of the target at two points in the visual field—centrally and more peripherally (color is processed maximally at fixation so color should always be brighter centrally) or on both sides of the vertical meridian (Fig. 2–28). If one side is "dimmer," confirm the hemianopia by moving the

object horizontally and ask the patient to say when it changes color. If the color change occurs at the vertical meridian, the hemianopia is confirmed. Definite absence of a color differential across the vertical meridian is strong evidence that no hemianopia exists.

Confrontation fields performed in this manner are relatively gross and not easily quantified. Nevertheless, if visual acuity is normal, confrontation fields normal, color vision normal, and there is no afferent pupillary defect, it is very unlikely that a large visual field defect will turn up even with more elaborate testing.

Amsler grid testing. The Amsler grid is a squared-off grid with a central fixation dot (Fig. 2–29). held 14 inches from the patient. The patient is asked to fixate on the small dot and to draw out any area of blur or distortion. One eye is tested at a time. The grid measures 10 degrees on either side of fixation, approximately the area inside a circle determined by the inner edge of the blind spot. Thus, it tests only the central portion of the visual field. The Amsler grid is excellent for mapping small central scotomas, the congruity of visual cortex lesions, and macular sparing, and can also detect enlarged blind spots. In addition, it is especially sensitive to macular lesions that may be confused with neurogenic visual loss. Distortion of the squares is frequently a good indicator of macular disease, especially central serous retinopathy. The Amsler grid may also be used by the patient at home to follow the evolution of small central field defects. However, as it tests only the central 10 degrees of the field, results are dependent on good fixation and cooperation.

Tangent screen. Using a tangent screen (a black screen stitched to delineate the points of fixation, the

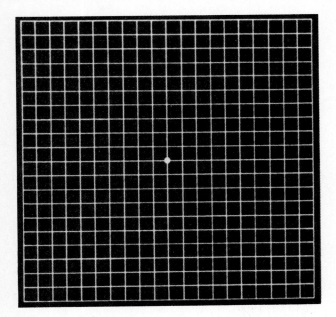

Figure 2–29. Amsler grid. The patient is instructed to maintain fixation on center dot throughout test. If the patient cannot identify it, an X drawn along the diagonals of the grid through the center may be of assistance. The patient is first asked whether all four corners and borders of the grid can be seen, and then whether there are any gaps or blurred areas in the field, and finally whether all horizontal and vertical lines appear straight and parallel. Any defects in the field can be drawn on the grid paper and placed in the patient's record. (*From Beck RW, Smith C. The neurologic exam.* Neurol Clin. *1983;1:807–830, with permission.*)

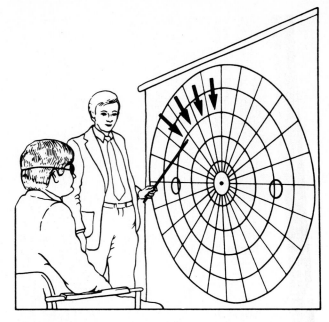

Figure 2–30. Visual fields performed on a tangent screen. The patient is seated 1 meter from the screen with one eye covered and is asked to look at the button at the center of the screen. The examiner looks at the patient to monitor fixation. A test object (eg, a 1-mm diameter white sphere) held on a black wand is moved slowly from nonseeing into seeing areas along multiple meridia and in the blind spot, and the patient is asked to signal as soon as it comes into view. (*From Gittinger JW Jr.* Ophthalmology: A Clinical Introduction. *Boston: Little, Brown, 1984, with permission.*)

blind spot, and 5-degree concentric circles; Fig. 2–30) is an excellent way to test the central visual field. Usually only the central 30 degrees is tested; the periphery is not evaluated. Utilizing test targets of various sizes, the field can be mapped fairly quickly and accurately. The examiner stands at the side of the screen and moves a test target on the end of a wand from the periphery toward fixation, marking the outer dimensions of the visual field. Any scotomas are mapped with movement in several directions. The sensitivity of the method can be increased by moving the patient farther away from the tangent screen or using a smaller target (eg, use a 1-mm target at 2 meters).

Tangent screen testing is especially effective for defining small scotomas (which appear "larger") or slit defects associated with slit defects in the retinal nerve fiber layer. If the patient is moved closer to or farther from the screen and the size of the test object changed accordingly, the angle occupied by any real visual field defect does not alter. Thus, the defect should appear larger when the patient is seated far from the screen and smaller when the patient is seated near the screen. Functional (hysterical or malingering) visual field defects often do not conform

to this physiologic change in scotoma size. In order to do the most accurate tangent screen evaluations, the brightness of the test targets and the lighting under which the testing is done must be carefully controlled. Monitor fixation closely while you are mapping out the visual field.

Goldmann perimetry. Goldmann perimetry remains the "gold standard" of visual field testing. Especially when done by an accomplished perimetrist, it gives extremely accurate and reproducible results. (However, as automated perimetry gains in popularity, perimetrists with the skills necessary to perform a good Goldmann field are becoming rarer.) In this test, the patient's head is stabilized in a bowl perimeter (Fig. 2–31). The luminance of the perimeter as well as the size and brightness of the test objects are controlled. The examiner monitors fixation accurately through a telescope at the back of the bowl.

The Goldmann field tests both central and peripheral fields and allows for reproducible and accurate follow-up of visual field defects. Patients generally find it the method of field testing most to their liking. Goldmann field testing is a kinetic field test in which the target is moved by the examiner. As

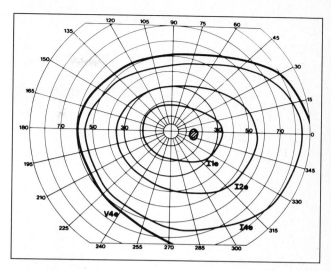

Figure 2–32. Goldmann plot. A normal field in a young person obtained on a Goldmann perimeter. Four isopters are represented: V4e, I4e, I2e, and I1e. The blind spot—a scotoma where no stimulus is seen—is hatched. (*From Gittinger JW Jr. Ophthalmology: A Clinical Introduction. Boston: Little, Brown, 1984, with permission.*)

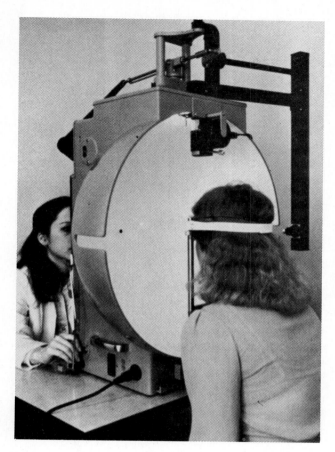

Figure 2–31. Goldmann perimeter. The patient is on the right and the perimetrist on the left. (*From Beck RW, Smith C. The neurologic exam. Neurol Clin. 1983;1:807–830, with permission.*)

in all types of visual field testing, several isopters (central, intermediate, and peripheral; Fig. 2–32) need to be tested to determine the nature of any defect (contracted versus depressed, absolute versus sloping). Spot testing for scotomata hiding between isopters also must be done. Testing the blind spot gives important information not only as to the size of the blind spot (increased with papilledema and other disc swelling and with depressed fields) but also as to the cooperativeness and reliability of the patient.

A specific note should be made about the patient's reliability. This information is often helpful in later interpretation of the visual field and in comparison with future fields. Goldmann field testing is somewhat time consuming (although usually more rapid than automated perimetry) and may be less sensitive to small defects in the central area than Amsler grid testing, tangent screen testing, or automated perimetry. Small variations from one test to the next are difficult to evaluate statistically as can be done with automated perimetry.

Static perimetry is done manually on the Goldmann and Tübingen perimeters. In contrast to kinetic testing where the target moves, static perimetry tests the sensitivity of the visual field at a given point, usually tested by placing the target at one point and increasing its intensity until it is just seen by the patient. This gives a precise evaluation of the contour of visual sensitivity (Fig. 2–33). It also allows very accurate follow-up. However, it is extremely time consuming, fatiguing for the patient, and somewhat difficult for the less experienced interpreter of visual fields; it does not give the total picture at a glance.

Automated (computerized) perimetry. Computerization allows the "automation" of visual field testing. Utilizing the computer, a set-testing paradigm can be used, eliminating most of the variability attributed to testing methodology. Quality of fixation is automatically recorded.

In a bowl perimeter, as for Goldmann and static perimetry, stimuli are presented in random locations. Two general strategies are used, threshold and suprathreshold testing. In *suprathreshold testing*, the target exceeds the threshold. Although reasonable for screening, suprathreshold testing lacks sensitivity. For more accurate visual field evaluation of both central and peripheral field and for comparison of fields over time, *threshold testing* is necessary. When performed in this manner, the incremental change in the intensity of the stimulus is varied. Differences

Kinetic Perimetry

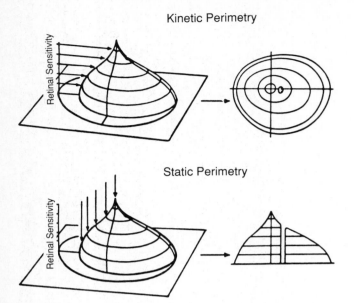

Static Perimetry

Figure 2–33. Two methods of measuring Traquair's "island of vision." In conventional kinetic perimetry (**top**), a moving test spot of fixed contrast to the background approaches the island (arrows). Isopters, lines connecting all points of equal sensitivity to light, encircle the island. In static perimetry (**bottom**), the island is approached from above; a stationary test object measures elevation (sensitivity) at selected points by increasing in contrast until detected by the subject. (*From Ellenberger C. Perimetry. In: Ophthalmol. Clinics, vol 17(1):1–38, Karp J. Burde RM, ed.* Clinical Neuro-ophthalmology: The Afferent Visual System. *Boston: Little, Brown, 1977, with permission.*)

Right

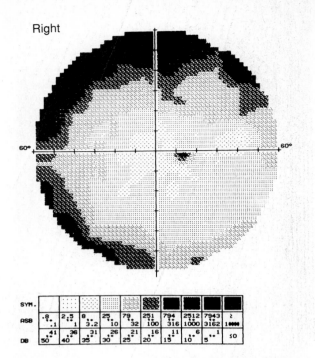

Figure 2–34. Gray scale. A normal visual field (Humphrey Field Analyzer). The visual field out to 60 degrees is represented on greytone and threshold value (decibel) printouts. Note that on the nasal side the absolute edge of the field is reached (zero values for some points at the upper left). (*From Anderson DR. Perimetry: With and Without Automation.* 2nd ed. St. Louis: Mosby, 1984, with permission.)

from a standard "normal" field, from fields of patients of similar age, or from previous fields of the same patient are derived statistically.

Because discrete points are tested, however, there is always need for some interpolation between various points. Unless testing strategies are chosen appropriately for the type of visual defect shown by the patient, some confusion may result. Thus, complete evaluation of a field, especially one with several scotomas, becomes very time consuming. To save time and spare the patient, automated perimetry often is limited to the central fields. Although very few neurologic defects are totally missed by 30-degree fields, they frequently are not well characterized and need to be further studied by testing the peripheral field or by kinetic perimetry. The usual output of automated perimetry is a gray scale plot (Fig. 2–34), although numerical data can be given as well.

As more and more experience is gained with automated perimetry, it may replace Goldmann testing as the "gold standard." Currently, it is certainly preferable where the Goldmann perimetry is performed by an inexperienced perimetrist. It is better for close following of scotomata in the central field,

as in glaucoma. However, it seems to be poorer than kinetic perimetry for the differentiation of functional from organic visual loss, because isopters are not depicted clearly.

The representations of these common methods of visual field testing are diagrammed in Figure 2–35. Newer methods of visual field evaluation hold promise. Acuity perimetry, sine wave gratings, high-pass resolution targets, and flicker stimuli each show advantages. High-pass resolution targets (the "ring test"), in particular, have several advantages: patient preference, speed, and low test-retest variability. The ideal visual field test should control the parameters mentioned above (patient and examiner variations, stimulus conditions, and so forth), and be rapid (so as not to fatigue the patient), sensitive, and easily compared with norms (for the population or for the patient). It has yet to be developed.

Visual Field Testing in the Hysterical or Malingering Patient. See also the visual field section in Chapter 20.

Examination of eye movements. See Chapters 11 and 15. **Slit-lamp examination:** Examination at the slit-lamp allows observation of the tissues

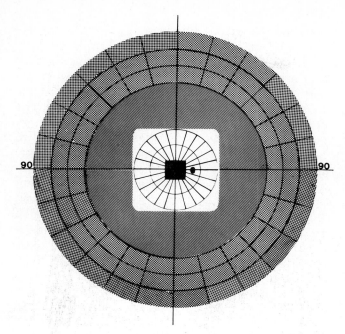

Figure 2–35. Drawing of types of visual field testing superimposed. The Amsler grid subtends 20 degrees (10 degrees to each side of fixation), the tangent screen and standard automated perimetry 60 degrees, and the Goldmann field 180 degrees.

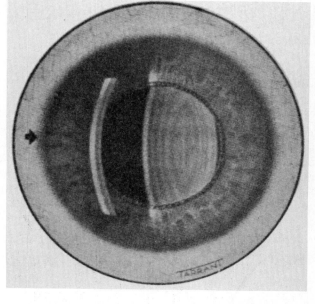

Figure 2–36. Slit-lamp optical section. The light (arrowed) comes from the left and in the beam of the slit-lamp the sections of the cornea and the lens are clearly evident. (*From Peter Hanse. In Duke-Elder S. System of Ophthalmology. London: Kimpton, 1961; 2; with permission.*)

around the eye and the anterior segment of the eye under binocular conditions with superb illumination and magnification. The same transparency of the eye that allows light to enter and start the visual process allows us to view the ocular structures. The anterior part of the eye may be examined by a handlight; however, use the slit-lamp to look for details on the lids, conjunctiva, cornea, and within the anterior chamber, iris, lens, and vitreous. With appropriate lenses, the fundus may also be examined.

The slit-beam produces an optical cross section of the structures viewed, allowing abnormalities to be accurately localized in depth (Fig. 2–36). The clarity and disorders of the media and tissues may be evaluated. Ocular disorders that decrease visual acuity, such as keratoconus and subtle cataracts, should be carefully sought out.

If no slit-lamp is available, a great deal of information may be obtained by utilizing a hand light and a magnifying lens or loupe.

The Ophthalmoscopic Evaluation

Examination of the fundus is another cornerstone of neuro-ophthalmic evaluation.

The ophthalmoscopic examination should *always* be done through a dilated pupil in order to observe fine details in the posterior pole and to be able to see the periphery. Details of small vessels and

the nerve fiber layer cannot be adequately evaluated through the diffraction caused by small pupil. If dilation is started after examining the pupil, it will be well underway by the time you finish the remainder of the exam. Use of a cycloplegic makes examination with bright light somewhat less uncomfortable for the patient.

It is a common concern that mydriatic drops will precipitate an attack of closed-angle glaucoma in anatomically predisposed eyes. To avoid this, grade the depth of the chamber angle with a hand light to detect eyes that are likely to suffer angle closure. However, precipitating such attacks is extraordinarily rare. In addition, there is probably no better place for a closed-angle glaucoma attack to be discovered than in the physician's office, where it can be instantaneously treated. Thus, apparently narrow angles are not a contraindication to dilating the pupil. Any potential risk of angle closure is significantly outweighed by the value of a meticulous fundus exam, which can be accomplished only through a dilated pupil. (I use Mydriacyl 0.5% and Neo-Synephrine 2.5%.) In addition, the cycloplegia, by paralyzing the patient's accommodation, also allows for a double check of the patient's true refraction. Although the fastest-acting cycloplegic, Mydriacyl, supposedly wears off in 1.5 to 3 hours, it is not rare to have a patient complain of effects lasting into the next day. Adding a sympathomimetic agent directly stimulates the dilator and speeds up dilation; it makes the dilation more complete and the pupil less likely to constrict during the examination.

The Optic Disc

The normal optic disc. The optic disc is composed of neural, vascular, and connective tissue components, arranged into functional columns. Alterations in the disc will manifest themselves by changes in these components seen ophthalmoscopically as alterations in one or more of the following: contour, color, cup size, or vascularity. The changes at the edge of the disc related to variations in the extent of the surrounding tissue layers will be discussed later in this chapter.

The cup to disc ratio. The optic cup is that portion of the optic disc that is relatively recessed and more pale than the surrounding neuroglial rim. The size of the cup is usually expressed as a fraction of the horizontal disc diameter and is 0.3 or less in 85% of normal individuals. Variation greater than 0.2 between right and left eyes occurs in less than 1% of normals. The size of the cup appears to be genetically determined. There is controversy as to whether or not the cup size increases with age, although it is likely that it does because central nervous system and optic nerve tissue are lost with aging.

Optic atrophy, seen as optic nerve pallor and accompanied by attrition of the nerve fiber layer and small nutrient vessels, represents damage to the optic nerve. Evaluation of disc color or its counterpart, pallor, is extremely difficult; there are no good objective measurements. Judgment must take into account the significant normal variations in color, effects of lens opacification, media alterations, relative brightness and whiteness of the ophthalmoscope light, and background pigmentation of the patient. Thus, assessment of mild degrees of pallor is especially difficult. When the atrophy is uniocular, comparison between the two eyes can be very helpful. Unfortunately, the degree of pallor and the visual acuity do not correlate closely; for example, following optic neuritis, it is not unusual for the optic disc to be stark white and the visual acuity 20/20 or even 20/15.

Which specific disc components contribute to the appearance of optic disc pallor remains somewhat unclear. Although the ratio of blood vessels to neural cells does not change in optic atrophy, the neural tissue is replaced with astrocytes. This substitution itself or a concomitant change in the optical properties of the restructured disc causes the appearance of pallor.

Kestenbaum's Rule. Clinicians count small vessels at the disc margin as an estimate of optic atrophy. The mean number of small vessels crossing the disc margin is 9.47. Ninety-five percent of patients has more than 8 when viewed with the ophthalmoscope and more than 7 when counted on a photograph. The number of small vessels decreases with age. The average number in the second decade is 10.5, and in the eighth decade 8.6. Less than 7 indicates optic atrophy.

In **glaucomatous optic atrophy** the loss of neurons is manifested by loss of the nerve fiber layer, enlargement of the optic cup (loss of the neuroglial rim tissue), and nerve fiber bundle defects in the visual field. In contrast to most other types of optic atrophy, the remaining neuroglial rim retains relatively normal color until the end stage. Although extensive cupping is characteristic of glaucoma, cupping occasionally occurs in nonglaucomatous neuropathies, such as ischemia, toxic neuropathy, and compression (Chapter 5).

The Macula

The macula lies two disc diameters temporal to the disc and slightly below the horizontal. It is a slightly deeper red than the surrounding fundus, with a bright yellow reflex marking the foveal pit. A circular halo reflex surrounds the parafoveal area (Fig. 2–37). In most disorders that affect the macula, the normal foveal and circular reflexes are lost early. Another early macular change is a disruption of the smooth pigmentation.

Specific macular disorders cause various patterns of degeneration, edema, exudation, pigment alteration, and detachment. These are associated with decreased visual acuity, metamorphopsia (distor-

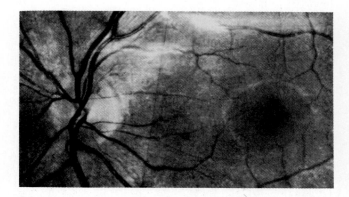

Figure 2–37. Circular macular reflex. Fundus photograph of normal macula with annular and foveal reflex. (*From Ballantyne AJ, Michaelson IC. Textbook of the Fundus of the Eye. 2nd ed. London: Livingstone, 1970, with permission.*)

tion), and central field defects. Unless the damage is profound, an afferent pupillary defect is unusual. The Amsler grid may show small scotomas, blur, or distortion. If macular disease is suspected but not obvious on ophthalmoscopic evaluation, use the indirect ophthalmoscope, slit-lamp, and appropriate fundus lenses to examine the macula with magnification and with stereopsis.

The Retinal Vessels

The retinal vessels radiate from the optic nerve head, dividing dichomatously. Note their caliber, regularity, and reflexes. There should be bright, even, longitudinal light reflexes off the top of the vessels and also from the internal limiting membrane as it makes a bend from the vessel to the retina. The vessel walls should be transparent and the blood column of the arteries a brighter red than that of the veins. Note sheathing and opacity as well as the branching pattern, especially at the disc. The diameter of the arteries should be approximately two thirds that of the veins. Look for abnormalities such as telangiectasia, aneurysms, angiomas, feeding vessels, and arteriovascular malformations. Other abnormal findings include emboli, abnormal vessels, and newly formed vessels. Neovascular changes occur in the retina (intraretinal microangiopathy, IRMA) or extend into the vitreous (proliferative retinopathy).

Venous pulsations at the disc are present in 80%

of normal eyes and are often lost with increased intracranial pressure. When they have been noted previously, their disappearance may indicate increased intracranial pressure.

Examination of the Retinal Nerve Fiber Layer

The nerve fiber layer of the retina originates in the ganglion cells and converges on the optic disc. It is the most anterior of the retinal layers, the closest to the ophthalmoscope.

The normal retinal nerve fiber layer has fine radial striations, best seen in the peripapillary region within 1.5 disc diameters of the disc and as they cross the disc margins. As they pass over blood vessels, they interrupt light reflexes on the larger vessels and partially bury smaller vessels, making them appear to be discontinuous. Finer fibers in the papillomacular bundle and the nasal retina are more difficult to evaluate (Fig. 2–38). The nerve fiber layer normally has a slightly gray, translucent cast that obscures details of the retinal pigment epithelium and choroid. Gunn's dots are bright spots (probably reflections from the insertions of Müller fiber footplates into internal limiting membrane) that come and go as the ophthalmoscope beam moves (Fig. 2–39).

Retinal nerve fiber layer observation is aided by an ophthalmoscope with a bright white light source, preferably halogen; a widely dilated pupil; clear media; a darkly pigmented choroid or retinal pigment epithelium; and increased contrast, usually in the form of "red-free" light. Polaroids, and photo-

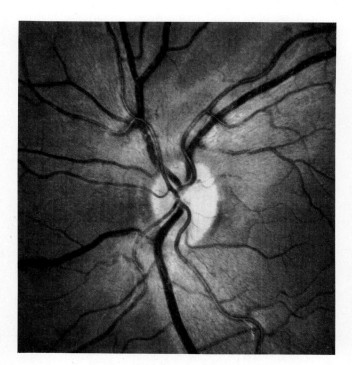

Figure 2–38. Retinal nerve fiber layer.

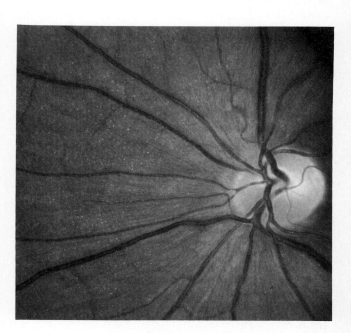

Figure 2–39. Gunn's dots.

graphic or computerized enhancement of images (discussed later in the chapter), can be useful as well. However, most important to the examination of nerve fiber layer detail is a skilled observer. Amazingly, in today's technological era, this relatively simple art of observation provides a rapid, inexpensive, and very sensitive method for study of the visual pathways.

A damaged axon undergoes both anterograde and retrograde degeneration; the retinal nerve fiber layer, therefore, is affected by any damage to the anterior visual pathways between the ganglion cells and the lateral geniculate body. The consequent axonal dropout frequently is visible ophthalmoscopically.

Between the onset of retrobulbar tertiary neuron damage and the appearance of nerve fiber layer alterations, there is a time lag. Thus, in acute optic nerve, chiasm, tract, and lateral geniculate lesions, the retinal nerve fiber layer and optic disc may appear to be totally normal, yet visual acuity may be decreased (as, for example, with retrobulbar neuritis).

Later, axonal changes, both atrophic and intrinsic, become ophthalmoscopically obvious (Chapter 3) and are important clues to neuro-ophthalmic diagnoses.

FURTHER TECHNIQUES FOR CLINICAL EVALUATION OF THE VISUAL AFFERENT PATHWAYS

The procedures discussed above should be performed for all patients without exception. Those described below (Table 2–6) confirm or rule out visual loss; some suggest a specific etiology. They also are useful as a battery of tests for the patient suspected of hysteria or malingering; for these patients the more tests utilized, the more chance there is to demonstrate a positive pattern of nonphysiologic inconsistencies.

Photostress (glare recovery, macular dazzle) test. This test, particularly sensitive to macular problems, is excellent for differentiating optic nerve from macular disease, especially central serous retinopa-

thy. First, record the patient's best corrected visual acuity. Then have the patient look directly at the light of an ophthalmoscope or penlight held close to the eye for 10 seconds. Subsequently, record the time to recover to one line less than best corrected visual acuity. Normally, vision will recover within 40 seconds and with less than 10 seconds difference between the two eyes. In neurogenic disease, the recovery time should be normal. In macular disease, the recovery time is prolonged; with some disease processes, such as central serous retinopathy, recovery can take minutes. The test is most accurate in patients with only mildly decreased visual acuity and is probably not valid if visual acuity is worse than 20/100.

Contrast sensitivity testing. Gratings or figures with a spectrum of spatial frequencies or contrast are presented to the patient (Fig. 2–40). Many patients with minimally decreased visual acuity and somewhat equivocal abnormalities on other types of testing have significant abnormalities in contrast sensitivity. Contrast sensitivity is also a broader test of visual function than visual acuity, which measures spatial resolution only at high contrast. Although results vary in different reports, some studies suggest that some disease processes primarily affect perception of particular frequencies—such as low spatial frequency loss in demyelinating disease and high spatial frequency loss in glaucoma. However, despite its sensitivity, we currently cannot reliably distinguish between optic nerve and macular disease nor distinguish between the many types of optic neuropathies. Nevertheless, contrast sensitivity testing is useful, especially if it confirms an abnormality when other tests are equivocal. It may be the earliest

TABLE 2–6. MORE OFFICE/BEDSIDE METHODS OF EXAMINATION

Photostress (glare recovery, macular dazzle) test
Contrast sensitivity test
Optokinetic nystagmus test
Stereoacuity test
Neutral-density filter test
Four-diopter prism test
Pulfrich stereo illusion test

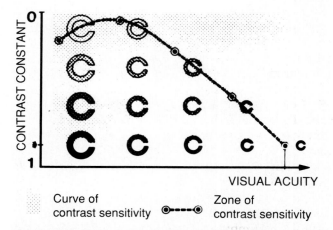

Figure 2–40. Contrast sensitivity. (Relation of contrast sensitivity to visual acuity). (*From Explorations du nerf optique. In: Hamard H, ed.* Neuropathies optiques. *Paris: Fr Soc Ophtal et Masson, 1986, with permission.*)

loss in the chronic papilledema of pseudotumor cerebri. It can be especially effective in malingerers, because as a less frequently used test the "correct" end point is difficult to anticipate. It is diminished universally following optic neuritis, explaining the persistent complaints of patients even when 20/20 vision returns.

Optokinetic nystagmus testing. Chapters 10, 11, 12, and 14 explain more fully optokinetic nystagmus (OKN) testing as it is used most often to evaluate ocular motility. However, optokinetic testing is useful to estimate visual acuity in preverbal children, in others unable to respond to the standard test charts, and in malingerers. Movement in response to movement of the tape or drum indicates a visual acuity corresponding to the angle subtended by the contrasting stripes.

Stereoacuity testing should correlate with best-corrected visual acuity. For example, if stereoacuity measures 40 seconds, visual acuity should approximate 20/20; 60 seconds, 20/40; 150 seconds, 20/200; and so forth. Obviously, a patient with true visual loss should not show stereo resolution finer than letter resolution. Lack of stereopsis appropriate for the visual acuity may differentiate amblyopia from acquired neurogenic visual loss and suggests early onset visual loss, amblyopia, strabismus, or anisometropia.

Neutral-density filter testing. The use of a neutral-density filter can differentiate among visual loss due to refractive error, optic nerve disease, and amblyopia. If a neutral-density filter (Kodak 149-6413, neutral density 2.0) is placed before a normal eye, visual acuity will be reduced about two lines (from 20/20 to 20/40, 20/40 to 20/60). The reduction will be much more severe, perhaps 20/20 to 20/100 or 20/200 in neurologic visual loss (or with posterior subcapsular cataract!). In contrast, in mild amblyopia (eg, in the monofixation syndrome) there is minimal or no reduction of visual acuity. Thus, a combination of decreased stereoacuity and minimal reduction in visual acuity through a neutral-density filter strongly suggests amblyopia rather than neuro-ocular visual loss.

Four diopter prism test. A prism bends light; thus, if a prism is held before a fixing eye, to maintain fixation on the same target, the eye will need to move. If the patient fixes a line of letters that can be read with either eye and a prism is introduced in front of the eye suspected to have neurogenic visual loss, a nonamblyopic eye will move in response to displacement of the image by the prism. If the patient has an amblyopic scotoma or any other central scotoma, the eye will not move. This test is also useful in testing malingerers, because if the eye moves when the patient views targets smaller than the

claimed visual acuity, the patient can see at least that well. Four diopter prism, stereoacuity, and neutral density filter testing help distinguish amblyopia from neurogenic visual loss.

Pulfrich stereo illusion. The Pulfrich stereo illusion describes the apparent elliptical path followed by a swinging pendulum if the luminance in one eye differs from that in the other. Swing a target on a pendulum back and forth, perpendicular to the visual axis. If a patient with asymmetric neurogenic visual loss observes the pendulum with both eyes, the target will appear to describe an ellipse, whereas with equal vision in both eyes, the pendulum merely moves from right to left (Fig. 2–41). This illusion may be demonstrated by placing a neutral-density filter (or a moderately dark sunglass) before one eye and viewing a pendulum. The precise physiologic basis of this test is not understood. The aberration may result from decreased stimulus value transmitted by the damaged optic nerve (as if a neutral density filter is present) or from delayed conduction. Both decreased simulus intensity and conduction delay produce increased latency of cortical evoked potentials.

The Pulfrich illusion is a useful companion to testing for color acuity, afferent pupillary defects, and

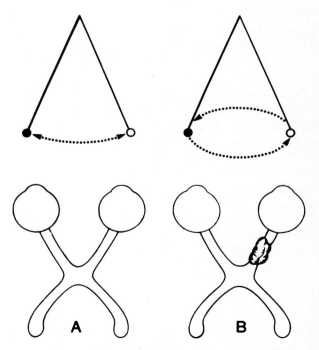

Figure 2–41. Clinical use of the Pulfrich stereo illusion. **A.** Normal appearance of pendular movement. **B.** Apparent elliptical movement of pendulum with unilateral optic nerve damage. (*From Newman NM. The prechiasmal afferent visual pathways. In: Karpe J., Burde, RM., (eds). International Ophthalmology Clinics, vol. 17(1):1–38. Clinical Neuro-ophthalmology: The Afferent Visual System. Boston: Little, Brown, 1977, with permission.*)

brightness sensation. It is easily appreciated by most patients with true neurogenic visual loss (as long as visual acuity allows the pendulum to be seen!). It is most dramatic when the conduction velocity is slowed significantly as in demyelinating optic neuritis. The results also help to explain complaints of disorientation and noncoordination in kinetic visual tasks voiced by patients with optic nerve disorders.

LABORATORY EVALUATION OF THE VISUAL AFFERENT PATHWAYS

Most of the tests considered here (Table 2–7) require sophisticated equipment not always available in a practitioner's office. They fall into three general categories: (1) electrophysiology; electroretinograms (ERG); electro-oculograms (EOG); pattern electroretinograms (PERG) and visual evoked potential testing (VEP); (2) psychophysics, dark adaptation, Vernier acuity; and (3) imaging techniques: fundus photography and fluorescein angiography, ultrasonography (A, B and Doppler), and plain x-rays,

TABLE 2–7. LABORATORY EVALUATION OF THE VISUAL AFFERENT PATHWAYS

Electrophysiology
  Visual evoked potential (VEP, VER)
  Electroretinography (ERG)—including oscillatory potentials, flicker
  Focal electroretinography (FERG)
  Pattern electroretinography (PERG)
  Electro-oculography (EOG)

Psychophysics
  Visual fields (see above)
  Interferometry
  Vernier acuity (hyperacuity)
  Dark adaptation (DA)
  Contrast sensitivity (see above)

Imaging
  Ophthalmoscopy
  Photography
    Color fundus
    Retinal nerve fiber layer
    Fluorescein angiography
  Ultrasound
    A- and B-modes
    Biometry
    Doppler, duplex (DCS)
  Neuro-imaging
    Plain films
    Computer tomography (CT)
    Magnetic resonance imaging (MRI)
    Single photon emission computed tomography (SPECT)
    Positron emission tomography (PET)
    Digital subtraction angiography (DA)
    Selective cerebral angiography

computed tomography and magnetic resonance scanning (MR); digital subtraction and angiography (DSA) and positron emission tomography (PET) and single photon emission computed tomography (SPECT).

Electrophysiology

Visual Evoked Potentials. The visual evoked potential (VEP) or visual evoked response (VER) testing measures the electrical activity of the visual afferent pathways. Visual impulses are transmitted as electrical energy from the retina to the optic nerve, chiasm, tract, radiations, and visual cortex. As the electrical response of the cortex is of very small amplitude, it is recorded by scalp electrodes and separated from background noise by computer averaging techniques. For most clinical studies, the electrodes are placed in positions O_1 and O_2 (international electroencephalography convention) on the occiput. The responses recorded from separate stimulation of each eye, and the responses over each hemisphere, are dependent on the integrity of the entire visual pathway. However, clinically VEP testing is most useful in diseases affecting the optic nerves. The precise sources of the electrical signals that are averaged are not known and must include input from association areas and from the opposite hemisphere, as occasionally even patients with complete homonymous hemianopias have relatively well-developed evoked responses on both sides. Hemifield stimulation with large checks improves the diagnostic accuracy of the VEP in chiasmal and postchiasmal diseases.

A number of stimuli (usually about 100) is averaged to produce the waveform. Initially, the stimulus was a light flash, but responses to checkerboards and sine-wave grating stimuli were found to yield more reproducible and standardized results. The alternating checkerboard has become the standard clinical test (pattern-reversal evoked potential or PREP).

To flash stimuli, the normal response usually shows an early wave and a W-shaped following wave. To pattern stimuli, there is usually a predominant positive wave at approximately 100 msec (the P_{100}). Its latency is the measurement most frequently evaluated (Fig. 2–42).

The visual evoked response is affected profoundly by lesions of the prechiasmal visual afferent pathways. Most of the changes are not pathognomonic; however, fragmentation and delay are seen both on flash and pattern stimulation in approximately 90% of patients with demyelinating disorders. Of course, if abnormalities are found on stimulation of each eye, when the patient has visual

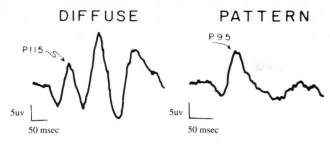

DIFFUSE   **PATTERN**

Figure 2–42. Conventional evoked potentials. The discrete averaged responses to a diffuse flash and to pattern reversal of black and white checks 1 degree square are illustrated. The first major positive-going peak at 95 to 115 msec is loosely termed the P_{100} component. This potential is known to be related to basic visual thresholds of interest for assessing visual performance. It is also used to define eye-to-brain latency. Positive is upward deflection. *(From Kupersmith MJ, Siegel IM. Electrophysiological testing in neuro-ophthalmology. In: Karpe J., Burde, RM. (eds). International Ophthalmology Clinics. 17(1):1–38. Neuro-ophthalmology. The Afferent Visual System. Boston: Little, Brown, 1986, with permission.)*

loss in only one eye, the findings become more significant, because they may indicate lesions disseminated in time and space as with multiple sclerosis. The changes found with ischemic and compressive lesions are not as distinctive and tend to affect the amplitude of the response more than the latency. During episodes of severe acute demyelinating visual loss, the visual evoked response may be nearly extinguished. The marked delay characteristic of demyelinating processes may persist as other measures of visual function improve or return to normal.

By using different-sized checks, the pattern-reversal visual evoked response can estimate refractive errors and visual acuity in nonverbal subjects. It also is very effective in documenting the integrity of the visual pathways in patients who dishonestly or hysterically profess a significant visual loss. In this case, a totally normal response can usually be trusted to be an indicator of virtually intact visual afferent pathways. However, especially in testing with pattern stimuli, the patient can ignore or stare through the pattern, producing a spuriously abnormal response. In such cases, an abnormal response in a patient with an otherwise normal neuro-ophthalmic examination does not necessarily indicate an organic defect. In these cases, the "abnormal" response usually consists of decreased amplitude with minimal change in latency, and the flash-evoked visual potential may be of particular value as it is harder to subvert.

During surgical procedures on the visual afferent pathway (in the orbit or cranium), intraoperative monitoring by VEP can demonstrate compromise or effective decompression. Additionally, in severe ocular and orbital trauma—where the integrity of the

optic nerve is in question, especially when the eye is filled with blood—a bright-flash VEP, analogous to bright-flash electroretinogram, may demonstrate integrity of the optic nerve and a reasonable prognosis following vitrectomy.

Flash Electroretinography (ERG). The electroretinogram (ERG) measures the integrity of the outer retinal layers (Fig. 2–43A). It is especially well suited to detecting diseases of the retinal receptors and pigment epithelium that diminish or abolish the response. A subnormal response typically is seen in tapeto-retinal degenerations (eg, retinitis pigmentosa). Whereas disease of photoreceptors renders the retina incapable of generating a normal electrical reaction to light, lesions of the inner retinal layer spare the electroretinogram. It is normal in ganglion cell, optic nerve, and higher visual pathway disease that does not affect the outer retinal layers; for example, the ERG is normal in central retinal artery occlusion and Tay-Sachs disease.

To obtain an ERG, an electrode is placed in contact with the cornea. After dark adaptation, the electrical response to a light flash is then recorded with respect to an indifferent electrode. The normal response shows a small negative A-wave (which probably arises from the activity of the rods and cones) and a larger positive B-wave (which probably relates to activity in the intermediate layers of the retina including the bipolar cells and Müller cells). A later C-wave arc, S-waves, and oscillatory potentials are less commonly studied but do provide evidence about the integrity of the inner retinal layers, especially in vascular diseases such as diabetes (Fig. 2–43B).

When the visual media are obscured (especially with dense vitreous hemorrhage), a bright-flash ERG (using brighter than normal flashes and a greater number of stimuli) may reveal the integrity of the outer retinal layers.

A dim or blue flash generates a scotopic ERG, a shallow and more extended wave obtained in dark adaptation that reflects the activity of the rods. Stimulation with fast (30/sec) flicker or red light isolates the cone response, because cones are sensitive to longer wavelengths and higher frequencies.

One disadvantage of the ERG is that it measures a mass response, the response of all the outer retinal layers. Some differentiation is obtained by concentrating on cone responses (which reflect central events) and rod responses (which reflect peripheral events). However, clinically this is generally not useful for localization beyond giving an estimate of the relative degree of involvement of rods and cones.

Focal Electroretinography. Focal electroretinography (FERG), in which only a very select area of the retina is stimulated, can be useful for localization,

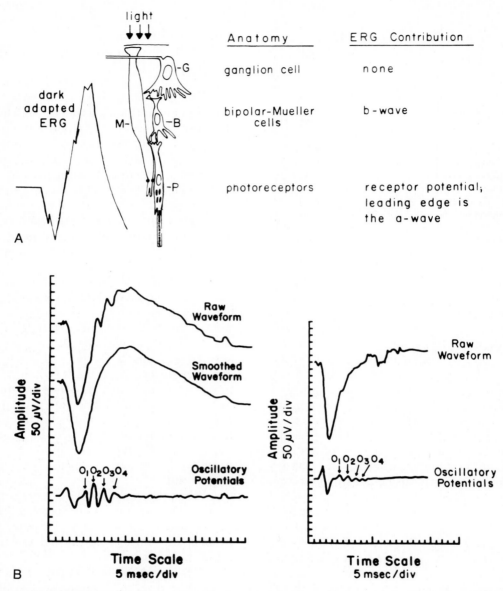

Figure 2–43. A. The ERG. The ERG waveform evoked by a diffuse flash of light represents a combination of separate components, each generated from a different retinal layer. The clinically recorded ERG in response to a diffuse flash is a composite of waveforms derived from different layers of the retina. Photoreceptors generate the a-wave, which is the leading edge of the receptor potential, and midretinal layer structures produce the b-wave via Müeller-cell activation. The figure correlates the different ERG components with the retinal structures that are associated with their generation. **B.** Oscillatory potentials. ERG produced by a photoflash stimulus showing the early receptor potential and oscillatory potentials. **Left.** Digital subtraction of digitally smoothed waveform (center tracing) from raw waveform (*top tracing*) to yield waveform with faster oscillatory potentials (*bottom tracing*). Data are from a control subject who is aged 34 years and is nondiabetic O_1, first oscillatory potential; O_2, second oscillatory potential; O_3, third oscillatory potential; O_4, fourth oscillatory potential. **Right.** Raw waveform (*above*) and digitally filtered waveform (below) from electroretinogram of a patient with proliferative retinopathy (DRS-High Risk Characteristics). Note severely reduced oscillatory potentials in both waveforms. (**A.** *from Kupersmith MJ, Siegel M, Cracco RQ, Bodis-Wollner I, eds. Electrophysiological evaluation of visual loss in ophthalmology using the ERG and VEP. In:* Evoked Potentials: Frontiers of Clinical Neuroscience. *New York: Liss, 1986; 3; with permission.* **B.** *From Bresnick GH. Background diabetic retinopathy. In: Ryan SJ, ed.* Retina. *St. Louis: Mosby, 1989; 2; with permission.*)

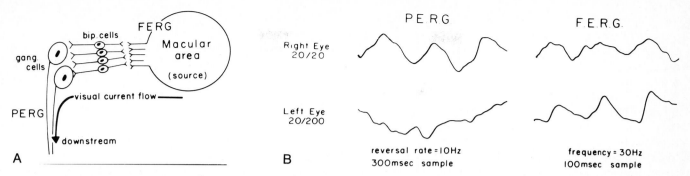

Figure 2–44. A. FERG/PERG testing. The focal electroretinogram (FERG) initiates light-induced activity in the cones and bipolar cells of the macula. The electrical activity of the ganglion cell layer of the retina can be detected using a pattern-reversal stimulus (pattern ERG or PERG). **B.** FERG/PERG testing. A patient with left-sided optic neuritis. The normal right eye has normal luminance on focal (FERG) and pattern (PERG) electroretinograms. The affected left eye has a normal FERG, since the outer and midretinal layers are intact, but shows an absent PERG response because of the ganglion cell involvement. (**A.** *From Kupersmith MJ, Siegel IM: Electrophysiological testing in neuro-ophthalmology. In: International Ophthalmology Clinics. Neuro-ophthalmology. Boston, Little, Brown, & Co.; 1986; 26(4); with permission.* **B.** *from Kupersmith MJ, Siegel IM: Electrophsiological testing in neuro-ophthalmology. In: International Ophthalmology Clinics. Neuro-ophthalmology. Boston, MA: Little, Brown, 1986, 26(4); with permission.*)

but is more difficult to perform, time consuming (especially if the affected area is not already defined), and not readily available (Fig. 2–44A).

Pattern electroretinography. Pattern electroretinography (PERG) measures the ERG response to patterned stimuli (usually an alternating checkerboard as in VEP testing), which derives from the inner retinal layers and preganglionic retinal elements (Fig. 2–44B). The PERG is reduced in inner retinal layer, optic nerve, and early macular disease. It seems to be particularly sensitive in early cases of Stargardt's disease, being diminished early while visual acuity is near normal. This is an unexplained paradox, as Stargardt's disease is thought to affect outer retinal layers only. It is also sensitive to retinal vascular occlusive processes.

Electro-oculography (EOG). There is a steady potential difference of approximately six millivolts between the cornea and the charged membranes of the posterior portion of the eye (Fig. 2–45), the pigment epithelium and receptor elements. This standing potential acts as a dipole oriented between the cornea and the posterior pole. Thus, if two electrodes are arrayed at the inner and outer canthi, the potential difference can be measured, as the eyes move back and forth. When the eye is illuminated, the standing potential increases to a maximum, the "light peak." As the light intensity diminishes, the potential decreases until it reaches a minimum, the "dark trough." For electro-oculography (EOG) the subject is asked to make eye movements of 30 to 40 degrees to either side of the midline. The potentials generated are recorded, first under conditions of dark adaptation to obtain the dark trough, and then with room illumination to obtain the light peak. The ratio of the

potential at the light peak to the potential at the dark trough is the test result. The average result is about 2.5; anything less than 1.5 is definitely abnormal. The use of the ratio eliminates variability generated by the differences that arise from individual variability in standing potentials, skin conductivity, type of electrode, and electrode placement.

The EOG reflects the presynaptic function of the retina and is abnormal in diseases interrupting interaction between the retinal pigment epithelium and the photoreceptors. Decreased peak-to-trough ratios occur in retinitis pigmentosa, choroideremia, vitamin A deficiency, toxic retinopathies, and retinal detachment, along with other diseases of the retina.

Psychophysics

The first two tests described below are used to estimate the "retinal acuity" behind media opacities (eg,

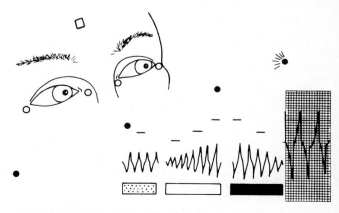

Figure 2–45. EOG. (*From Explorations de nerf optique. In: Hamard H, ed.: Neuropathies optiques, IV. Paris: Fr Soc Ophtal et Masson; 1986, with permission.*)

for approximating the potential for visual improvement following cataract extraction). Although one can get a fairly good estimate of visual potential by applying the adage "the view in equals the view out," some patients can see surprisingly well through media opacities that seem quite severe; at other times, visual acuity is degraded much more than one estimates when viewing the fundus. Thus, it is useful to have objective measurements. These tests also can be helpful in determining the true acuity in patients suspected of hysteria or malingering.

Interferometry. In these tests, interference fringes are projected onto the retina. They are generally able to penetrate through "windows" in cataracts and corneal opacities and thus measure the acuity of the retina. Although these tests are resistant to retinal image degradation by media opacities, sometimes no windows are found and the test is not effective.

Vernier acuity. This measures the ability of the retina to resolve dots or lines minimally displaced one from the other. Because of the extreme precision of Vernier acuity, it is sometimes called "hyperacuity"; it can resolve 3 seconds of arc, which is approximately one tenth of the intercone spacing in the human fovea, the theoretical limit of ocular resolution. This is interesting in and of itself because it implies additional information processing, probably centrally mediated. It has been shown that this test is very robust and that "hyperacuity" is not significantly degraded by media opacities. Thus, Vernier acuity is an excellent test of foveal function in the presence of ocular opacities.

Vernier tests also are useful in the evaluation of amblyopia, as it has been shown that amblyopes of different etiologies show different patterns of Vernier acuity loss.

Dark Adaptation (DA) measures the increase in ocular sensitivity as the eye goes from the light-adapted (photopic) to the dark-adapted (scotopic) state. The Goldmann-Weekers adaptometer is a small bowl into which the head of the subject is inserted (Fig. 2–46). First, a bright light condition is maintained for 10 minutes. Then all lights are extinguished and measurement of the light threshold is made at 30-second intervals. The resulting graph shows an initial steep slope (the cone limb) lasting about 10 minutes and representing adaptation of the cones. A subsequent, more gradual and lengthy slope lasting about 20 minutes represents the adaptation of the rods. In cone disorders, the first portion of the slope is abolished, but normal rod thresholds may eventually be obtained. In general, diseases of the outer retinal layers and retinal pigment epithelium (especially retinitis pigmentosa) severely affect the response. Dark adaptation testing is rarely used in isolation to evaluate possible neurogenic visual loss. However, in the setting of unexplained visual loss, dark adaptation frequently complements electroretinography in establishing the diagnosis of outer retinal layer disease, particularly retinitis pigmentosa.

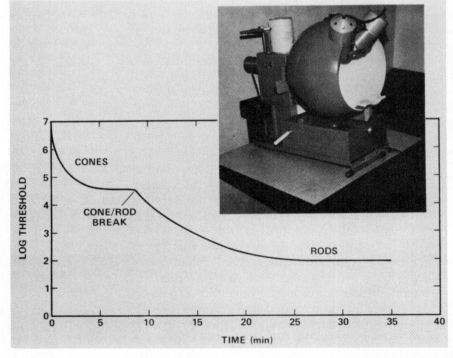

Figure 2–46. Dark adaptation. Dark adaptation testing with a Goldmann-Weekers adaptometer. Subject looks at test light within dome, while recording drum keeps continuous record of patient's responses. Dark adaptation curve represents response of normal observer following five to seven minutes preadaptation to light. If only foveola were tested, using a very small test spot, cone plateau would be maintained and there would be no rod limb to curve. (*From Peyman G, Sanders D, Goldberg M, eds. Principles and Practice of Ophthalmology. Philadelphia, WB Saunders; 1980; II; with permission.*)

Diagnostic Imaging

Not surprisingly, much evaluation of vision and motility disorders is visually oriented. The most anterior portions of the afferent visual pathways are accessible to examination by the eye, ophthalmoscope, and camera as are no other portions of the central nervous system and very few parts of the other major bodily systems.

Thus, imaging modalities play a significant role in detection and differential diagnosis of neuro-ophthalmic disorders; they are important in documenting baseline status as well as evolution of disease processes. Studies of visible portions of the visual afferent pathway are done by ophthalmoscopy, fundus photography, and fluorescein angiography. Modalities that allow us to study structures not accessible to the eye include ultrasonography, plain x-rays, computed tomography (CT), magnetic resonance imaging (MRI), positron emission tomography (PET), single photon emission computed tomography (SPECT), digital subtraction angiography (DSA), and selective cerebral angiography (Table 2–8).

Ophthalmoscopy. Meticulous examination of the ocular fundus is a key examination skill for evaluation of ocular and neurologic disease and many systemic illnesses with ocular manifestations (eg,

TABLE 2–8. COMPARATIVE ADVANTAGES OF IMAGING TECHNIQUES

	Ultrasound	CT[a]	MRI[b]	Angiography
Eye	+ + +	+ +	+ +	(Fluorescein) + + +
Craniofacial				
Skeleton		+ +		
Soft tissue	+ +	+ +	+ +	
Orbit				
General	+ +	+ + +	+ +	+
Mass	+	+ +	+ +	
Optic nerve	+ +	+ +	+ +	
Bones		+ + +	+	
Extraocular muscles	+ + +	+ +	+ +	
Intracranial				
Optic nerve		+	+ +	
Chiasm		+	+ +	
Sella		+	+ +	
Pituitary tumor		+ +	+ +	
Suprasellar mass			+ +	+
Basal Structures		+	+ +	
Cranial vessels, aneurysm		+ +	+ +	
Nerves		+ +	+ +	
Brain Stem, Cerebellum, Intrinsic Hemisphere Lesions		+	+ + +	
Mass		+ +	+ + +	
Hemorrhage (extrinsic, too)				
Acute		+ +	+	
Chronic			+ + +	
AVM		+	+ + +	
Demyelinating plaques			+ + +	
Vascular				
Infarction		+	+ +	+
Aneurysm		+	+ +	+ +
Thrombosis		+	+ + +	+ + +
Fistula		+	+ +	+ + +
CNS Malformation		+	+ + +	

[a] CT—better for study of very small lesions due to spatial resolution.
[b] MRI—evolving rapidly. Use of contrast, more experience will only augment its current potential.

sarcoid, diabetes, temporal arteritis, and the phako-matoses). (See Chapter 3.)

Ocular photography. Color photography of the fundus documents pathologic processes. It allows objective comparisons over time, especially of aberrations that are diagnostic but difficult to quantify, such as changes in disc configuration or color in optic neuropathy. It is a good idea to give the patient a copy of the photos for use in medical care away from your office. The young boy with "swollen discs" from optic nerve head drusen who ends up in the emergency room after minor head trauma could well be saved a CT, MRI, or even a burr hole.

When there is particular interest in the retinal nerve fiber layer, *"red-free" photography* accentuates the visibility of the ganglion cell axons.

Fluorescein angiography is especially helpful in the diagnosis of subtle vascular alterations not easily visible with the ophthalmoscope, such as subretinal neovascular membranes, minimal telangiectatic changes, and areas of decreased capillary perfusion. Fluorescein dye is injected intravenously and its progression through the retinal circulation studied by rapid-sequence photos taken through a fundus camera. Sodium fluorescein absorbs light between 485 and 500 nanometers, and emits light between 525 and 530 nanometers. Using appropriate excitatory and barrier filters to excite the dye and transmit only the fluorescence, transit of dye is photographed over a 30- to 45-minute period.

The contrast between the bright fluorescence of the dye and the dark background of the fundus allows visualization of vascular detail and aberrations. The normal choriocapillaris allows the dye to leak freely, whereas the normal retinal capillaries with their tight epithelial junctions do not. Thus, leakage of dye into the retina indicates either disruption of Bruch's membrane and/or the retinal pigment epithelium or pathology of the retinal vasculature. Newly formed vessels, which in the retina are always abnormal, also leak dye. In papilledema, papillitis, and other inflammatory swelling of the nerve head, the vessels on the disc leak, especially in the late stages of the fluorescein study. In contrast, congenitally full discs, discs in Leber's optic neuropathy, and discs with optic nerve head drusen do not leak. Leakage also occurs from inflamed vessels.

Adverse reactions (nausea and vomiting in 4%, urticaria or pruritis in 0.3% of patients) occur in about 5% of injections. Serious anaphylactic and other morbid complications are very rare.

Ultrasonography. Ultrasonography (echography) records ultrasonic pulses reflected from ocular and orbital tissues as high-energy sound waves are directed from a transducer into the eye or orbit. The ultrasound beam acts like a light ray in many ways; it traverses the structures of the eye and orbit; it is reflected, refracted, and absorbed within the tissues, and finally is reflected back to the transducer, which then transforms the sound waves into an electrical pulse. The electrical pulse is amplified and displayed on a video screen.

There are two major ways in which these echoes are presented, A-mode and B-mode (Fig. 2–47). In *A-mode* the signals are presented as spikes, with the height of the spike representing the strength of the echo. Thus, in tissues that have few echoes the spike height will be very low; those that are very echogenic will generate very high spikes. By and large, as with light rays, an echo occurs when there is a difference in the refraction of the beam. In the eye, refraction occurs at interfaces between media of differing acoustic properties; the echoes occur when the beam

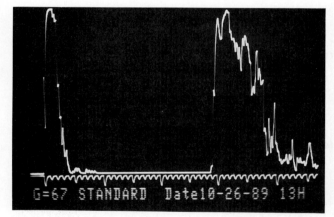

A

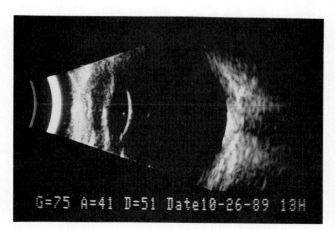

B

Figure 2–47. Ultrasonography. **A.** A-scan of a normal eye. **B.** B-scan of a normal eye. The cornea is to the left and the retina to the right.

enters the cornea from the air, the anterior chamber from the cornea, and so forth. With all modes of ultrasonography, unless an immersion bath is used, there are a few millimeters of dead space before the echoes are recognized.

A-scan echography has the distinct advantage of providing accurate quantification of tissue reflectivity and is useful in differential diagnosis. However, because the picture presented by the spikes is not familiar, its use and interpretation remain difficult and require considerable experience.

B-mode ultrasonography provides a type of echotomography. A cross section of the object scanned by to-and-fro movement of the transducer is projected on the screen. Here, the brightness of the points on a gray scale corresponds to the echogenic quality of the tissue (as does the height of the echoes on A-scan). The transducer moves to obtain successive cuts through the globe and orbit, which reconstructs a three-dimensional mental picture of the tissues examined. Echography is important for the examination of eyes with opaque media. It has absolutely no adverse effects on tissue at diagnostic energy levels.

In ophthalmology, **A-scan ultrasonography** can also be used for *biometry*, for calculation of lens power for intraocular lens implantation, quantification of intraocular tumor dimensions, corneal thickness, and optic nerve and nerve sheath diameter. In the orbit, it works well for localizing masses and to some degree for differential diagnosis. Ultrasound reliably detects orbital lesions; *quantitative A-scan echography* reliably differentiates most tumors, inflammation, and foreign bodies of the orbit. *Kinetic echography* can demonstrate the compressibility of hemangiomas and blood flow within them (even when the blood movement is not seen with angiography or magnetic resonance imaging), the enlargement of an orbital varix with the Valsalva maneuver, and enlarged superior orbital veins in carotid–cavernous fistulae (MRI is good for them, too). However, ultrasound is limited to the orbit itself, as it does not penetrate intact orbital walls. Ultrasound (especially A-scan) is less effective than CT and MRI in the orbital apex, where so many tissues are jammed together. CT is especially good where there is invasion of bone or the periorbital cavities are involved; MRI is excellent for intraocular extension of orbital processes and orbital extension of intraocular disease (Tables 2–9 and 2–10).

Quantitative A-scan echography is also particularly useful in evaluation of the optic nerve and the perioptic meningeal space. The optic nerve is a compact and relatively homogenous tubular structure surrounded by layers that provide excellent contrasting echoes (cerebrospinal fluid, meningeal sheaths,

TABLE 2–9. INDICATIONS FOR ULTRASOUND

Ocular
Opaque media (eg, dense cataract, vitreous hemorrhage)
Trauma
Retinal or choroidal detachment
Intraocular masses
Foreign bodies
Optic nerve head drusen
Biometry

Orbit
Ex(en)ophthalmos—r/o pseudoexophthalmos (eg, high myopia, buphthalmos)
Optic nerve lesions
Orbital inflammation
Thyroid orbitopathy (quantification of muscle size)
Foreign bodies
Orbital masses

and orbital fat). Both A- and B-scans demonstrate enlarged optic nerves. By quantitative A-scan, low reflectivity reportedly is characteristic of a glioma and medium reflectivity of a meningioma. In my hands the distinction is less complete than the literature indicates. If the nerve is of normal width and the CSF space enlarged, an inflammatory process in the orbit (pseudotumor) or optic nerve itself (optic neuritis) is suggested. The sensitivity of the determination is increased by the "30-degree test," where the width of the vaginal spaces is measured first in primary position and then with the eye turned 30 degrees eccentrically. Normally, the sheaths are compressible and the space should decrease in diameter. If they do not, increased fluid or fluid pressure is demonstrated, suggestive of optic neuritis, increased intracranial pressure, trauma, central retinal vein occlusion, or arachnoid cyst (sometimes these form an-

TABLE 2–10. ULTRASONOGRAPHIC CHARACTERISTICS OF SOME OCULAR AND ORBITAL LESIONS

Ultrasound Finding	Type of Lesion
High reflectivity	Calcium (retinoblastoma, pthisis, optic nerve head drusen), metallic foreign body
Medium reflectivity	Mixed tumor lacrimal gland, meningioma
Low reflectivity	Malignant melanoma, lymphomas, inflammation
Extra low reflectivity	Cysts (eg, mocecele)
Blood movement	Vascular structures—some malignant melanomas, orbital and choroidal hemangiomas, enlarged draining vessels in carotid–cavernous fistulas

terior to sheath meningiomas). In gliomas, the 30-degree test shows no compression.

Two of the most important roles for ultrasound in neuro-ophthalmic diagnosis are recognition and follow-up of enlarged extraocular muscles in thyroid orbitopathy (probably the most common cause of unusual limitations of ocular motility) and detection of reflective optic nerve head drusen.

This noninvasive test causes minimal discomfort and no risk to the patient, and thus may be utilized repetitively for both initial diagnosis and for monitoring ocular and orbital lesions.

Doppler Ultrasound: In the evaluation of patients with signs or symptoms of extracranial vascular occlusive disease, especially of the internal carotid artery, the optimum diagnostic paths, like the optimum therapy, remain controversial (see Chapter 8). Duplex carotid sonography (DCS, conventional B-scan ultrasonography plus range-gated, pulsed-wave Doppler analysis) has an important role as a noninvasive method.

DCS is the combination of high-resolution, real-time, B-mode echography and pulsed-Doppler sonography. B-mode is used to image the arterial structures, and to assess the extent and nature of plaques and the degree of stenosis (Fig. 2–48). The principles are the same as for ultrasound of the eye and orbit; in fact, ophthalmic B-scan equipment images carotid and vertebral arteries very well.

In the Doppler mode, the sound signal is scattered by moving red blood cells, causing a shift in frequency. In stenotic vessels, red blood cell velocity increases in an attempt to maintain flow. At 50 to 70% stenosis (critical or hemodynamically significant stenosis) the increased velocity can no longer be sustained. The change in the Doppler waveform caused by the change in velocity and the associated turbulance are sensitive indicators of the status of the vessels (Fig. 2–49). It is most accurate (> 90%) in detecting stenoses greater than 50% (Table 2–11).

Color Doppler Imaging (CDI) adds semiquantitative color encoding to the Doppler measurements. CDI allows more accurate and rapid detection of the point of maximal stenosis, especially when caused by anechoic plaque which may be difficult to differentiate otherwise. It may be of value in imaging ocular and orbital blood flow velocity. This has potential value for the evaluation of vascular occlusion and mass lesions of the eye and orbit.

Duplex scanning is indicated in asymptomatic carotid bruits and retinal emboli, other possible ischemic events likely to have a carotid etiology, follow-up of patients following carotid endarterectomy, and presurgical evaluation of patients scheduled to undergo major vascular surgical procedures.

Transcranial Doppler (TCD) imaging is effective in monitoring blood velocities in large intracranial arteries. It detects severe stenosis and vasoconstriction in the major basal arteries and assesses patterns of flow in patients with stenosis, occlusion, or arteriovenous malformations.

Computerized Imaging

Computerized scanning has almost completely replaced the use of plain skull x-rays (and **has** completely displaced some invasive procedures such as pneumo-encephalography) because the same information may be obtained with more accuracy, less invasion, and lower or no x-ray exposure.

Computed tomography (CT), now overshadowed by magnetic resonance imaging for most intracranial processes, remains the most sophisticated modality available to many. Thus, it retains its place in neuro-ocular imaging and remains the premier test when thin sections are needed and for many orbital studies, especially when calcified structures need study. For conditions that need to be followed sequentially, the clinician should also remember that x-rays are cataractogenic and the lens of an infant may not tolerate more than 450 rads and that of an adult more than 700 rads. (A single conventional skull x-ray delivers a dose of approximately 5 rads.) In CT scanning, even when direct axial and coronal scans are both made, the dose remains less than 10 rads by most protocols—it may be greater if multiple thin sections and/or direct coronal or saggital scans are performed.

Computed Tomography. In CT scanning, a collimated x-ray beam is directed through the tissue and then received by a detector, minus radiation absorbed by the tissue. The array of tubes then rotates and the scan is repeated until all tissue is studied, either by two 180-degree rotations or one 360-degree

Figure 2–48. Normal duplex carotid sonography. **A.** sagittal image of the common carotid artery (CCA) (curved arrows). Internal carotid artery (ICA) (short solid arrows) and ECA (open arrows). The ICA and external carotid artery (ECA) are imaged in the same plane, as shown here, only in about 20% of cases. **B.** Cursor in the "distal" (4 cm from origin) ICA.

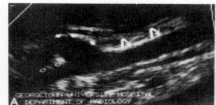
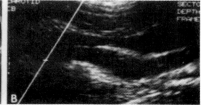

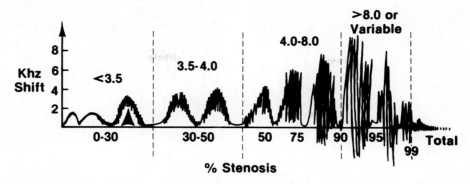

Figure 2–49. Doppler ultrasound. Artist's drawing showing Doppler spectral appearance as a function of internal carotid artery (ICA) diameter stenosis. The "window" under the waveform (arrowhead) is gradually filled in as turbulence increases with increasing stenosis. Note the difference in waveform appearance between a 95 and 99% stenosis and a stenosis below 30%. (*From Jacobs N, et al. The role of duplex carotid sonography, digital subtraction angiography, and arteriography in the evaluation of transient ischemic attack and the asymptomatic carotid bruit. Med Clin North Am. 1984; 68:1423–1450, with permission.*)

rotation. Attenuation values (the difference between the energy emitted and that received) are calculated between each small segment of tissue. These are then converted to a gray scale and displayed on a CRT or TV screen.

In addition to the usual axial planes studied for most neurologic problems, several methods are especially effective in enhancing CT scanning for orbital or neuro-ophthalmic evaluation. **Coronal scanning** shows the orbital structures in great detail and allows for easy comparison between the contents of the two orbits. This can be especially helpful in detecting multiple enlarged extraocular muscles in thyroid orbitopathy or comparing the size of the optic nerves (Fig. 2–50). It is also helpful in evaluating the chiasm and pituitary fossa. **Reformatted images**—for example, along the sagittal plane or the plane of the optic nerve—are also useful but the image quality suffers in the reformation process. **Scan-**

ning in the neuro-ocular plane (the plane of the visual pathways from the cornea to the calcarine fissure, oriented at − 7 degrees to the orbitomeatal line) images the orbits and intracranial visual paths at the same time (Fig. 2–51). For studies of visual loss, the initial scan can be limited to this plane, and thus the total visual afferent pathway can be studied yet the dose of radiation and scan time are decreased. Use of this angulation may be the key to a good study in a youngster or uncooperative patient.

Intravenous contrast is helpful in the differential diagnosis of vascular lesions (eg, aneurysm, meningioma); MRI seems to be better for most of these lesions, however. For most purposes, a very limited series of scans without contrast, followed by thin overlapping section scans of the critical areas, is a good first strategy. As diagnostic methods become more and more sophisticated, we look for smaller and smaller lesions; therefore, thin sections should

TABLE 2–11. CRITERIA FOR STENOSIS BY DUPLEX CAROTID SONOGRAPHY

Diameter of Stenotic Occlusion	KHz Shift	Spectral Broadening and Waveform: HRS
Normal–30%	<3.5	HRS useful to differentiate stenosis <30% from normals.
30–50%	3.5–4	Systolic window under waveform half to two thirds filled in. HRS helpful, particularly in occasional cases of a smooth stenosis at the carotid bulb where Doppler criteria may fail.
50–90%	>4, <8	Window usually two thirds filled in, waveform recognizable.
>90%	>8	Window filled in, waveform becoming distorted.
Usually >95%	Variable (can be <4)	Waveform very distorted, window filled in.
Total occlusion	0	No waveform. Series of dots seen along baseline.

From Jacobs N, Grant E, Schellinger D, Cohan S, Byrd M. The role of duplex carotid sonography, digital subtraction angiography, and arteriography in the evaluation of transient ischemic attack and the asymptomatic carotid bruit. Med Clin North Am. 1984;68:1423–1450.

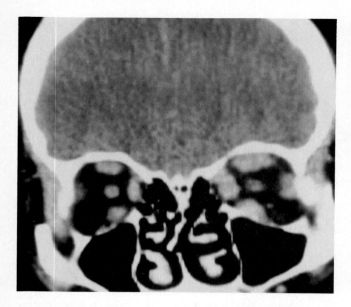

Figure 2–50. Coronal CT through the orbits showing the extraocular muscles, optic nerves, middle cranial fossa, ethmoid sinuses and nasal spaces and maxillary sinuses.

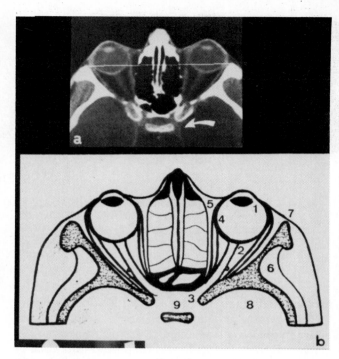

Figure 2–51. CT through orbit in the neuro-ocular plane 1. lens, 2. optic nerve head, 3. optic canal, 4. sclera, 5. medial canthus, 6. temporalis muscle, 7. lateral canthus, 8. middle cranial fossa, 9. dorsum sellae. (lens, optic papilla, optic canal). (*From Cabanis EA, Pineau H, Iba-Zizen MT, et al. CT scanning in the "neuro-ocular plane"; the optic pathways as a "new" cephalic plane.* Neuro-ophthalmology *1981;1:237–252, with permission.*)

almost always be obtained. Although thin-section scans provide the spatial resolution to detect small lesions in thin section, structures show variations (eg, hypodense areas in the optic nerves) due to volume averaging. Obviously, better scans can be obtained with less radiation if the neuro-radiologist knows precisely where to look. It is your job to guide the radiologist! You should have localized the lesion and have a pretty good differential diagnosis *before* referring the patient.

CT scanning remains the procedure of choice for many orbital processes (excepting optic nerve lesions), especially small lesions and processes in the orbital apex, but it is rather limited for ocular lesions for which ultrasound usually provides a better diagnostic study. Foreign bodies and calcified structures (for example, the bony orbit, craniopharyngiomas, and optic nerve head drusen) are seen well both by ultrasound and CT. The ability to compare simultaneous images of both orbits is a great advantage of both CT and MRI, as is the ability to evaluate the orbital contents, peri-orbital tissues, and intracranial cavity at the same time.

Magnetic Resonance Imaging. Magnetic resonance imaging (MRI) uses the radiowaves emitted by protons in a powerful magnetic field. The effect of turning on the huge magnet causes the nuclei to resonate at different frequencies depending on their magnetic spin properties. After the magnetic pulse ceases, the protons return to their original orientations. The receptors of the scanner are tuned to specific atoms (usually the hydrogen nucleus) and detect the location of the atoms, their rate of movement, and their molecular environment. By computerized techniques, a display similar to that obtained with CT scanning is generated.

The MR signal detected depends on the sequence of exciting pulses. In clinical MRI, the pulse sequences are chosen to enhance differences between tissues. This is done by manipulating the signal to emphasize T_1 (the time necessary for individual nuclei to recover 63.2% of original longitudinal magnetization), T_2 (the time necessary for dephasing to cause a 63.2% loss of signal), T_2^* (dephasing due to external field inhomogeneities), and proton density. The aim is to minimize T_2^* and maximize the other parameters. This is done in part by manipulating the delay between the pulses and the repetition time (TR).

The ability to do direct multiplane image formation (avoiding the image degradation of reformatted CTs) is a great advantage of MRI. Magnetic resonance imaging also visually portrays the inherent contrast of gray and white matter in the central nervous system. Cerebral spinal fluid and flowing blood appear black, providing good blood vessel detail without the need for contrast injection. Especially with stronger magnets, MRI is extremely sensitive to plaques of demyelination. MRI avoids radiation exposure and thus is an excellent modality for lesions that need repeated follow-up (eg, small meningiomas, microadenomas of the pituitary gland, and phakomatoses).

MRI is much superior to CT for imaging parenchymal abnormalities. This is especially true in the posterior fossa and brain stem, where the proximity of dense bony structures and low contrast resolution make CT relatively ineffective. MRI is the imaging modality of choice for pathologies of the hypothalamus, other suprasellar structures, and extrasellar extension of pituitary tumors, especially in evaluating arterial encasement by parasellar tumor. On the other hand, calcified structures are not well imaged by MRI, and processes that are expected to alter bony structure (eg, skull fractures) or contain calcium (craniopharyngiomas) may be better studied by CT. In addition, as mentioned above, CT scanning currently remains preferable for the orbit because thinner sections can be obtained, better detecting most small lesions. However, MRI is better for the intracranial optic nerve and fluid in distended optic nerve sheaths (although A-scan ultrasonography may be better yet for optic nerve sheath fluid).

The use of surface coils, fat-suppression paradigms, higher-energy magnets, and varied scan strategies in MRI is producing scans nearly as detailed as the best CT scan. As the signal-to-noise ratio is improved and better resolution achieved with less scan time, MRI probably can achieve at least the same spatial resolution in the orbit as CT and become the preferred modality for all but bone lesions.

The special sensitivity of MRI for demyelinating lesions demonstrates these lesions in a large percentage of cases where they cannot be observed on CT. Moreover, 1.5-Tesla machines have demonstrated the acute optic nerve lesions of optic neuritis for the first time. Thus, MRI is a very sensitive method for detecting multiple sclerosis, although not quite as sensitive as VEP testing; however, it is the best method for establishing cerebral alterations and for demonstrating dissemination in space.

The signals generated by blood, both within vascular structures and in tissues, vary significantly with rate of flow, clotting, or change to hemosiderin, especially in high field strength (1.5-Tesla) machines; thus, the evaluation of a non-hemorrhagic or vascular lesion is facilitated by MRI. In occult (sometimes to both CT and angiography!) arteriovenous malformations, MRI may show circumscribed regions of low intensity (hemosiderin deposits). Irregular signal patterns suggest fibrotic regions and hematomas in various stages of resolution. In the first week following intracranial hemorrhage, there will be central hypodensity on T_2-weighted images; sub-

acutely (after 1 week to 1 month) there is peripheral hyperintensity on both T_1 and T_2 images, and chronic hematomas are hyperintense. Yet, for fresh hemorrhage, CT scan with contrast may still be best. Most arteriovenous malformations are supratentorial, usually subcortical or periventricular, and not infrequently occipital, and thus can often appear in the neuro-ophthalmic differential diagnosis.

On appropriate T_1- and T_2-weighted studies, many metastases and malignant melanomas also present very characteristic combinations of images.

Using gradient echo techniques with short echo times, excellent magnetic resonance angiograms (MRA) of the carotid arteries and intracranial vasculature are achieved. In some instances such as subadventitial internal carotid artery dissection (as opposed to the commoner sub-intimal dissection) MRA is the optimal diagnostic modality. MR spectroscopy shows promise for detecting metabolic abnormalities in tumors and other pathological processes.

Disadvantages of MRI. Less sensitive to calcium than either CT or ultrasound, MRI shows bone detail less well. The chemical shift phenomenon, especially without fat suppression, produces potentially confusing shadowy artifacts in the orbit along the optic nerve and muscles where they abut the orbital fat. The scan time is long. So, to avoid movement distortion, the patient must be very cooperative (especially for orbital studies where eye movements must be held to a minimum for best results). The gantry tunnel is narrow and some patients get claustrophobic.

Exciting vistas exist for the future: The use of contrast agents (Gadolinium is now used extensively and other agents will add additional dimensions in the future), scanning for magnetic particles other than protons, and the ability to characterize intracellular components (DNA) and metabolic products. The latter ability already allows differentiation of neuroblastomas with malignant potential from those more benign! Gadolinium, the first MRI contrast agent approved for clinical use, is a marker for blood–brain barrier integrity and behaves similarly to iodinated contrast agents in CT. It helps to differentiate tumor from edema, assess biologic activity, and detect extra-axial lesions (eg, acoustic neuroma) and metastases with a high degree of sensitivity. Gated acquisition to eliminate movement also improves the sensitivity of all modalities of computerized imaging—CT, MRI, PET, and SPECT.

Positron Emission Tomography. By the use of ultrasensitive detectors of radioactive emission, positron emission tomography (PET) is able to present striking pictures of the brain in action and thus provide a dynamic image of neural processes.

The production of these images requires sophisticated computed processing as well as precise control of environment. At the moment, considerable patient exam time is needed in addition to facilities able to prepare suitable radioactive isotopes. This imaging technique allows simultaneous monitoring of many neurons in the intact brain. Thus, it has given us the first pictures of the spatial organization of neuronal responses and truly understandable maps of brain function. We are just learning to recognize responses to specific stimuli. Currently, the research uses of this magnificent new tool have exceeded its clinical utility. The ability to study specific pathways, their action and interaction to given stimuli, and changes after various lesions, is unprecedented. However, so far, PET scanning on a clinical level has been most useful for a few structural lesions and for the demonstration of decreased function, predominantly in vascular lesions (Fig. 2–52). Single photon emission computed tomography (SPECT) scanning similarly detects radioactive emissions. This methodology can employ isotopes with longer half-lives and is less expensive. It may be the most sensitive means for detection of cerebral infarction in the first 48 hours.

Digital Subtraction Angiography. Detailed studies of vascular structures still necessitate angiography. Digital subtraction angiography (DSA) allows electronic computerized techniques to amplify data and subtract distracting details, such as bone, and thus makes possible the use of smaller amounts and concentrations of contrast material. It also enables theaortic arch and great vessels to be imaged at the same time as the carotid vessels; however, the head and neck cannot be imaged at the same time on most systems. When this can be done, it significantly decreases the time for the study.

Initially it was thought that intravenous injection could be used, but large amounts of contrast were necessary for sufficient resolution, and overlapping structures made interpretation difficult. Currently, transfemoral arterial catheterization with smaller doses of contrast than in conventional angiography is usually used for digital subtraction. For the localization and identification of most lesions, this is sufficient, but it does not provide adequate spatial resolution for highly detailed studies of extra and intracranial vessels. Additionally, because of the limited field of view in most systems and the lack of biplane capability, a larger number of injections or combination with selective injections and film techniques may be needed. When precision is necessary for planning of treatment or surgery, conventional angiography still is necessary.

Selective Cerebral Angiography. Selective cere-

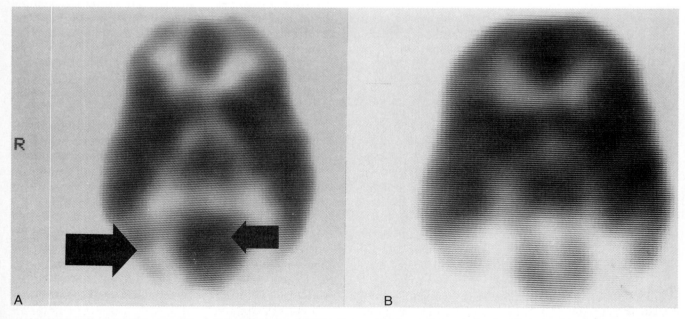

Figure 2–52. A. PET scan using fluoro-2-deoxyglucose (FDG) with head inclined at an angle of −20 degrees to the orbitomeatal line. Image is at level of thalami and calcarine cortex with darker areas showing greater glucose uptake. The patient's right is on the left of this image. Small arrow points to left striate cortex, large arrow points to right visual association cortex. Uptake is normal and symmetric in this image. **B.** FDG PET scan on a patient with bilateral optic neuritis without visual recovery resulting in visual acuity of 20/400 OU. Images at roughly the same level as **A.** through the thalami and primary visual cortex. Patient's right is at the left of the image. Note strikingly decreased glucose uptake in calcarine cortex and visual association cortex of both hemispheres. (*Courtesy of Thomas M. Bosley, M.D.*)

bral arteriography remains the most accurate means to evaluate many extra- and intracranial vessels, although duplex ultrasonography may be more as sensitive to arteriosclerotic changes in accessible vessels (especially the internal carotid artery [ICA]). The increased spatial resolution of angiography makes it the only means to study small intracranial vessels reliably. Arteriography carries a small but definite risk of morbidity and mortality: a 5% risk of any complication (50% of these are nonsignificant hematomas) and a 2% risk of subclinical renal failure. There is also a 0.2% risk of permanent neural damage and a 0.4% chance of a major systemic reaction.

BIBLIOGRAPHY

General

Cogan D. *Neurology of the Visual System*. Springfield, IL: Thomas, 1967.

Glaser J, et al. Chapters 1–20 in: Duane T, ed. *Clinical Ophthalmology*. Hagerstown, MD: Harper & Row, 1976.

Miller N, ed. *Walsh & Hoyt's Clinical Neuro-ophthalmology*. 4th ed. Baltimore: Williams & Wilkins, 1982; 1.

Visual Acuity

Frisén L, Frisén M. How good is normal visual acuity? *Arch Klin Exp Ophthalmol*. 1981; 215:149–157.

Color

Pokorny J, Smith VC. Eye disease and color defects. *Vis Res*. 1986; 26:1573–1584.

Afferent Pupillary Defect

Folk JC, Thompson HS, Farmer JG, et al. Relative afferent pupillary defect in eyes with retinal detachment. *Ophthalmic Surg*. 1987; 18:757–759.

Johnson LN, et al. Correlation of afferent pupillary defect with visual field loss on automated perimetry. *Ophthalmology. 1988; 95:1649–1655*.

Brightness Sense

Sadun AA, Lessell S. Brightness-sense and optic nerve disease. *Arch Ophthalmol*. 1985; 103:39–43.

Photostress (Macular Dazzle)

Baillart JP. L'examen fonctionnel de la macula. *Bull Soc Ophthalmol France*. 1954; 4:52–58.

Vernier Acuity

Essock EA, Williams RA, Enoch JM, et al. The effects of image degradation by cataract on vernier acuity. *Inv Ophthalmol*. 1984; 25:1043–1050.

Levi DM, Klein S. Hyperacuity and amblyopia. *Nature*. 1982; 298:268–270.

Fields

Anderson DR. *Perimetry: With and Without Automation*. 2nd ed. St. Louis: Mosby, 1987.

Harrington DO, Drake MV. *The Visual Fields: A Textbook and Atlas of Clinical Perimetry*. 6th ed. St. Louis: Mosby, 1989.

Leventhal AG, Ault SJ, Vitek DJ. The nasotemporal division in primate retina: The neural bases of macular sparing and splitting. *Science*. 1988; 240:66–67.

Reed H, Drance SM. *The Essentials of Perimetry: Static & Kinetic*. London: Oxford, 1972.

Traquair HM. *An Introduction to Clinical Perimetry*. 6th ed. St. Louis: Mosby, 1949.

Trobe JD, Acosta PC, Shuster JJ, et al. An evaluation of the accuracy of community based perimetry. *Am J Ophthalmol*. 1980; 90:654–660.

Fields—Newer Methods

Frisén L. High-pass resolution targets in peripheral vision. *Ophthalmology*. 1987; 94:1104–1108.

Neiman D, LeBlanc R, Regan D. Visual field defects in ocular hypertension and glaucoma. *Arch Ophthalmol*. 1984; 102:1042–1045.

Smith TJ, Baker RS. Perimetric findings in functional disorders using automated techniques. *Ophthalmology*. 1987; 94:1562–1566.

Optic Disc

Armaly MF. Genetic determination of cup to disc ratio of the optic nerve. *Arch Ophthalmol*. 1971; 85:224–226.

Armaly MF. Interpretation of tonometry and ophthalmoscopy. *Invest Ophthalmol*. 1972; 11:75–79.

Balazsi AG, et al. The effect of age on the nerve fiber population of the human optic nerve. *Am J Ophthalmol*. 1984; 97:760–766.

Henderson G, Tomlinson BE, Gibson PH. Cell counts in human cerebral cortex in normal adults through life using an image analyzing computer. *J Neurol Sci*. 1980; 46:113.

Quigley HA, Anderson DR. The histologic basis of optic disc pallor in experimental optic atrophy. *Am J Ophthalmol*. 1977; 83:709–717.

Repka MX, Quigley HA. The effect of age on normal human optic nerve fiber number and diameter. *Clin Neuro-ophthalmol*. 1989; 9:219.

Snydacker D. The normal optic disc. *Am J Ophthalmol*. 1964; 58:958–964.

Veith NW, Sacks J. Enumeration of small vessels on the optic discs in normal eyes. *Am J Ophthalmol*. 1973; 26: 660–661.

Duplex Scanning

Goodson SF, et al. Can carotid duplex scanning supplant arteriography in patients with focal carotid territory symptoms? *J Vasc Surg*. 1987; 5:551–557.

Jacobs N, et al. The role of duplex carotid sonography, digital subtraction angiography, and arteriography in the evaluation of transient ischemic attack and the asymptomatic carotid bruit. *Med Clin North Am.* 1984; 68: 1423–1450.

Lewis BD, James EM, Welch TJ. Current applications of duplex and color Doppler untrasound imaging: Carotid and peripheral vascular system. *Mayo Clin Proc.* 1989; 64:1147–1157.

CT Scanning

Bresnick GH. Background diabetic retinopathy. In: Ryan SJ, ed. *Retina.* St. Louis: Mosby, 1989; 2.

PET Scanning

Kushner MJ, et al. Cerebral metabolism and patterned visual stimulation: A positron emission tomographic study of the human visual cortex. *Neurology.* 1988; 38:89–95.

MRI

Ross JS, Masaryk TJ, et al. Magnetic resonance angiography of the extracranial carotid arteries and intracranial vessels: A review. *Neurology.* 1989; 39:1369–1376.

CHAPTER 3

DISORDERS OF THE FUNDUS OCULUS

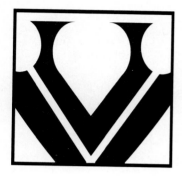

RETINAL DISORDERS

Like neuro-ophthalmologic diseases, retinal disorders cause loss of visual acuity and visual field. In addition, the same vascular and systemic disorders may affect the retina, the optic nerve, and the central nervous system. Thus, the retina is often an important signpost to optic nerve and central nervous system disease—for example, in neurodegenerative diseases, phakomatoses, central nervous system malformations, infections, and vascular disease.

Retinal Vascular Disease

The **cardinal manifestations of retinal vascular disorders** are abnormalities of the vessels themselves, exudates, hemorrhages, cotton-wool spots or larger areas of axoplasmic stasis, and retinal nonperfusion. A small area of axoplasmic stasis is seen as a *cotton-wool spot* (Table 3–1). Typically, cotton-wool spots are seen in hypertension, diabetes mellitus, collagen vascular disease, and in the retinopathy of AIDS. With occlusion of larger retinal vessels, larger areas of the retina become opaque. In chronic ischemia, vessels in ischemic areas frequently become sheathed and areas of nonperfusion are seen.

Chronic ischemia, nonperfusion, and vascular stasis or incompetence leads to retinal microaneurysms, neovascularization (usually adjacent to areas of capillary closure), and exudation.

Chronic ischemia stimulates an angiogenic factor that causes *neovascularization*, the proliferation of vessels within the retina (intra-retinal microangiopathy, IRMA) and on the retinal surface, into the vitreous, and on the iris (rubeosis iridis). Subsequently, posterior vitreous detachment or contraction of fibro-vascular strands may produce repetitive

vitreous hemorrhages by traction on these fragile vessels, distortion of retinal and vitreal anatomy, organization of the vitreous, and ultimately, retinal detachment. Progression of iris neovascularization leads to angle closure and neovascular glaucoma. Although typical of proliferative diabetic retinopathy and retinal venous occlusions, neovascularization occurs as the end stage of diverse destructive retinal vascular processes (Table 3–2).

Damage to the outer retinal layers, particularly Bruch's membrane, is associated with another type of neovascularization, the subretinal neovascular membrane (SRNVM). These membranes originate from choroidal vasculature, which unlike retinal vessels does not have tight junctions; thus, like new-formed retinal vessels, SRNVMs leak and are well seen on fluorescein angiography. In fact, fluorescein can be the only way to clearly demonstrate subtle subretinal membranes.

Retinal exudates. When vascular integrity is lost, exudation of serum occurs, often from capillaries deep in the retina, in the outer plexiform layer. In most of the retina, exudates are confined by the vertical Müller cells and form small yellowish masses. Even when the primary vascular anomaly is in the periphery (as in the hemangioma of von Hippel–Lindau disease) or at the disc (as in neuroretinitis), exudates have a predilection for the posterior pole, where they often form a star figure defined by the radiating fibers of Henle's layer (Fig. 3–1). When exudates are subretinal, they form a circinate pattern in the perimacular area. More massive exudation leads to even larger yellowish masses that can actually cause retinal detachment (Fig. 3–2).

Retinal hemorrhages. If the loss of vascular integrity is so severe that red blood cells escape, hem-

TABLE 3–1. SUMMARY OF SYSTEMIC ASSOCIATIONS WITH COTTON-WOOL SPOTS IN 24 PATIENTS

Systemic Abnormality	Number of Cases
Diabetes mellitus	5
Systemic hypertension	5
Collagen vascular disease	4
Cardiac valvular disease	2
Radiation retinopathy	2
Carotid artery obstruction	2
Dermatomyositis	1
Systemic lupus erythematosus	1
Polyarteritis nodosa	1
Giant-cell arteritis	1
Leukemia	1
Trauma	1
AIDS	1
Intravenous drug abuse	1
Metastiatic carcinoma	1
Partial central retinal artery obstruction	1
None found	1

From Brown GC, et al. Cotton-wool spots. Retina. 1985;5:206–214.

orrhages are seen, either alone or in combination with exudates. Their size and shape are determined by the vascular bed that bleeds, the amount of bleeding, and its location (Fig. 3–3). Small superficial hemorrhages are *flame-shaped* because they are confined by the retinal nerve fiber layer. Small hemorrhages deeper within the retinal layers are seen as "dots" and "blots."

Large superficial hemorrhages obscure the retinal nerve fiber layer. Preretinal hemorrhages, limited by the internal limiting membrane, not infrequently show a fluid level, and may break through into the

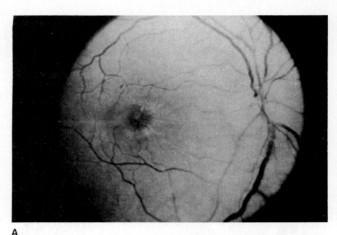

A

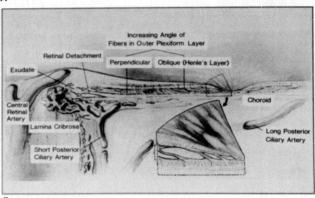

B

Figure 3–1. Retinal exudates. **A.** Fundus photograph shows typical appearance of Leber's idiopathic stellate neuroretinitis, demonstrating stellate pattern of macular exudate in association with papillitis. **B.** Anatomic drawing of retina and optic nerve demonstrates origin of macular exudate from prelaminar disc capillaries and indicates its pathway through outer plexiform layer of retina. Leaking fluid has also caused peripapillary limited neurosensory retinal detachment. (*From Parmley VC, Schiffman JS, Maitland CG, et al. Does neuroretinitis rule out multiple sclerosis? Arch Neurol. 1987;44:1045–1048, with permission.*)

TABLE 3–2. RETINAL NEOVASCULARIZATION

Central	Diabetes
	Hypertension
	Retinal venous occlusion
	Myelinated nerve fibers (rare)
Central and Peripheral	Arteriolar occlusion—carotid occlusion, temporal arteritis, radiation retinopathy, Takayasu arteritis
	Chronic inflammation—sarcoid retinopathy, Still's disease, Behcet's disease, talc retinopathy, other embolic particles, homocystinuria, blood dyscrasias, hyperviscosity, dysproteinemias
Peripheral	SC/SS/S thalassemia, and other hemoglobinopathies
	Retinopathy of prematurity
	Eales' disease
	Coats'/Leber's disease
	Pars planitis
Subretinal Neovascular Membranes (SRNVM)	Age-related macular degeneration
	Chronic disc swelling, optic nerve head drusen, chronic papilledema
	Angioid streaks
	Choroidal rupture, chorioretinal scars
	Photocoagulation
	High myopia

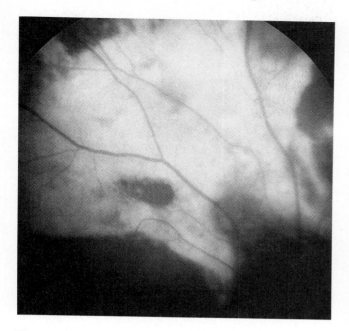

Figure 3–2. Massive retinal exudates in Coats' disease.

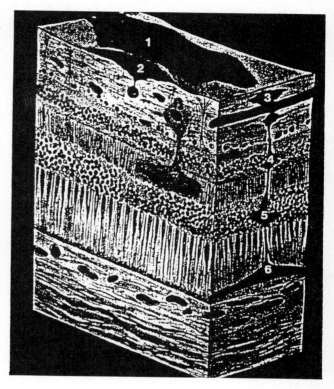

Figure 3–3. Artist's cross-sectional drawing shows potential locations of hemorrhage and exudate: 1, preretinal; 2, subretinal lining membrane; 3, nerve fiber layer; 4, inner nuclear layer; 5, outer nuclear layer; 6, subretinal; 7, outer plexiform layer. (*From Wessing A.* Fluorescein Angiography. *St. Louis, MO: Mosby; 1969, p. 42.*)

vitreous. Hemorrhages in the perifoveal area can form a star-shaped figure as do exudates.

In several diseases, including hypertension, blood dyscrasias, and anemia, hemorrhages with white centers are seen. These *Roth's spots*, once thought to be pathognomonic of subacute bacterial endocarditis (SBE), are now recognized as associated with many etiologies (Table 3–3).

Retinal vascular sheathing. Damage to vascular walls can be caused by systemic diseases (hypertension, diabetes); local infectious or inflammatory processes (sarcoid, Behcet's syndrome); ischemia, multiple sclerosis, Eales' disease, or emboli. The damage leads to hyalinization, seen as opacification along the sides of the vessels (sheathing); (Table 3–4); increased reflexes on the vessels; and when the arteries are involved, crossing changes obscuring the underlying veins.

Retinal telangiectasia is prominent in many retinal angiopathies and dystrophies; the possible association with retinal metabolic abnormalities is intriguing (Table 3–5).

From a neuro-ophthalmic standpoint, three processes associated with retina telangiectasia are notable. The first two, Leber's optic neuropathy and toxic amblyopia, are discussed in detail elsewhere (see Chapter 5). Their similarities include optic disc swelling, centrocecal scotomas, initial dropout of the papillomacular bundle, and posterior-pole telangiectasia, as well as a potential relationship to cyanide metabolism. The telangiectatic changes in asymptomatic relatives of Leber's patients, and the disappearance of telangiectasis with the evolution of optic atrophy in both Leber's optic neuropathy and "toxic" amblyopia, suggest that telangiectasia is a response to disordered retinal metabolism.

It is not difficult to imagine a similar mechanism in the third process, cone-rod dystrophy, which in addition to telangiectasia, may show disc swelling and pseudoneurogenic visual field defects.

Occlusive Retinal Vascular Lesions

Occlusive disease of the retinal arteries causes visual field defects with configurations determined by the portion of the arterial supply occluded. Retinal arterial occlusions divide into two large categories: embolic and nonembolic. *Emboli* usually are composed of cholesterol, fibrin–platelet aggregations, or calcified bits that arise within the vascular tree, mostly from the carotid artery or the heart (from valves or mural thrombi). Rarer emboli include cardiac myxomas, fat (Purtscher's retinopathy and pancreatitis), air, amniotic fluid, and particles injected by IV drug abusers. In 70 patients with evidence of retinal emboli, cholesterol formed 50% of emboli;

TABLE 3–3. CAUSES OF ROTH'S SPOTS

Infection
  Subacute bacterial endocarditis
  Candida
  Acquired immune deficiency syndrome (AIDS)
  Legionella
  Rocky Mountain spotted fever
Anemia
  Especially after transfusion
Dysproteinemia
Leukemia
Hypertension
Systemic lupus erythematosis and other collagen–vascular disease
Diabetes mellitus (rarely)
Emboli
  Cardiac sources
  Carotid stenosis
  Talc injection and periocular steroids
  Fat emboli from long-bone fracture
  Pancreatitis (acute)
Trauma
  Birth trauma
  Battered children
  Intracranial hemorrhage

From Hedges T III. Consultation in Ophthalmology. *Toronto: Decker, 1987.*

TABLE 3–5. OPTIC DISC AND RETINAL TELANGIECTASIA

Optic Disc	Cone-rod dystrophy[a]
	Rod-cone dystrophy
	Choroideremia
	Usher's syndrome
Peripapillary	Leber's optic neuropathy[a]
	Toxic amblyopia[a] (acute stage, temporal vascular arcades)
	Congenital telangiectasia
	Systemic hypertension
Peripheral	Coats' disease (with exudates), Coats'-type retinal pigmentary degeneration
	Leber's (with miliary aneurysms) retinopathy
	Eales' disease
	Fabry's disease
	Pigmented paravenous chorioretinal atrophy
Syndromes	Osler-Weber-Rendu syndrome
	Angiomatosis retina
	Rare syndromes:
	1. With retinalschisis and retinal detachment
	2. In paramacular area of young males, unilateral, associated with cystoid macular edema
	3. Fascioscapulohumeral muscular dystrophy (mostly peripheral microvascular alterations)

[a] Especially characteristic.

cholesterol and fibrin–platelet aggregations together 79%, fibrin–platelet aggregations alone 4%, and calcium 9%. Twenty-nine percent showed only sheathing (Arruga and Sanders).

Nonembolic retinal arteriolar occlusion occurs in systemic diseases (primarily diabetes, hypertension, and vasculitides); in diseases that cause hyperviscosity; in association with inflammation of the retinal vessels; in association with abnormal vasculature; and in ocular migraine.

Central retinal artery occlusion. (Table 3–6) Occlusion of the central retinal artery causes sudden severe visual loss and a classic fundus picture: opaque posterior retina around a macular cherry-red spot (Fig. 3–4). The fovea and peripheral retina, thinner and effectively nourished by the choroidal circulation, maintain a near-normal color. The retinal opacity is caused by blockage of axoplasmic transport in the ischemic area.

In the fortunate patient with one or more cilioretinal arteries to nourish the macula and papillomacular bundle (Fig. 3–5), central vision may be preserved despite central retinal artery occlusion.

TABLE 3–4. SHEATHING OF RETINAL VESSELS

Inflammation/infection
  Sarcoid, syphilis, AIDS, Behcet's syndrome
Vascular disease
  Systemic hypertension, Eales' disease, Coats' disease, ischemia, emboli
Retinal degenerations
  X-linked retinoschisis, Wegener's vitreoretinal degeneration
CNS disorders
  Multiple sclerosis
Pseudosheathing
  Retinal nerve fiber layer atrophy (heightened reflexes along vessels in posterior pole)

TABLE 3–6. CAUSES OF CENTRAL RETINAL ARTERY OCCLUSION

Arteritides, vasculitides
Blood dyscrasia with hyperviscosity
Cardiac disease
Connective tissue disease
Diabetes mellitus
Emboli
Fabry's disease
Glaucoma
Hemoglobinopathies
Homocystinuria
Hypertension
Inadvertent intra-arterial injection (steroid, retrobulbar), IV drug abuse (esp. talc emboli)
Loaiasis
Migraine
Oral contraceptives
Sydenham's chorea
Syphilis
Temporal arteritis
Trauma, orbit and ocular

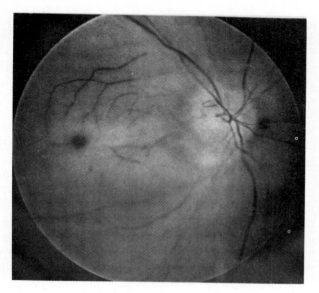

Figure 3–4. Macular cherry-red spot. Acute central retinal artery obstruction. Whitening, or opacification, of the superficial retina is present, and a cherry-red spot can be seen centrally. The opacification is most pronounced in the peripheral fovea, where the retina is the thickest. Narrowing of the retinal arteries is also evident. (*From Brown GC. Retinal arterial obstructive disease. In: Ryan SJ, ed.* Retina. *St. Louis: Mosby, 1989; 2; with permission.*)

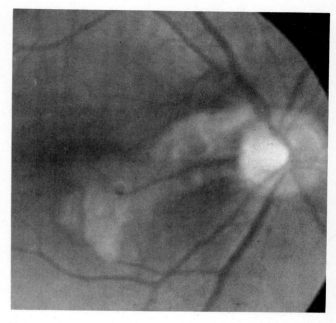

Figure 3–6. Cilioretinal artery occlusion causing ischemia of the papillomacular bundle.

Conversely, a cilioretinal artery occlusion (Fig. 3–6) may cause a central defect, usually a centrocecal scotoma, with a spared peripheral field.

About 20% of central retinal artery occlusions is due to emboli; most others are arteriolarsclerotic in

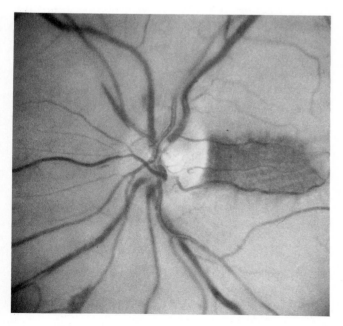

Figure 3–5. Papillomacular bundle sparing by a patent cilioretinal artery in central retinal artery occlusion.

nature. Rarely, in internal carotid occlusion, the thrombus will extend to occlude the central retinal artery; or in orbital trauma, retrobulbar optic nerve sheath hemorrhage will compress the central retinal artery and cause occlusion.

An avoidable iatrogenic cause of central retinal artery occlusion occurs in operative procedures in which the patient is positioned prone. Pressure on the face from the headrest may obstruct vascular flow. The patient awakes from anesthesia blind or with severe loss of visual acuity. If the occlusion also involves the ophthalmic artery, there may be an associated retrobulbar ischemic optic neuropathy, choroidal infarcts, ophthalmoplegia, ptosis, or a combination of these.

Branch artery occlusions present similarly with sudden visual loss that corresponds to the area of ischemic retina distal to the occlusion. Altitudinal hemianopias result from occlusion of the major superior or inferior branches and quadrantic defects from occlusion of superior and inferior nasal or temporal branches. Temporal branches are involved in almost all cases. Frequently, the macular area is spared and visual acuity relatively normal so the visual field defect may be the major symptom. The involved nerve fiber layer is opaque but there is no cherry-red spot.

The major causes of branch artery occlusion are emboli and arteriolarsclerosis as in central artery occlusion, but the frequency is reversed. Emboli are the more frequent cause of branch artery occlusion, whereas arteriolarsclerosis is the more frequent cause of central retinal artery occlusion.

If you see the patient within the first hour or so following an embolic occlusion, the fundus may look astonishingly normal. Slow flow may segment the blood in the narrowed retinal arterioles, giving a "boxcar" appearance, but fluorescein angiography shows some blood flow to be present.

The most frequent cause of the obstruction, a *cholesterol embolus*, usually has broken up and moved on. If present, cholesterol emboli appear as bright, mobile, refractile plaques often at a bifurcation and not obstructing blood flow. Most cholesterol emboli (68%) originate from an ulcerated plaque in the ipsilateral internal carotid artery.

Fibrin-platelet emboli come from the great vessels or the heart and form soft white emboli several times the size of a cholesterol embolus, often molding themselves into both branches at an arteriolar bifurcation. Usually, both cholesterol and fibrin–platelet emboli are multiple; they may occur together. *Calcific emboli* usually (67%) originate from diseased heart valves (aortic and mitral) and appear as bright, white irregular densities. They are nearly always single, unilateral, and located in vessels on or near the optic disc.

All emboli show a preference for the temporal vasculature of the posterior pole. Calcific and platelet–fibrin emboli cause infarction; cholesterol emboli, although more common, less frequently produce permanent retinal damage. The majority of the cholesterol emboli is asymptomatic; others cause classic transient ischemic attacks (TIAs), which are rarely caused by calcium and fibrin–platelet emboli (see Chapter 8 for more details).

Even if the embolus has moved on by the time the patient is examined, there is frequently a calling card left behind: segmental arteriolar narrowing and a periarterial sheathing. After several months, only the sheathing may persist.

Other causes of emboli. Extensive traumatic long-bone fractures cause fat emboli, which can also occur in pancreatitis. IV drug abusers frequently show *talc retinopathy* (tiny, glistening "crystals" in small arterioles predominantly in the perifoveal arcades). Occasionally, papillary neovascularization and peripheral neovascular changes similar to those of sickle cell retinopathy occur in talc retinopathy.

Septic emboli associated with endocarditis—both bacterial and nonbacterial (marantic)—often cause white-centered hemorrhages (Roth's spots). Similar white-centered hemorrhages are found in leukemia and other blood disorders, subacute bacterial endocarditis (SBE), disseminated intravascular coagulation, and AIDS. Other rarer emboli originate from cardiac myxomas, metastatic tumors, amniotic fluid, air, and corticosteroids (especially after "sub-Tenon's" injections), as well as from artificial heart valves, synthetic vascular implants, and cardiac bypass machinery.

Nonembolic causes of retinal artery occlusion. Nonembolic causes of major retinal artery occlusion include arteriolarsclerosis and inflammatory and occlusive disease of the retinal arteries.

Retinal arterial disease may be primary or associated with systemic inflammatory disease. Contributing processes include hypertension, diabetes mellitus, sarcoidosis, fungi, systemic lupus erythematosus (SLE), temporal arteritis, Takayasu's arteritis, hypersensitivity angiitis, Behcet's syndrome, Wegener's granulomatosis, hypercoagulable states associated with a multitude of systemic disorders (such as dysproteinemia and multiple myeloma), and hyperviscosity (polycythemia vera and leukemia). However, hyperviscose states more often cause venous than arterial occlusion (Table 3–7).

In children and young adults, many retinal arterial occlusions are associated with migraine and coagulation disorders (Table 3–8). Sickle hemoglobinopathies should be sought in the appropriate population. Increased IOP associated with trauma is another prominent cause of retinal arterial occlusion in young patients and also occurs in older patients.

Hypertension. Retinal arterioles respond to elevated systemic blood pressure by arteriolar narrowing and irregularity, telangiectasia, alterations of the light reflex, obscuration of the arterial blood column, and arteriovenous crossing changes. More severe involvement causes arteriolar necrosis, retinal edema,

TABLE 3–7. RETINAL ARTERIAL AND VENOUS OCCLUSIVE DISEASE

Antiphospholipid antibody syndrome
Behcet's syndrome
Crohn's disease
Diabetes mellitus
Fungal infection
Hypercoaguable states
Hypertension
Disorders of clotting mechanism
Dysproteinemia
Hyperviscosity
Leukemia
Polyarteritis nodosa
Polycythema vera
Sarcoid
Syphilis
Systemic lupus erythematosus
Rarer vasculitides
Wegener's granulomatosis
Whipple's disease

retinal infarcts (cotton-wool spots), and flame-shaped hemorrhages. Severe hypertension is associated with encephalopathy and ischemic swelling of the optic disc. Whereas focal arteriolar irregularity is the hallmark of hypertensive retinopathy, other changes overlap arteriolarsclerotic alterations. Arteriolar constriction is most obvious in young individuals without significant arteriolarsclerotic change. Less frequently noted than hypertensive retinopathy, hypertensive choroidal changes include pigmented spots deep to the retina (Elschnig's spots) and pigmented streaks (Siegrist's streaks). Elschnig's spots result from necrosis of the retinal pigment epithelium.

The modified Keith-Wagener-Barker classification (Table 3–9) is used to categorize and follow hypertensive retinal vascular changes and to establish 10-year survival rates. These decrease significantly as the severity of the hypertensive retinal changes increases: Group 1 has a 71% 10-year survival rate; group 2, 51%; group 3, 35%; and group 4, 21%. However, direct ophthalmoscopy is not clinically useful in assessment of mild to moderate hypertension where only focal narrowing of arterioles is associated with the elevated blood pressure.

Diabetic retinopathy is an increasingly prevalent cause of visual loss. The retinopathy is uncommon in the first 10 years of diabetes, but affects nearly 90% of individuals who have been diabetic for 30 years or more (Table 3–10).

In diabetes, the vascular abnormalities are confined primarily to the posterior pole of the eye (especially in the macular area between the vascular arcades), in contrast to the midperipheral changes of the "ischemic eyeball" (discussed later in the chapter) or more peripheral changes seen in other vasoocclusive disorders such as Coats' disease, Eales'

disease, or sickle retinopathy (also discussed later). The major vessels are spared in diabetes, in contrast to their involvement in embolic occlusive disease and von Hippel–Lindau disease.

A very similar, but usually more limited, retinopathy may follow irradiation. Hemorrhages are less common and there is frequently a predilection for the inferior macular area.

Other retinopathies. Retinopathies are seen in anemia and acute blood loss. Anterior ischemic optic neuropathy and Roth's spots may be part of the picture. Paradoxically, the retinopathy may become evident days to weeks after the blood loss; the pathophysiologic mechanism is not understood. As in many retinopathies, unless the macula is involved, the patient may be asymptomatic. If the ischemia has

TABLE 3–9. MODIFIED KEITH-WAGENER-BARKER CLASSIFICATION

Vascular Change	Group 1	Group 2	Group 3	Group 4
Sclerosis	<1	1 or >	0–4	0–
General arteriolar narrowing	0–4	0–4	0–4	0–
Focal arteriolar narrowing	0–4	0–4	0–4	0–
Hemorrhage	—	=	=	=
Exudate	—	—	+	=
Papilledema	—	—	—	+

0–4 depends on amount or extent of vascular change.
+, present; —, absent.
From Walsh J. Hypertensive retinopathy: Description, classification and prognosis. Ophthalmology. 1982;89:1130.

TABLE 3–8. RETINAL ARTERIAL OBSTRUCTION IN YOUNG PATIENTS (N = 43)

Migraine	8
Coagulation abnormality	8
Intraocular abnormality	6
Increased IOP	3
Optic nerve head drusen	2
Prepapillary arterial loop	1
Trauma/surgery	5
Hemoglobinopathy	3
Oral contraceptives/ pregnancy	5
Cardiac disorders	2
Systemic lupus erythematosus	1
Talc Emboli	1
?	4

Modified from Brown GC, et al. Retinal arterial obstruction in children and young adults. Ophthalmology. 1981;88:21.

TABLE 3–10. RETINAL VASCULAR PATHOLOGY IN DIABETIC RETINOPATHY

Location	Disorder
Capillary	Occlusion
	Dilation
	Microaneurysms
	Abnormal permeability
Arteriole	Narrowing of origin of terminal arterioles
	Occlusion
	Sheathing
Vein	Dilation
	Beading
	Reduplication
	Looping, kinking
	Branch vein occlusion
	Central vein occlusion

From Bresnick G. Diabetic retinopathy. In: Peyman G, et al, eds. The Principles and Practice of Ophthalmology. Philadelphia: Saunders, 1980;2.

been mild and the optic nerves spared, recovery is usually complete.

Other Arteriolar Vascular Occlusive Diseases

Primary occlusion of the retinal arteries occurs in Takayasu's disease ("pulseless disease"), an arteritis of the great vessels predominantly affecting young Japanese women in association with fever, leukocytosis, and an increased sedimentation rate. The proximal arterial occlusion often causes an "ischemic eyeball" (discussed later in the chapter). In temporal arteritis, central retinal artery occlusion occurs; branch arterial occlusions are rare (see section on temporal arteritis in Headache chapter and on arteritic AION in Optic Disc Disorder chapter).

The retinopathy of systemic lupus erythematosus (SLE) usually shows occlusion of small retinal arterioles leading to very prominent cotton-wool spots. There is less hemorrhage and exudation than in many other vasculopathies. Occasionally, the central retinal artery and larger vessels are occluded and massive neovascularization may develop. In systemic lupus erythematosus (and presumably other collagen diseases), occlusion is due to necrotizing disease of the arterial wall, which may be compounded by systemic hypertension and antiphospholipid antibodies. Polyarteritis nodosa has a predilection for choroidal involvement. Rarely, cells in the vitreous signal a uveitis. Neovascularization is extremely rare.

Lupus anticoagulant factor unassociated with SLE also causes a severe vaso-occlusive retinochoroidopathy characterized by intraretinal hemorrhage, sheathing, neovascularization, and vitreous hemorrhage. Antiinflammatory and immunosuppressive drug therapy and panretinal photocoagulation or vitrectomy may be necessary to preserve vision. Other rarer alterations in blood factors may also cause vaso-occlusive processes (Table 3–11).

TABLE 3–11. BLOOD FACTORS TO CONSIDER IN VASO-OCCLUSIVE PROCESSES

Abnormal hemoglobins
Abnormal plasminogen
Antiphospholipid antibodies
Antithrombin III deficiency
Defective fibrinolysis
Dysfibrinogenemias
Elevated factor V
Elevated factor VIII
Factor XII deficiency
Hypoplasminogenemia, abnormal plasminogen, plasminogen activator deficiency
Lupus anticoagulant
Protein C deficiency
Protein S deficiency

Systemic inflammatory disorders such as Behcet's syndrome, sarcoid, Whipple's disease, and the reaction to giardiasis, are usually associated with vitreous cells, if not a frank uveitis, and opacification (axoplasmic stasis?) of the retina adjacent to the vasculopathy. These are important diseases to consider and diagnose because they all are treatable.

Sarcoid retinopathy: Ocular involvement (uveitis, chorioretinitis, periphlebitis, choroidal granulomas, or invasion of the optic nerve) occurs in nearly 50% of patients with sarcoidosis. The uveitis frequently obscures peripheral retinal neovascular changes that can form seafans similar to those seen in sickle cell disease. Associated central nervous system abnormalities are found in about one third of the patients with ocular sarcoid; cranial neuropathies are frequent manifestations. Evaluation includes chest x-ray, appropriate conjunctival or lacrimal gland biopsy, and determination of angiotensin-converting enzyme and lysozyme levels. With neurological findings, a spinal fluid examination and neuroimaging should be performed.

Behcet's syndrome is a multisystem inflammatory disorder characterized by oral and genital ulceration. Most patients are young males (20 to 30 years) from Turkey, other Mediterranean countries, and Japan. Seventy-five percent has ocular symptoms, the presenting symptoms in 20% of cases. Most frequent is recurrent hypopyon uveitis. Sequellae are very serious, including blindness, vena cava obstruction, central nervous system disorder, and paralysis. The primary therapy is steroids, although some believe fibrinolytic agents are helpful, free of side effects, and may allow the steroid dose to be substantially reduced. Antimetabolites, especially chlorambucil and cyclosporin, may also be helpful.

Recent increases in sexually transmitted diseases have led to an increase in *ophthalmic complications of syphilis* and the recognition that standard treatment protocols for syphilis may not be adequate to prevent the development of neurosyphilis (with which arteritic occlusion and optic nerve involvement are not unusual). In the retina, syphilis usually causes a perivasculitis, but arterial occlusion, chorioretinitis, and uveitis also occur. The treatment is penicillin (see Chapter 5 for therapy of neurosyphilis and serologic testing).

Retinal vascular changes (white spots and hemorrhages) are also among the most frequent *manifestations of AIDS*, and occur in about 75% of those affected. Recent studies suggest HIV-induced vascular alterations result in arteriolar occlusion. In general, the changes are evanescent and benign, but the small, apparently benign hemorrhage or cotton-wool spots seen today may be the forme fruste of a devastating cytomegalic virus retinitis.

Frosted branch angiitis causes sudden and severe bilateral visual loss, diffuse retinal edema, and unusual venous sheathing without systemic symptoms. Dye leakage is seen with fluorescein angiography. The ERG response is absent but recovers. Systemic steroid therapy is usually successful in returning vision to normal.

Arteriolar Spasm

The role of arteriolar spasm in the pathogenesis of retinal vascular disorders remains controversial, but is blamed by some for vaso-occlusion in systemic hypertension and eclampsia (here the choroid is also involved), migraine, and in the adverse effects on both the retina and optic nerve of the abuse of nasal sprays, cocaine, and amphetamines (Table 3–12). On rare occasions fluorescein angiography documents spasm leading to ischemia or thrombosis. High oxygen tension and ergot preparations also cause arterial spasm.

The roles of platelet changes and complement-mediated leukocytosis remain inadequately elucidated in retinal vascular spasm and occlusive disease.

Abnormal Vasculature

Many disorders of the vascular tree associated with vascular incompetence and occlusion have already been mentioned. Others include primary retinal vascular abnormalities, Wyburn-Mason arteriovenous malformation (see Chapter 21), retinal macroaneurysms, congenital tortuosity of the retinal vessels (a benign variant), and retinal telangiectasia.

DIAGNOSTIC EVALUATION

The diagnostic evaluation of embolic and occlusive retinal arterial disease includes evaluation for sources of emboli and primary vascular disease (see Chapter 8). Because patients with concomitant ciliary artery obstruction have the worst visual prognosis, a decreased a-wave on the electroretinogram indicates outer retinal layer damage and a poorer

TABLE 3–12. SYSTEMIC MEDICATIONS ASSOCIATED WITH RETINAL ARTERIOLAR OCCLUSION

Chloroquine
Nose sprays
Amphetamines
Cocaine
Ergotamine
O_2
Quinine

prognosis. Abnormalities of choroidal filling on fluorescein angiography have a similiar significance.

Fluorescein angiography is necessary for the evaluation of vascular disorders of the eye, especially in unexplained visual loss. It not only reveals obvious vascular changes, it also often differentiates between microaneurysms and small-dot hemorrhages; demonstrates unsuspected microvascular abnormalities and nonperfusion; and makes visible distended, irregular, and telangiectatic capillary beds, arteriovenous shunts of all sizes, and the leakage characteristic of subretinal neovascular membranes and newly formed and inflamed vessels (normal retinal vessels do not leak).

Optic atrophy, high myopia, carotid occlusive disease, glaucoma, and extensive chorioretinal scarring often seem to protect against the development of new vessels. Clinically, this means that a patient with vascular proliferative disease in only one eye needs thorough evaluation for these factors, especially for carotid occlusive disease on the opposite ("good") side.

TREATMENT

Treatment of completed occlusion. Retinal arterial occlusion, especially central retinal artery occlusion, has no truly effective treatment. The manipulations employed attempt to increase blood flow by removing the obstruction, causing vasodilation, and decreasing intraocular pressure. Beyond that, efforts should be made to define the cause of the obstruction and to prevent further emboli or progression of vascular occlusive disease.

Generally, with central retinal artery occlusion, place the patient in the Trendelenburg position. Give retrobulbar anesthesia (without epinephrine!), ocular massage, and IV acetazolamide, glycerin, or isosorbide; institute inhalation of carbogen (5% CO_2, 95% O_2); and do an anterior chamber paracentesis. These measures aim to decrease intraocular pressure and hopefully, increase perfusion. Although emboli may be seen to move into the periphery after paracentesis, they do this spontaneously as well. Because fluorescein angiography usually demonstrates that some blood flow is present, evidence for a beneficial effect of any of these treatments is not overwhelming.

Irrigation of heparin into the arterial system via cannulation of the frontal arteries has been reported to be of use, and a similar approach may be more effective with the development of increasingly effective and better-tolerated fibrinolytic agents. Theoretically, placing the patient in a hyperbaric chamber might also increase oxygen saturation, especially in the choroidal blood supply, and preserve visual acuity.

Nevertheless, despite all therapies, the majority of patients with central retinal artery occlusion has a dismal prognosis. After approximately 20 minutes, the damage is permanent; optic atrophy, loss of the nerve fiber layer, and marked constriction of the arteries ensues. When first seen, 94% of patients has count fingers or worse vision; significant visual recovery is rare; only 28% ever sees better.

Control of atherosclerosis and sources of emboli are usually the most important steps to take in the aftermath of the occlusion. Systemic atherosclerosis and cardiovascular disease pose the greatest threat to the patient's longevity; stroke is relatively rare (about 10%), although four to five times more frequent than in a control population. (Medical therapy is discussed in Chapter 8.)

The "ischemic eyeball". Retinal changes also are concomitants of proximal vascular occlusive disease, especially carotid occlusive disease. The profound decrease in ocular blood flow in the ischemic eye leads to poor retinal **and** choroidal perfusion. Externally, one can see dilation, tortuosity, and congestion of the episcleral vessels. Cell and flare appear in the anterior chamber; the iris may be boggy or affected by neovascularization (rubeosis) and the pupil sluggish. Intraocular pressure may be high due to angle closure; low because of decreased ciliary blood flow and aqueous production; or normal, because these two factors balance each other out. In contrast to similar retinopathies in vein occlusion or background diabetes, attentuated arteries, dilated or constricted veins, and dot and blot hemorrhages are usually maximal in the **midperiphery** rather than in the posterior pole.

PERIPHERAL RETINAL VASCULAR OCCLUSIVE DISEASE AND ABNORMALITIES

Because it occurs in an area of relative visual insensitivity, peripheral retinal vascular disease may be entirely asymptomatic, detected only on examination or when complications occur. As in many vascular processes already discussed, there can be retinal nonperfusion and ischemia, endothelial incompetence, neovascularization, exudation (sometimes massive), and/or hemorrhage into the retinal and subretinal space, which may produce retinal detachment.

Symptoms occur with exudation into the posterior pole; exudative retinal detachment; and/or vitreous hemorrhage, which if minor may cause blurred vision or floaters, and if major may cause significant visual loss. As with all vascular proliferative disorders, the major causes of serious visual loss include repeated vitreous hemorrhages; vitreous organization and traction retinal detachment and/or exudative retinal detachment; rubeosis iridis; neovascular glaucoma; cataracts; and a blind, painful eye (phthisis) leading to enucleation.

Some of the diseases affecting the peripheral retinal vessels also affect the central retinal vessels (eg, talc or sarcoid retinopathy). Others seem to have a predilection for the retinal periphery: Coats', Leber's, and Eales' diseases; sickle cell disease, thalassemia, and retinopathy of prematurity. The capillary hemangiomas of von Hippel–Lindau disease and cavernous hemangiomas frequently involve the peripheral retina.

Sickle hemoglobin retinopathy. Retinopathies occur in association with several types of sickling hemoglobin and thalassemia. In SC sickle cell disease the retinopathy is much more severe than that of SS sickle cell disease; in SS disease, systemic manifestations predominate. The predilection of the retinal vascular abnormalities for the retinal periphery is thought to result from very high oxygen extraction in the retina, subsequent decreased oxygen tension in the peripheral capillaries, and sickling of the abnormal hemoglobin in the red blood cells, which produce arterial occlusions. This results in a panoply of vascular changes ranging from relatively prosaic neovascularization and angioid streaks to dramatic proliferations within the vitreous ("seafans"), choroidal infarcts ("black sunbursts"), and retinal hemorrhages ("salmon patches"). Fluorescein angiography reveals occlusions of the small peripheral arteries, tortuous veins, and arteriovenous shunts in addition to areas of nonperfusion and the more dramatic abnormalities mentioned above.

Coats'/Leber's disease. Coats' disease is a congenital retinal vascular anomaly, a coarse net of dilated arterioles and capillaries and aneurysmal swelling that leads to fluorescein leakage. When the disease is predominantly central in location, and the changes are relatively quiescent (telangiectasia and microaneurysm without much exudation), the picture describes Leber's miliary aneurysms. On the other hand, when more peripheral retinal and subretinal exudation predominates with lipid deposition, cystoid macular edema (CME) and hemorrhage, or retinal detachment, the changes are described as Coats' disease.

Most contemporary authors think these are variations of the same process because they tend to occur predominantly in young males and to involve one eye only. The disease progresses in fits and starts with some spontaneous regression. Frequently, symptoms are first caused by exudation in the posterior pole or vitreous hemorrhage. Massive transudation and retinal detachment lead to secondary glaucoma, phthisis, and leucocoria. Leucocoria always necessitates ruling out retinoblastoma as the cause of the abnormal reflex (Table 3–13). In contrast to retinoblastoma, Coats' disease is seen in older boys (around 8 years old) rather than infants and shows prominent telangiectasis. Leber's disease usually presents in still older patients.

Eales' disease. Eales' disease is an idiopathic peripheral vasoproliferative disease characterized by extensive nonperfusion. It may be unilateral or bilateral. Typically, young, healthy adults present with recurrent vitreous hemorrhages, which are more frequent in this disease than in other peripheral perivasculitis. Traction retinal detachment with consequent loss of vision is frequent. Staining of vessel walls is commonly seen with fluorescein angiography. Some authors consider Eales' disease an idiopathic inflammatory process in continuum with pars planitis, which can also show neovascular changes. When massive exudation occurs, it too enters into the differential diagnosis of leucocoria.

Retinopathy of Prematurity (Retrolental Fibroplasia). In retinopathy of prematurity (ROP), also known as retrolental fibroplasia (RLF), vasoproliferative tissue forms as the response of the immature retina to increased oxygen tension, usually in premature infants who are placed in a high-oxygen environment in order to survive. Its severity is usually proportional to the oxygen concentration used and the period over which it was used. The more severe the fibroplasia, the less likely is significant regression. Severe fibrous change results in traction on the posterior pole, causing heterotopia of the macula and disc tissues (the so-called "dragged macula" and "dragged disc"). The displacement of the macula results in pseudoexotropia as the eye turns out to align the laterally displaced macula with the visual axis. More advanced stages lead to recurrent vitreous hemorrhages, retinal detachment, gliosis, and a poor visual prognosis.

TABLE 3–13. LEUKOCORIA: DIFFERENTIAL DIAGNOSIS

Astrocytic hamartoma of tuberous sclerosis
Colobomas of posterior pole
Complete retinal detachment
Congenital cataract
Congenital retinal folds
Exudative retinal detachment Coats'/Leber's, Von Hipple–Lindau and Eales' diseases
Incontinentia pigmenti
Massive retinal fibrosis
Morning glory syndrome
Myelinated nerve fibers
Nematode endophthalmitis
Norrie's disease
Persistent hyperplastic primary vitreous
Retinal dysplasia of trisomy 13
Retinoblastoma
Vitreous abscess

Peripheral retinal angiomas. Capillary hemangiomas occur in 50% of the patients with von Hippel–Lindau disease (see Chapter 21); although they develop throughout the patient's lifetime, they usually are detected in early adulthood. The lesions start out as small capillary abnormalities that increase in size. Larger lesions develop a prominent, tortuous feeding artery and vein and arteriovenous sheathing. In fact, noticing a central exudate or a large abnormal artery and vein with funduscopy may lead to detection of the angioma (Fig. 3–7).

Symptoms occur because of edema, retinal or vitreous hemorrhage, exudation, and occasionally retinal detachment or glaucoma. Even in peripheral lesions, there may be massive posterior pole exudates.

Treatment of early lesions by photocoagulation is very successful; thus, it is worthwhile to follow patients with this disease closely by examination of the periphery with fluorescein angiography or angioscopy. The larger lesions can be very difficult to destroy, and when treated may cause a greater amount of exudation and even exudative or serous retinal detachment.

Cavernous hemangiomas appear as clusters of saccular vessels filled with dark venous blood and are usually located posterior to the equator. These angiomatous lesions do not leak fluorescein dye and need no treatment until they cause symptoms. They occur in isolation or associated with central nervous system and cutaneous hemangiomas.

RETINAL VENOUS OCCLUSION

Central retinal vein occlusion causes visual loss. Occasionally the visual loss follows a few hours or days of fluctuating visual acuity and photopsias. Usually, vision is very poor (20/400, LP), but may be somewhat better when the macula is spared. The occlusion usually occurs at or behind the lamina cribrosa. The ophthalmoscopic picture is one of massive hemorrhage obscuring many retinal details, tending to conform to the retinal nerve fiber layer pattern where less severe, and accompanied by a variable degree of ischemia and cotton-wool spots. The veins are tortuous, dark, and distended. The optic disc is swollen but often the swelling is camouflaged by retinal hemorrhages that obscure the disc margins.

Branch vein occlusions cause hemorrhages spread out in a pie-shaped sector beyond the area of occlusion (usually an arteriovenous crossing). Branch vein occlusions are three times as frequent as central retinal vein occlusions and most commonly involve the supratemporal vein. Visual acuity depends on the extent of macular involvement with hemorrhage, opacity, and/or edema.

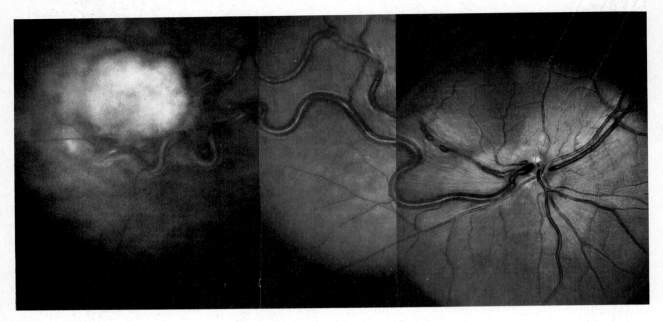

Figure 3—7. Peripheral retinal angiomas.

Arteriolarsclerosis is important in the pathogenesis of venous occlusions, which also are more frequent in patients with hypertension (75% of retinal vein occlusions), glaucoma (15%), diabetes, and systemic diseases associated with hyperviscosity.

Often spontaneous recovery of good visual acuity occurs after 6 to 12 months when the macula is healthy (50% ends up with 20/50 or better). The hemorrhages resorb, the cotton-wool spots disappear, and the edema of the disc and retina subsides. The veins gradually resume their normal dimensions. Frequently, collateral vessels form around the obstruction.

Neovascularization with the threat of neovascular glaucoma, vitreous hemorrhage, and macular edema are the major vision-threatening complications; neovascularization occurs in 25% of central retinal vein occlusions and 20% of branch vein occlusions. When neovascular glaucoma occurs, at least 20% of the eyes becomes blind; many become painful and must be enucleated.

Panretinal photocoagulation, and/or focal photocoagulation to areas of nonperfusion, seem to be effective in preventing neovascularization and neovascular glaucoma. Be careful not to treat collateral shunt vessels! The presence of an afferent pupillary defect; decreased electroretinogram amplitude, S-waves, flicker, and/or oscillatory potentials; or decreased PERG amplitude are indicative of ischemia and predictors of neovascular complications.

Papillophlebitis may simulate a central retinal vein occlusion with a swollen disc, engorged veins, and sometimes macular edema; but it usually occurs in a younger patient with better collateral circulation, shows much less hemorrhage and ischemia, and has a better prognosis. Visual acuity is usually normal. This entity may be associated with circulating immune complexes and is considered in more detail in the section on the swollen disc.

CHOROIDAL OCCLUSIVE DISEASE

Choroidal occlusive disease often is overshadowed by more extensive retinal changes. Generally, arterial occlusion of larger choroidal vessels is caused by atherosclerosis and of smaller vessels by hypertension; other occlusive processes, such as periarteritis, are unusual.

Large occlusions result in wedge-shaped areas of pigmentary change and nonperfusion, corresponding to the anatomy of the long posterior ciliary arterial branches (Fig. 3—8).

Smaller vessel occlusion is more spotty, corresponding to the central arterioles of choroidal lobules, (see vascular anatomy, Ch 1), and occurs predominantly in hypertension and toxemia, resulting in Siegrist's streaks and Elschnig's spots.

Similar changes may be seen after closed-eye operations with fluid infusion (cataract extraction, vitrectomy) that causes excessively elevated intraocular pressure. The outer retina becomes white and opaque. Lesions in the posterior pole are confluent, the midperiphery shows spotty changes, and the retinal vessels and periphery are normal. The lesions correspond to the distribution of the choroidal vas-

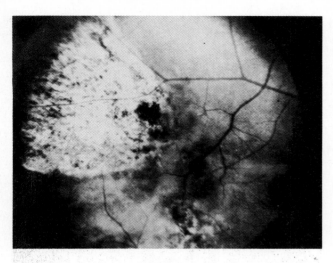

Figure 3–8. Choroidal occlusive disease. Triangular chorioretinal lesion in peripheral part of right eye of 68-year-old man with temporal arteritis, anterior ischaemic optic neuropathy, and no perception of light. (*From Hayreh SS. Acute choroidal ischemia. Trans Ophthal Soc UK. 1980;100:409; with permission.*)

culature. Visual acuity transiently decreases but returns nearly to normal with persistent paracentral scotomas.

MACULAR DISORDERS

Macular disease is also easily confused with neurogenic visual loss, especially if the physical findings in the macula are minimal and the visual loss takes the form of a central scotoma similar to that seen in optic nerve disease.

In addition to decreased visual acuity, macular disease may present with distortion (metamorphopsia) and color-vision loss. However, for the same level of visual loss, the color deficit and central scotoma are less evident than when associated with optic nerve disease.

A number of macular degenerations needs to be distinguished from neurogenic visual loss; many are hereditary and some are associated with central nervous system degeneration. Thus, it is critical to take a good family history, not only for visual difficulties but for associated neurologic illness. If the macular problem is a hereditary dystrophy, keep in mind the variable expressivity of the disorder. Most hereditary dystrophies are bilateral, relatively symmetrical, and begin subtly. This presentation is less common in optic nerve disease.

The nondystrophic macular disorders most likely to be confused with optic nerve disease include central serous retinopathy, cystoid macular edema, solar retinopathy, retinal pigment epithelial detachment, and subretinal neovascular membranes.

Central serous chorioretinopathy. Patients with central serous chorioretinopathy (CSR; Fig; 3–9) complain of blurred vision and, frequently, metamorphopsia. They have a central scotoma. It is characteristically a positive scotoma, frequently colored a pinkish or purplish hue, which interferes between the patient and the object viewed (rather than a "negative scotoma," which is just an absence of the object observed). The serous detachment of the neurosensory retina, a clear dome of elevation usually in the perifoveal area, caues a relative increase in hyperopia, an associated decrease in uncorrected visual acuity, and alters the internal limiting membrane reflexes.

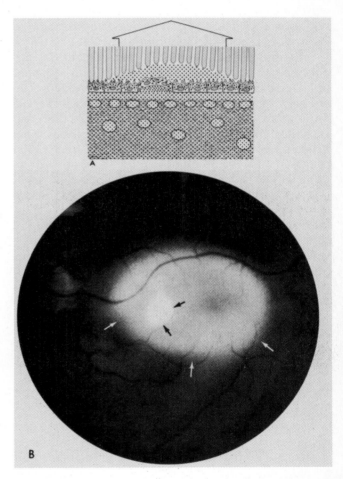

Figure 3–9. Central serous chorioretinopathy. Hyperfluorescence in patient with central serous chorioretinopathy. **A.** Accumulation of fluorescein (black dots) between the neurosensory retina and the retinal pigment epithelium (RPE). There is also a small focal detachment of the RPE that is filled with fluorescein. **B.** Area of hyperfluorescence corresponding to serous detachment of neurosensory retina that has filled with fluorescein (white arrows). Within this area is a smaller, more hyperfluorescent site (black arrows) resulting from small focal detachment of the RPE. (*From Federman J. Fluorescein angiography. In: Duane T, ed. Clinical Ophthalmology. Hagerstown, Harper & Row, 17; 1976; with permission.*)

The disease predominantly affects males, in a ratio of approximately 9:1, usually in the third and fourth decades. It may be related to primary disease of the retinal pigment epithelium through which serum leaks into the retina. Because of the separation of the retinal sensory elements from the retinal pigment epithelium, metabolism is slowed, resulting in positive photostress tests. CSR is self-limiting; usually there is complete remission within 6 months. Some distortion may persist. If the symptoms are particularly bothersome, laser photocoagulation may decrease the time for resolution. However, in order to qualify for treatment the leaking point should be at least 300 μ from the fovea. Rarely, following treatment, patients complain of visual illusions.

On fluorescein angiography, the leak from the choroidal vasculature shows as a small puddle of fluorescein, frequently with a wick-like extension to the area of retinal pigment epithelial leak.

Retinal pigment epithelial detachment. In retinal pigment epithelial detachment (Fig. 3–10), central visual acuity is less frequently involved. The etiology is sometimes similar to that of central serous retinopathy with an apparent leak of serous fluid that separates the retinal pigment epithelium from Bruch's membrane. The elevation of the retina causes a change of refraction in the hyperopic direction, which causes an apparent decrease of visual acuity. The natural history is variable; some resorb and some increase in size. Rarely, there is an associated subretinal neovascular membrane. If the lesion is not in the fovea, it probably should be watched. If in the macular area and enlarging toward the fovea, or if associated with a subretinal neovascular membrane, laser photocoagulation may be indicated.

Fluorescein angiography often shows a "hot-cross bun" configuration, with bright fluorescein bands crossing the darker bullous areas of the detachment.

Cystoid macular edema. Cystoid macular edema (CME) can cause an insidious visual loss, and if allowed to persist, permanent loss of vision. Often CME is associated with intraocular inflammation and hypotony; it may follow cataract extraction; it is associated with retinal angiopathies (diabetes and retinal vein occlusions), retinitis pigmentosa, Goldman-Favre syndrome, and nicotinic acid toxicity. Fluorescein angiography demonstrates a petalloid pattern of staining caused by fluid accumulation in Henle's layer (Fig. 3–11). Laser photocoagulation or cryotherapy of vascular abnormalities may cause the fluid to resorb. Treatment of vitreous bands causing traction, inflammation, or hypotony is indicated. Where no obvious cause exists, as in many cases that follow cataract extraction, there have been some reports of successful treatment with antiinflammatory

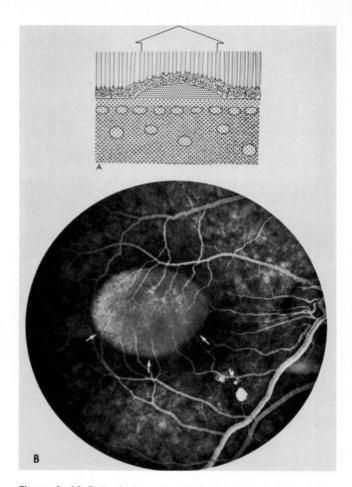

Figure 3–10. Retinal pigment epithelial detachment. Hyperfluorescence in patient with detachment of the retinal pigment epithelium (RPE). **A.** Accumulation of fluorescein (black dots) in localized serous detachment of RPE. **B.** Localized area of hyperfluorescence (arrows) due to accumulation of dye under the RPE. (*From Federman J. Fluorescein angiography. In: Duane T, ed.* Clinical Ophthalmology. *Hagerstown: Harper & Row; 4:16; with permission.*)

agents, but most cases of cystoid edema resolve or persist independent of treatment efforts.

Solar retinopathy. Staring at the sun or an eclipse without adequate protection produces a foveal burn. When done inadvertently, the lesions frequently are bilateral. Those that occur in an effort to avoid something unpleasant, such as military service, or as part of yoga exercise, are usually uniocular. If seen immediately following the burn, there is a small area of retinal edema. Over time, this becomes a small pigmented area with a brownish to reddish color. It must be distinguished from other causes of a macular cherry-red spot (see Chapter 23). If it is precisely in the fovea, visual acuity may be significantly affected by the apparently minuscule lesion. Although the appearance, especially if bilateral, is relatively characteristic, many other pigmentary al-

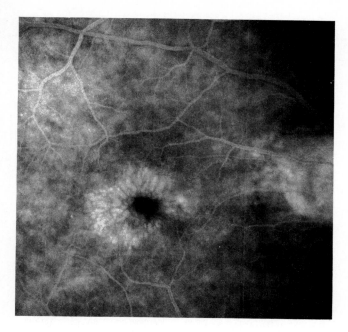

Figure 3–11. Cystoid macular edema as demonstrated by fluorescein angiograhy.

terations can look similar; the best way to make the diagnosis is to obtain the appropriate history.

Optic-disc-related subretinal neovascular membranes. Chronic disc swelling, papilledema, and optic nerve head drusen may also be associated with peripapillary subretinal neovascular membranes.

Other dystrophic macular processes are listed in Table 3–14 and macular disorders associated with systemic disease are tabulated in Chapter 23.

DIFFUSE RETINAL DEGENERATIONS AND DYSTROPHIES

This grab bag of retinal disorders is characterized primarily by alterations in retinal pigmentation. They may involve the entire retina or affect either the central retina or the peripheral retina predominantly. The prototype disorder is retinitis pigmentosa, and many of the disorders discussed below are frequently mentioned as retinitis pigmentosa variants. For clarity, "retinitis pigmentosa" will refer to diseases inherited in the described patterns and possessing typical findings. Other disorders will be termed "RP-like" or "pigmentary retinal disturbances," especially because many of them present with flecks, areas of depigmentation, and crystalline deposits rather than typical bone spicule pigmentation. A different approach to classification (by age of onset, severity, and association with nonocular abnormalities) might be more useful than description by fundus appearance and electroretinogram status, nonspecific end products of many degenerative processes.

Retinitis pigmentosa. Retinitis pigmentosa is a hereditary progressive retinal degeneration characterized by nyctalopia (night blindness), progressive loss of visual field, and a depressed to absent electroretinogram. The fundus shows bone spicule pigmentary changes, "waxy" pallor of the optic disc, and attenuation of arterioles (Fig. 3–12). A posterior subcapsular cataract often is associated. Optic nerve head drusen occasionally occur within the substance of the optic disc or, in a pattern unique to retinitis pigmentosa, in the peripapillary area. Heredity is autosomal dominant, autosomal recessive, or sex-linked recessive.

Classically, the electroretinogram and peripheral visual field are affected early. The prototypical visual field defect is a ring scotoma, while central vision remains normal for a long time. Variants include central retinitis pigmentosa in which the macular area is predominantly affected, sector retinitis pigmentosa, and unilateral retinitis pigmentosa. Occasionally, the classic bone spicule pigmentation is not seen (retinitis pigmentosa sine pigmento). Unless the other findings are absolutely typical or there is a consistent family history, some of these cases actually may be other entities.

The patterns of visual field loss vary and when the retina is disproportionately affected in various sectors, the field defects may mimic optic nerve defects (inferonasal field loss), chiasmal field defects (bitemporal defects), and vascular optic neuropathies (altitudinal field defects). However, if several isopters of the fields are examined carefully, it will be found that the defects disregard the strict alignment along horizontal and vertical meridians characteristic of neurogenic visual loss.

Cone dystrophies. Cone dystrophies are the primary retinal degeneration most often confused with neuro-ophthalmic disease. The classically described varieties usually present at an early age with significantly decreased visual acuity, achromatopsia, and nystagmus. There is a positive family history. The scotopic electroretinogram is nonrecordable.

However, this more common form does not cause diagnostic confusion. Cone dystrophies range from a severe type with early onset described above to minimal changes presenting in the elderly. The type frequently referred for neuro-ophthalmic workup presents in the first or second decade with a central visual field defect, a relatively normal looking fundus and a decreased B wave on the electroretinogram. There are difficulties in bright light often described as photophobia or glare; in elderly patients, these symptoms are so similar to those associated with posterior subcapsular cataracts that the underlying retinal dystrophy may not be detected until cataract extraction results in a less than optimal result.

Digitalis toxicity, when it presents with diffuse

TABLE 3–14. HEREDITARY MACULAR DYSTROPHIES

Retinal Layer Affected	Macular Changes	Other Retinal Changes	Symptoms
Nerve Fiber Layer			
X-linked juvenile retinoschisis	Foveal retinoschisis and macrocysts (wheel-like spokes)	Peripheral retinoschisis in 50%, vascular sheathing, vitreous hemorrhage, vitreous veils, pigmentary alterations	VA approximately 20/60
Sensory Retina, Receptors			
Cone dystrophy	Bull's-eye lesions, macular atrophy sometimes	Temporal pallor of disc, peripheral pigmentary changes late	Decreased VA, decreased color vision, photophobia
Retinal Pigment Epithelium			
Fundus flavimaculatus (Stargardt's disease)	Sometimes macular atrophy, pigment changes	Yellow-white flecks	Decreased VA with macular changes (20/80–20/20 eg. w/20c)
Vitelliform dystrophy	Early: "Sunny-side-up egg" (may be multiple) Later: "scrambled egg"		VA good until "egg" scrambles
Butterfly dystrophy	Pigment clumping and atrophy		VA more or less normal
Hereditary drusen	Yellow deposits	May have RPE, choroidal atrophy	VA normal early, decreased 4th to 5th decade
Miscellaneous			
Dominant progressive foveal dystrophy	Drusen-like changes Choroidal atrophy		Decreased VA Central scotoma

AD, autosomal dominant; AR, autosomal recessive; DA, dark adaptation; EOG, electro-oculogram; ERG, electroretinogram; VA, visual acuity; XLR, X-linked recessive.

Heredity	Onset	ERG	EOG	Other
XLR	Birth, slow progression	Decreased B-wave	Normal early, progressing to abnormal	Late strabismus, nystagmus DA normal early, decreased rate
AD	2nd decade	Decreased photopic flicker	Normal early progressing to abnormal	Late nystagmus, decreased DA
AR	End 1st decade	Initially normal, becoming abnormal	Decreased late	Decreased PERG early, DA decreased late; "silent" choroid on fluorescein angiogram
AD	1st decade normal, decreased VA 4th decade	Normal	Decreased	DA normal
AD		Normal	Decreased	DA normal
AD		Normal	Normal	DA normal
AD	As early as 5 mo	Normal	Normal	DA normal

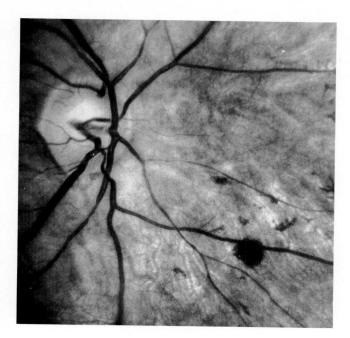

Figure 3–12. Retinitis pigmentosa.

TABLE 3–15. CLASSIFICATION OF CONGENITAL AND EARLY-ONSET RETINITIS PIGMENTOSA

Group 1
Uncomplicated LCA[a]
Typical LCA
LCA with macular colobomas
Group 2
Systemic disorders
Zellweger syndrome
Saldino-Mainzer syndrome
Senior-Loken syndrome
Multiple neurologic abnormalities
Others
Group 3
Juvenile RP
Group 4
Early-onset RP
Autosomal recessive
Autosomal dominant
X-linked recessive

[a] Leber's congenital amaurosis.
From Foxman SG, et al. Classification of congenital and early-onset retinitis pigmentosa. Arch Ophthalmol. 1985;103:1505.

difficulty in color vision rather than a specific distortion of color acuity, can present a very similar picture.

Some of the cone-rod dystrophies show prominent telangiectasia in the disc and peripapillary areas, pseudo-disc edema, and pseudoaltitudinal visual field defects.

Leber's congenital amaurosis. In Leber's congenital amaurosis (LCA), a rare and heterogeneous congenital disorder (Table 3–15), vision is severely limited (<20/200) and the electroretinogram is extinguished or nearly so. The disc may be hypoplastic and the retina show a salt-and-pepper-type pigmentary abnormality, which tends to become more obvious with age. Neurologic, renal, and skeletal abnormalities may be associated. The inheritance pattern is autosomal recessive. There may be a subgroup associated with high hyperopia and lack of neurologic abnormality (Table 3–16). Many exhibit the oculodigital sign and eventually develop enophthalmus.

These patients develop nystagmus or wandering eye movements at the age of 2 to 3 months. Typically these oculomotor manifestations of very poor visual acuity bring the child to medical attention. Early diagnosis is important in order to provide genetic counseling. However, rule out other retinal syndromes that may present similarly: congenital stationary night blindness, achromatopsia, infantile-onset retinitis pigmentosa, Joubert's syndrome, Zellweger's syndrome, Alström's syndrome, and in-

fantile Refsum's disease (in infants with nystagmus and decreased vision). Unusual refractive errors, the oculodigital sign, and photophobia and a normal anterior segment suggest a retinal disorder.

Other syndromes that include retinitis pigmentosa or retinitis-pigmentosa-like manifestation are listed in the tables in Chapter 23. Toxic retinopathies are listed in Table 3–17.

RETINAL NERVE FIBER LAYER DISORDERS

Changes in the retinal nerve fiber layer can be categorized into two large groups: (1) atrophic changes (loss of nerve fibers) and (2) changes that appear to be intrinsic within the nerve fibers themselves.

Atrophic Changes

Atrophic nerve fiber layer changes all are characterized by loss of the normal striated pattern of the nerve fiber layer. Where the gray translucent fibers are lost, so are the striations, and the retina takes on a rather dull, mottled appearance because one is looking directly at the surface of the inner retina, retinal pigment epithelium, and choroid. The retinal blood vessels seem to stand out in stark relief; reflexes appear along their borders, probably from draping of the internal limiting membrane over the vessels (Fig. 3–13).

Small areas of focal nerve fiber layer atrophy show up as *slit or rake-like defects*, which are best seen one to two disc diameters from the optic disc in the superior and inferior temporal arcades, where

TABLE 3–16. DIFFERENTIAL DIAGNOSIS OF CONGENITAL AND EARLY-ONSET RETINITIS PIGMENTOSA (RP) AND OF LEBER'S CONGENITAL AMAUROSIS (LCA)

Findings on Initial Examination	Uncomplicated LCA (Group 1)	Complicated LCA (Group 2)	Juvenile RP (Group 3)	Early-onset RP (Group 4)
Onset of symptoms	Prior to 6 mo	Difficult to determine	Prior to 2 years	At approximately 4 years
Visual acuity	Poorer than 20/400	Poorer than 20/400	Better than 20/100	Better than 20/60
Refractive error	More than 4 diopters hyperopic	Variable	Slightly hyperopic	Slightly hyperopic
Nystagmus	Searching	Searching	Occasionally latent	Absent
Pupillary reaction	Sluggish	Sluggish	Normal	Normal
Systemic abnormalities	None	Neurologic, renal, skeletal	None	None
Electroretinographic responses	Extinguished	Extinguished or minimally recordable	Extinguished	Extinguished or minimally recordable
Fundus appearance	Normal or mild pigmentary changes	Normal or mild pigmentary changes	Variable	Typical peripheral pigmentary abnormalities
Family history	Autosomal recessive	Dependent on syndrome	Unknown	X-linked recessive, autosomal recessive, autosomal dominant
Visual fields	Unable to determine	Unable to determine	Constricted	Mild to moderate constriction

From Foxman SG, et al. Classification of congenital and early onset retinitis pigmentosa. Arch Ophthalmol. 1985;103,1505.

the nerve fiber layer is thicker (and gives more contrast between relatively normal nerve fiber layer and the atrophic defects) (Fig. 3–14). These defects become slightly wider as they progress away from the optic disc and may be associated with notching or narrowing of the neuroglial rim in the corresponding disc meridian. Sometimes the defects are contiguous with the notch, but not always.

These rake-like defects must be differentiated from "*pseudodefects*," which are normal reflections from the internal limiting membrane. In contrast to the true defects, pseudodefects tend to fork and fuse,

be wider, and do not correspond to the pattern of the nerve fiber layer for all of their length (Fig. 3–15). Also, unlike true nerve fiber layer defects, if the ophthalmoscopic beam is moved slightly, due to parallax, the pseudodefects move.

Large areas of atrophy, which correspond to large areas of damage or to coalescence of slit defects, form various types of *sector defects*. Characteristic types of sector defects are seen in atrophy of the papillomacular bundle (Fig. 3–16A), as in nutritional amblyopia; these are usually associated with central or centrocecal scotomas. Sector defects in the

TABLE 3–17. RETINAL DRUG TOXICITY

Drug	Fundus Appearance and Other Changes
Canthaxanthine	Bull's-eye maculopathy
Chloroquine and related drugs	Macular mottling, bull's-eye maculopathy
	Peripheral pigment patches (pigment in lens and cornea, too)
	Narrow vessels, optic atrophy
	Decreased electroretinogram **but** dark adaptation normal (unlike retinitis pigmentosa); usually stops if drug stopped, but may progress
Colchicine	Optic atrophy
Indomethacin	Retinal thinning, pigment mottling, bull's-eye maculopathy on fluorescein angiography
Methoxyfluorane	Oxalate crystals, flecked retina
Niacin	Cystoid maculopathy (small cystic space, no stain with fluorescein angiography), reversible early
Nicotinic acid	Maculopathy—atypical cystoid macular edema, improves if drug stopped
Phenothiazine	Granular pigmentation of retina; pigmentation of skin, conjunctiva, cornea, lens
Quinine	Optic atrophy
Synthetic retinoids	Electroretinogram decreased
Tamoxifen	White fleck-like retinopathy (products of axoplasmic degeneration?)

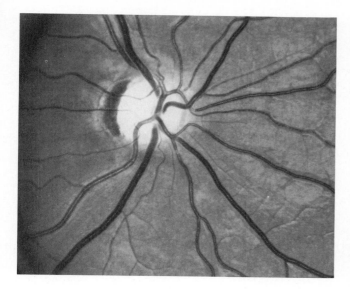

Figure 3–13. Atrophic nerve fiber layer changes.

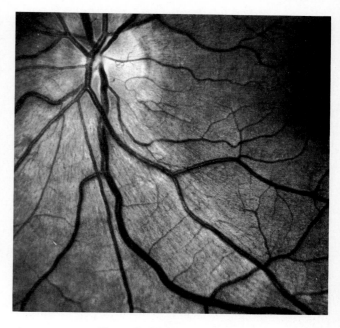

Figure 3–15. Pseudodefects.

temporal arcades may be found in glaucoma and are associated with Bjerrum's scotomata (Fig. 3–16B). *"Bow-tie" atrophy* is a specific type of sector defect (Fig. 3–16C), the ophthalmoscopic counterpart of an ipsilateral temporal hemianopic defect; it is seen most often in optic tract lesions, occasionally with chiasmal lesions, and rarely with lesions of the retrogeniculate visual afferent pathways arising early in development and allowing transsynaptic degeneration.

Photocoagulation, especially if performed in a focal manner, will frequently cause nerve fiber layer atrophy and ophthalmoscopically visible nerve fiber defects (Fig. 3–17).

Defects in the retinal nerve fiber layer also occur in a number of diseases thought to affect predominantly the outer retinal layers (eg, retinitis pigmentosa, cone-rod dystrophies, Stargardt's disease, vitelliform degeneration, and choroideremia; Fig. 3–18). In these diseases, either transsynaptic degeneration occurs within the retina, or—although the disease appears localized to the outer retinal layers on ophthalmoscopy—many retinal layers are involved. From a practical standpoint, this means that patients who present with subtle nerve fiber defects and no clear history or findings suggesting neurogenic visual loss should be evaluated for heredo-degenerative retinal problems.

When the atrophic alterations in the nerve fiber are less discrete, generalized attrition or total atrophy of the nerve fiber layer occurs. In *generalized attrition*, reflexes along the vessels are heightened, but the striations of the nerve fiber layer are less visible and the retina has a somewhat dark appearance. Small vessels, especially in the peripapillary area, are bared by the atrophy of the nerve fiber layer. The borders of the optic discs are more sharply seen than usual (Fig. 3–19). If the nerve fiber layer in the contralateral eye is normal, the contrast between the two can help to identify this somewhat subtle picture of nerve fiber loss.

The picture of *total atrophy* shows a dark fundus

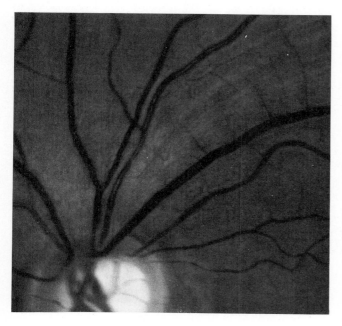

Figure 3–14. Slit or rake-like defects.

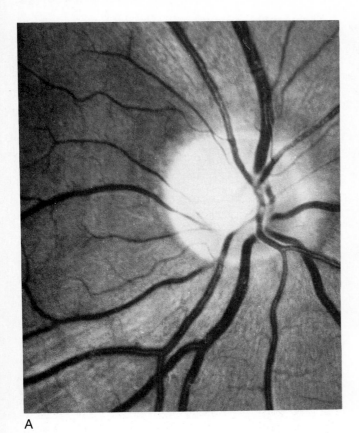

A

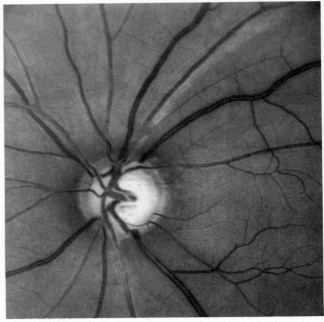

B

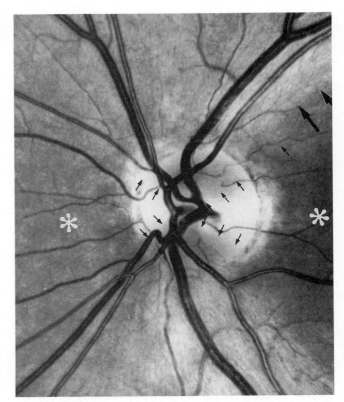

C

Figure 3–16. Sector defects.
Figure 3–16. **A.** Papillomacular bundle defect in "toxic" amblyopia.
B. Bjerrum scotomas with corresponding superior and inferior wedge
defects in glaucoma. **C.** "Bow-tie" atrophy (arrows) in traumatic
chiasmal transection. Areas of nerve fiber loss contrast with normal
appearance of nerve fibers in the temporal arcades.

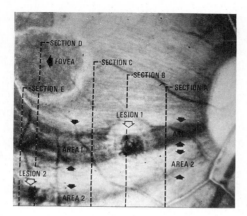

Figure 3–17. Photocoagulation scar and resultant nerve fiber layer atrophy in a monkey. (*From Frisch GC, et al. Remote nerve fiber bundle alterations in the retina as caused by argon laser photocoagulation. Nature. 1974;248:433, with permission.*)

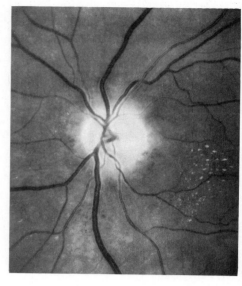

Figure 3–19. Generalized attrition, baring borders of optic disc (following anterior ischemic optic neuropathy; same patient as Fig. 3–22, 1 month later).

with a granular appearance because one looks directly at the choroid and retinal pigment epithelium. The disc margins are sharply outlined and there is obvious draping of the internal limiting membrane over the retinal vessels. The small vessels in the peripapillary area are very well defined because they are no longer obscured by the nerve fiber layer.

In *papilledema*, the immediate peripapillary area is darkened and void of normal striations. This

is probably the earliest change. Thereafter, increased opacity of the axons occurs at the disc margin, first at the superior and inferior poles. Vessels in the immediate peripapillary area lose their normal reflexes

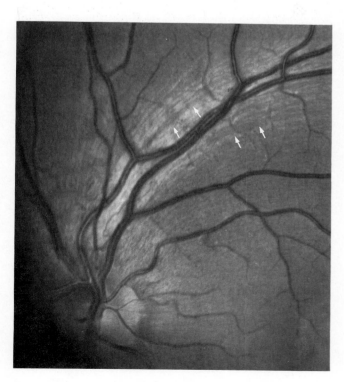

Figure 3–18. Nerve fiber layer defects in outer retinal layer dystrophy (vitelliform).

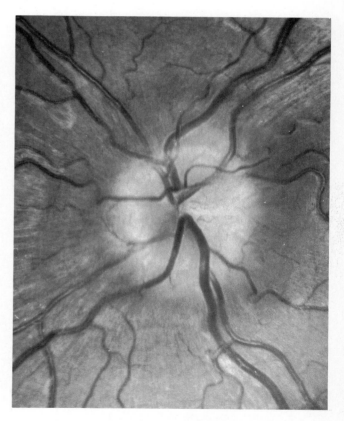

Figure 3–20. Papilledema.

and may be obscured by the engorged nerve fibers (Fig. 3–20). More peripherally, the normal reflexes of the internal limiting membrane are heightened, frequently forming a band of circular reflexes approximately one disc diameter from the disc, especially in young patients. There may be hemorrhages, cotton-wool spots, and loss of venous pulsations.

In *pseudopapilledema*, caused by buried *optic nerve head drusen*, the peripapillary retina may be normal or atrophic with respect to the nerve fiber layer, but does not show opacity—an extremely important differential point. Some subclinical optic nerve damage occurs in optic nerve head drusen; as the patient becomes older, nerve fiber defects and generalized atrophy usually are associated with visible drusen of the optic disc (Fig. 3–21).

Intrinsic Changes

Increased opacity of the nerve fiber layer: Especially in the acute stages of ischemic processes (eg, anterior ischemic optic neuropathy, but also with other processes leading to nerve fiber layer atrophy, such as demyelination and nutritional toxic amblyopia), the nerve fiber layer assumes a somewhat glistening appearance with heightened opacity. The opaque retina of central retinal artery occlusion and the white spots seen with focal retinal infarction, both of which represent obstruction of axoplasmic flow, are extreme examples of this phenomenon. White spots are also seen in the retinopathy of AIDS, and may represent patches of HIV-infected ganglion cells. Other processes that slow or halt axoplasmic flow (eg, optic neuritis, neuroretinitis, and ischemia) cause a similar but less obvious increase in the retinal opacity (Fig. 3–22).

Leber's optic neuropathy in the presymptomatic and early symptomatic stages is almost always associated with a considerably heightened opacity of the nerve fiber layer and telangiectatic vessels in the peripapillary area (Fig. 3–23). A similar appearance is found in asymptomatic relatives of these patients.

DARK RETINAL SPOTS

The differential diagnosis of dark spots in the retina is important primarily to rule out malignant mela-

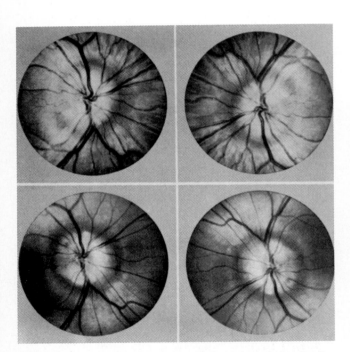

Figure 3–21. Pseudopapilledema. Bilateral drusen of optic disc. **Top.** Buried intrapapillary drusen producing anomalous disc elevation ("pseudopapilledema") in 4-year-old boy with hypermetropia of 7 diopters. **Bottom.** Optic discs of same patient 10 years (!) later, indicating exposed intrapapillary drusen, especially on nasal side of disc, and in some places "moth-eaten" appearance of pigment epithelium surrounding disc. Good demonstration of gradual exposure of buried drusen over period of 10 years. Left illustrations correspond to right eye, and right illustrations to left eye. Note loss of nerve fiber layer striations in later photos. (*From Huber A. Eye Symptoms in Brain Tumor. 3rd ed. Edited and translated by Blodi FC. St. Louis: Mosby, 1976, with permission.*)

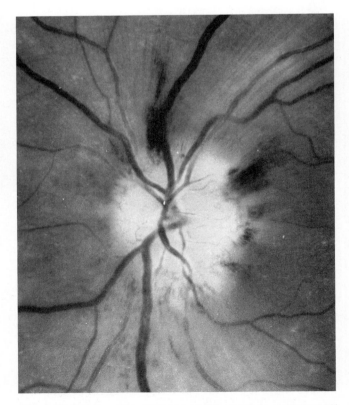

Figure 3–22. Opacity of the nerve fiber layer in superior and inferior temporal arcades in anterior ischemic optic neuropathy.

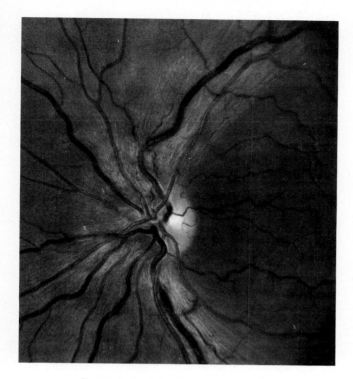

Figure 3–23. Leber's optic neuropathy.

noma, the commonest intraocular tumor in adults (Table 3–18). It is also important to recognize grouped pigmentation, the so-called "bear tracks," which are a congenital hypertrophy of the retinal pigment epithelium. These are benign hamartomas, but when bilateral and multiple, they are absolute

TABLE 3–18. DARK RETINAL SPOTS (R/O MALIGNANT MELANOMA)

Nevus

Flat, ovoid, less than three disc diameters, **no change over time;** overlying drusen, best seen with indirect ophthalmoscopy

Grouped Pigmentation (Bear Tracks)
Congenital hypertrophy of retinal pigment epithelium: when stationary and unilateral are benign; when bilateral and multiple (>4) are pathognomonic of Gardner's syndrome (colonic adenomatous polyposis—colonic adenocarcinoma always occurs if untreated-benign soft tissue and bony tumors, dental abnormalities, desmoid tumors, extracolonic carcinoma, autosomal dominant, 100% penetrance)

Malignant Melanoma
Commonest intraocular tumor of adulthood
Raised, larger than nevi, grow, metastasize especially to liver
Therapy: enucleation, photocoagulation, radiation

Melanocytoma
Arise at disc, **very** dark, small, flat
Locally invasive only, vision rarely affected severely

indicators of the abnormal gene for Gardner's syndrome. Recognition is critical because these patients develop colonic polyposis, which if untreated always progresses to adenocarcinoma of the colon.

In contrast, metastatic lesions to the choroid and retina are not usually pigmented; they present as choroidal masses with or without an associatred retinal detachment.

INFLAMMATION AND INFECTION OF THE OUTER RETINAL LAYERS

The outer retinal layers, retinal pigment epithelium, and choroid may be disrupted by poorly understood inflammatory entities. Their pathogenesis often is attributed to nonspecific inflammation, an autoimmune response, or virus infection. Changes are manifest by discoloration of the deep retinal layers and, ultimately, pigment disruption and migration. Frequently the changes are asymptomatic except for associated signs of inflammation (eg, uveitis or vasculitis). Symptoms occur with involvement of the macula, papillitis, or vasculitis. Photoreceptor dysfunction causes nonspecific flashes or sparks, a common manifestation of outer retinal layer inflammation. The multiple evanescent white-dot syndrome may be associated with an enlarged blind spot that may persist after the retinal changes are resolved.

TABLE 3–19. CLINICAL FEATURES OF APMPPE

Age group: 15–40 yr (mean 27 yr)
Sex: M, F
Self-limited disease
Ophthalmologic manifestations:
  1. Bilateral visual acuity and visual field loss with corresponding retinal lesions
  2. Uveitis
  3. Papillitis
  4. Serous retinal detachment
  5. Episcleritis
  6. Peripheral corneal thinning
Neurologic manifestations
  1. Headache
  2. Transient ischemic attacks
  3. Fixed neurologic deficit
Systemic manifestations
  1. Thyroiditis
  2. Asymptomatic renal disease (active phase)
Laboratory findings
  1. Cerebrospinal fluid
    a. Elevated protein levels
    b. Lymphocytic pleocytosis
  2. Electroencephalographic evidence of diffuse slowing
  3. Urinary casts in the active phase
  4. Arteriographic evidence of a diffuse cerebral vasculitis

From Smith CH, et al. Acute posterior multifocal placoid pigment epitheliopathy and cerebral vasculitis. Arch Neurol. 1983;40:50.

One of these disorders, **acute multifocal placuoid pigment epithelitis** (APMPPE; Table 3–19), is often part of a more widespread inflammatory process including (1) changes in the cerebrospinal fluid, lymphocytic pleocytosis and an increase in cerebrospinal fluid pressure with or without cerebral vasculitis; (2) abnormal urinary sediment; and (3) associated ocular changes—papillitis, serous retinal detachment, episcleritis, and corneal thinning.

A similar disorder, clearly vascular in etiology, consists of a microangiopathy affecting the retinal arterioles, a subacute encephalopathy, and associated sensoral neural hearing loss. The changes appear to be confined to the eye, ear, and central nervous system. No systemic vasculitis has been detected. It appears to affect young women exclusively and is an occlusive vasculopathy rather than a vasculitis.

Birdshot chorioretinopathy shows diffuse changes in the outer retinal layers, retinal pigment epithelium, and possibly choroid. It is associated with a specific HLA antigen (HLA-A_{20}) present in 90% of the affected population as opposed to 8% of the normal population.

Recently, a multifocal chorioretinitis and retinal epithelial disturbance characterized by a punctate, outer retinitis has been attributed to the *Epstein-Barr virus* (even in patients with no history of mononucleosis). There frequently are cells in the vitreous.

TABLE 3–20. CHOROIDAL DYSTROPHIES

Area Affected	Macular Changes	Other Retinal Change	Symptoms	Onset/Course	ERG	EOG	Heredity	Other
Segmental								
Central areolar atrophy	Atrophic macular lesion	—	Decreased VA	20–50 years	Normal	Normal		Central scotoma, normal peripheral visual field, possible association with glaucoma
Peripapillary atrophy	—	—	VA Normal	Adult onset	Normal	Normal		
Malignant myopia	Fuch's spot	Diffuse thinning	VA normal to severely decreased	Adult onset	Decreased (Rarely)	Decreased (Rarely)		
Diffuse								
Choroideremia	Minimal	Progressive RPE Atrophy; choroid present in submacular area only	VA normal until about 20 years old	Childhood/ progressive	Decreased	Decreased	XLR	Males only; female carrier—night blindness in first decade
Gyrate atrophy	Late	Equatorial choroidal atrophy expands Circumscribed atrophic areas Attenuated vessels	VA normal until late	20–50 y/o	Decreased	Decreased	AR	Myopia, dark adaptation decreased, night blindness, ring scotoma
Aicardi syndrome	Congenital	Disc coloboma Lacunes	?	Congenital	?	?	Not familial	Infantile spasms, agenesis corpus callosum, female only

AR, autosomal recessive; EOG, electro-oculogram; ERG, electroretinogram; NLP, no light perception; RPE, retinal pigment epithelium; VA, visual acuity, XLR, X-linked recessive.

Vogt-Koyanagi-Harada syndrome (VKH) is a uveomeningeal syndrome of uveitis, poliosis, vitiligo, deafness, meningeal signs, and pleocytosis. The uveitis is predominantly posterior, and as it resolves, leads to episodes of choroiditis and exudation, profound pigmentation, and pigmentary disturbance. Fluorescein angiography usually reveals a striking staining and leakage of retinal vessels. Treatment is by corticosteroids.

It appears that other diseases, in addition to syphilis, are vying to acquire reputations as great mimics. This includes another disease caused by a spirochete, *Lyme disease*, manifestations of the human immunodeficiency viruses (HIV) including the AIDS virus, and disorders attributed to Epstein-Barr virus. The latter causes a multifocal chorioretinal punctate outer retinitis, a picture similar to AMPPE, and a chorioretinopathy with sword-like lesions.

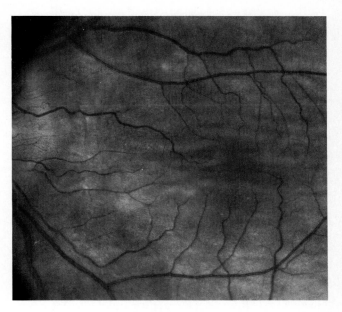

Figure 3–24. Choroidal folds.

CHOROIDAL DISORDERS

Many disorders that affect the choroid have already been mentioned, including vascular diseases that affect both the retinal and choroidal vasculature (eg, systemic hypertension and toxemia cause choroidal vascular occlusion, Elschnig's spots, and Siegrist's streaks); and pigmented lesions—choroidal nevi, malignant melanoma, retinal pigment epithelial hypertrophy, and melanocytoma. Many choroidal disorders may be masked by simultaneous retinal pathology; sometimes fluorescein angiography will reveal the alterations, especially acute perfusion and other vascular deficits.

Choroidal dystrophies are listed in Table 3–20.

Choroidal folds are mentioned in Chapter 18, but are also associated with other entities (Table 3–21), and in many cases no etiology is found. They appear as alternating lines of increased and decreased color in the posterior pole (Fig. 3–24). At times, they are visible only on fluorescein angiography, where they appear early and become less obvious in the later stages of the study.

The choroid may also be involved by the phakomatoses—for example, with a hemangioma in Sturge-Weber's disease.

BIBLIOGRAPHY

AIDS

Pomerantz RJ et al. Infection of the retina by human immunodeficiency virus type I. *N Engl J Med.* 1987;317:1643–1647.

Arterial Occlusion

Brown GC, et al. Retinal arterial obstruction in children and young adults. *Ophthalmology.* 1981;88:18–25.

Duker J, Brown GC. Iris neovascularization with obstruction of the central retinal artery. *Ophthalmology.* 1988;95:1244–1250.

Kleiner RC, et al. Vaso-occlusive retinopathy associated with antiphospholipid antibody (lupus anticoagulant retinopathy). *Ophthalmology.* 1989;96:896–904.

McLeod D, et al. The role of axoplasmic transport in the pathogenesis of cotton-wool spots, *Br J Ophthalmology.* 1977;61:177–191.

Monteiro MLR, et al. A microangiopathic syndrome of encephalopathy, hearing loss and retinal arteriolar occlusions. *Neurology.* 1985;35:1113–1121.

Newman NM, DiLoreto DA, Ho JT, et al. Bilateral optic

TABLE 3–21. ETIOLOGIES OF CHOROIDAL FOLDS

Associated with retinal detachment
Hypermetropia
Hypotony
Macular degeneration
Ocular inflammation (scleritis, uveitis, choroiditis)
Ocular tumor
Orbital tumors
Papillitis
Sinusitis
Thyroid disease
Trauma
Unknown
Uveal effusion
Venous occlusion

neuropathy and osteolytic sinusitis. Complications of cocaine abuse. *JAMA.* 1988;259:72–74.

Scott JA, et al. Treatment of dural sinus thrombosis with local urokinase infusion. *J Neurosurg.* 1988;68:284–287.

Vine AK, et al. Recombinant tissue plasminogen activator to lyse experimentally induced retinal arterial thrombi. *Am J Ophthalmol.* 1988;103:266–270.

Emboli

Arruga J, Sanders MD. Ophthalmic findings in 70 patients with evidence of retinal embolism. *Ophthalmology.* 1982;89:1336–1347.

Frosted Branch Angiitis

Watanabe Y, Takeda N, Adachi-Usami E. A case of frosted branch angiitis. *Br J Ophthalmol.* 1987;71:553–558.

Systemic Disease

Aaberg TM, O'Brien WJ. Expanding ophthalmologic recognition of Epstein-Barr virus infections. *Am J Ophthalmol.* 1987;104:420–423.

Dimmitt SB, et al. Usefulness of ophthalmoscopy in mild to moderate hypertension. *Lancet.* 1989;1:1103–1105.

Gass JDM, Pautler SE. Toxemia of pregnancy pigment epitheliopathy masquerading as a heredomacular dystrophy. *Tr Am Ophthalmol Soc.* 1985;83:114–130.

Mullaney J, Collum LMT. Ocular vasculitis in Behcet's disease: A pathologic and immunohistochemical study. *Int Ophthalmol.* 1985;7:183–191.

Traboulsi EI, et al. Prevalence and importance of pigmented ocular fundus lesions in Gardner's syndrome. *N Engl J Med.* 1987;316:661–667.

Macula

Kivlin JD, Sanborn GE, Myers GG. The cherry red spot in Tay Sachs and other storage diseases. *Ann Neurol.* 1985; 17:356–360.

Retinal Degeneration

Foxman SG, et al. Classification of congenital and early onset retinitis pigmentosa. *Arch Ophthalmol.* 1988;103: 1502–1506.

Heckenlively JC, Martin DA, Rosales TD: Telangiectasia and optic atrophy in cone-rod degenerations. *Arch Ophthalmol.* 1981;99:1983–1991.

Vasculitis

Andrews BS, et al. Circulating immune complexes in retinal vasculitis. *Clin Exp Immunol.* 1977;29:23–29.

Fitzsimons RB, Gurwin EB, Bird AC. Retinal vascular abnormalities in fascioscapulohumeral muscular dystrophy. *Brain.* 1987;110:631–648.

AMMPE

Wilson CA, et al. Acute posterior multifocal placoid pigment epitheliopathy and cerebral vasculitis. *Arch Ophthalmol.* 1988;106:796–800.

Retinal Nerve Fiber Layer

Newman NM, Stevens RA, Heckenlively JR. Nerve fiber layer loss in diseases of the outer retinal layer. *Br J Ophthalmol.* 1987;71:21–26.

Retinal Toxicity

Brown RD, Gratton CEH. Visual toxicity of synthetic retinoids. *Br J Ophthalmol.* 1989;73:286–288.

Retinal Inflammation

Kimmel AS, et al. The multiple evanescent white dot syndrome with acute blind spot enlargement. *Am J Ophthalmol.* 1989;107:425–426.

CHAPTER 4

DISORDERS OF THE OPTIC DISC

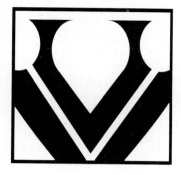

VARIANTS OF THE NORMAL OPTIC DISC

Variants of the disc can be divided into two general categories: remnants of embryologic development (which normally disappear by the time of birth) and anomalous development (anomalies of the optic nerve head as it inserts into the globe, anomalies of the scleral canal, and congenital anomalies of ocular tissues). The majority of these variants is clinically innocuous, and all but the most extreme have no functional significance for the patient. However, because they may be associated with visual field defects, they must be distinguished from pathologic optic discs, particularly neurogenic disc swelling and glaucomatous cupping. The patterns of the field defects associated with disc anomalies are variable; however, the visual field defects themselves should **not** change (the disc appearance should also be stable). If the field defect is noted to progress or if the disc appearance changes, it should **not** be attributed to a mere structural variant.

Remnants of Bergmeister's papilla and the hyaloid system. These remnants of the embryonic primary vitreous normally atrophy prior to birth. Yet residua of these tissues are present in nearly 30% of autopsy eyes in two forms, glial and vascular. Glial remnants—somewhat bright, fibrotic membranes—occur on the disc surface or more peripherally in the retina, although they usually appear in the posterior pole, frequently along blood vessels. Vascular remnants arise along the path of the fetal primary hyaloid vessels—for example, attached to the back of the lens (Mittendorf's dot); less frequently they occur in midvitreous or at the disc as an empty or filled blood vessel or twisted loop. In rare cases, the midvitreous alterations cast shadows on the retina, as floaters do; otherwise they are asymptomatic. Even more rarely, the preretinal loops bleed.

In **persistent primary hyperplastic vitreous** (PHPV) there is more extensive persistence of the primary vitreous forming retrolental or prepapillary masses that occasionally proliferate. In PHPV visual loss usually is significant and the leukocoria must be differentiated from retinoblastoma (Table 4–1).

Congenital falciform folds and **retinopathy of prematurity** (ROP, retrolental fibroplasia) accompany various degrees of fibrous proliferation at the disc. The fibrovascular bands may produce traction that "drags" the disc and macula temporally. ROP is a pathologic reaction of immature retina to high oxygen tension.

Abnormalities of insertion of the optic nerve into the globe. Commonly seen in myopic eyes, these changes range from the very common myopic crescent to more extensive abnormalities of the retina or other ocular layers. Their ophthalmoscopic appearance depends on termination of retinal tissues relative to the scleral opening at the optic disc. If the tissues all terminate at the same place, the disc has a normal appearance. If the tissues of the retina do not extend as close to the disc as the retinal pigment epithelium, a darkly pigmented crescent results (Fig. 4–1). When all tissues including the retinal pigment epithelium fall short of the disc margin, a white scleral crescent results (Fig. 4–2). These appearances also vary according to the position of the embryonic fold and variations in pigmentation.

Tilted and dysverted discs result from more extreme alterations. These variations occur most frequently in the inferonasal portion of the globe (Fig. 4–3) and are considered defects in the closing of the fetal fissure. In contrast, the myopic crescents discussed above are usually located temporally. In addition to recognizing these variants, be aware of their association with pseudo-bitemporal hemianopic field defects, which differ from true bitemporal

TABLE 4–1. PSEUDORETINOBLASTOMAS

Hereditary Conditions	Norrie's disease
	Congenital retinoschisis
	Incontinentia pigmenti
	Familial exudative vitreoretin-
	opathy
	Retinal folds in trisomy 13
Developmental Anomalies	Persistent hyperplastic primary
	vitreous
	Cataract
	Coloboma
	High myopia
	Retinal dysplasia
	Congenital retinal fold(s)
	Myelinated nerve fibers
	Morning glory syndrome
	Congenital corneal opacities
Inflammatory Conditions	Uveitis
	Nematode endophthalmitis
	(toxocara)
	Congenital toxoplasmosis
	Congenital cytomegalovirus
	retinitis
	Herpes simplex retinitis
	Peripheral uveoretinitis
	Metastatic endophthalmitis
	Orbital cellulitis
	Cysticercosis
	Vitreous abscess
Tumors	Retinoblastoma
	Retinal astrocytoma
	Medulloepithelioma
	Glioneuroma
	Choroidal hemangioma
	Retinal capillary hemangioma
	Combined retinal hamartoma
Miscellaneous	Retinal telangiectasia with
	exudation (Leber's or
	Coats' disease)
	Retinopathy of prematurity
	(retrolental fibroplasia)
	Retinal angioma/von Hippel–
	Lindau disease
	Rhegmatogenous retinal de-
	tachment
	Vitreous hemorrhage
	Perforating ocular injuring and
	other trauma
	Massive retinal fibrosis

Adapted from Shields JA, Augsburger JJ. Current approaches to the diagnosis and management of retinoblastoma. Surv Ophthalmol. *1981;25: 348.*

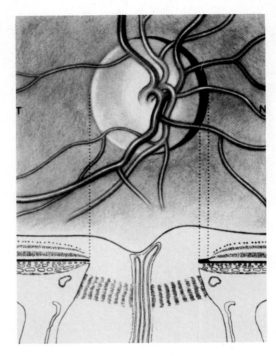

Figure 4–1. Drawing of a pigment crescent as seen ophthalmoscopically and correlated with a histologic section. (C, choroidal; N, nasal; PE, pigment epithelium; R, retina; S, sclera; T, temporal). (*From Hogan M, Alvarado G, Weddell J.* Histology of the Human Eye. An Atlas and Textbook. *Philadelphia: Saunders, 1971:530, with permission.*)

visual field defects. For small isopters, the "hemianopic" margin slants across the vertical meridian (Fig. 4–4), rather than adhering to it as does a true hemianopic defect. Part of this defect may be due to ectasia and eliminated by refraction. These discs may be associated with changes in the VEP.

More extreme abnormalities in the closing of this fissure result in a *true coloboma,* with defects in retinal and/or choroidal tissue; or a staphyloma, an inferonasal ectasia of the sclera. These more extensive defects not infrequently are associated with colobomas of the ciliary body, iris, and lens, and even defects in the cornea.

Myelinated nerve fibers occur in 1% of the population and are the one abnormality associated with prolonged growth of normal tissue elements. Myelination usually proceeds from the lateral geniculate body toward the eye and ceases in the retrolaminar optic nerve. When it progresses into the eye, the myelinated fibers appear as white patches with typical "feathered" edges, usually in proximity to the disc but also as isolated, more peripheral patches (Fig. 4–5). They may cause visual field defects when their opacity blocks the transmission of light through the retina. Occasionally, they dramatically disappear in association with optic nerve atrophy; rarely neovascularization occurs in the region of the myelinated fibers.

Other variants of the optic nerve head include **pits of the optic nerve head.** Defects within the substance of the nerve head, these may be seen any-

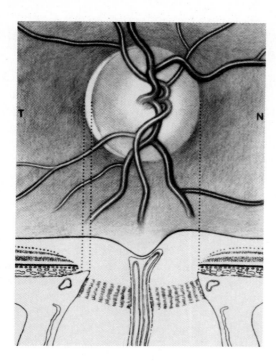

Figure 4–2. Drawing of a scleral crescent as seen ophthalmoscopically and correlated with a histologic section. (C, choroidal; N, nasal; PE, pigment epithelium; R, retina; S, sclera; T, temporal). (*From Hogan M, Alvarado G, Weddell J. Histology of the Human Eye. An Atlas and Textbook. Philadelphia: Saunders, 1971:530, with permission.*)

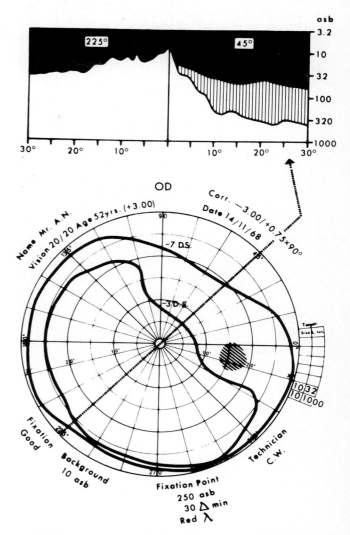

Figure 4–4. Pseudotemporal field defect in myopia. Visual field of a patient with −3D myopia. A baring of blind spot and contraction in the upper temporal quadrant is present with the patient's own correction. There is some ectasia of the sclera below the optic disc and more concave lenses are necessary to expand these isopters. Similar changes can be seen on the static profiles along the 45-degree meridian. (*From Reed H, Drance SM. The Essentials of Perimetry: Static and Kinetic. 2nd ed. London: Oxford, 1972:166, with permission.*)

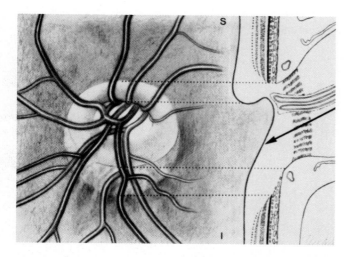

Figure 4–3. Inferior oblique nerve. Drawings showing the varying direction of the optic nerve through the canal. The arrows depict the axis of the nerve. (I, inferior; N, nasal; S, superior; T, temporal.) (*From Hogan M, Alvarado G, Weddell J. Histology of the Human Eye. An Atlas and Textbook. Philadelphia: Saunders, 1971:531, with permission.*)

where along the neuroglial rim; they may even be multiple. Central pits (about 20% of pits) must be differentiated from glaucomatous cupping. Usually pits are found in the inferotemporal quadrant, where they appear as slightly dark to grayish, oval depressions in the disc substance. This appearance is accentuated on fluorescein angiography (Fig. 4–6). Sometimes there is an associated nerve fiber defect

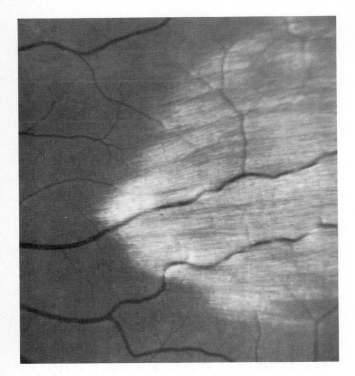

Figure 4-5. Myelinated fibers.

fanning out from the neuroglial rim in the region of the pit and a concomitant visual field defect. Optic pits may be associated with serous detachment of the macula (in 50% of cases), the most frequent cause of visual decrease in these patients.

ABNORMALITIES OF THE OPTIC NERVE HEAD ASSOCIATED WITH ALTERATIONS IN THE SIZE OF THE SCLERAL CANAL

Small scleral canals. When the scleral canal is small, the optic nerve head may range from frankly hypoplastic (usually associated with severe visual field defects and decreased visual acuity) to the common "small, full discs" with normal function. Hypoplastic discs occur with increased incidence in babies of diabetic mothers, young mothers, mothers who abuse alcohol and other drugs, and mothers who have taken quinine or anticonvulsants. Frequently, small full discs with blurred margins mistakenly are thought to be "swollen" (discussed later in the chapter). They apparently carry an increased risk for anterior ischemic optic neuropathy in later life.

The **frankly hypoplastic disc.** These discs are very small with visual acuity that ranges from normal to nil. Frequently, when actual nerve tissue is minimal, the scleral canal or the termination of the retinal structures can be seen as a grayish crescent or doughnut surrounding the nubbin of nerve tissue (Fig. 4-7).

Hypoplastic discs, especially if bilateral, are associated with a spectrum of developmental problems of the central nervous system. Their detection mandates a thorough evaluation—accurate visual acuities and visual fields, even in young children, and neuroimaging studies to rule out visual afferent pathway tumors (particularly gliomas and craniopharyn-

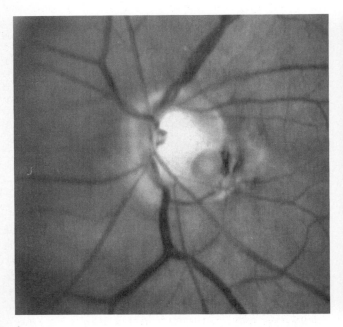

A

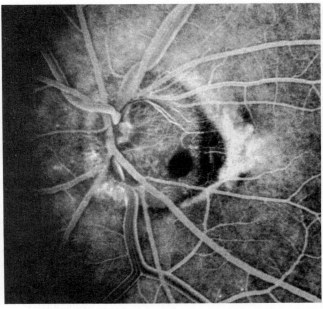

B

Figure 4-6. **A.** Pit of the optic nerve head. **B.** Fluorescein angiogram.

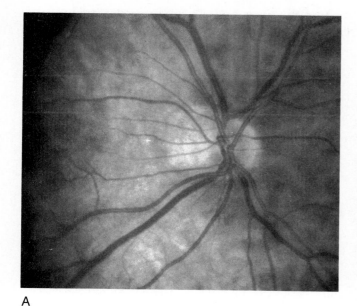

A

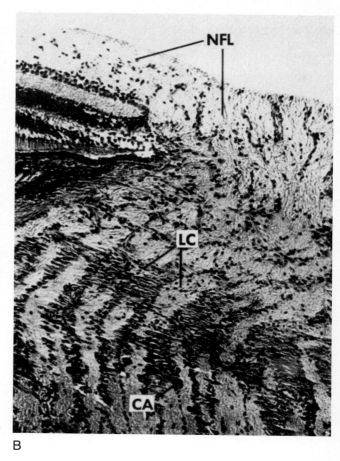

B

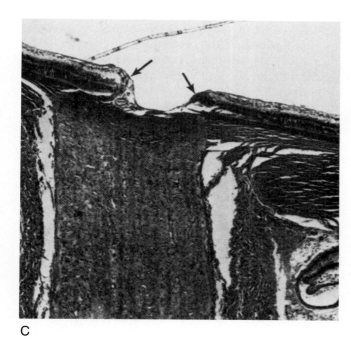

C

Figure 4–7. A. Frankly hypoplastic disc. **B.** Normal optic nerve with a relatively shallow physiologic cup (*upper right*) and slight posterior bowing of the lamina cribrosa (*LC*), which has two parts: the anterior pars choroidalis and the posterior pars scleralis (CA, corpora amylaces; NFL, nerve fiber layer.) **C.** Optic nerve hypoplasia. Retinal ganglion cells and nerve fiber layer are absent, and there is no passage of axons from the retina into the nerve (*arrows*). Compare with B. (*From Apple DJ, Rabb MF, Walsh PM. Congenital anomalies of the optic disc. Surv Ophthalmol. 1982;27:3–41, with permission.*)

giomas) and associated midline malformations (Table 4–2).

Associated CNS malformations. These include DeMorsier's syndrome: septo-optic dysplasia, hypoplastic discs, absence of the septum pellucidum, and a frequently treatable growth hormone deficiency. The treatable hormonal deficiency is the major reason to make this diagnosis, because there is not much to be done about the other problems.

Sometimes small discs are associated with basal encephaloceles that appear as orbital, frontal, nasal, or pharyngeal masses.

Disc anomalies due to a larger-than-normal scleral canal also are associated with midline malformations. Failure of closure of the fetal fissure results in colobomas that may include the optic discs; encephaloceles may be an associated anomaly. Megalopapilla and the morning glory syndrome are other disc dysplasias associated with large

TABLE 4–2. FINDINGS ASSOCIATED WITH OPTIC NERVE/DISC HYPOPLASIA

Ocular	Decreased visual acuity; severity of deficit is variable
	Nystagmus, especially if bilateral
	Albinism
	Aniridia
	Colobomas
	High myopia
Central Nervous System	Encephalocele
	Cerebral palsy
	Mental retardation
	Seizures
Systemic—Endocrine/ Hypothalamic Dysfunction	Septo-optic dysplasia and other midline anomalies, with or without treatable growth hormone deficiency
	Hypothyroidism and other hormonal deficiencies
	Sexual infantilism
	Sexual precocity
	Diabetes insipidus
	Hyperprolactinemia
	Neonatal hypoglycemia
	Hypoadrenalism
Radiologic (Usually With Bilateral Hypoplasia)	Midline anomalies—absent septum pellucidum, encephaloceles
	Central nervous system maldevelopment—anencephaly, porencephaly, etc
	Occasional CNS tumor—craniopharyngioma, childhood glioma
Syndromes	Duane's
	Median cleft face
	Klippel-Trenaunay-Weber
	Goldenhar's
	Epidermal Nevus
	Chondrodysplasia punctata
	Meckel's
	Hypertelorism
	Hemifacial atrophy
	Blepharophimosis
Toxic Causes	Maternal use of dilantin quinine, phentoin, LSD, PCP, ETOH (occurs in 48% of fetal alcohol syndrome); other maternal and possibly paternal substance abuse (?)
Maternal Associations	Diabetes mellitus
	Young mothers

From Lambert SR, et al. Optic nerve hypoplasia. Surv Ophthalmol. 1987;32: 1–9.

scleral canals. The latter contains abnormal mesodermal elements.

In all of these midline problems there may be associated treatable hormonal deficiencies. The hormonal deficits may also occur in association with the disc anomalies and without obvious other structural CNS problems. It is critical to keep in mind the treatable conditions.

Morning glory discs, enlarged, with central glial hyperplasia and vessels that exit radially, show peripapillary pigment disruption (Fig. 4–8). They may be bilateral and hereditary and are also associated with retinal detachment. When the anomaly is bilateral, visual function is only moderately disturbed. When unilateral, visual acuity is 10/200 or less with a central or centrocecal scotoma, a Marcus Gunn pupil, strabismus, or both, are always present. As in retinopathy of prematurity and PHPV, progressive alterations in the fibrovascular tissues may produce traction on the disc and macula.

Cupping of the optic disc. In general, the normal variation in disc diameters correlates with the normal variation in cup-to-disc ratio. A patient with a congenitally deep or broad cup has a minor anomaly due to overextensive resorption of Bergmeister's papilla. Other variants of the normal optic disc—such as those that occur with myopia, tilted discs, colobomas, and optic pits—also need to be differentiated from true glaucomatous cupping (Table 4–3). In most of these variants, the associated visual field defects differ from the typical Bjerrum scotomas of glaucoma and correspond to the areas of the disc that are malformed. These visual field defects do not progress.

Low-tension glaucoma is so named because characteristic glaucomatous visual field defects,

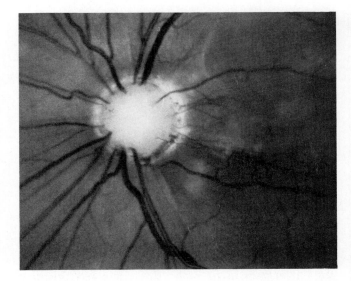

Figure 4–8. Morning glory disc. (*Courtesy of H. Shatz, M.D.*)

TABLE 4–3. CONGENITAL ANOMALIES THAT MAY MIMIC OR HIDE GLAUCOMATOUS CHANGES IN THE OPTIC DISC

1. Congenital deep cup (genetic influences)
2. Anomalous embryonic hyaloid glial-vascular remnants
   a. Congenital deep cup due to extensive resorption of Bergmeister's papilla
   b. Epipapillary membranes (remnants of Bergmeister's papilla) producing a deceptively shallow optic cup
   c. Vascular loops mimicking optociliary shunt vessels
3. Myopia, usually with conus
4. Coloboma of the optic nerve
5. Tilted disc
6. Optic pit

From Apple DJ, et al. Congenital anomalies of the optic disc. Surv Ophthalmol. 1982;27:4.

which correspond to notches in the neuroglial rim, are associated with nerve fiber layer defects in the temporal arcades despite relatively normal intraocular pressure. There is still debate as to whether or not this is a variant of chronic open-angle glaucoma. Patients with low-tension glaucoma seem to show an abnormally high incidence of vasomotor instability and migraine.

Cupping also occurs in a small percentage (approximately 6%) of patients with compressive lesions of the anterior visual pathway. Changes commonly associated with glaucomatous cupping—baring of circumlinear vessels, erosion of the temporal rim, the "overpass phenomenon," temporal unfolding, and "polar notching"—all occur in this group of patients, and suggest that these signs are indicators of acquired optic neuropathy and tissue loss within the disc substance and are not peculiar to glaucoma. Further, the nerve fiber layer defects in this group of patients **are not glaucomatous.** Frequently, nasal nerve fiber loss corresponds to bitemporal visual field defects associated with compressive chiasmal lesions. Afferent pupillary defects are present, but in these patients with compressive lesions there is not the marked asymmetry of cupping usually found when an afferent defect occurs in glaucoma.

Also, the area of pallor is consistently greater than the area cupped, while the loss of Snellen acuity is far out of proportion to the extent of the cupping; in true glaucoma, the cupping is usually extreme by the time that central vision is diminished and the pallor limited to the cupped portion of the optic disc.

Optic atrophy. Optic atrophy, a nonspecific consequence of damage to the pregeniculate visual afferent pathway, will not be covered in detail here. Specific causes of optic atrophy are covered separately.

THE SWOLLEN DISC

Discussions of optic disc swelling (Table 4–4) can be quite confusing. In the older literature, many causes of disc swelling were indiscriminately lumped together. Thus, demyelinating papillitis, ischemic optic neuropathy, and true papilledema were all described as optic neuritis, papilledema, papillitis, or any of the other terms used to describe disc elevation. Much of the confusion resulted because it was not understood how multiple etiologies of disc swelling each caused a clinically similar appearance.

Many studies explored pathophysiologic mechanisms involved in disc swelling. However, until the phenomenon of axoplasmic flow became understood, the true physiology of disc swelling remained unclear. Axoplasmic stasis at the scleral lamina cribosa is the common basis of all forms of disc "edema," regardless of etiology. Thus, in ischemic optic neuropathy, demyelinating papillitis, hypotony, or acute glaucoma, the swollen disc is the visible manifestation of axoplasmic stasis. The exact relationship of this common pathway to each individual etiology is less clear. Perhaps best understood is the effect of ischemia on axoplasmic flow (see Chapter 3).

Because optic disc swelling has many causes (Table 4–5, Fig. 4–9), each type of disc swelling deserves as precise a description as possible.

Most neuro-ophthalmologists reserve the term "papilledema" for bilateral swelling of the optic disc associated with increased intracranial pressure. All other types should be described as a swollen disc, disc edema, or disc swelling. However, be aware that many use the term "papilledema" in a less restrictive manner.

The extreme importance of finding a swollen disc lies in the frequent association of papilledema due to increased intracranial pressure with life-threatening intracranial pathology. Thus, it is critical to distinguish true papilledema from other causes of disc swelling.

This necessity for accurate differential diagnosis of the swollen disc leads to intense evaluation of these patients. Of course, the presence of disc swelling *can* signify ominous intracranial processes, but in most ophthalmic and neuro-ophthalmic practice the swollen disc is relatively benign.

The Swollen Disc Without Decreased Visual Acuity

The ophthalmoscopic differential diagnosis between papilledema and other causes of bilateral "swollen

TABLE 4–4. DIFFERENTIAL DIAGNOSIS OF DISC SWELLING

	Nearly Always Bilateral				Syphilitic Perineuritis (ONHD)	Papillitis	AION/TA	Nearly Always Unilateral			
	True PE	Chronic Atrophic PE	Acute Leber's Optic Neuropathy	Pseudo PE				Ocular Hypotony / Inflammation	CRVO, BBSS	Vasculitis	ON Tumor
SYMPTOMS											
Decreased VA	O, + obscurations	+/-	+++	+/-	+/-	Acute +++	Acute ++	With vitritis +	+/-	Rarely, with mac. changes	+
Decreased color vision	O	+/-	+++	+/-	+/-	+++	+/++	+/-	O	O	+
Visual field	Enlarged BS	Enlarged BS, NFBDs	Centrocecal scotoma	Enlarged BS, NFBDs	Enlarged BS, occas. NFBDs	Central scotoma	Alt. VFD	Can be N	Enlarged BS	Enlarged BS	NFD or contract.
Pain	HA	O/HA in PTC	O	O	O	With eye movement	Usually precedes	Photophobia	O	O	O
Onset	Insidious to abrupt	Subacute	2nd eye follows in 2–3 months	Congenital	Insidious	Acute	Acute	Often insidious on awakening	Subacute	Subacute	Insidious
Systemic symptoms/disease	HA, N, V	Occas. neurol.	Cardiac arrhythmia	RP +/-	AIDS	MS?	R/O ASHD	+/-	Increased blood pressure	Rarely arteritis	In NF
SIGNS											
APD	O	+/-	++	(rare)	O/+O	+++	+	O	O	O	+
Bilateral	++	+	++ (2nd eye later)	++	+	Rare	Rare/+++ (untreated)	Rare	O	O	Rare
Disc/vessels	Obscured at disc margins	Narrowed	Peripap. telangiectasia	Late branching	Occas. sheathing	N	Narrow	Depends on etiology	Engorged	N or engorged	Optociliary shunt (?)
Disc margins	Swollen	Shaggy	Swollen	Lumpy if drusen exposed	Low grade swelling	Swollen	Pallid swelling	Swollen	Swollen	Swollen	N or swollen
Cupping	O	O	Decreased	O	O	Small cups	+/-	+/-	+/-	+/-	+/-
NFL	Dull, loss of striation	Attrition	Opaque	Mild atrophy NFBDs, ok around disc	N early	N acutely Slit defects(?), indicate previous involvement	Slightly opaque	N	N	N	Atrophy
Hemorrhages	NFL, often WS	Rare	Rare	Occas., esp. subretinal, peripap.	Rarely	Occas. NFL	A few NFL	O	NFL, may be passive	Rare	O
Disc color	Often plethoric	Pale to N	Slightly plethoric	N/occas. pale	N	Plethoric, pale	Pale	N, less often hyperemic	Plethoric	Usually N	Pale
Fluorescein angiography	Capillary dilation	Late stain	Telang.	Autofl.	Stain	Disc leak	Disc leak	May leak	Disc leak +/- mac. edema	Disc leaks/late stain	Nonspecific

TABLE 4–4. DIFFERENTIAL DIAGNOSIS OF DISC SWELLING (*Continued*)

	Nearly Always Bilateral							Nearly Always Unilateral Ocular Hypotony			
	True PE	Chronic Atrophic PE	Acute Leber's Optic Neuropathy	Pseudo PE	Syphilitic Perineuritis (ONHD)	Papillitis	AION/TA	Inflammation	CRVO, BBSS	Vasculitis	ON Tumor
			OTHER					OTHER			
Family history	O	O	+++	++	---	O	O	O	O	O	O
Age	Any	Any	Teens	Full disc, congen. drusen appear +/–10 y	Any	Most 20–40	45–65/65–85	Any	CRVO older	10–40	Any
Treatment	Treat cause	Treat cause	None known	None needed	Penicillin & steroids	None proven	None known/ steroids	Primary disease	Steroids if mac. involved	Treat ocular systemic inflammatory disease	Rx tumor
Prognosis for VA	Good if not chronic	+/–	Poor (20/100 to 2/400)	Decreased VA rare	Very good if treated promptly	90% return to at least 20/30	2nd eye affected in 30%/in 80% without treatment	Treat primary diagnosis	CRVO: depends on extent of ischemia	excellent BBS	that of type of tumor

O, none or absent; +, sometimes present; ++, common; +++, very common; +/–, possible; –/+, less possible; N, normal; VA, visual acuity. AION/TA, anterior ischemic optic neuropathy/temporal arteritis; ASHD, arteriosclerotic heart disease; BBSS, big blind spot syndrome; BS, blind spot; CRVO, central retinal vein occlusion; HA, headache; MS, multiple sclerosis; NFBD, nerve fiber bundle defect; NFD, nerve fiber defect; NFL, nerve fiber layer; ONHD, optic nerve head drusen; ON T, optic nerve tumor; CWS, cotton wool spots; PE, papilledema; PTC, pseudotumor cerebri; RP, retinitis pigmentosa or retinal pigmentary degeneration; VA, visual acuity; VFD, visual field defect

TABLE 4–5. ETIOLOGY OF THE "SWOLLEN" DISC

Congenital	Anomalous elevation
	Drusen (hyaline bodies)
	Gliotic dysplasia
	Small, full disc
Ocular Disease	Uveitis
	Hypotony
	Vein occlusion
	Inflammation
Metabolic	Dysthyroidism
	Juvenile diabetes
	Hypoparathyroidism
	Hyperparathyroidism
Inflammatory and Infectious	Papillitis
Optic Nerve Disease	Neuroretinitis
	Papillophlebitis
	Perineuritis
Infiltrative	Lymphoma, leukemia
	Reticuloendothelial
	Metastatic
	Meningeal carcinomatosis
Systemic Disease	Anemia
	Hypoxemia
	Hypertension
	Uremia
	GI—Crohn's disease, Whipple's disease
Disc Tumors	Hamartomas
	Hemangioma
	Glioma
	Metastatic
Vascular	Ischemic neuropathy
	Arteriosclerotic
	Arteritic, cranial
	Arteritic, collagen, associated with other vaso-occlusive processes and coagulation abnormalities
	Embolic
	Hypertension
	Proliferative retinopathies
	Diabetes mellitus
	Arterial spasm (?)
	Migraine
	Hypertension
Orbital Disease	Perioptic meningioma
	Glioma
	Sheath "cysts"
	Retrobulbar masses
	Inflammatory and infectious orbital conditions, including thyroid and nonspecific orbital inflammatory disease (orbital pseudotumor)
Sinus Disease	Sinusitis
	Tumor
CNS Disease	Meningitis
	Carcinoma
Increased Intracranial Pressure	Mass lesion
	Pseudotumor cerebri
	Hypertension
Toxic	(See Table 5–6)

discs'' is a challenge; common factors outnumber distinguishing characteristics.

"Swollen Discs" That Should Not Be Confused With Papilledema. The **small full disc** can be considered a true variant of normal. It has slightly indistinct disc margins, late-branching central vessels, and no central cup. All measures of visual function are normal.

Pseudopapilledema. This term refers to small full discs with presumed buried drusen. Obvious drusen with calcification are found in approximately 4% of the adult population and are usually bilateral. Infants do not have optic nerve head drusen; the definitive abnormality is usually detected in the latter part of the first decade.

Clinically, most discs with drusen have an irregular nodular appearance (Fig. 4–10); the elevation is confined to the disc, in contrast to the extension of axoplasmic stasis to the retina in papilledema. Optic nerve head drusen arise within the confines of the small full disc. Drusen are almost never found in a disc with a large cup and are almost always associated with a late-branching pattern of the retinal vessels on the disc. Drusen frequently transilluminate; additionally, they may autofluoresce in preinjection frames on fluorescein angiography.

Some years ago, it was noted that ligation of the optic nerve of rabbits to simulate a small scleral canal caused formation of globules of axoplasm within the optic nerve head. It was postulated that over years in the congenitally small, full disc, chronic obstruction of axoplasmic flow leads to degeneration and death of ganglion cell axons. These degenerated axons calcify, producing optic nerve head drusen. This hypothesis also is compatible with other changes frequently associated with optic nerve head drusen: loss of the nerve fiber layer, visual evoked potential changes, and visual field defects. Luckily, these dysfunctions usually are minor and rarely are symptomatic.

Hoover's recent study of children with optic nerve head drusen revealed that, on average, the children were first examined at 10 years of age and discrete hyaline bodies noted at 12 years. In 25% of children, visual fields were abnormal (enlarged blind spots and inferior altitudinal nerve fiber defects each accounted for 50% of the visual field defects). Eighty percent of adults with optic nerve head drusen has field defects; the lower incidence in children supports the hypothesis that the optic neuropathy of optic nerve head drusen is progressive.

As with other chronic crowded or swollen discs, optic nerve head drusen may be associated with subretinal neovacular membranes and peripapillary hemorrhage. Usually these hemorrhages are asymp-

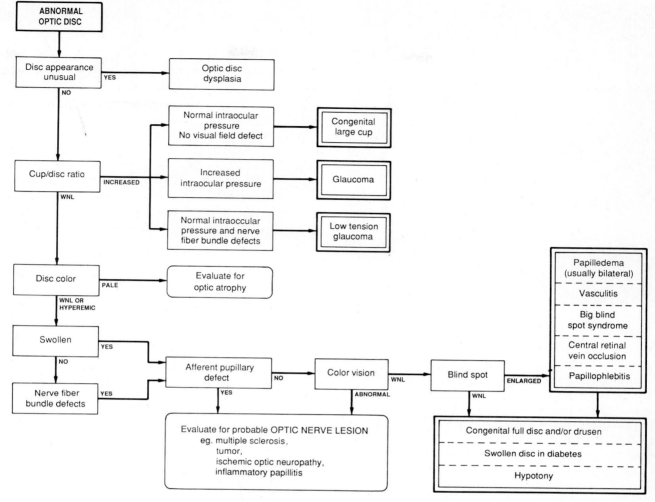

Figure 4—9. Differential diagnosis of the abnormal disc.

As with other chronic crowded or swollen discs, optic nerve head drusen may be associated with subretinal neovacular membranes and peripapillary hemorrhage. Usually these hemorrhages are asymptomatic and discovered incidentally, but if they involve the macula or break into the vitreous, visual acuity is affected. More often they lead to pigment disruption in the peripapillary area that is detected on ophthalmoscopic examination.

Slow progression of visual field defects (often nasal, usually an increased blind spot, and occasionally an arcuate or other nerve fiber bundle defect); changes in visual evoked potentials; and nerve fiber layer dropout are frequent; but loss of central visual acuity is rare.

When a patient presents with "swollen discs," headache, or visual field defects, making a definitive diagnosis of optic nerve head drusen may save a great deal of time, money, and anxiety and obviate the search for a brain tumor. Calcified drusen are easily detected by both ultrasonography and CT scanning. Whether "buried drusen" can be detected reliably by either of these methods while still hidden from ophthalmoscopic view, and possibly uncalcified, remains in doubt.

Certainly whenever other symptoms suggest that optic nerve head drusen alone may not explain the clinical picture, a complete neuro-ophthalmic and neuro-imaging workup is indicated. Because optic nerve head drusen are common, they will occur in association with unrelated central nervous system pathology. In addition, changes resembling drusen may occur in patients with chronic papilledema. These bright masses are superficial and generally smaller in size than optic nerve head drusen; they appear in discs with chronic papilledema (Fig. 4–11).

Because optic nerve head drusen are familial,

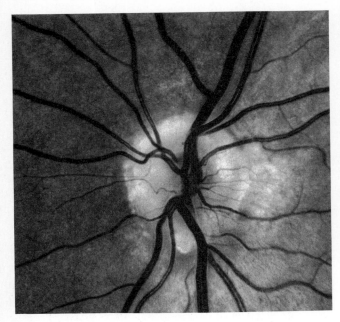

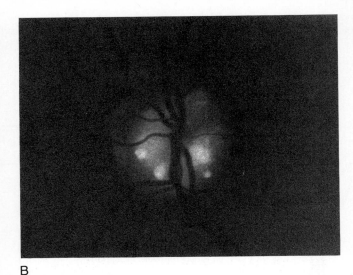

A   **Figure 4–10. A.** Optic nerve head drusen (red free photo). **B.** Autofluorescence of drusen (fluorescein angiogram).

plasmic stasis, which occurs as increased intracranial pressure is transmitted along the optic nerve sheaths to the retrobulbar nerve and lamina. Axonal flow decreases and intracellular debris and cytoplasmic organelles accumulate and cause swelling. Once the axonal distention has occurred, varying degrees of venous stasis and other vascular obstructive pro-

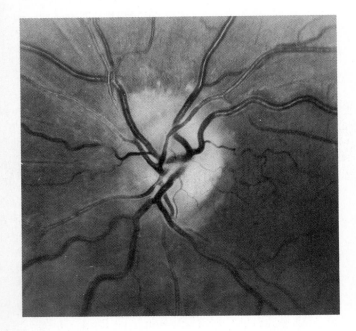

Figure 4–11. Drusenoid changes in chronic papilledema.

cesses produce interstitial edema, microinfarcts, and hemorrhages. True papilledema usually is bilateral and symmetric unless some anomaly of the optic nerve sheath prevents the transmission of pressure or if there is a lack of axoplasm to swell, as in preexisting unilateral optic atrophy. Distension of the optic nerve sheaths on ultrasound, computed tomography, or magnetic resonance imaging investigation can be an important concomitant finding; bilateral sheath distention is essentially pathognomonic of increased intracranial pressure.

Usually, the disc swelling of true papilledema is considerable and the disc is plethoric with venous distension and dilation of the capillaries on the optic nerve head. Depending on the degree of associated ischemia there may be areas of pallid swelling; nerve fiber layer and blot hemorrhages occur on the disc and in the peripapillary area. The nerve fiber layer itself is dusky and its details are lost in the immediate peripapillary area. The axonal swelling also obscures vessels as they cross the disc margin (Fig. 4–12). These are the best early signs of papilledema. Heightened internal limiting membrane (ILM) reflexes occur more peripherally. The optic cup (if there is one) will *not* disappear in *early* papilledema. Also, in early papilledema, the superior and inferior poles of the disc are the first areas to swell, followed by the nasal and then the temporal rims. The absence of spontaneous venous pulsations helps establish the diagnosis only if they were known to be present previously (approxi-

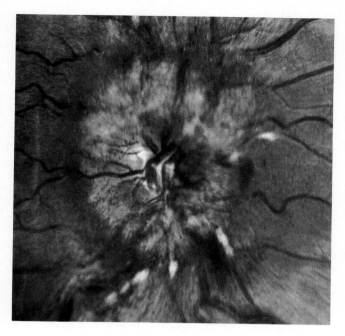

Figure 4–12. True papilledema.

mately 20% of normals have no spontaneous venous pulses).

True papilledema with increased intracranial pressure is *not associated with visual loss* until the disc swelling has become chronic and atrophy begins. The ophthalmoscopic signs are much more dramatic than the visual symptoms; there can be mammoth swelling and no visual symptoms whatsoever—the only sign may be an increased blind spot on visual field testing. The only symptom may be obscurations or momentary episodes of visual blur (see Chapter 8). The pupil is always normal in early papilledema. Thus, if a patient has definite visual loss and equivocal disc swelling, the diagnosis is *not* papilledema. Obviously, visual loss *can* occur in association with papilledema (as in craniopharyngiomas or optic nerve compression by intracranial tumors) or when papilledema coexists with macular edema or exudation.

As papilledema becomes chronic, some of the distended axons atrophy and gliosis occurs, which leads to increasing disc pallor and shaggy disc margins. The disc vessels may become sheathed.

Nerve fiber layer hemorrhages and retinal exudates arise both in papilledema and papillitis. Venous stasis, hyperemia, and late-stage fluorescein staining may be present in early central retinal vein occlusion and papillitis. However, true papilledema is almost always bilateral, whereas the majority of disc swellings are unilateral. Thus, it becomes ever more critical to distinguish pseudopapilledema. Disc anomalies are often bilateral, whereas pathologic cases of disc swelling other than papilledema are generally unilateral.

Some ophthalmoscopic findings frequently emphasized as significant in the differential diagnosis of papilledema really are not useful. An enlarged blind spot may be present with any disc swelling regardless of etiology. Absence of physiologic cup is much more typical of pseudopapilledema. Venous tortuosity may be a normal variant; late-branching vascular patterns and tortuosity are characteristic of pseudopapilledema. In addition, papilledema is associated with normal visual acuity, normal color vision, and normal pupillary reactions, and has as its only field defect an enlarged blind spot until atrophy develops. Most of the pathological entities with which it may be confused are associated with other visual field defects.

Aside from implying a mass lesion, brain swelling, or both, papilledema is an important sign of pseudotumor cerebri, either idiopathic or associated with venous sinus thrombosis. The swollen discs in pseudotumor cerebri are the only significant risk factors for disability and need to be carefully followed (see Chapter 19). Other causes of increased intracranial pressure are also associated with papilledema (Table 4–6).

Differential Diagnosis of Papilledema. Syphilitic perineuritis also produces bilateral disc swelling without decreased visual acuity and must be differentiated (positive fluorescent treponcemal antibody-absorption test or HATTS). It is thought to represent inflammation of the perineural meningeal sheaths that spares the nerve itself (a true neuritis is more common, however). Even rarer causes of bilateral optic disc swelling with normal visual acuity are sarcoid, viral meningoencephalitis, and Lyme disease, which may cause a similar perineuritis, a neuritis, a neuroretinitis, or pseudotumor cerebri.

Unilateral Disc Swelling. The big blind spot syndrome. Nearly always unilateral, the swollen disc is seen most frequently in teenagers and young adults, often following a viral syndrome (could it be a viral optic meningitis?). Visual function is normal unless the macula is involved. The swollen disc is usually surrounded by very prominent retinal light reflexes and the retina may show evanescent small white dots. BBSS is thought to be of inflammatory origin, although there may be a vascular component; occasionally arteritides are associated with this type of disc swelling. When not associated with a generalized disease process, BBSS is benign and needs no

TABLE 4–6. KNOWN CAUSES OF PAPILLEDEMA AND INCREASED INTRACRANIAL PRESSURE (EXCLUDING SPACE-OCCUPYING LESIONS)

Renal Disease	Chronic uremia
Developmental Diseases	Syringomyelia, craniostenosis, aqueductal stenosis (adult type)
Toxic Conditions	Heavy-metal poisoning: lead, arsenic; hypervitaminosis A; tetracycline therapy; nalidixic acid therapy; prolonged steroid therapy; steroid withdrawal
Allergic Diseases	Serum sickness, allergies
Infectious Diseases	Bacterial: subacute bacterial endocarditis, meningitis, chronic mastoiditis (lateral-sinus thrombosis)
Radical Neck Surgery	
Viral Diseases	Poliomyelitis, acute lymphocyte meningitis, coxsackie B virus encephalitis, inclusion-body encephalitis, recurrent polyneuritis, Guillain-Barré syndrome
Parasitic Diseases	Sandfly fever, trypanosomiasis, torulosis
Metabolic Endocrine Conditions	Eclampsia, hypoparathyroidism, Addison's disease, scurvy, oral progestational agents, diabetic ketoacidosis, menarche, obesity, menstrual abnormalities, pregnancy
Degenerative Diseases	Schilder's disease, muscular dystrophy
Head Trauma	
Miscellaneous Causes	Gastrointestinal hemorrhage, lupus erythematosus, sarcoidosis, syphilis, subarachnoid hemorrhage, status epilepticus, Paget's disease, optic-ochiasmatic arachnoiditis
Neoplastic Conditions	Carcinomatous "meningitis", leukemia, spinal-cord tumors
Hematologic Diseases	Infectious mononucleosis, idiopathic thrombocytopenic purpura, pernicious anemia, polycythemia, iron-deficiency anemia, hemophilia
Circulatory Causes	Congestive heart failure, mediastinal neoplasm, congenital cardiac lesion, hypertensive encephalopathy, pulmonary emphysema, dural-sinus thrombosis, chronic pulmonary hypoventilation

Modified from Buchheit WA, Burton C, Haag B, et al. Papilledema and idiopathic intracranial hypertension: Report of a familial occurrence. N Engl J Med. 1969;280:938.

treatment. If the swelling extends into the macula, the process often responds promptly to oral prednisone, 60 mg qAM.

BBSS serves to remind us how little we really know of the causative factors in disc swelling. Although the typical syndrome in young adults is moderately well defined, it overlaps significantly with a host of other disc swellings that are better understood, or at least better recognized, syndromes. To confuse things further, BBSS may exist without disc swelling. **Diabetes,** especially in juvenile diabetics, is known to be associated with disc swelling without visual loss, as well as a presumed anterior ischemic optic neuropathy with decreased vision. One patient presented with disc swelling of essentially identical appearance in his two eyes. One eye showed no visual loss whatsoever and the other a central scotoma, afferent pupillary defect, and moderate loss of color vision! It is now recognized that there is an anterior "pre"-ischemic optic neuropathy, an asymptomatic swollen disc. Over a period of a few months, this may evolve into the classic picture of anterior ischemic optic neuropathy. *Hypertension,* especially in younger patients, also may be associated with asymptomatic disc swelling. *Syphilitic perineuritis,* which classically is bilateral, has now been described as a unilateral condition in a BBSS-like syndrome.

Most of these entities are associated with alterations in the disc arterioles; other swollen discs merge imperceptibly into syndromes associated with obstruction of venous outflow. The BBSS, if a component of venous stasis is added, would then appear as *papillophlebitis* in which the disc swelling is associated with venous engorgement and asymptomatic small hemorrhages. If the macula is involved, vision is decreased; photopsias often are reported. Papillophlebitis usually resolves over months and has a good prognosis unless it progresses to a frank central retinal vein occlusion. Fluorescein angiography shows a prolongation of venous transit. Most observers consider papillophlebitis a forme fruste of central retinal vein occlusion occurring in younger individuals who are able to cope with and eventually overcome the venous obstruction.

Other swollen discs unassociated with visual loss include a host of disc swellings with poorly understood mechanisms. A swollen disc may be associated with ocular hypotony or uveitis without hypotony. In these cases, the swelling may be related to the imbalance of pressures at the nerve head or inflammation.

Systemic maladies including pulmonary insufficiency (chronic obstructive pulmonary disease, Pickwickian syndrome, sleep apnea) and cyanotic heart disease produce swollen discs without decreased visual acuity. In these cases, hypoxemia, hypercarbia, hypercapnia, increased venous pressure, secondary polycythemia, and acidosis are blamed. Pseudotumor cerebri may or may not occur. *Metabolic imbalances* (thyroid, parathyroid, and diabetes) may also be associated with disc swelling without loss of vision, as may *anemias* and *infectious diseases*. Rocky Mountain spotted fever and diabetes may also be associated with true ischemic swollen discs and visual loss.

Disc Swelling Associated With Decreased Visual Acuity (Usually Unilateral)

Papillitis. Swelling of the disc associated with loss of central vision (usually a central scotoma), relatively profound decrease in color vision, afferent pupillary defect, and pain on movement, are manifestations of papillitis. Further fundus findings may include a few cells in the vitreous overlying the optic disc and peripheral sheathing of retinal venules.

The visual loss usually develops suddenly over hours to days and recovers within 3 to 6 weeks. It is thought to be the anterior variant of retrobulbar optic neuritis that, by virtue of presentation at the disc, causes swelling. On magnetic resonance imaging, short-time inversion recovery (STIR) sequencing shows bright plaques in 84% of optic neuritis patients. The lesions associated with papillitis are either retrobulbar or within the optic canal.

Although papillitis usually is a disease of young patients (the diagnosis should be made with caution in those over 45 years), in children it has a slightly different presentation: It is more often bilateral, more frequently preceded by an obvious viral illness or vaccination, and frequently associated with neuroretinitis or the peripapillary retina and macula. The exudates can form a star figure. This disorder generally is benign; almost all patients with neuroretinitis *and* papillitis, regardless of age, recover good visual acuity. The incidence of multiple sclerosis or other demyelinating or central nervous system disease is low. Thus, papillitis associated with neuroretinitis or a macular star figure represents an entity separate from optic neuritis related to multiple sclerosis.

In addition, papillitis occurs in isolation, analogous to "isolated optic neuritis"; and as one of multiple neurologic symptoms displaced in time and space—multiple sclerosis. Thus, the patient with papillitis always needs close examination of the nerve fiber layer of the other eye for nerve fiber bundle defects that document a second lesion. Visual evoked potentials are advised. If the other eye is clinically involved but shows minimal optic atrophy or nerve fiber layer defects, or if there are bilateral changes in the visual evoked potentials, lesions disseminated in time and space have been documented, and it may be presumed that the patient has multiple sclerosis rather than an isolated optic neuritis or papillitis.

The validity of the latter diagnosis has been called into question with the advent of magnetic resonance imaging (MRI). Even without STIR sequence imaging, as many as 75% of cases with "isolated optic neuritis" (eg, without other neurologic symptoms or previous episodes suggesting demyelination) have been found to have bright spots on MRI that are presumed to be other areas of demyelination. Unfortunately, although some intriguing recent studies suggest there may soon be effective treatments for multiple sclerosis (interferon, plasmapheresis, antimetabolites), the risk–benefit ratio for these modalities is high; probably too high to advocate their use for optic neuritis alone (see Chapter 5 for a discussion of treatment and what to tell the patient).

A recent study by Rizzo and Lessel with prolonged follow-up of patients with a true "isolated" optic neuritis shows an increasing number (74% of women and 34% of men) develops other neurologic symptoms. However, no study has yet looked closely at the degree of disability suffered by these patients. It may be that as our diagnostic technology becomes increasingly sophisticated, asymptomatic demyelination will be found to be common and debilitating disease uncommon. The impression given is that in those patients with a truly isolated optic neuritis who present to a neuro-ophthalmologist, the incidence of disabling disease is low. In the study mentioned, only 17% of their patients became moderately or severely disabled.

Anterior ischemic optic neuropathy (AION; Table 4–7) presents with sudden unilateral decrease in visual acuity frequently noted on awakening. There is usually pallid, sometimes sectoral, swelling of the optic nerve head, and often a variable number of nerve fiber layer hemorrhages at the edge of the disc or in the immediate peripapillary area. Examination shows an afferent pupillary defect, decrease in color vision, and nerve fiber bundle type visual field defects, very often altitudinal. This clinical syndrome is usually divided into two categories: nonarteritic and arteritic. Because there are many syndromes that produce a similar but not always identical clinical picture, it is useful to divide the anterior ischemic optic neuropathies into a classic anterior ischemic optic neuropathy, arteritic ischemic optic neuropathy, and other ischemic optic neuropathies.

The **classic, nonarteritic anterior ischemic optic neuropathy** is a disease of middle-aged individuals, the 45- to 65-year age group; it affects men more frequently than women.

Although the onset is usually sudden and the

TABLE 4–7. CAUSES OF ANTERIOR ISCHEMIC OPTIC NEUROPATHY

Vasculitides	Temporal arteritis
	Polyarteritis nodosa
	Systemic lupus erythematosus
	Berger's disease
	Allergic vasculitis
	Postviral vasculitis
	Postimmunization
	Syphilis
	Radiation necrosis
	Herpes zoster
	Rheumatoid arthritis
Systemic	Hypertension
	Hypotension, hypoxia, shock
	Atherosclerosis
	Diabetes mellitus
	Migraine
	Takayasu's disease
	Carotid occlusive disease
	Behcet's disease
	Hypertension
	Emboli
	Relapsing polychondritis
Hematologic	Anemia
	Polycythemia vera
	Sickle cell disease (trait)
	G6PD deficiency
	Hyperviscosity
	Protein C deficiency (?)
	Antithrombin III deficiency (?)
	Increased antiphospholipid antibodies ?
Ocular	Postcataract
	Low-tension glaucoma (?)

From Causes of anterior ischemic optic neuropathy. In: Miller N, ed. Walsh and Hoyt's Clinical Neuro-ophthalmology. 4th ed. Baltimore: Williams & Wilkins, 1982;1:212.

visual loss is frequently present on awakening (related to nocturnal hypotension?), there may be prodromal headache or orbital ache. Occasionally there are visual symptoms prior to the ictal event, a sensation of a veil, a shadow, or an episode similar to a transient ischemic attack. Usually the visual loss is complete by the time the patient reaches you, but occasionally it may progress over several days.

Generally, the disc swelling is pallid and frequently sectoral, with the fine nerve fiber layer hemorrhages mentioned above (Fig. 4–13). In contradistinction to papillitis, a macular star or other hard exudates are rare and seen most frequently in young people who have an associated systemic vascular disease such as systemic lupus erythematosus. Orbital pain often precedes the visual loss and, unlike the pain associated with optic neuritis, is not associated with eye movement. The visual field defects are altitudinal in the large majority of cases.

Once stable, recurrence in the same eye is very uncommon; however, the chance of the other eye

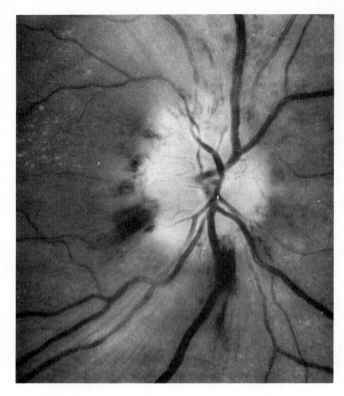

Figure 4–13. Anterior ischemic optic neuropathy.

becoming involved within months to years approximates 35%.

The risk for involvement of the second eye is greater in younger individuals and in diabetics. Rarely is the second eye involved at the same time as the first. However, cases have been noted in which an asymptomatic second eye had a swollen disc. Within a few weeks, that eye developed classic AION. What variations in pathyphysiology allow the second eye to show axoplasmic stasis, but no conduction defect, are not understood. As mentioned earlier, the asymptomatic disc swellings merge into the big blind spot syndrome and diabetic disc swelling.

Following cataract extraction, AION—thought to be caused by increased intraocular pressure—occurs in the immediate postoperative period (within hours to days of the procedure). The patient never develops normal visual acuity. These patients have a high risk of similar visual loss in the second eye if cataract extraction is undertaken. For surgery on the second eye, pretreatment with acetazolamide and timolol is suggested. The treatment should be continued for 1 week following surgery in an attempt to avoid increased intraocular pressure and AION. Of course, it is not surprising that AION develops in patients who have had cataract extraction, many of whom fall into the susceptible age group. If the visual loss occurs more than 2 months following the ocular procedure, it may be a coincidence.

The etiology of the classic anterior ischemic optic neuropathy is thought to be arteriosclerotic occlusion of the ciliary circulation. The prognosis for significant recovery of vision is poor; there is no known effective treatment, although a recent report suggests that optic nerve decompression may improve vision in the subset of AION patients whose visual loss deteriorates progressively over 1 to 4 weeks after the onset of symptoms. Surgery was performed between 4 and 30 days after the onset of symptoms. The timing of the surgery and the visual outcome were not related.

AION occurs with increased incidence in subjects with small, full discs. Diabetes, increased blood pressure, and perhaps increased intraocular pressure also are thought to be risk factors. An immediate erythrocyte sedimentation rate (ESR) test should always be done on these patients to rule out the possibility of arteritic ischemic optic neuropathy.

The **Foster-Kennedy syndrome** connotes optic atrophy in one eye and a swollen disc in the other, originally described with subfrontal tumors and usually associated with anosmia. The **pseudo-Foster-Kennedy syndrome,** which is much more common, refers to the occurrence of a swollen disc from classic AION in the second eye when the other eye already is atrophic from previous AION. Pseudo-pseudo-Foster-Kennedy syndromes are described with cocaine abuse and orbital meningioma.

Arteritic ischemic optic neuropathy is associated with poor visual acuity, usually 20/400 or worse; more extensive field loss than in classic AION; and, occasionally, premonitory intermittent visual loss. The typical altitudinal field defect of classic AION is uncommon. Most of these patients are more than 80 years old and have classical symptoms of temporal arteritis, polymyalgia rheumatica, or both. Even in occult temporal arteritis, when these symptoms are not obvious, the involvement of the whole disc with massive pallid swelling as well as obvious involvement of other portions of the ciliary tree (cilioretinal artery, areas of poor choroidal filling on fluorescein angiography), suggest the diagnosis. An immediate ESR test should always be done, steroid therapy instituted, and a temporal artery biopsy scheduled. (See Chapter 19 for more details and discussion of temporal arteritis and polymyalgia rheumatica.)

The prognosis for visual recovery is even poorer than in classic AION. More importantly, the second eye is usually lost within a week if not promptly treated. Thus, institute immediate steroid treatment to preserve vision in the second eye.

In all cases of optic disc and retinal ischemia, vasoconstrictors, hypotensive agents, nose drops, and cocaine must be used with great caution. Anterior ischemic optic neuropathy has been precipitated by the use of ergotamine to treat the AION-associated headache (misinterpreted as migraine) or nasal vasoconstrictors given for "sinus" headache. Amphetamines have been described as causing similar problems, as has cocaine abuse. Of course, ocular migraine itself can cause optic disc infarction.

Similarly, misinterpretation of headache as occurring from increased blood pressure (it rarely does; see Chapter 19) and excessively energetic efforts to decrease systemic blood pressure, result in visual loss all too often. The loss of vision can be from occipital lobe infarction, but also may be due to anterior ischemic optic neuropathy—in this case, unfortunately, often bilateral.

Hypotension or hypoxemia, associated with cardiac bypass procedures, renal dialysis, shunt, profound rapid blood loss, or profound anemia, have also been associated with AION.

Interestingly, AION does not appear to be positively associated with carotid occlusive disease or cerebral ischemia.

Other ischemic optic neuropathies. Infectious and inflammatory diseases such as sarcoidosis, syphilis, Lyme disease, cytomegalic, Epstein-Barr, and herpes virus infections can also give an ischemic appearance.

The differential diagnosis of a unilateral swollen disc with decreased visual acuity includes ischemic optic neuropathy; the usual arteritic and vasculitic processes; infectious processes including syphilis, herpes, sarcoidosis, systemic lupus; tumors presenting at the optic disc; tumors compressing the optic nerve in the orbit; and infiltration of the nerve by leukemia, reticulum cell sarcoma, and meningeal carcinomatosis. A similar picture also occurs with peripapillary inflammatory processes.

Other etiologies present a clinical picture similar to, if not identical, to anterior ischemic optic neuropathy. The disc swelling associated with hypertensive encephalopathy appears to be a form of AION (not papilledema, as previously thought), even though visual loss may be less than in classical AION and cotton-wool spots more prevalent. A similar picture occurs in systemic arteritis, particularly systemic lupus erythematosus; however, in these cases concomitant retinal vascular involvement and cotton-wool spots are frequent and the patients are younger.

Invasion of the optic nerve head by tumor may be associated with infarction, but usually is preceded by a more slowly progressive visual loss and disc swelling. Papillitis affects a very different age group, and usually is associated with denser color-vision defects and a central scotoma, rather than altitudinal or nerve fiber bundle type defects.

Diseases that increase blood viscosity and coaguability produce venous stasis syndromes and disc infarction.

The evaluation of these patients includes a search for treatable systemic disorders. Care should be taken not to lower blood pressure or control diabetes too precipitously when they are found.

Leber's Optic Neuropathy. This fascinating neuropathy has an inheritance suggesting a sex-linked recessive pattern; but pedigrees do not conform to Mendelian principles, because it is inherited with mitrochondrial, not chromosomal, DNA. In acute Leber's optic neuropathy, the hyperemic swollen disc is associated with heightened opacity of the peripapillary retinal nerve fiber layer and telangiectatic microvascular changes within the posterior pole (Fig. 4–14). During the acute phase, in contrast to papilledema, fluorescein angiography shows no leakage of dye from disc vessels. Almost always, the disc is small and full and the arterioles are tortuous from early childhood.

The visual loss is usually associated with a relatively dense central or centrocecal scotoma, sometimes with more dense islands; it progresses significantly over a period of days to months. Usually, within a few months, the other eye becomes similarly affected. Nerve fiber bundle defects appear in the temporal arcades, generalized nerve fiber layer attrition ensues, the microangiopathy disappears, and profound optic atrophy results.

This disorder typically affects young men in the second decade. There is almost always a family history, although this is sometimes suppressed by the relatives. When a family history is present, the disease may anticipate from one generation to another. Occasionally, other central nervous system symptoms are present. Once the diagnosis is established, appropriate genetic counseling is advised.

A metabolic abnormality in the mitochondria of skeletal and heart muscle of Leber's families explains an increased incidence of heart disease in these patients and their relatives. This should be sought for carefully; however, the metabolic abnormality of the muscles appears to be asymptomatic, as it may be in other mitochondrial syndromes (see Chapter 21).

Telangiectatic microangiopathy is also found in asymptomatic family members (always in the female line) and may indicate an increased risk for the syndrome.

Analysis of mitochondrial DNA indicates that a single nucleotide change, a specific point (at position 11,778) mutation, is present in a large number of patients with Leber's hereditary optic neuropathy. The result is a marked decrease in the activities of complex I of the mitochondrial electron-transport chain. The diagnosis of Leber's optic neuropathy now can be made by analysis of mitochondrial DNA, although the possibility remains that other mutations also may be found in association with LON as only 50–60 percent of patients has the 11,778 mutation.

These recent discoveries not only provide a fascinating glimpse into the new concept of mitochondrial inheritance, but also suggest a link between Leber's optic neuropathy and another optic neuropathy, so-called "toxic" or nutritional amblyopia. The similarities include peripapillary telangiectasia, an acute to subacute onset, presence of centrocecal scotoma, and continuing controversy about the possible role of cyanide in the genesis of the optic neuropathy.

Although most researchers have discredited the role of a systemic cyanide toxicity in both of these diseases, it is fascinating to consider the possibility of a more localized effect. Rhodanese (thiosulphate-sulphur-transferase) is a mitochondrial enzyme that catalyzes detoxification of cyanide; it is decreased in the liver of Leber's patients. Cyanide is a known inhibitor of complex I, already markedly decreased in these patients. Future study will clarify the role of this and other enzymes in optic neuropathies, as well

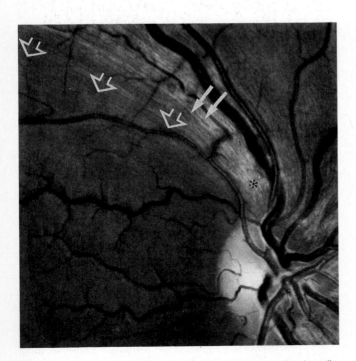

Figure 4–14. Leber's optic neuropathy. Papillomacular bundle atrophy (*thick arrows*). Rare defects in superior temporal arcade (*thin arrows*).

as other mitochondrial metabolic disorders—the mitochondrial myopathies and encephalopathies including the MELAS (myopathy, encephalopathy, lactic acid, and stroke) syndrome, Leigh's syndrome, Kearns-Shy syndrome, and myoclonic epilepsy with "ragged red" fibers. The treatments recommended previously on the assumption that cyanide toxicity contributed to the morbidity of Leber's optic neuropathy—hydroxycobalamin, cystine, and sodium thiosulphate—are benign and could, theoretically, be of some help.

OPTIC NERVE AND NERVE SHEATH TUMORS

Tumors often present as gradually progressive unilateral disc swelling and visual loss. The most common tumors are optic nerve gliomas and meningiomas of the perioptic nerve sheaths. The nerve sheaths may also be affected by cysts, especially arachnoid cysts (occasionally found in association with meningiomas). Visual acuity is usually decreased, optociliary shunts may be present, especially in nerve sheath meningioma, and a thorough neuro-imaging workup is in order. With time, the disc swelling proceeds to atrophy. Proptosis is a late development (see Chapter 5 for more details).

Primary tumors of the optic nerve head are somewhat unusual and include vascular tumors such as hemangioma and hemangioblastoma and pigmented tumors such as melanocytoma. These rarely are confused with neurogenic disc swelling. The capillary hemangiomas are circular, reddish, and may be associated with retinal hemangiomas and Von Hippel–Lindau disease. Cavernous hemangiomas may be associated with cerebellar hemangiomas and seizures. The "giant drusen" and other hamartomas associated with tuberous sclerosis and sometimes other phakomatoses also rarely are confounded with papilledema or even optic nerve head drusen. They are translucent in children and in older individuals become calcified (like optic nerve head drusen) and assume a mulberry-like appearance. Unlike drusen, they often are at least partly anterior to the retinal vessels. The rare optic disc glioma appears to be a harbinger of NF-2 (bilateral acoustic neuro fibromatosis).

Tumors metastatic to the optic nerve head run the usual gamut of metastatic tumors; breast carcinoma in women and lung carcinoma in men are most frequent. Certainly this diagnosis should be suspected in anybody known to harbor a primary tumor elsewhere in the body. Meningeal carcinomatosis also may produce a swollen nerve head (see Chapter 17), as may other infiltrative processes (sarcoidosis, leukemia, lymphoma, fungi).

BIBLIOGRAPHY

Normal Variants and Developmental Abnormalities

Apple DJ, Rabb MF, Walsh PM. Congenital anomalies of the optic disc. *Surv Ophthalmol.* 1987;27:3–41.

Bass SJ, Sherman J. Visual evoked potential (VEP) delays in tilts and/or oblique entrance of the optic nerve head. *Neuro-ophthalmology.* 1988;8:109–122.

Beyer W, Quencer R, Osher RH. Morning glory syndrome. *Ophthalmology.* 1982;89:1362–1367.

Fantes FE, Anderson DR. Clinical histologic correlation of human peripapillary anatomy. *Ophthalmology.* 1989;96:20–25.

Lambert SR, Hoyt CJ, Narahara MH. Optic nerve hypoplasia. *Surv Ophthalmol.* 1987;32:1–9.

Roth AM, Foos RY. Surface structure of the optic nerve head/epipupillary membranes. *Am J Ophthalmol.* 1972;74:977–985.

Optic Nerve Head Drusen

Carter JE, Merren MD, Byrne BM. Pseudodrusen of the optic disc. Papilledema simulating buried drusen of the optic nerve head. *J Clin Neuro-ophthalmol.* 1989;94:273–276.

Hoover DL, Robb RM, Petersen RA. Optic disc drusen in children. Scientific poster 170, American Academy of Ophthalmology, November 1987.

McLeod D, et al. The role of axoplasmic transport in the pathogenesis of cotton-wool spots. *Br J Ophthalmol.* 1977;61:177–191.

Newman NM, et al. Image-dense optic nerve head drusen (in preparation).

Big Blind Spot Syndrome

Fletcher WA, et al. Acute idiopathic blind spot enlargement: A big blind spot syndrome without optic disc edema. *Arch Ophthalmol.* 1988;106:44–49.

Papillitis

Parmley VC, et al. Does neuroretinitis rule out multiple sclerosis? *Arch Ophthalmol.* 1987;44:1045–1048.

Magnetic Resonance Imaging in Optic Neuritis

Miller DH, et al. MR Imaging of the optic nerve in optic neuritis. *Neurology.* 1988;38:175–179.

Risk of Multiple Sclerosis in Optic Neuritis

Rizzo JF, Lessel S. Risk of developing multiple sclerosis after a complicated optic neuritis. *Neurology.* 1988;38:185–190.

Foster-Kennedy Syndrome

Gelwan MJ, Seidman M, Kupersmith MJ. Pseudo-pseudo Foster-Kennedy syndrome. *J Clin Neuro-ophthalmol.* 1988;8:49–52.

Newman NM. Pseudo-pseudo Foster-Kennedy syndrome. In: Smith JL, Katz R, eds *Neuro-ophthalmology Enters the Nineties.* Hialeah, FL: Dutton Press, 1989.

Low-tension Glaucoma

Drance SM, et al. Response of blood flow to warm and cold in normal and low tension glaucoma patients. *Am J Ophthalmol.* 1988;105:35–39.

Leber's Optic Neuropathy

Hotta Y, Hayakawa M, et al. Diagnosis of Leber's optic neuropathy by means of polymerase chain reaction am-plification. *Am J Ophthalmol.* 1989;108:601–602. Letter.

Singh G, et al. A mitochondrial DNA mutation as a cause of Leber's hereditary optic neuropathy. *N Engl J Med* 1989;320:1300–1305.

Uemura A, et al. Leber's hereditary optic neuropathy: Mitochondrial and biochemical studies on muscle biopsies. *Br J Ophthalmol.* 1987;71:531–536.

Optic Disc Tumors

Dossetor FM, Landau K, Hoyt W. Optic disc glioma in neurofibromatosis type 2. *Am J Ophthalmol.* 1989;108: 602–603. Letter.

CHAPTER 5

DISORDERS OF THE OPTIC NERVE

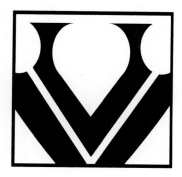

Disorders of the optic nerve can present subtly or dramatically, in isolation or in association with other signs and symptoms.

When a full-blown syndrome is present, the diagnosis of a specific optic neuropathy is not difficult. However, before there is obvious optic atrophy, it may be difficult to distinguish between subtle macular disease and early optic neuropathy. Table 5–1 lists some helpful points in this differential diagnosis.

OPTIC NEURITIS

Inflammation of the optic nerve causes **optic neuritis,** an acute to subacute decrease in central vision usually with a central scotoma. Visual acuity ranges from 20/15 to no light perception; color vision is significantly diminished, as are brightness sensation and contrast sensitivity. Nearly always there is an afferent pupillary defect. In 80% of patients pain on movement of the eye occurs and occasionally antedates the visual symptoms. More women than men are affected. *Optic neuritis is the most frequent cause of neurogenic visual loss in patients less than 50 years old.* In fact, nearly all patients have their initial attacks as young adults; the diagnosis of acute optic neuritis is unlikely in anyone over 45.

Although loss of acuity may be minimal to profound, the patient usually complains vociferously about *visual dysfunction.* Frequently, the loss of color vision and decline in contrast sensitivity are much more troublesome to the patient than the change in visual acuity. Patients describe a sensation of dimness, as if the rheostat were turned down. In unilateral optic neuritis, the Pulfrich phenomenon (see Chapter 2) is usually present and may explain some of the spatial disorientation that patients recount.

Optic neuritis is often a manifestation of demyelination—idiopathic or a harbinger of multiple sclerosis (MS), Schilder's disease or other leukodystrophy. Demyelination is the most frequent cause of optic neuritis, and MS is the most frequent cause of demyelination. Optic neuritis is the first symptom in 20% of MS patients; it occurs at some time in 75%.

In the large majority (70 to 90%) of patients, visual acuity recovers to 20/30 or better within 6 to 8 weeks, but the patients may still complain of a disproportionate and real loss of visual function. This is explained by the considerable and persistent defects in color vision, contrast sensitivity, and conduction. It is not unusual for the patient to have a stark white disc and relatively normal visual acuity.

If repeated episodes of optic neuritis occur in the same eye (as they do in 20 to 30% of cases) with each episode the chance of complete recovery declines. The reported likelihood that disseminated disease, MS, will develop in the patient with a truly isolated optic neuritis (unassociated with any history, symptoms, or findings of MS) varies from 17 to 90%. If patients are followed closely and meticulously examined, the percentage who will develop disseminated findings is probably greater than 50%. If bright spots on magnetic resonance imaging (MRI) are accepted as evidence for MS, the percentage may be even higher.

Associated Signs and Symptoms

Ask the patient about a decrease in visual function during exercise, hot baths, and so forth (Uhthoff's phenomenon, related to conduction block within the optic nerve with increased bodily temperature); ask about electric sensations in the arms and legs when the neck bends (Lhermitte's sign); ask about photopsias, light or movement induced. In contrast to

TABLE 5–1. DIFFERENTIAL DIAGNOSIS OF DECREASED VISUAL ACUITY WITH A "NORMAL" FUNDUS

	Ophthalmos-copy	NFL	Pinhole with refraction	color	VF	Pupil	Subj. MG	VEP	Photostress
Ocular Disorders									
Refractive error	N	N	VA N	N	N with correction	N	N	N	N
Keratoconus	Distorted?	N	VA N	N	N w/correction early	N	N	N	N
Macular Disorders									
CSR	Dome in macula	N	Increased hyperopia	+/– N	Amsler distorted, scotoma	N	N	Slightly decreased	Prolonged
CME	Cysts in macula		No change	Slight decrease	Slight centrocec.	N	N	Slightly decreased	Slightly prolonged
RPE detachment	Gray dome in mac. area	N	No change	+/– N	Local depression	N	N	Slightly decreased	Slightly prolonged
SRNVM	Elevation in mac. area	N	No change	+/– N	Local depression	N	N	Slightly decreased	Slightly prolonged
Age-related	Pigment changes	N	No change	+/– N	Central depression	N	N	Slightly decreased	Slightly prolonged
Retinal Dystrophy									
Cone-rod	Macular changes, telangiectasia	+/– Rakes	No change	Decreased	Central scotoma	APD	N	Decreased VEP	Slightly increased
Stargardt's/Fundus Flavimaculatus	Macular changes, flecks	+/– Rakes, PMB loss	No change	Slight decrease	Central scotoma	APD	N	Decreased PERG	Slightly increased
Other Retinal Syndromes									
CAR syndrome	N early	N early	No change	Decreased	Varies, abnormal	ERG low, VEP decreased	?		
Optic Nerve Disease									
Demyelination	NFL defects	Decreased, rakes	No change	Decreased	Central scotoma/NFD	++ APD	++	Delay ++ frag.	N
Ischemia	Slight OA	Alt defects	No change	Decreased	Alt defect	+ APD	+	Decreased amplitude	N
Compression	Slight OA	Diffuse loss	No change	Decreased	Constriction	+ APD	+	Decreased amplitude	N
Intrinsic optic nerve tumor	Slight OA Cilioret. shunt	Diffuse loss	No change	Decreased	Constriction	+ APD	+	Decreased amplitude	N
Malingering/Hysteria	N	N	N	*a*	Spiral field, abnormal 1+2 meter tangent screen	*a*	N	*a*	N if patient co-operates
Amblyopia	N	N	No change	N	N	N	+/– N	N	N

a All subjective tests may be abnormal, often nonphysiologic.

alt, ??; APD, afferent pupillary defect; CAR, carcinoma associated retinopathy; CME, cystoid macular edema; CSR, central serous retinopathy; ERG, electroretinogram; N, normal; NFL, nerve fiber layer; OA, optic atrophy; PH, pin hole; RPE, retinal pigment epithelium; SRNVM, subretinal neovascular membrane; Subj. MG, subjective Marcus Gunn; VA, visual acuity; VEP, visual evoked potential; VF, visual field.

the worsening of symptoms with increased body temperature, lowering the temperature can improve symptoms. Other factors are effective but not well understood. In fact, one report described a patient with retrobulbar neuritis whose visual acuity improved after drinking beer. The improvement occurred even if the beer was warm! The responsible elements remain to be elucidated. These frequent concomitants of demyelinating lesions, although not present exclusively in MS, are characteristic.

Other signs of dissemination include Charcot's triad: (1) nystagmus, ataxia, and dysarthria; (2) bowel and bladder problems; and (3) paraesthesias. Demyelination may be a manifestation of systemic disease such as systemic lupus erythematosus, other autoimmune diseases, or adrenal insufficiency and demyelination (Schilder's disease).

Fundus findings range from minimal to dramatic. In an initial retrobulbar neuritis, the fundus may be entirely normal; whereas if there have been previous attacks or if there is an insidious or occult onset, optic atrophy and/or nerve fiber bundle defects are found. When papillitis occurs, the anterior portion of the nerve is involved, frequently with a few cells in the vitreous overlying the disc; the lesion is retrobulbar or in the optic canal. More rarely, there is frank uveitis or periphlebitis. Occasionally, the onset is insidious with slow visual loss that produces very few symptoms, yet nerve fiber layer loss and subtle disc pallor may be evident. Acutely, fluorescein angiography may show leakage at the disc (more common in papillitis) and will highlight venous sheathing.

In children and teenagers, the affliction is often bilateral with inflammation extending into the retina in the form of a neuroretinitis with or without macular exudation. A history of preceding viral disease or vaccination is common; the subsequent development of MS is rare whenever neuroretinitis occurs.

Following the loss of vision, over several weeks nerve fiber bundle defects appear in the temporal arcades and papillomacular bundle; the latter defect is the neurologic concomitant of the central scotoma. Optic atrophy ensues if visual recovery occurs.

Visual field defects. A central scotoma is classic in optic neuritis. Other nerve fiber patterns of visual field loss do occur; however when other patterns of field loss exist, rethink the diagnosis.

Evaluation of patients with possible optic neuritis. All patients who present with an optic neuritis should have the second eye carefully examined for nerve fiber defects and optic atrophy in a search for evidence of disseminated disease. Finding evidence of two separate anatomic lesions separated in time of occurrence establishes a diagnosis of multiple sclerosis. Visual evoked potential testing is very

sensitive to the conduction delay associated with demyelination and shows a characteristic fragmentation and delay on both pattern and flash tests. It remains the single most useful test for MS because of its sensitivity and stability.

When all the clinical characteristics, the patient's age, and everything else are typical of optic neuritis, limit the workup to a neuro-ophthalmologic evaluation, red-free photography of the nerve fiber layer, visual evoked potentials, fluorescein angiography, and contrast sensitivity studies as a baseline. Although the latter two examinations infrequently add much diagnostic help in demyelination, they often yield very important clues to less common causes of optic neuritis. Visual evoked potentials that are not delayed suggest another cause of the optic nerve dysfunction. Fluorescein studies may show profound leakage, vascular irregularity, or micro-occlusions associated with inflammatory or arteritic processes.

When patients have minimally symptomatic and insidious visual loss, acuity that does not recover significantly, progressive visual loss, persistent pain, atypical visual field defects, or other courses not typical of optic neuritis, they deserve further workup. Other indications of atypical optic neuritis are onset in patients older than 45 years, unusual visual field defects, bilateral and simultaneous onset in adults, or a history of vasculitis or recent sinusitis. **Never** accept a diganosis of chronic optic neuritis without further evaluation.

In the atypical case, the further workup includes complete blood count, erythrocyte sedimentation rate test, serologic tests for collagen disease, serum fluorescent treponemal antibody-absorption (FTA-Abs) or HATTS test for syphilis, serum B_{12} and folate tests, and tests for human immunodeficiency virus, Epstein-Barr virus, and Lyme disease.

After these studies, proceed with neuro-imaging of the orbits and chiasmal region. If MRI is available, it is the optimal imaging modality for establishing a diagnosis of MS (visual evoked response testing is still more sensitive in symptomatic patients) and also for detecting other parenchymal CNS abnormalities. MRI detects many more demyelinating plaques than does computed tomography (CT) scanning. Nevertheless, a definite diagnosis of MS should not be made on the basis of a single scan. If orbital inflammation, sinus infection, and so forth, are suspected, because of better spatial and bone resolution, a thin-section CT study is the choice, as it is if MRI is not available.

Long term follow-up is needed not only to detect signs and symptoms of disseminated disease but also to evaluate disability suffered by the patients. It is my impression that patients who present with truly isolated optic neuritis rarely become debilitated with the disease. In a study by Rizzo and Lessell, only 17% was mild to moderately disabled. As our diagnostic technology becomes increasingly sophisticated, we may find that demyelination is common and that debilitating disease is only an extreme manifestation.

The precise role and significance of associated changes in the cerebrospinal fluid (such as light chains, oligoclonal bands, and myelin basic protein); T-cell ratios; genetic markers (eg, HLA haplotypes); or the possible association of previous infections, particularly viral diseases; remain to be clarified. Nevertheless, the sensitivity of modern examination methods leads to a real dilemma: today it is possible to find evidence of dissemination at the first presentation in a large percentage of patients.

Although some intriguing recent studies suggest there may soon be effective treatments (interferon, plasmapheresis, antimetabolites), there is currently no recognized treatment for MS. Until our ability to treat these patients is proportionate to our ability to diagnose them, there is no clinical reason for an extensive workup of the patient with an isolated optic neuritis; no need to search for symptomatic lesions. Because we have no therapy to offer, the decision to discuss frankly the possibility of MS with a patient with "isolated" optic neuritis must rest on evaluation of the potential benefit and harm to the patient. However, as the patient population becomes increasingly medically sophisticated, many patients (or their relatives or friends) will ask about the association with MS, and I find it best to approach this subject directly with most patients. It is reasonable that patients be allowed to plan for their futures and, frankly, many will have considered the possibility of MS prior to seeing you.

The majority of patients who will develop severe disseminated disease suffers another symptom within 2 to 4 years of the first. Certainly, many demyelinating plaques are asymptomatic; histopathologic studies in MS patients without optic nerve symptoms show 100% of optic nerves contains demyelinating plaques.

Most demyelinating optic neuritis is either idiopathic or associated with MS. **Other rarer causes of demyelination** include **Devic's syndrome** (bilateral optic neuritis and transverse myelitis), in which the second eye is usually involved within a short time. In addition to more severe visual loss and bilaterality in contrast to MS, Devic's syndrome is associated with significant pleocytosis in the cerebrospinal fluid. Nevertheless, it is often considered an MS variant rather than a separate entity, although the associated pathologic changes may be quite different. In the past, the prognosis for significant neurologic or

visual recovery has been quite poor. Although the visual results remain rather dismal, it seems that more patients now survive this very debilitating type of demyelination but remain paraplegic. The precise role of more aggressive treatment—such as interferon therapy, plasmapheresis, and treatment with antimetabolites—in achieving a better prognosis remains to be fully elucidated.

Schilder's disease (adrenoleukodystrophy; ALD) usually presents as severe cerebral demyelination associated with Addison's disease. It is an inherited sex-linked disorder with relentless progression to decorticate spastic quadriparesis. Adrenomyeloneuropathy (AMN) is a milder, more slowly progressive form of ALD with later onset. The adrenal insufficiency and white matter changes on MRI may precede neurologic deterioration. Because dietary treatment with fatty acids shows promise in the treatment of these previously relentless disorders, evaluate every male with renal insufficiency for ALD and AMN. Neonatal adrenoleukodystrophy, Zellweger's syndrome and hyperpipecolicacidemia are biochemically indistinguishable recessively inherited demyelinating disorders separate from Schilder's. All are peroxisomal disorders (see Chapter 21).

Systemic lupus erythematosus (SLE) can affect the optic nerve, both by arteritis or ischemia (of the optic nerve head, retina, choroid, or optic nerve itself) or as true demyelination. At times SLE affects other portions of the central nervous system and produces a picture very much like that of MS.

Other causes of optic neuritis include inflammatory and infectious diseases, especially sarcoid, contiguous sinus disease, syphilis, herpes, and a host of infectious agents (Table 5–2). Idiopathic optic neuritis seems to occur following viral illnesses and vaccination more frequently than would be expected by chance, especially in children. Apparently typical inflammatory optic neuritis (as well as anterior ischemic optic neuropathy) may also be associated with inflammatory bowel disease, such as Crohn's disease, ulcerative colitis, and Whipple's disease.

An autoimmune optic neuritis has been described, as well as a paraneoplastic optic neuritis that may occur independently or in association with paraneoplastic photoreceptor degeneration (carcinoma associated retinopathy syndrome; see Chapter 22 and paraneoplastic encephalomyelitis.

Obviously, the appropriate studies to rule out these processes depend on the history you have elicited from the patient. For neurosyphilis, the (VDRL and rapid plasma reagin in the serum may be negative. Therefore, it is most efficacious to start off with an FTA-Abs (or HATTS) test, which if negative rules out neurosyphilis as well. Nevertheless, where

TABLE 5–2. ETIOLOGIES OF OPTIC NEURITIS

Idiopathic
Demyelinating
  Multiple sclerosis
  Devic's disease
  Adrenoleucodystrophy (Schilder's disease)
Viral, paraviral, postviral, postvaccination:
  Measles, rubella, mumps, chickenpox, influenza, polio, coxsackie, viral encephalitis, Herpes zoster
Infectious mononucleosis/Epstein-Barr virus
Other Infections: Toxoplasmosis, histoplasmosis, syphilis, Lyme disease, tuberculosis, sarcoid, *Cryptococcus*, cat scratch fever
Inflammatory
  Sinusitis, meningitis, orbit infection and inflammation
  Introcular infection—nematode, cysticercus
  Acute Multifocal Placoid Pigment Epitheliopathy
  Birdshot chorioretinopathy
Associated with systemic disease
  GI—Whipple's disease, Crohn's disease, ulcerative colitis
  Behcet's syndrome
  Reiter's syndrome
  Autoimmune disorders, including systemic lupus erythematosus (SLE)

clinical findings and history are especially suggestive of syphilis, dark-field examination should be done whenever possible. If the FTA-Abs is positive, a lumbar puncture should be done. Neurosyphilis is diagnosed if any two of the three following criteria are fulfilled: (1) positive cerebrospinal fluid VDRL, (2) increased protein, and (3) greater than 5 white blood cells/10 mL. Lumbar puncture is indicated in any patient with optic neuritis or disc edema plus a positive VDRL or FTA-Abs test. Although the FTA-Abs test is most sensitive for documenting syphilitic infection, when active infection is to be treated, the VDRL provides the best means to follow the effect of treatment (see Chapter 22).

Treatment: We currently have no effective treatment for demyelination. Goals should be to hasten and improve recovery from each event and to decrease the recurrence rate. Steroids have been used in almost every possible form, but there is as yet no large double-blind study that proves either their efficacy or the advantage of one route or dose over another. Many smaller studies do, however, suggest a trend, at least for quicker improvement if not for better final outcome of visual acuity. In cases with somewhat atypical optic neuritis, profound loss of visual acuity or poor vision in the "normal" eye, some consultants now advocate high-dose prednisone (1000 mg q12h × 10). Paradoxically, however, a dramatic response to steroids is suspect; in general, nondemyelinating inflammation, infection, and tumors respond much better to steroids than does demyelinating optic neuritis.

Antimetabolites and other treatments such as copolymer 1 (Cop_1), which alter immune status, are currently used for debilitating disease. Again, no large double-blind studies are available, but there are suggestions that plasmapheresis, interferon treatment, and antimetabolites (eg, cyclophosphamide) may be helpful. For the moment, the morbidity associated with these treatments relegates their use to patients with severe disseminated disease.

The differential diagnosis of optic neuritis (Table 5–3) includes other optic neuropathies (ischemic, toxic, and hereditary); optic nerve compression; tumorous compromise either by primary optic nerve tumors or secondarily by thyroid orbitopathy, metastatic tumor, carcinomatous meningitis, or paraneoplastic effects of distant tumor; and primary ocular conditions such as cone dystrophies, buried optic nerve head drusen, glaucoma (especially low-pressure glaucoma), and nonorganic visual loss.

ISCHEMIC OPTIC NEUROPATHIES

Retrobulbar ischemia (RBION) is uncommon in comparison with anterior ischemic optic neuropathy (AION). It is a diagnosis of exclusion in patients who present with a sudden decrease in vision. The diagnosis should be made with caution, especially in patients without obvious risk factors for ischemic optic nerve disease, such as other arterial disease (hypertension, diabetes, or vascular occlusive disease). The only other common acute and occult cause of retrobulbar visual loss is optic neuritis; in contrast to RBION, optic neuritis affects a younger group of patients, is associated with a central scotoma rather than an altitudinal visual field defect, and recovers in 6 to 8 weeks. In the often insidious ischemic visual loss, the differential diagnosis with prechiasmal compressive lesions is quite difficult, even though an insidious onset is more common with RBION than anterior ischemic optic neuropathy (Fig. 5–1). As with anterior ischemic optic neuropathy, symptoms of temporal arteritis should be sought for and an erythrocyte sedimentation rate obtained. Other vascular pathologies must be ruled out.

Findings on examination are nonspecific, although occasionally on fluorescein angiography slow or patchy choroidal filling suggests diffuse posterior ciliary artery disease and helps to substantiate the diagnosis.

In addition to idiopathic ischemic optic neuropathy, trauma has been implicated in ischemic disease of the optic nerve. In many cases of posttraumatic, transient decrease in visual acuity, there is poor perfusion on fluorescein angiography. In other cases, evidence of vascular compromise is

TABLE 5–3. DIAGNOSIS OF 421 PATIENTS (424 DIAGNOSES) WITH REFERRAL DIAGNOSIS OF OPTIC NEURITIS, UNEXPLAINED OPTIC NEUROPATHY, OR VISUAL FAILURE OF UNCERTAIN CAUSE

Optic neuritis of unknown etiology	71
Neuronal and choroidal lesions	46
Optic neuritis associated with multiple sclerosis	42
Ischemic optic neuropathy	34
Toxic and deficiency optic neuropathy	28
Compressive lesion of nerve or chiasm	26
Optic atrophy of unknown etiology	23
Hysterical amblyopia	19
Optic neuropathy of unknown etiology	10
Congenital disc anomaly	10
Drusen of nerve head	8
Glaucoma	8
Leber's disease	7
No disease	7
Traumatic optic neuropathy	6
Amblyopia of unknown etiology	6
Congenital optic atrophy	6
Juvenile diabetes mellitus and optic atrophy	5
Chiasmal syndrome of unknown etiology	4
Hereditary optic atrophy	4
Hypoplasia of optic nerve	4
Uveitis	3
Acute optic neuropathy due to drusen	3
Disc edema due to peripheral uveitis	3
Optic neuritis due to viral disease	3
Optic neuropathy with endocrine exophthalmos	3
Optic atrophy due to meningitis	2
West Indian amblyopia	2
Chronic atrophic papilledema	2
Cirsoid aneurysm retina	2
Retinal vasculitis	2
Optic neuropathy due to orbital tumor	2
Homonymous hemianopia	2
River blindness	1
No diagnosis	1
Cataract	1
Optic atrophy due to congenital CNS malformation	1
Myopia	1
Pseudotumor of orbit	1
Tolosa-Hunt syndrome with retinopathy	1
Alexia	1
Visual agnosia	1
Papillophlebitis	1
Migraine	1
Opticochiasmatic arachnoiditis	1
Cortical blindness	1
Optic atrophy due to Paget's disease	1
Devic's disease	1
Optic nerve pit with central serous retinopathy	1
Central retinal vein occlusion	1
Convergence insufficiency	1
Optic neuritis due to Guillain-Barré syndrome	1
Optic neuritis due to encephalitis	1
Amblyopia due to strabismus	1
Traumatic chiasmal syndrome	1

From Lessell S. Toxic and deficiency optic neuropathies. In: Smith JC, Glaser JS, eds. Neuro-ophthalmology. St. Louis: Mosby, 1973;7.

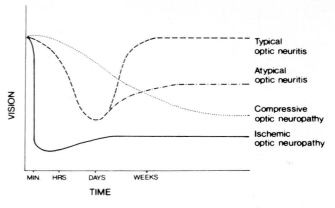

Figure 5–1. Time courses of optic neuritis, anterior ischemic optic neuropathy. (*From Hedges TR III. The neuro-ophthalmic examination. In:* Consultation in Ophthalmology. *Toronto: Decker, 1987;3; with permission.*)

not present and a vascular etiology cannot be differentiated from primary, evanescent, neural compromise.

One other cause of occlusive vascular disease deserving mention is the vasculopathy associated with radiation therapy or chemotherapy. This can affect the optic nerve, retina, or both within weeks, months, or several years after treatment. Its occurrence is predictable with high doses of radiation (greater than 60 to 70 Gy), especially in patients who are treated concomitantly with chemotherapy. In these patients, some decrement in visual function, although subtle, is almost universally present. Occasionally, the diagnosis can be established by the presence of radiation retinopathy that looks like diabetic retinopathy, but more frequently involves the inferior portions of the retina. More commonly, radiation optic neuropathy presents on its own.

Infiltrative diseases, such as amyloid, may wreak havoc either by direct infiltration of the nerve or compromise of its blood supply.

HEREDITARY OPTIC NEUROPATHIES

Of the panoply of neurologic, metabolic, and other hereditary diseases that compromise optic nerve and retinal function (see Table 5–4), relatively few affect the optic nerve in isolation. These include Leber's hereditary optic neuropathy (a multisystem mitochondrial disorder that may be monosymptomatic), dominant optic atrophy, and congenital recessive optic atrophy.

Leber's hereditary optic neuropathy presents with a papillitis-like swollen disc; the degree of visual loss is usually more profound, however, though

TABLE 5–4. HEREDITARY OPTIC ATROPHIES

	Age at Onset	Visual Acuity	Progression	Nystagmus	Disc Appearance	Color Vision	Other
Isolated							
Dominant juvenile	4–8 years	20/40–200	Minimum	Rare	Temporal pallor	Decreased blue-yellow discrimination	Rare
Recessive early infantile	3–4 years	20/200–hand motions	None	+ +	Marked optic atrophy	Severely decreased	–
Mitochondrial							
Leber's optic neuropathy	Teens	20/200–20/400	Over months	None	Swollen disc, temporal atrophy progressing to optic atrophy	Severely decreased	Almost all males, cardiomyopathy/arrhythmias
Associated With Systemic Disease	(See Chapters 21–23)						

much more gradual, and the scotoma is more centro-cecal than in papillitis. In addition, almost invariably the second eye is affected, within weeks to months. Men are afflicted almost exclusively. Usually, young men are affected in their late teens or early 20s; however, all ages may be affected and there may be anticipation within a given family. Leber's optic neuropathy is transmitted by mitochondrial inheritance via the female lines (egg cytoplasm).

Early in its course, Leber's optic neuropathy is distinguished by a pathognomonic appearance of the fundi. Initially, the discs are hyperemic and swollen and the surrounding nerve fiber layer appears to have increased opacity. There are telangiectatic and microvascular abnormalities at the posterior pole. Nearly always, the discs are small and full with late-branching vessels. (A similar appearance has also been found in many family members of Leber's patients.) With time, nerve fiber layer defects occur, especially in the temporal arcades and papillomacular bundle; they progress steadily until the nerve fiber layer is totally atrophic. At this point, the findings are similar to those of any other severe optic neuropathy. Unfortunately, unlike papillitis, the prognosis for improvement of vision is not good. Very few patients are reported to recover.

Associated neurologic findings, usually mild, may occur concomitantly or briefly after the onset of visual loss. Rarely, these are quite severe, making it difficult to distinguish Leber's disease from multiple sclerosis or Devic's disease, especially if the patients are not examined early, when the pathognomonic fundus changes are present.

Associated systemic findings include a cardiac myopathy with preexcitation syndrome (an EKG must be done!) and histologic changes in systemic musculature (but without clinical myopathy). The alterations are typical of other known mitochondrial myopathies, and thus give credence to the assumption that similar biochemical changes cause Leber's optic neuropathy. Unfortunately, there is no effective treatment (see Chapter 4 for details of heredity and diagnosis by DNA analysis).

FAMILIAL OPTIC ATROPHIES

Table 5–4 summarizes hereditary optic atrophies discussed here.

Dominant Optic Atrophy

When optic atrophy occurs in an infant with a strong family history, there is little problem in making a diagnosis of dominant optic atrophy. Nystagmus develops early and is the finding that brings the patient to medical attention. Of course, all other causes of bilateral optic atrophy must be ruled out. Frequently the family history is suppressed or the patients are ignorant of it. Because the visual loss starts in the first decade of life and many patients may never experience normal vision, the patient usually cannot date the onset of visual loss. Dysfunction is usually relatively mild, in the range of 20/40 to 20/60, and severe visual loss is exceptional. Vision in the two eyes may vary somewhat.

Visual fields most often show a central scotoma, but paracentral or cecocentral scotomas are also found. Loss of color acuity is disproportionately marked for blue. Vision usually stabilizes by the end of the second decade.

Early infantile recessive optic atrophy: This form of optic atrophy presents at a very early age, is usually discovered before 3 or 4 years, and is associated with much more severe visual damage, ranging from very poor to no light perception. Because severe visual loss is present in early infancy there is nystagmus almost invariably. The discs are very atrophic and frequently deeply cupped.

In very young children, the differentiation between these syndromes and Leber's congenital amaurosis or other tapeto-retinal degenerations is made by electrophysiology; the electroretinogram is severely involved or diminished in tapeto-retinal degenerations and normal in optic atrophies.

Hereditary Optic Atrophies Associated with Other Findings

Many optic atrophies are associated with other sense organ disorders, central and peripheral neurologic disease, and multisystem disorders. As it is impossible to cover the classification of these somewhat confusing and overlapping syndromes in detail here, they are presented in tabular form in Chapter 22. Only one will be mentioned in detail. The DIDMOAD syndrome usually brings the patient to the ophthalmologist in childhood when recognition of the syndrome can lead to appropriate treatment for its associated problems, diabetes and hearing loss.

DIDMOAD Syndrome. The diabetes insipidus, diabetes mellitus, optic atrophy, and deafness (DIDMOAD) syndrome begins in the first or second decade with visual loss and severe progressive optic atrophy. As a rule, the visual acuity is less than 20/200. The diabetes requires insulin and is very similar to type I juvenile diabetes. Diabetes insipidus is critical to the diagnosis of the syndrome. In contrast to the severity of the other portions of the syndrome, the hearing loss may be subtle and must be tested for; it tends to be a mild high-frequency loss. Gonadal dysfunction also occurs. This syndrome is inherited as an autosomal recessive trait with incomplete penetrance.

OPTIC NERVE TUMORS

Optic nerve tumors may be divided into primary tumors of the optic nerve (the gliomas and nerve sheath meningiomas), metastatic tumors, tumors of the orbit and ocular adnexae, and nonneoplastic masses

(see Chapter 18). Most present with slowly progressive visual loss, although transient visual aberrations do occur occasionally.

Optic nerve gliomas: Optic nerve gliomas include (1) astrocytic tumors of the anterior visual pathway, occurring predominantly in prepubertal children; and (2) the rare, malignant glioma (glioblastoma) of adulthood.

The **childhood gliomas** usually present with unilateral visual loss, proptosis, disc pallor and/or swelling, and strabismus. Approximately one third of the tumors is associated with neurofibromatosis, and thus café-au-lait spots should be searched for. Since these spots may not pigment until after puberty, however, they may be overlooked in the typical patient, a young child. As many as 15 to 20% of patients with VRNF-1 have asymptomatic visual pathway gliomas.

Because of the tumor's presentation in young children, the visual loss may not be recognized until proptosis develops. In older children, the visual loss usually is noted prior to obvious exophthalmos.

Optic nerve gliomas may be asymptomatic and are compatible with practically normal visual function. Approximately 15% of NF-1 patients without visual abnormality harbors optic gliomas. Neither orbital pain nor inflammatory signs are associated with optic nerve glioma. Approximately half the patients have a stable clinical course (NF-1 is associated predominantly with this group); the others suffer progressive enlargement of their tumors.

Patients with an optic nerve glioma have abnormal visual evoked potentials. Because **rarely** treatable or benign disorders appear identical to optic nerve gliomas on neuro-imaging, there is the question of whether all these tumors should be biopsied prior to making a therapeutic decision. MRI scanning potentially will differentiate most of the vascular lesions and help to decrease the numbers of potentially confusing lesions (Table 5–5).

TABLE 5–5. CAUSES OF OPTIC NERVE ENLARGEMENT ON IMAGING STUDIES

ON Tumors	Glioma (fusiform)
	Meningioma (fusiform or excrescent)
	Metastasis
	Leukemic infiltrate
	Rarer optic nerve tumors
Other	Increased intracranial pressure
	Arachnoid cyst
	Central retinal vein occlusion
	Optic neuritis
	Orbital pseudotumor
	Sarcoid
	Idiopathic inflammation

Chiasmal gliomas are considered in Chapter 6.

Although theoretically the differential diagnosis of optic nerve glioma runs the gamut of optic nerve and orbital diseases, there is only one serious alternate consideration, the optic nerve sheath meningioma. Although optic nerve gliomas tend to present in children and nerve sheath meningiomas in adults, there is a significant overlap in the teenage years. It is especially important to make the differential diagnosis correctly in this age group, as many authors feel that sheath meningiomas are much more malignant in this age group than in older individuals. The stable group tends to show optic atrophy and the progressive group shows papilledema and restriction of eye movement.

The appropriate evaluation of these patients, in addition to ascertaining the presence or absence of neurofibromatosis, is a neuro-imaging workup. The characteristic fusiform shape of the glioma, optic canal enlargement if the tumor extends out of the orbit, and associated abnormalities of the sphenoid ridge, are demonstrable on both CT and MRI scanning. On CT imaging, the overlap in appearance between the tumors still leaves a good deal of question. Obvious bends are typical of a glioma whereas contrast enhancement and a "railroad track" appearance are frequent in meningiomas. Both ultrasound and MRI are somewhat more helpful in making a differential diagnosis, but no single methodology or combination of methodologies has yet proven absolutely effective. This inability to establish a firm diagnosis adds to the controversy about appropriate management of these tumors.

Treatment: The appropriate treatment of optic nerve gliomas remains controversial. Recent evidence implies that the cell kinetics of optic nerve gliomas follow those of a neoplasm, rather than an hamartoma, as has been suggested. Yet the major problem associated with optic nerve gliomas is not the precise pathologic characterization but the most prudent management.

When the tumor is limited to the orbit and visual acuity is poor, most would agree that the appropriate course is to extirpate the tumor anterior to the chiasm. If visual acuity is good and there appears to be a clear demarcation between the tumor and chiasm, many would wait and watch. Others would biopsy the mass to eliminate the possibility of a meningioma or other rare pathology (Fig. 5–2). Chiasmal tumors cannot be extirpated, but some of their associated signs—nystagmus, diabetes insipidus, and the diencephalic syndrome—may be ameliorated by radiotherapy. High-dose radiotherapy also appears to have some effect on many gliomas, but the potential complications must be weighed against potential risks, especially in very young children.

Malignant gliomas of adulthood: This rare tumor may present as an optic neuritis with unilateral visual loss. However, it usually progresses relatively rapidly (in a few months) to total blindness. The contralateral optic nerve becomes involved in a few months. Death ensues within a year. This tumor is analogous to malignant glioblastoma in the central nervous system. A recent report suggests some amelioration by radiation and chemotherapy.

Primary meningiomas of the optic nerve sheaths: Classically, nerve sheath meningiomas present in middle-aged women with insidious and often minor visual loss. With time, proptosis and optociliary shunts at the nerve head may develop (Fig. 5–3). The tumor expands within the dural sheaths compressing the optic nerve.

Evaluation: Again, neuro-imaging will usually show the typical railroad track enlargement of the optic nerve shadow, sometimes associated with calcification on both CT and MRI. Fat-suppression paradigms and the use of the paramagnetic contrast agent gadolinium increase the detection rate of meningiomas. The intracranial portions of sheath meningiomas enhance more readily than the orbital portions. On ultrasonography, meningiomas and gliomas have only slightly different levels of reflectivity and, in my experience, overlap too much to make for comfortable differential diagnosis.

Pneumosinus dilatans—enlarged aerated spaces within the posterior ethmoids, sphenoid sinuses, and anterior clinoids—is very suggestive of the presence of a meningioma.

Management: Occasionally visual loss is arrested in tumors arising close to the globe by decompressing or unfolding the tumor surrounding the optic nerve. However, usually there is slow unrelenting progression. Again, management is somewhat controversial. As usual, the decision is somewhat easier in a patient who has lost vision. Because these are slowly progressive tumors, if the patient is older than 40 and a woman and if the tumor can be removed en toto, it should be done when the tumor encroaches on the optic canal. This can be done by orbitotomy, or, if the tumor extends through the optic canal, with a combined orbitocranial approach. More anterior tumors may be observed at 3- to 6-month intervals. When visual acuity is good or when the tumors are bilateral, as occasionally happens, the management decisions are more difficult. Most surgeons agree that an ipsilateral tumor that has extended intracranially should be removed as completely as possible. Radiotherapy may slow the progression of visual loss. In young patients, particularly in males, these tumors are more aggressive. Those younger than 30 should have transcranial removal of the tumor. Those between 30 and 40 should

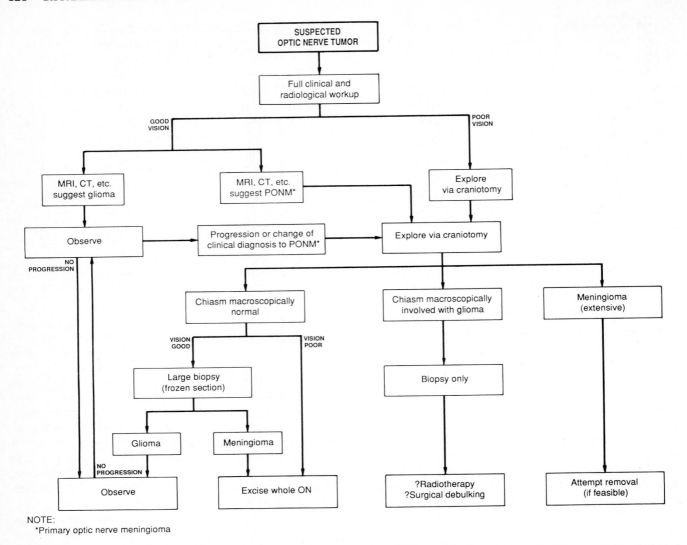

Figure 5–2. Flowchart of recommended management of optic nerve tumors in young patients. (*From Wright JE, McNab AA, McDonald W. Optic nerve glioma and the management of optic nerve tumors in the young.* Br J Ophthalmol. *1989;73:967–974, with permission.*)

have careful observation and surgery if the tumor seems aggressive (Fig. 5–2).

Rarely, ectopic meningeal tissue will give rise to an ectopic meningioma within the orbit. Rarer tumors such as schwannomas occur in orbital nerves and affect the optic nerve even more rarely.

Meningiomas originating intracranially may involve the optic nerve, either by invasion along its sheaths or by compression. Intracranial meningiomas arise from the planum sphenoidale and tuberculum sella areas as well as the sphenoid ridge. **Sphenoid ridge meningiomas** are frequently divided into three types that can be differentiated on the basis of their clinical signs and symptoms.

Meningiomas of the outer third of the sphenoid ridge and pterion. These tumors include pterional meningiomas and en plaque meningiomas. **Pterional**

meningiomas grow very large before they produce neuro-ophthalmic signs and symptoms. Patients usually present with headache, papilledema, or both.

En plaque meningiomas occur predominantly in women of 40 to 60 years of age. They form a thin layer of tumor that infiltrates in the region of the outer third of the sphenoid ridge. Accompanying hyperostosis may be massive and sometimes is seen on external examination as fullness in the temporal fossa. As these tumors spread medially, they may involve the optic nerve. At this point they produce symptoms similar to those of inner-third meningiomas. The massive hyperostosis often causes significant proptosis often with chemosis, vascular engorgement, and enlargement of the extraocular muscles. Some of these cases have been misdiagnosed as thyroid orbitopathy. The diagnosis of thyroid orbitopathy should always be

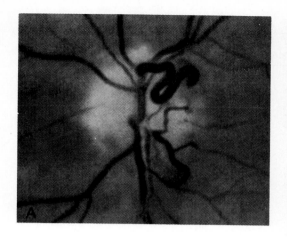 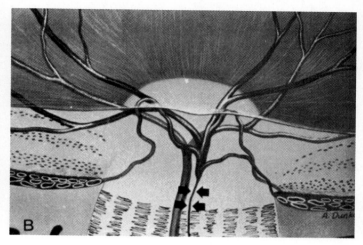

Figure 5–3. Appearance of optociliary shunt vessels. **A.** Optociliary shunt vessels in a 55-year-old woman with a spheno-orbital meningioma. **B.** Drawing of optociliary shunt vessels showing that they represent veins that shunt blood between the retinal and choroidal venous circulations. Retinal venous blood cannot exit the eye via the central retinal vein because it has been compressed (eg, by tumor). Collateral channels that normally exist between the retinal and choroidal venous circulations subsequently enlarge so that the retinal venous blood is shunted to the choroidal venous circulation to exit the eye via the vortex veins. (*From Miller N, ed. Diagnosis of tumors and related conditions. In:* Walsh and Hoyt's Clinical Neuro-ophthalmology. *4th ed. Baltimore: Williams & Wilkins, 1985;3; with permission.*)

considered with suspicion if there is not bilateral orbital involvement.

Middle-third meningiomas usually cause no symptoms until they enlarge significantly. At this point, the clinical picture is similar to that of an inner third meningioma, including possible extension into the optic canal or superior orbital fissure.

Inner-third meningiomas produce a multitude of symptoms involving the optic nerve and orbit, depending upon which structures are involved and in which order. If the optic canals and optic nerves are involved early, visual loss may be the presenting sign. On the other hand, if the tumor extends through the superior orbital fissure, combinations of cranial nerve palsies and proptosis may precede the visual loss. If the tumor becomes large, it may present as the Foster-Kennedy syndrome: anosmia, unilateral optic atrophy, and contralateral "papilledema." However, the Foster-Kennedy syndrome is more classically associated with subfrontal masses, especially olfactory groove meningiomas.

Usually, meningiomas are easily diagnosed by neuro-imaging. If the symptoms warrant, the treatment is surgical. However, because of their insidiously infiltrative nature, it is rarely possible to effect complete removal. Thus, one must temper one's desire to achieve a total removal with the risk of damage to the structures that are usually intimately involved: the optic nerve, cavernous sinus, and carotid artery.

Other tumors of neurogenic origin are much rarer. One that needs mentioning is the plexiform neuroma associated with neurofibromatosis. Massive enlargement of nerves within the orbit frequently occurs coexistent with enlargement of nerves within the cavernous sinus. The orbital masses can cause proptosis and must be differentiated from optic nerve glioma. A typical wormy plexiform neuroma in the lid of the affected orbit usually suggests the abnormal plexiform involvement of the orbit; this concomitant of neurofibromatosis is independent of an optic nerve glioma, but both may occur in the same patient.

The optic nerve may also be compressed by many other masses arising in or invading the orbit, cranial cavity, or skull. These entities, including the neuropathy associated with thyroid orbitopathy, are considered in Chapter 18.

TOXIC OPTIC NEUROPATHIES

Toxic optic neuropathies (Tables 5–6 and 5–7) are associated with gradual painless, nearly always bilateral, and relatively symmetrical visual loss. Centrocecal scotomas are the commonest visual field defect, although central scotomas and generalized constriction of the fields may occur also. Early in the course, the fundus may appear normal, but eventually nerve fiber layer dropout occurs, especially in the papillomacular bundle. Visual loss may progress to hand motions, but virtually **always** remains hand motions or better. *The patient with total blindness does not have toxic optic neuropathy.* Dyschromatopsia is a frequent early manifestation.

TABLE 5–6. TOXIC OPTIC NEUROPATHIES

Drugs	Optic Disc Swelling	Central Scotoma	Peripheral Visual Field Constriction
Amantidine			
Amoproxan	+	+	
Antibiotics			
Chloroamphenial, sulfonamides,			
Ethambutol, isoniazide,			
Streptomycin			
Arsenicals			
Barbiturates		+	
Chemotherapeutic agents			
Vincristine, methotrex-			
ate,			
BCNU, Cis-platinum			
Chloramphenical	+	+	+
Chlorpropamide		+	
Corticosteroids	+		
Desferoxamine			
Digitalis		+	
Disulfiram			
Emetine	+	+	
Enterovioform			
Ergot preparation		+	+
Ethambutol	+	+	+
Ethchlorvynol (Placidyl)		+	
Hexamethonium			
Hexachlorophene			
Hydroxyquinalones			
Chloroquin			
Diiodohydroxyquin			
Enterovioform			
Hydroxychloroquin		+	
Iodochlorhydroxyquin			
Ibuprofen			
Iodides			
Iodoform	+	+	
Iodopyrocet (Diodrast, IV)			
Isoniazid	+		
Minoxidil	+		
Motrin			
Octamoxin			
Oral contraceptives	+		
Penicillamine	+		
Placidyl			
Phenozone			
Phenipyrazine			
Phenothiazine		+	+
Quinine			+
Streptomycin	+		
Sulfonamides	+	+	
Tolbutamide			
Triparasamide			
Vincristine			

Vitamins			
Decreased			
A			
B_1, B_2, B_6, B_{12}		+	
Folic acid	+	+	
Niacin			
Increased			
A			
D			

TABLE 5—7. TOXIC OPTIC NEUROPATHIES

Environmental Agents	Optic Disc Swelling	Central Scotoma	Peripheral Visual Field Constriction
Aniline dyes	+	+	+
Antimony			+
Arsenic			+
Aspidium			+
Bee sting			
Carbon bisulfide		+	+
Carbon monoxide			
Carbon tetrrachloride			
Cobalt chloride			
DDT			
Dintrobenzyl			
Dinitrotoluene			
Ethylene glycol	+		
Favism	+		
Fluoride	+		
Ketogenic diet			
Lead	+	+	+
Lysol	+		
Mannioc			
Mercury			
Methyl alcohol	+	+	
Organic arsenicals			
Organophosphates	+		
Permanent wave solution	+		
Radiation			
Styrene			
Sulfa drugs	+	+	
Thallium		+	
Tin			
Toluene	+	+	
Trichlorethylene	+		
Wasp sting			

The commonest toxic amblyopia seen in the United States is *nutritional (tobacco or alcohol) amblyopia*. Although originally ascribed to toxic effects of alcohol or tobacco, nutritional amblyopia probably is a vitamin deficiency due to lack of cobalamin (vitamin B_{12}) in the diet. Folic acid, vitamin B_1, vitamin B_6, and niacin deficiencies are also implicated separately or together as causes of nutritional amblyopia. Thus, if patients with toxic amblyopia continue drinking and smoking, but eat well with B-vitamin supplements, visual acuity may improve.

A history of significant alcohol intake is not always easy to obtain. Patients sometimes are more willing to describe their diets than their drinking habits, and so a detailed history of intake of vegetables, salads, and so forth, should be taken. Although the prognosis for recovery of significant vision in this disease is not good (in contrast to some other types of toxic exposure), IM vitamins should be administered immediately and the patient instructed in a proper diet. The presence of bilateral centrocecal scotomas is very rare in optic nerve disease, aside from toxic or nutritional amblyopias. Leber's optic neuropathy is the one other neuropathy characterized by centrocecal scotomas (see the earlier discussion for the differential diagnosis and fascinating similarities).

In most other toxic neuropathies, elimination of the toxin, treatment, or both, usually leads to recovery, although occasionally the recovery may not start for many months after the exclusion of the offending substance.

Leopold suggests zinc sulfate be administered (100 to 250 mg PO TID) if ethambutol, diiodohydroxyquin, or iodochloroxyquine are the toxic substances. Pyridoxine may prevent the toxic side effects of isoniazid and is also thought to be helpful in toxicity associated with monamine oxidase inhibitors.

Aside from "nutritional" amblyopia, the only

toxic amblyopia I have seen in significant numbers is due to ethambutol for treatment of tuberculosis. In ethambutol toxicity, in addition to the early onset of dyschromotopsia, there frequently is the sensation of "pinkness" of vision. If the ethambutol is withdrawn early in the process, the changes are usually reversible. The incidence of this complication is decreasing as awareness of the toxic potential increases and as doses are tailored to the individual patient. It is rare to find significant ocular side effects unless a dose of 15 mg/kg per day is exceeded for several months or drug clearance is impeded by renal tuberculosis.

Methyl alcohol toxicity. Depending upon the amount of alcohol ingested, visual loss occurs within hours to days. Color vision is severely impaired and there are bilateral central scotomas. Early in the course there may be some optic disc swelling, but generally the discs are normal at the time of presentation. If the exposure is minimal, there may be recovery; however, because the exposure is frequently significant, there is more often an inexorable progression to profound optic atrophy and very severe bilateral visual loss. If caught in time, treatment with ethyl alcohol that displaces the methyl alcohol in the metabolic pathways may save vision.

It is obviously impossible to deal with all of the substances thought to be toxic to the optic nerve, their mechanisms, circumstances, toxicity, and treatment. Thus, Tables 5–6 and 5–7 provide a list of substances reported to cause optic nerve toxicity or papilledema. Use the list to double-check for iatrogenic or environmental toxic exposure and then verify the details in the references listed in the Bibliography.

BIBLIOGRAPHY

Optic Neuritis

Alvarez SL. Visual changes mediated by beer in retrobulbar neuritis—an investigative case report. *Br J Ophthalmol.* 1986;70:141–146.

Boghen D, Sabag M, Michaud J. Paraneoplastic optic neuritis and encephalomyelitis. *Arch Neurol.* 1988;45:353–356.

Dutton JJ, et al. Autoimmune retrobulbar neuritis. *Am J Ophthalmol.* 1982;94:11–17.

Hammond SR, et al. The epidemiology of multiple sclerosis in three Australian cities: Perth, Newcastle, and Hobart. *Brain.* 1988;111:1–26.

Killian JM, et al. Controlled pilot trial of monthly IV cyclophosphamide in multiple sclerosis. *Arch Neurol.* 1988;45:27–30.

Miller DH, et al. MRI of the optic nerve in optic neuritis. *Neurology.* 1988;38:175–179.

Rizzo JF, Lessell S. Risk of developing multiple sclerosis after uncomplicated optic neuritis. *Neurology.* 1988;38:185–190.

Rudick RA, et al. Relative diagnostic value of cerebrospinal fluid kappa chains in MS: Comparison with other immunoglobulin tests. *Neurology.* 1989;39:964–968.

Syphilis in HIV-infected persons. *San Francisco Epidemiol Bull.* January 1989;5(1).

Tumors

Albers GW, et al. Treatment response in malignant optic glioma of adulthood. *Neurology.* 1988;38:1071–1074.

Alvord C, Lofton S. Gliomas of the optic nerve or chiasm: Outcome by patient's age, tumor site and therapy. *J Neurosurg.* 1988;68:85–98.

Clark WC, et al. Primary optic nerve sheath meningiomas. *J Neurosurg.* 1989;70:37–40.

Kennerdell JS, et al. Management of optic nerve sheath meningiomas. *Am J Ophthalmol.* 1988;106:450–457.

Listernick R, Charrow J, Greenwald M, Esterly N. Optic gliomas in children with neurofibromatosis type 1. *J Pediatr.* 1989;5:788–792.

Wright JE, McNab AA, McDonald WI. Optic nerve glioma and the management of optic nerve tumours in the young. *Br J Ophthalmol.* 1989;73:967–974.

Wright JE, McNab AA, McDonald WI. Primary optic nerve sheath meningioma. *Br J Ophthalmol.* 1989;73:960–966.

Toxicity

Blondel M, et al. Onze cas de neuropathie a l'almitrine dont une avec neuropathie optique. *Rev Neurol.* 1986;142:683–688.

Fraunfelder FT: *Drug-Induced Ocular Side Effects and Drug Interactions.* 2nd ed. Philadelphia: Lea & Feibiger, 1982.

Gombos G: Bilateral optic neuropathy following minoxidal administration. *Ann Ophthalmol.* 1983;15:259–262.

Grant WM. *Toxicology of the Eye.* 3rd ed. Springfield, IL: Thomas, 1986.

Hamburger HA, Beckman H, Thompson R. Visual evoked potentials and ibuprofen (Motrin) toxicity. *Ann Ophthalmol.* 1984;16:328–329.

Knox DL, et al. Nutritional amblyopia, folic acid, vitamin B_{12} and other vitamins. *Retina.* 1982;2:287–293.

Leopold IH. Optic nerve: Drug-induced optic atrophy. In: Fraunfelder FT, Roy FH, eds. *Current Ocular Therapy.* Philadelphia: Saunders, 1980.

Lessel S. Toxic and deficiency optic neuropathies. In: Smith JL, ed. *Neuro-Ophthalmology.* St. Louis: Mosby, 1973;7.

Miller N, ed. *Walsh and Hoyt's Clinical Neuro-ophthalmology.* 4th ed. Baltimore: Williams & Wilkins, 1982;2.

Olivieri NF, et al. Visual and auditory neurotoxicity in patients receiving subcutaneous desferoxamine infusions. *N Engl J Med.* 1986;314:869–873.

Heredofamilial Disorders of the Optic Nerve

Glaser JS. The eye and systemic disease. In: Goldberg, ME ed. *Goldberg's Genetic and Metabolic Eye Disease.* Boston: Little, Brown, 1986.

CHAPTER 6

DISORDERS OF THE CHIASM, PITUITARY FOSSA, AND PARASELLAR REGION

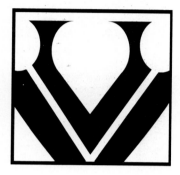

ANATOMY, PHYSIOLOGY, AND EVALUATION

Disorders of the chiasmal region, even those lesions not intrinsic to the visual pathways, frequently cause visual symptoms (Table 6–1). Thus, it is important to understand the anatomy and physiology of chiasmal structures, the best methods for their evaluation, and the important considerations in treating the offending pathology.

The optic chiasm is formed by the junction of the two optic nerves. Within its body occurs the hemidecussation (only the nasal fibers from each retina decussate) of the visual fibers by which each hemisphere occupies itself with the visual environment of the opposite side. This critical structure lies at an angle 45 degrees to the horizontal, approximately 1 cm above the diaphragma sella. It forms a convex lump in the anterior inferior third ventricle, between the infundibular and chiasmatic recesses (Fig. 6–1). It is surrounded by the circle of Willis, which is superior to the chiasm anteriorly and inferior to the chiasm posteriorly. The arterial optic chiasm of the supply is from multiple contiguous arteries, the superior anterior aspects of the chiasm being supplied by the internal carotid, anterior cerebral, and anterior communicating arteries and the inferior portion by the anterior carotid, meningohypophyseal trunk, and other arteries. Some postulate that because this inferior blood supply is by far the more ample and supplies the median raphe of the chiasm especially well, interference with this supply causes the characteristic bitemporal field defects of chiasmal disorders.

Pituitary tumors, the most frequent cause of chiasmal compression, arise from the pituitary fossa, which lies below the chiasm, bordered laterally by the cavernous sinuses. Within the cavernous sinuses pass the internal carotid artery and, in the body of the sinus, the sixth cranial nerve. The third and fourth nerves with the first and second divisions of the trigeminal nerve lie in the walls of the sinus.

Beneath the pituitary fossa is the sphenoid sinus. Both the optic nerves and the carotid arteries may protrude into the body of the sinus, uncovered by any bony protection, an important consideration in transsphenoidal surgery.

Within the visual afferent pathways the macular fibers are proportionately so much more prevalent than others that these pathways may be considered as macular conduits. Within the chiasm the macular fibers tend to cross posteriorly and superiorly where they are at risk in pathology of the anterior third ventricle (eg, ectopic pinealoma) and with dilation of the third venticle in hydrocephalus. In these cases, a central hemianopic bitemporal scotoma is often seen (Fig. 6–2).

Accurate measurements of pituitary hormones in the peripheral blood and computerized scanning have substantially altered the manner in which many patients present to the specialist for medical care. Historically, the majority of patients with pituitary adenomas presented to ophthalmologists with visual field defects. Now, those with secreting tumors or endocrinologic signs and symptoms (eg, the galactorrhea/amenorrhea syndrome, acromegaly) are frequently diagnosed when the tumors are micro-

TABLE 6–1. CAUSES OF CHIASMAL VISUAL LOSS

Malformations and Congenital Anomalies	Encephalocele
	Craniopharyngioma/Rathke pouch cysts
Masses	Extrinsic
	Pituitary tumor
	Meningioma—sphenoid ridge, cavernous sinus
	Ectopic pinealoma
	Intrinsic
	Glioma
Infection and Inflammation	Chiasmal arachnoiditis
	Sarcoid
	Meningitis
Vascular	Compression by aneurysm, dolichoectatic vessels
	Radiation necrosis
Other	Hydrocephalus and dilated anterior third ventricle
	Empty sella syndrome
	Multiple sclerosis and other demyelination
	Trauma

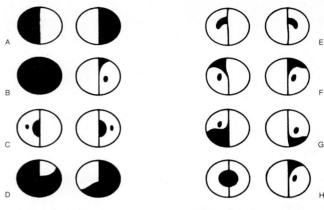

Figure 6–2. Chiasmal field defects. (*From Mills R. Disorders of the visual system. In: Swanson PD, ed. Signs and Symptoms in Neurology. Philadelphia: Lippincott, 1984, with permission.*)

adenomas (less than 1 cm) because we can measure the responsible hormones and detect the small tumors in situ with computed tomography (CT) and magnetic resonance imaging (MRI) scans. Because these tumors are too small to reach up to the optic

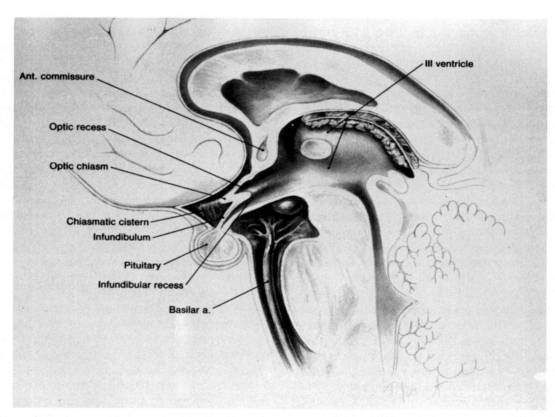

Figure 6–1. Midsagittal section through the cerebral hemispheres, showing the position of the optic chiasm relative to the third ventricle and basal cisterns. (*From Miller N, ed. Walsh and Hoyt's Clinical Neuro-ophthalmology. 4th ed. Baltimore: Williams & Wilkins, 1982;1; with permission.*)

chiasm, these patients rarely have visual field defects. Thus, it is now the patient with the nonsecreting tumor who usually presents first to the ophthalmologist with visual loss, because the endocrinologically silent tumor grows larger before causing symptoms.

The **bitemporal field defect** is the classic visual field defect of chiasm lesions. **Binasal field defects** occur rarely in chiasm lesions. *Much* more frequently, optic nerve lesions (eg, chronic papilledema and optic nerve head drusen) cause the binasal defects.

Relatively complete hemianopias can produce unusual visual symptomatology. Because these symptoms can sound so bizarre, awareness of their occurrence and underlying mechanisms can be quite helpful.

Hemifield slide. In relatively total bitemporal or binasal defects, the remaining normal fields abut along the vertical meridian. Thus, any disturbance in ocular motility—even a minimal phoria—will cause displacement of the field. This can cause a gap in the center of the field through which whole portions of cars, buildings, and other objects may disappear, sometimes with frightening perceptions for the patient (Fig. 6–3). In addition, only a small area of binocular vision remains between the patient's eyes and the point of fixation. Consequently a large scotoma, an area of *postfixational blindness*, exists beyond this point (Fig. 6–4). Patients with complete bitemporal hemianopias may complain of things suddenly disappearing, tilting, or doubling, and of loss of depth perception. Conversely, with binasal field defects there is an area of prefixational blindness and preservation of a wedge of binocular vision beyond fixation.

Disc anomalies are associated with pseudobitemporal field defects (Table 6–2; also Chapter 2). In these cases, careful field testing using several isopters will reveal that the smaller isopters tend to slant obliquely across the vertical meridian, in contrast to true bitemporal field defects in which not only do the defects align reliably along the vertical meridian, but also do so increasingly well as smaller isopters are tested (see Chapter 2). Again, it is worth remembering that when the visual field defects are atypical, as occurs with pre- and postfixed chiasms, a search for bitemporal desaturation of colored targets can be extremely useful and may define bitemporal visual field defects poorly characterized by more "sophisticated" testing.

Other diagnostic considerations. Although visual evoked potential testing cannot indicate the etiology of a chiasmal lesion, recordings made from both hemispheres will sometimes clearly demonstrate the predominant involvement of the crossed fibers that is the concomitant of the bitemporal visual field defect.

Evaluation of pituitary hormones will be covered below as each type of hypersecreting adenoma is considered.

The most powerful methods for evaluation of this region are the scanning modalities.

CT scanning. *Intrinsic lesions of the chiasm* deform the characteristic flat appearance of the chiasm. In *chiasmatic gliomas*, this is frequently a bulbous distension. Where the glioma involves the visual pathway extensively, the chiasm will be swallowed into a large mass that may involve not only the chiasm, but also the optic nerves, optic tracts, hypothalamus, and radiations. Rarely, a craniopharyngioma will invade and distend the optic chiasm and optic nerves.

Pituitary microadenomas generally present as lucent areas within the pituitary fossa, whereas larger adenomas are characterized by upward convexity of the diaphragma sella and even larger adenomas extend beyond the confines of the pituitary fossa. Any abnormal density or enhancement with contrast media may indicate a tumor. When the tumors are quite small, CT scanning with thinner sections and greater spatial resolution may be more sensitive than MRI scanning. Prolactinomas and growth hormone (GH) producing tumors frequently produce asymmetries of the pituitary fossa.

CT scanning is preferable for those lesions where the presence of calcium has diagnostic significance. The presence of calcium suggests a meningioma, aneurysm, or craniopharyngioma. Hyperostosis is especially characteristic of meningiomas.

Eccentric lesions are more likely to be meningiomas or aneurysms. Although most of these masses will cause distortion and molding of bone if they have been present for a long time, actual bone destruction characterizes metastatic lesions. Encasement of the internal carotid artery (ICA) occurs in meningiomas, pituitary adenomas, and chordomas.

CT with intrathecal metrizamide is useful in evaluation of chiasmal syndromes. When plain CT shows a normal sella turcica or is unable to distinguish between an extrinsic and intrinsic lesion, cerebrospinal fluid analysis is often useful in diagnosing inflammatory and infectious disorders.

Angiography plays a role in the diagnostic and presurgical evaluation of both vascular and nonvascular lesions in this area. **Digital subtraction** studies may be adequate to rule out the presence of an aneurysm, verify the exact position of the carotid arteries and other arteries of the region, or locate dolichoectatic vessels and arteriovenous malformations in surgical planning. When detailed views of

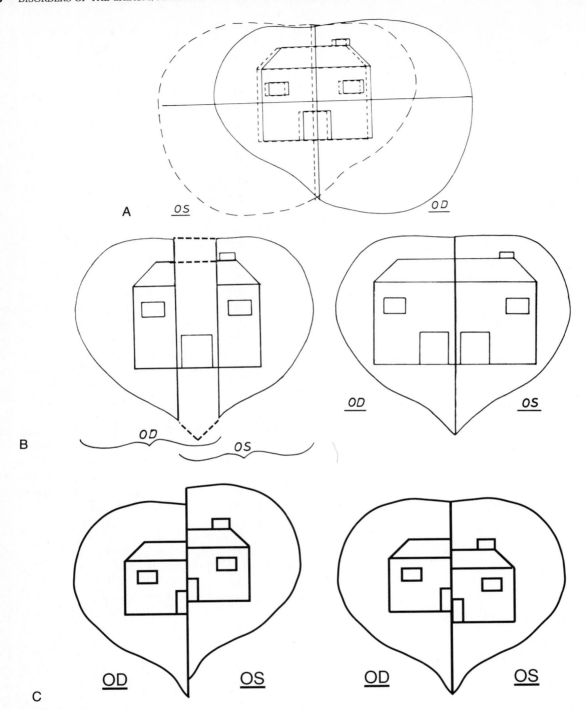

Figure 6–3. Hemisfield slide. Vertical displacement of nasal fields. *(From Nachtigaller H, Hoyt WF. Störungen des Scheindrucks bei bitemporaler Hemianopsie und Verschiebung jeder Schachsen. Kl Mbl Augenheilk. 1970;156:821–836.)*

the lesions are desired, the increased spatial resolution of standard arteriography is necessary.

Motility disorders associated with chiasmal region lesions. Large lesions of this region can extend into or distort the brain stem, with the expected effects on ocular motility. Obviously, lesions extending into the cavernous sinus or arising within the cavernous sinus can affect the third through sixth cranial nerves with resultant palsies and motility disorders. In addition, two unusual types of dissociated nystagmus occur with lesions in this region, a predominantly monocular nystagmus, spasmus nutans, and seesaw nystagmus.

Spasmus nutans is an asymmetric, small-amplitude, jerky, dissociated movement of the eyes that usually presents in early childhood, lasts for

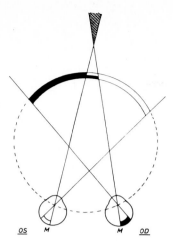

Figure 6–4. Post fixation blindness. The binocular visual field in bitemporal hemianopia. **A.** Orthophoria. *(From Van Balen A. Diplopia in concomitant strabismus and other disturbances of fusion. In: Sanders EACM, et al. eds. Eye Movement Disorders. Hingham, MA: Kluwer Boston, 1987;11; with permission.)*

months to years, and disappears. The abnormal eye movements are associated with a head turn. The etiology is not well understood; there is *no optic atrophy*. However, an acquired nystagmus that is very similar, if not identical, is also seen with chiasmal gliomas, at times associated with the diencephalic syndrome. The triad of acquired monocular nystagmus, the diencephalic syndrome, and optic atrophy is pathognomonic for a chiasmal or hypothalamic glioma.

Seesaw nystagmus results from lesions that extend to or involve by vascular compromise the anterior pretectal region (in the vicinity of the rostral interstitial nucleus of Cajal), usually in combination with a bitemporal field defect. In this most unusual type of nystagmus, one eye rises and intorts while the other depresses and extorts.

PATHOLOGIC CONDITIONS OF THE CHIASMAL REGION

Malformations and Congenital Anomalies

Developmental abnormalities in the chiasmal region not infrequently are associated with dysfunction of

TABLE 6–2. CAUSES OF NONCHIASMAL PSEUDO-BITEMPORAL FIELD DEFECTS

Tilted optic discs
Inferior nasal coloboma
Sector retinitis pigmentosa
Cecocentral scotomata
Gross papilledema, optic nerve head drusen
Overhanging eyelid skin
Drugs (eg, chloroquine)
Bilateral retinal detachments
Hysteria (very rare)

the visual afferent pathways. Hypoplastic and tilted discs, the morning glory syndrome, and other disc anomalies mentioned previously (Chapter 4) may occur not only in association with malformations such as encephaloceles, but also may have associated pseudobitemporal field defects.

Craniopharyngioma. The craniopharyngioma is an histologically benign epithelial mass, frequently with a cystic component, derived from vestiges of the hypophyseal stalk. Although the literature debates whether these tumors are histologically separate from Rathke pouch cysts and epidermoid cysts of this region, because they affect the visual afferent pathways similarly, they will be considered together.

As congenital tumors, they most frequently manifest in childhood but with a second peak of incidence in adulthood. The calcification characteristic of craniopharyngioma is seen more frequently in the tumors presenting in childhood. The frequently solid squamous papillary tumors form approximately one third of adult tumors, do not calcify, have fewer visual defects and more endocrine disorders, and have an excellent prognosis. Adamantinous tumors are usually cystic and recur more frequently. Craniopharyngiomas are the second most common parasellar tumor.

They represent close to 10% of childhood intracranial tumors and nearly half of suprasellar tumors in the pediatric age group. Twenty-seven percent occur in adults; 80% shows visual loss and about half of these will present first to the ophthalmologist.

They present in three ways:

1. Anteriorly protruding tumors push the chiasm back, elevate the anterior cerebral arteries, distort the optic nerves, and produce visual loss. The visual loss may be a bitemporal hemianopia, central or paracentral hemianopic scotoma, or with a more posterior origin and tract involvement, a homonymous hemianopia.
2. More posteriorly protruding tumors push the chiasm forward, fill the third ventricle, and produce hydrocephalus. These patients present with papilledema with or without chiasmal or optic tract visual field defects, depending upon the degree to which those structures are compressed.
3. Smaller tumors may not impinge on the visual afferent pathways, but may enlarge the sella turcica, impair endocrine function, and mimic pituitary adenomas.

Although these tumors usually are slow growing, their proximity to important hypothalamic structures and the visual afferent pathway may produce significant morbidity. Tumors that produce hydrocephalus are associated with headache and vomiting. Compression of the hypothalamus causes diabetes insipidus (rare in pituitary adenomas) and hypopituitarism. Rapid enlargement of the cystic component of the tumor or rupture of the cyst may produce a sudden exacerbation of symptoms or meningitic signs. Characteristic CT and MRI findings (a lobulated mass of nonhomogeneous tissue, frequently harboring a cystic component and calcification), the typical location, and presentation in childhood are nearly pathognomonic. In the adult form the findings are often more subtle and the tumor may become huge before its discovery.

Because of the cystic component, symptoms are often intermittent in craniopharyngioma. Thus, they have sometimes been misdiagnosed as an optic neuritis because of remitting visual loss. However, the age groups in which craniopharyngioma usually presents rarely develop optic neuritis. Craniopharyngiomas almost always are associated with a diffuse optic atrophy; recurrent optic neuritis more often exhibits focal slit-defects in the retinal nerve fiber layer. Although there may be some variability in visual acuity with craniopharyngiomas, there is rarely the complete or nearly complete resolution of visual loss that is the rule in optic neuritis. When appropriate neuro-imaging studies are done, the diagnosis is usually obvious.

The **management of craniopharyngiomas** continues to be controversial. Advances in imaging, microneurosurgery, ultrasonic aspiration, and laser surgery have significantly increased the technical ability to deal with these tumors. In the recent past, efforts to remove the tumors en toto have met with morbidity and some mortality; so-called total removals left deficits and had nearly a 50% recurrence rate. Currently in the hands of experienced neurosurgeons, mortality is very low and morbidity usually limited to diabetes insipidus. Whether surgical advances will further reduce the recurrence rate is uncertain at this point. Incomplete removal plus irradiation leads to a recurrence rate of only 6%. Total removal in experienced hands can achieve apparently complete removal in 90% of cases with a similar low recurrence rate. At this time, the optimum approach is probably the removal of as much tumor as possible without jeopardizing vital contiguous structures, possibly followed by irradiation.

Empty sella syndrome: The empty sella syndrome occurs when the subarachnoid space extends into the sella, remodeling the bone and enlarging the sella. The residual pituitary gland is flattened posteriorly. The *primary empty sella syndrome* is quite common (found in approximately 25% of autopsies) and theorized to result from transfer of cerebrospinal fluid pressure through a congenitally large opening in the diaphragma sella (40% of autopsy cases have an opening in the diaphragmatic sella larger than 5 mm). It is most frequent in multiparous women and elderly arteriosclerotic patients. In affected women there is sometimes concomitant benign intracranial hypertension. The *secondary empty sella syndrome* occurs following irradiation, pituitary surgery, or pituitary apoplexy. The presence of an empty sella does not rule out the coexistence of a pituitary adenoma.

Given the common occurrence of an empty sella, associated visual loss is rare. It is thought to relate to herniation of the suprasellar structures (optic nerves, chiasm, and third ventricle and anterior cerebral arteries) into the sella; or alternatively, scar tissue, fibrosis, and arachnoid adhesions, pulling the chiasm into the sella. Vascular compromise as a result of the distorted anatomy may contribute to the visual loss.

In some instances of the empty sella syndrome, the damage to the visual system is caused by a common etiologic factor such as radiation or arteriosclerotic vascular disease. In a study by Schatz and Schlessinger, for example, 16 of 22 patients with an ischemic chiasmal syndrome had an empty sella.

Most empty sellas are asymptomatic and unassociated with endocrinopathy. However, occasionally patients have a slightly elevated prolactin or other endocrinopathy, headache, or cerebrospinal fluid leak or rhinorrhea.

At times the bony changes may be indistinguishable from those of pituitary tumor, but MRI or CT scanning will reveal the pathognomonic cerebrospinal fluid density within the sella.

Tumors and Inflammation of the Chiasmal Region

Tumors of the chiasmal region comprise 50% of all brain tumors. Of these, 50% are pituitary tumors, 25% craniopharyngiomas, 10% meningiomas, and 5% gliomas.

Intrasellar lesions: Compression of the normal pituitary gland by masses produces hypopituitarism (Table 6–3). The systemic effects of secreted hormones characterize hypersecreting adenomas. Headache is also a frequent symptom of pituitary lesions thought to result from pressure on the diaphragma sella. With expansion of these lesions, the sella is ballooned. Lesions that extend more than 1 cm above the sella may compress the chiasm, interfere with the chiasmal blood supply, and cause visual loss and chiasmatic field defects.

By far the most common intrasellar lesion is a pituitary adenoma. On average, a general ophthalmologist will see 3 patients with chiasmal disorders

TABLE 6–3. ETIOLOGIC CLASSIFICATION OF HYPOPITUITARISM

Developmental Defects	Anencephaly
	Holoprosencephaly (cyclopia, cebocephaly, orbital hypotelorism)
	Midfacial anomalies (eg, hypertelorism)
	Basal encephalocele
	Septo-optic dysplasia (de Morsier's syndrome)
	Cleft lip and palate
	Solitary maxillary central incisor
	Hall-Pallister syndrome (hypothalamic hamartoblastoma, imperforate anus, polydactyly)
	Rieger's syndrome
Genetic Defects of GH (growth hormone) or GRF (growth releasing factor)	Fanconi's syndrome
	Isolated GH deficiency
	Autosomal recessive—type I
	Type 1A—deletion of gene for GH
	Type 1B
	Autosomal dominant—type II
	X-linked—type III
Destructive Lesions	Trauma
	Perinatal (trauma, anoxia, hemorrhagic infarction)
	Basal skull fractures
	Child abuse
Infiltrative Lesions	Tumors
	Histocytosis X
	Craniopharyngioma
	Hypothalamic tumors
	Germinoma
	Optic glioma
	Pituitary adenomas
	Sarcoidosis
	Hemochromatosis
	Tuberculosis
	Toxoplasmosis
	Irradiation (CNS, eyes, middle ears)
	Empty sella with enlarged sella
	Surgery
	Removal of pharyngeal pituitary
	Surgery for craniopharyngioma and other tumors
	Vascular
	Infarctions (eg, hemoglobinopathy)
	Aneurysm
	Autoimmune hypophysitis
Unresponsiveness to Growth Hormone	Insulin-like growth factor I deficiency
	Laron syndrome
	African pygmy
	Bioinactive growth hormone
Other Functional Deficiency	Hypothyroidism
	Psychosocial deprivation

Modified from Behrman RE, Vaughan VC, Nelson WE, eds. Nelson's Textbook of Pediatrics. 13th ed. Philadelphia: Saunders, 1987.

each year. Unfortunately, in one older large series, not one single case of pituitary adenoma was correctly diagnosed at presentation.

With the ability to measure pituitary hormones and to visualize microadenomas on CT and MRI scans, more and more adenomas are detected before suprasellar extension and therefore before visual symptoms and signs develop. In 1973, 70% of patients with pituitary adenomas presented with visual loss. In 1983, the figure was less than 10%. Those tumors that present to the ophthalmologist are likely to be nonsecreting tumors that have grown large enough to compress the chiasm without much in the way of systemic manifestation.

On the other hand, secreting tumors frequently make themselves known by their systemic symptoms. The three most frequent syndromes are (1) Cushing's disease, associated with increased adrenocorticotropic hormone (ACTH) corticotropin production; (2) acromegaly, associated with excess growth hormone production; and (3) infertility, amenorrhea, galactorrhea, and impotence, associated with prolactinemia (Table 6–4).

Thyrotropin and other glycoprotein (FSH, LH) secreting tumors are so rare, TSH secreting tumors and other glycoprotein secreting tumors went unrecognized until 1970. Because of unfamiliarity with them, their appropriate treatment is usually delayed even longer than that of other pituitary tumors. They manifest symptoms of their size: headache, visual loss, hypopituitarism. They frequently become so large that they are not amenable to complete surgical removal. However, recent discovery of a tumor marker elevated in all patients (n = 9) with thyrotropin-secreting tumors may lead to earlier detection. On radioimmunoassay most "non-functioning" tumors produce glycoprotein hormones. Bromocriptine appears to be minimally effective against these tumors. Effective treatment by radiotherapy has not been documented. However, short-term efficacy of a long-acting somatostatin analogue has been reported. Mixed-hormone-secreting tumors are even rarer.

Cushing's disease (corticotropin secreting adenomas). Cushing's disease of pituitary origin must be differentiated from rarer causes of ACTH hypersecretion, adrenal tumors, sources of ectopic ACTH production, and chronic alcoholosm (alcoholic pseudo-Cushing's) causing **Cushing's syndrome** (Fig. 6–5). Approximately 80% of noniatrogenic Cushing's disease cases are caused by microadenomas. But many of these tumors are small, intraglandular, and hard to find by the best of imaging efforts (MRI with gadolinium is most sensitive, detecting about 10% of corticotropin secreting tumors) or even at surgery. However, sampling of blood from the petrosal sinus for ACTH sometimes establishes the presence of a hypersecreting tumor, even when the CT doesn't show it. Prompt diagnosis is critical because of the life-threatening complications of Cushing's syndrome.

TABLE 6–4. TRANSSPHENOIDAL MICROSURGERY FOR PITUITARY ADENOMA[a]

Tumor	Number of Patients (Total = 968)
Prolactin (PRL) adenoma	394 (41%)
Null-cell adenoma ("Nonfunctioning")	262 (27%)
GH adenoma (acromegaly)	173 (18%)
ACTH adenoma (Cushing's disease)	105 (11%)
ACTH adenoma (Nelson's syndrome)	34 (3%)

[a] Mayo Clinic 1972–1983.
From Laws ER. *Management of Prolactin-secreting pituitary adenomas.* In: Johnson RT, ed. *Current Therapy in Neurologic Disease. Philadelphia:* Decker, 1985.

Since introduction of sensitive, high-resolution scanning techniques for identification of pituitary microadenomas, adrenalectomy for treatment of Cushing's syndrome now is rarely done. Consequently, Nelson's syndrome has become rare. Nelson's syndrome comprises chiasmal visual field defects and hyperpigmentation of the skin, the result of highly aggressive pituitary adenomas that proliferate after inappropriate adrenalectomy for Cushing's disease and secrete melanocyte-stimulating hormone.

Growth-hormone-secreting tumors. In adults, excess growth hormone (GH) results in acromegaly; in children, GH excess results in gigantism. Characteristic acromegalic features include enlargement of hands and skull, especially the jaw. Excess GH is associated with an increased incidence of cardiovascular disease, athritis, hypertension, diabetes, pulmonary infections, thyroud abnormalities (including toxic nodular and nontoxic goiter), cancer, and the carpal tunnel syndrome. Enlarged extraocular muscles also occur although actual exophthalmus is rare. Most GH-secreting tumors also secrete at least one other hormone.

Treatment is usually surgical, although a trial with dopaminergic drugs or somatostatin analogues may be worthwhile. Treatment goals include reducing tumor size, and restoring GH secretion to normal. Dopaminergic agents, however, are much less effective than in treatment of prolactinomas; endogenous GH usually decreases by 50% or more, but rarely becomes normal and tumor size is little affected. In contrast, somatostatin analogs such as octreotide often decrease tumor volume substantially.

Prolactinomas. A large number of pituitary tumors are prolactinomas. They predominate in women and are heralded by galactorrhea and amenorrhea. In men, they produce gonadal dysfunction, oligospermia, and decreased libido. Because of the obvious effects of hormone excess, most tumors detected in women are microadenomas; men more commonly come to diagnosis with large tumors causing headache and visual loss.

Elevation of serum prolactin itself is nonspecific; it is elevated in about 30% of hypothalamic pituitary region disorders other than pituitary adenoma (craniopharyngioma, meningioma, atypical teratoma, metastases, sarcoid, histiocytosis X, empty sella, aneurysm, and so forth Table 6–5); and by many drugs (Table 6–6); the elevation is nondiagnostic and relatively moderate (less than 100 μg/mL). Significant elevation of prolactin (between 100 and 1000 μg/mL) is indicative of prolactinoma. Massive elevations (levels exceeding 1000 μg/mL) of prolactin are frequently indicative of invasive adenomas.

Management of pituitary adenomas. Therapeu-

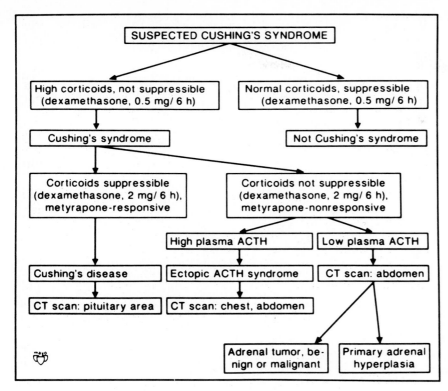

Figure 6–5. Evaluation of patients with suspected Cushing's syndrome. Because some medications alter ACTH production rate, patients should be medication-free before initiation of assessment. (*From Carpenter P. Cushing's syndrome—Update of diagnosis and management. Mayo Clinic Proc. 1986;61:51, with permission.*)

tic goals in pituitary adenomas include: (1) the control of compressive effects of expansive tumors, especially chiasmal compression; (2) preservation or restoration of fertility; (3) control of adverse effects of hypopituitarism; and (4) control of effects of hypersecretion. There are three principal modes of therapy: medical, surgical, and radiation. The therapies achieve these goals by eliminating tumor mass, normalizing hormone secretion, and preventing recurrence.

The development of pharmacologic agents, principally dopaminergic agents such as bromocriptine and somatostatin analogues, which effectively shrink the tumors and halt their hypersecretion, has radically altered the management of these tumors. These agents are most effective in prolactinomas but may also be effective in GH and corticotropin-secreting tumors.

Somatostatin analogues seem to have a role in treating TSH- and perhaps GH-secreting tumors as well. Ketoconazole, an antimycotic agent, is somewhat successful in treatment of corticotropin-secreting tumors.

When the only clinical problems are the adverse effects of excess hormone, treatment with these agents may be sufficient. When it is not, transsphe-

TABLE 6–5. CAUSES OF AMENORRHEA-GALACTORRHEA

1. Central
   - A. Functional
     1. Postpartum (Chiari-Frommel syndrome)
     2. Idiopathic (Ahumada-del Castillo syndrome)
   - B. Organic
     1. Pituitary
        - a. Prolactin-secreting tumor (Forbes' disease, Albright's disease)
        - b. Other tumors: meningioma, craniopharyngioma aneurysm, cysts, ectopic pinealoma
        - c. Inflammatory
        - d. Stalk section
        - e. Empty sella
     2. Hypothalamic
        - a. Neoplasm
        - b. Inflammatory
   - C. Drug Action
2. Peripheral
   - A. Metabolic/endocrine disorders
     1. Hypothyroidism, cirrhosis, renal failure, stress
   - B. Neoplasm
     1. Ectopic-prolactin-producing tumor
   - C. Neurogenic
     1. Chest wall trauma, surgery, or herpetic lesion
     2. Breast lesion
3. Pregnancy

From Young RL, Pruett KM. The amenorrha-galactorrhea syndrome. In: Smith JL, Katz RS, eds. Neuro-ophthalmology Enters the 90s. Miami: Dutton Press, 1989.

TABLE 6–6. DRUGS THAT INCREASE CIRCULATING PROLACTIN OR STIMULATE LACTATION

Phenothiazines
    Alpha-adrenergic receptor blockers
Rauwolfia
    Catecholamine storage depletion and receptor blockage
Tricyclic antidepressants
    Receptor blockers
Opiates (codeine, morphine, methadone)
    Block catecholamine reuptake
Methyldopa, carbidopa
    Inhibit metabolism of dopa to dopamine
Haloperidol (butyrophenone)
Thioxanthenes
    Receptor blockers
Thyroid-releasing factor
    Prolactin release
Sex steroids, including birth control pills
    Stimulate prolactin secretion (locally inhibit lactation)
Corticosteroids
    Action similar to sex steroids
Spironolactone
    Action similar to sex steroids
Piperoxane
    Alpha-adrenergic antagonist
Metoclopramide
    Dopamine antagonist
Neutral amino acids (alpha-methylotyrosine, alpha-methyldopa)
    Catecholamine metabolism inhibition
Pimozide, clonidine, phenoxybenzamine, phentolamine, propanolol, reserpine

From Smith JL, ed. Neuro-ophthalmology: Focus 1980. *New York: Masson, 1979.*

noidal removal is usually curative for microadenomas. This neurosurgical approach is also effective for many tumors that extend out of the sella. Only very massive tumors must be approached transcranially. The decision for a transcranial approach must be made cautiously, because of its increased morbidity. Frequently the transsphenoidal approach provides sufficient decompression to relieve symptoms even if total ablation of the tumor cannot be achieved. The beneficial results of surgical therapy are usually inversely proportional to the size of the tumor. Postoperative radiation is optional for residual tumor. Elderly or debilitated patients who cannot withstand surgery may be treated with primary radiation.

The therapeutic decisions become more complicated when prolactinomas occur in young women (Fig. 6–6). If the patient wishes to become pregnant, the same considerations pertain. If the tumor does not threaten the visual pathways or hypothalamus, the patient may be treated with bromocriptine and followed closely with serial visual fields. Prolactinomas have a bimodal growth pattern during pregnancy, enlarging prior to 14 weeks in patients with a

short history (less than 4 years) of amenorrhea and after 24 weeks in patients with a long (more than 10 years) history of amenorrhea. However, recent evidence suggests that pregnancy neither initiates prolactinoma formation nor accelerates their growth. Approximately 5% of microadenomas and 35% of macroadenomas will increase in size significantly during pregnancy. Should field loss ensue in a patient with a very small microadenoma that has been untreated or a patient with a macroadenoma, bromocriptine may be used safely in pregnancy. No adverse effects on either the fetus or the mother have been found. If the tumor still appears to be growing, further compromising the visual system or hypothalamus, transsphenoidal surgery can be done without sacrificing the pregnancy.

The effectiveness of bromocriptine is impressive. In 73% of cases it will acutely shrink the tumor; it will normalize prolactin in more than 95% of cases. Fertility will be restored in 80 to 90% of cases. However, the tumor may reexpand frighteningly if therapy is ever discontinued willingly or through patient noncompliance; on the other hand, growth of the tumor during bromocriptine therapy is very rare.

Following delivery, around 10% of the tumors autoablates and ovulatory cycles resume. Any visual field deficits that were present usually improve. If further pregnancy is desired, this is the time to consider surgery.

Regardless of the treatment modality chosen, these patients need continual follow-up as the hormonal abnormalities may recur even after apparent total tumor removal or may abate spontaneously.

The rare *invasive adenoma* is associated with very high hormone levels. These tumors usually invade the cavernous sinus, producing multiple cranial nerve palsies. Facial pain is especially characteristic.

Other intrasellar masses. The presence of any other mass within the sella is unusual. Those that do occur include tumors that are usually suprasellar, such as craniopharyngiomas, atypical teratomas, ectopic pinealomas, and metastases.

Metastases occur in about 17% of patients with disseminated carcinoma but are rarely detected antemortem. Metastatic carcinoma to the pituitary is associated with a 71% incidence of diabetes insipidus, an important clue to the diagnosis.

Arachnoid cysts occasionally present in the sella. Vascular structures (eg, dolichoectatic arteries, especially the basilar artery and aneurysms) may make their way into the sella as well; thus, it is obligatory to localize the major vessels of the region prior to any surgery. Of course, the contents of the sella may be involved by infectious and inflammatory processes, as may any other part of the body.

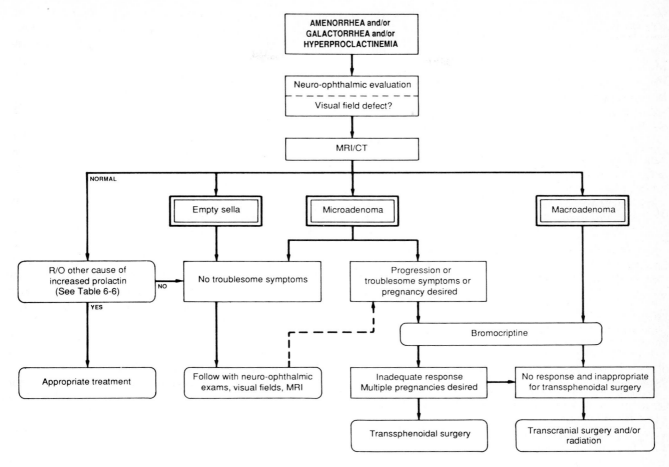

Figure 6—6. Management of hyperprolactinemia.

Pituitary abscess is diagnosed by discovering meningitis in combination with an enlarged sella, a known pituitary tumor, or a chiasmal field defect. The first line of treatment is antibiotics, but these frequently are not very successful; if there is no response within 48 hours, the abscess should be drained transsphenoidally.

Lymphocytic adenohypophysitis is diffuse lymphocytic infiltration of the hypophysis, thus far recognized nearly exclusively in women. Fifty-five percent of the time it is related to pregnancy, possibly to immune alterations during the pregnant state. Presenting as a pituitary mass, it can be differentiated from nonsecreting tumors only by biopsy. Other autoimmune afflictions of endocrine glands (eg, thyroiditis) are associated on occasion.

Pituitary apoplexy, one of few true neuro-ophthalmic emergencies, is characterized by the acute onset of neurologic, ophthalmologic, and endocrinologic symptoms. It is caused by hemorrhage into an adenoma (which occurs in about 15% of adenomas) and threatens both life and vision. Unfortu-

nately, it is rarely diagnosed promptly. The acute presentation of headache, cranial nerve palsies, and decreased vision suggests the diagnosis. Symptoms of the adenoma usually precede the apoplectic event but may not be elicited from the seriously ill patient. Acutely, these patients present to the emergency room and not the physician's office. Either CT or MRI scanning shows an enlarged sella and intratumoral, subarachnoid, or intraventricular bleeding. There are usually meningeal signs and CSF leukocytosis.

Untreated, many cases of pituitary apoplexy are fatal. Medical therapy includes administration of high-dose corticosteroids, hormonal replacement, and management of diabetes insipidus or inappropriate ADH as necessary. If the patient does not stabilize, or shows significant visual loss or depression of consciousness, surgical decompression may be lifesaving. Transsphenoidal surgery is possible, even in patients too ill to undergo transcranial surgery. The prognosis for recovery of vision and recovery from ophthalmoplegia is generally good if decompression is accomplished promptly.

Multiple endocrine neoplasia, type I (MEN I) is characterized by multifocal adenomatous proliferation involving the parathyroid glands, pancreatic island cells, anterior lobe of the pituitary gland, and other adenomatous tissues. The syndrome appears to be inherited through a dominant pleiotropic gene with variable expressivity. Primary hyperparathyroidism (which occurs in 97% of the patients) is the most frequent manifestation. The other abnormalities, including Zollinger-Ellison syndrome, occur with very variable rates; however, autopsy studies suggest that given sufficient time, parathyroid, pituitary, and pancreatic disease would develop in 100% of MEN I patients. Multiple lipomas and the carcinoid syndrome are also associated.

Multiple endocrine neoplasia, type II (MEN II) involves the thyroid most frequently and is also associated with pheochromocytomas and parathyroid adenomas, but not pituitary adenomas. Prominent corneal nerves are characteristic.

PARACHIASMAL AND PARASELLAR LESIONS

Suprasellar Lesions

Suprasellar lesions cause signs and symptoms of displacement or compression of optic nerves, the chiasm, and the optic tracts. The visual field defects may be typical of optic neuropathy, chiasm, or tract lesions, or may be combinations of these that are difficult to identify. There may be loss of visual acuity or optic atrophy. In addition, hypothalamic dysfunction is manifested by growth retardation, diabetes insipidus, or obesity; sleep disorders also may appear. If the mass is large, compression of the cerebrospinal fluid pathways may result in increased intracranial pressure, papilledema, and headache.

Chiasmatic glioma. The most frequent and significant intrinsic mass of the chiasm is the glioma. Gliomas usually present in childhood and are very-low-grade malignancies that do their damage by local invasion and compression. Most chiasmal gliomas present with decreased visual acuity and optic atrophy. Hypothalamic dysfunction is often present. Unique syndromes that may be present in association with chiasmal gliomas include the diencephalic syndrome with spasmus-nutans-like eye movements. Interestingly, the abnormal eye movements and diencephalic syndrome often resolve after irradiation, even though no change is apparent in the glioma. Seesaw nystagmus may also be present in lesions of this area.

Vascular lesions. Suprasellar aneurysms and dolichoectatic vessels may arise from any of the numerous arteries of the region, but most frequently involve the internal carotid artery, ophthalmic artery, and anterior communicating arteries. Occasionally, aneurysms arising from the basilar tip may extend into this region.

Aneurysms involving other arteries of this region may be either giant aneurysms or smaller aneurysmal ectasias that are more likely to rupture. When large enough to cause symptoms from mass effect, these are usually slated for surgical removal. Giant aneurysms are more difficult to attack and their surgical approach is somewhat more controversial; the decision to operate or attempt ablation using interventional radiology frequently depends upon the degree of associated symptomatology and proximity to contiguous structures that could be damaged by treatment.

Meningiomas. Meningiomas of this region arise from the tuberculum sella or sphenoid wing as well as within the cavernous sinus. The group most frequently affected is middle-aged women. If orbital involvement is massive, proptosis, chemosis, and engorgement of orbital vasculature ensues. CT scanning may better reveal the hyperostosis and calcification present in these tumors, although MRI portrays the tissue involvement better. Meningioma most frequently encases the internal carotid artery. When the tumors are extensive, decompression rather than total removal may be wisest. Meningiomas that predominantly involve the optic nerve are covered in Chapter 5. These tumors frequently cause loss of vision that occurs insidiously over a long period of time.

Rarer suprasellar masses. The histiocytic disorders (formerly Weber-Christian disease, Lederer-Siwe disease, and so forth) form a continuum of disease caused by a proliferation of Langerhans' cells, a subpopulation of the mononuclear phagocytic system; they are classified into unifocal eosinophilic granuloma of bone, multifocal eosinophilic granuloma of bone, or diffuse histiocytosis X. The orbit is a common site of involvement in eosinophilic granuloma but is less commonly involved in diffuse histiocytosis.

Prognosis is determined by the age at onset and, to some degree, by the histologic diagnosis. Eighty-seven percent of those who develop disease after age 2 survive, in contrast to 46% of those who develop it before then. Those tumors with more extensive involvement, more organs involved, and more organ dysfunction have a poorer prognosis. Pulmonary symptoms are particularly ominous, whereas bone lesions are associated with a more favorable course.

There is almost no mortality associated with unifocal eosinophilic granuloma, and many modalities of treatment are available. In multifocal eosinophilic granuloma with widespread lesions or lesions resistent to irradiation, systemic chemotherapy is often effective. However, in the diffuse multisite multisystem histiocytosis, even with cytotoxic therapy the prognosis is poor. Treatment with a thiamine extract has been reported to be somewhat effective.

Ectopic germinoma/pinealoma. These tumors have the same histologic appearance as pinealomas, present in the suprachiasmatic area, the hypothalamus, or the third ventricle and occur during the first and second decades. There is an equal predilection for boys and girls, whereas pinealomas predominantly affect boys. Diabetes insipidus is frequently the first symptom; visual field defects, optic atrophy, and hypophyseal dysfunction may be associated. Scanning shows an isodense, large, noncalcified mass. The children usually show growth retardation.

Rarely, these masses are part of the trilateral retinoblastoma syndrome, in which pineoblastomas and bilateral retinoblastomas are found as part of the hereditary blastoma picture. These patients all have a positive family history. The age of onset of their tumors is early relative to the average age of onset for either retinoblastoma or pineoblastoma. The retinoblastoma usually manifests before 6 to 8 months and the pineoblastoma before 10 years of age.

Other rare lesions, including malformations of the third ventricle and absence of the septum pellucidum and vellum cavi, may occasionally cause sufficient distortion to be symptomatic.

Infrasellar lesions. These lesions most frequently present with cerebrospinal fluid rhinorrhea and nasopharyngeal masses. Occasionally, infrasellar lesions such as sphenoid sinus mucocele and nasopharyngeal carcinoma invade upward, causing optic nerve or chiasmal involvement and cranial nerve palsies. In the case of nasopharyngeal carcinoma, it is the sixth nerve that is most frequently involved early.

Retrosellar lesions. These lesions, which often involve the optic tract, also cause memory loss due to involvement of the temporal lobes and mammillary bodies and, if large enough, brain-stem syndromes. Any of the cranial nerves transversing this area may be effected as well. Because of the tract involvement, these lesions will be covered in Chapter 7.

Parasellar lesions sometimes enlarge laterally to involve the temporal lobe and cause seizures, particularly uncinate fits. Other less common lesions are tumors of the base of the skull, chordomas, osteochordomas, gangliofibromas, aneurysmal bone cysts, and angiofibromas.

Intracavernous aneurysms. Intracavernous aneurysms occur most frequently in middle-aged women. They present with headache that may be abrupt in onset, and ophthalmoplegia. Nearly 20% of cavernous sinus syndromes is caused by these aneurysms. Possibly because of their investment by the surrounding sinus tissues, they are unlikely to rupture; their effect is predominantly that of a mass. On CT or MRI one can see ballooning of the cavernous sinus and bony expansion or destruction of the adjacent skull. Cavernous meningiomas, pituitary adenomas, or chordomas also cause expansion of the cavernous sinus but encase a carotid artery of relatively normal size.

Aneurysmal masses are easily identified on either CT or MRI scans unless they are totally thrombosed. New symptoms occur at the time of enlargement or thrombosis. The MRI scan usually will show changes in the composition of the blood contained within the aneurysm. The mass may enlarge the superior orbital fissure and erode into the orbit. If it extends upwards, it may undermine the optic canal and cause loss of vision, as do other masses growing in this region. Aberrant regeneration of the third nerve may ensue primarily or following the initial ophthalmoplegia. If the mass involves the trigeminal nerve, pain in the face frequently accompanies episodes of enlargement.

Infectious and inflammatory lesions such as sarcoid, tuberculosis, Lyme disease, Epstein-Barr virus, and syphilis, may involve chiasmal, sellar, or parasellar structures. Involvement is usually associated with meningeal thickening on contrast-enhancing CT or MRI scans. Sarcoid usually involves the hypothalamus primarily and is often associated with diabetes insipidus. Less frequently, tuberculomas and mycotic aneurysms present as mass lesions. Abnormalities of the cerebrospinal fluid may be helpful for diagnosis.

BIBLIOGRAPHY

Pituitary Adenomas

Adamson TE, Wiestler OD, et al. Correlation of clinical and pathological features in surgically treated craniopharyngiomas. *J Neurosurg.* 1990;73:12–17.

Anderson D, et al. Pituitary tumors and the ophthalmologist. *Ophthalmology.* 1983;90:1265.

Gesundheit N, Petrick P, et al. Thyrotropin-secreting pituitary adenomas: Clinical and biochemical heterogeneity. Case reports and follow-up of nine patients. *Ann Intern Med.* 1989;111:827–835.

Hollenhorst RE, Younge BR: Ocular manifestations produced by adenomas of the pituitary gland. In: Kohler PO, Ross GT, eds. *Diagnosis and Treatment of Pituitary Tumors.* New York: American Elsevier, 1973:53–68.

Klibanski Ann, Zervas Nicholas. Diagnosis and management of hormone-secreting pituitary adenomas. *NEJM.* 1991;324:822–831.

Laws ER. Management of prolactin-secreting pituitary adenomas. In: Johnson RT, ed. *Current Therapy in Neurologic Disease.* Philadelphia: Decker, 1985.

Oldfield EH, et al. Preoperative lateralization of ACTH-secreting pituitary microadenomas by bilateral and simultaneous inferior petrosal venous sinus sampling. *N Engl J Med.* 1985;312:100–103.

Scheithauer BW, Sano T, Kovacs K, et al. The pituitary gland in pregnancy: A clinicopathologic and immunohistochemical study of 69 cases. *Mayo Clin Proc.* 1990; 65:461–474.

Segal AJ, Fishman RS. Delayed diagnosis of pituitary tumors. *Am J Ophthalmol.* 1975;79:77–81.

Yasargil MG, Curcic M, et al. Total removal of craniopharyngiomas. Approaches and long-term results in 144 patients. *J Neurosurg.* 1990;73:3–11.

Empty Sella

Schatz NJ, Schlessinger NS. Noncompressive causes of chiasmal disease. *Trans New Orleans Acad Ophthalmol.* 1976;vol: p.

Hemifield Effects

Kirkham TH. The ocular symptomatology of pituitary tumors. *Proc Roy Soc Med.* 1972;65:517.

Nachtigaller H, Hoyt WF. Störungen des Scheindrucks bei bitemporaler Hemianopsie und Verschiebung jeder Schachsen. *Kl Mbl Augenheilk.* 1970;156:821–836.

Hypopituitarism

Behrman Re, Vaughan VC, Nelson WE, eds. *Nelson's Textbook of Pediatrics.* 13th ed. Philadelphia: Saunders, 1987.

CHAPTER 7

DISORDERS OF THE POSTCHIASMAL VISUAL AFFERENT PATHWAYS

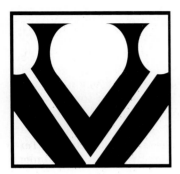

The hallmark of postchiasmal visual afferent pathways lesions is a homonymous hemianopic visual field defect. Homonymous defects align themselves along the vertical meridian and, unless bilateral, do not decrease visual acuity. A *total homonymous hemianopia has no localizing value;* in contrast, partial homonymous hemianopias often suggest the site of the lesion by their degree of congruity: the more congruous, the more posterior. Additionally, postchiasmal disorders are diagnosed by the character of the field defect, the history, and associated findings frequently caused by damage to contiguous structures (Table 7–1).

OPTIC TRACT LESIONS

Optic tract lesions are exceedingly rare, representing only about 3% of hemianopsias. When the hemianopsia is incomplete, tract hemianopsias usually are quite incongruous. In lesions present long enough for retrograde degeneration, there is associated optic atrophy, frequently in a horizontal band (bow-tie configuration) typical of the ipsilateral temporal field defect associated with a contralatral tract lesion (see Chapter 3). In contradistinction to lesions involving the parietal lobes, optokinetic nystagmus is normal.

Lesions that also involve the hypothalamus cause endocrine and autonomic disturbances. If the brain stem is involved, there are disturbances of consciousness and contralateral pyramidal tract signs; if the lesions extend laterally to involve the temporal lobe, there may be seizures. The contralateral pupil may be larger (Behr's sign—really an ipsilateral Horner's syndrome) and if the optic nerve is in-

volved, an ipsilateral afferent pupillary defect may also be present.

The optic tracts are susceptible to the same disorders that affect the chiasm. They may be involved by posterior extension of pituitary adenomas or intrinsic optic pathway lesions: chiasmatic and hypothalamic gliomas, craniopharyngiomas, aneurysms, and demyelinating disorders such as multiple sclerosis.

Infarcts, like demyelinating lesions, usually present suddenly. In contrast, compressive lesions such as tumors and aneurysms usually cause more insidious symptoms.

LESIONS OF THE LATERAL GENICULATE NUCLEUS

Lateral geniculate body lesions are even rarer than those of the optic tracts. They comprise about 1% of hemianopic lesions. Occasionally the lateral geniculate is involved by tumors, but more frequently lesions of this region are of vascular origin. A characteristic "keyhole" hemianopia is seen (Fig. 7–1), although this visual field is also caused by lesions of adjacent optic radiations.

LESIONS OF THE PARIETAL AND TEMPORAL LOBES

Lesions of the retrogeniculate visual afferent pathways are rarely associated with optic atrophy. (Congenital lesions or acquired lesions of long standing may cause transsynaptic degeneration.)

Temporal Lobe Lesions

Typically, the hemianopic defect of temporal lobe lesions begins in the upper quadrants, the "pie in the

TABLE 7–1. HOMONYMOUS HEMIANOPIA—ASSOCIATED FINDINGS

Temporal lobe	Parietal lobe	Occipital lobe
Field defect denser superiorly	Field defect denser inferiorly	Isolated hemianopia
Uncinate fits	Abnormal optokinetic nystagmus	Very congruous visual field defects
Hemiplegia	Aphasia	Alexia without agraphia (dominant hemisphere lesion)
Aphasia	Agraphia	Normal optokinetic nystagmus
Alexia	Acalculia Astereognosia	
Hemianesthesia	Right–left confusion	
Anosognosia	Extinction	
Normal optokinetic nystagmus	Construction/ dressing apraxias	

From Mills R. Disorders of the visual system. In: Swanson PD, ed. Signs and Symptoms in Neurology. Philadelphia: Lippincott, 1984.

sky" visual field defect. Again, the history and symptoms will frequently be the best clue to the nature of the causative lesion, with vascular and demyelinating lesions having a relatively acute onset and tumors a slower course. Occasionally, patients experience hallucinations that may be formed or uncinate, and

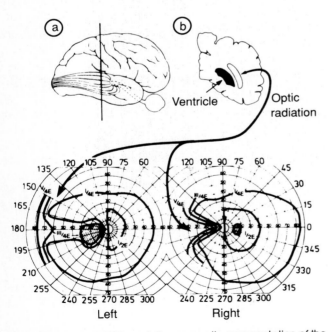

Figure 7–1. Visual fields and diagrammatic representation of the visual radiations seen from the side (**A**) and in cross section (**B**) of a patient with a "key-hole" hemianopia. The shaded area is the proposed site of the lesion. (*From Carter JE, O'Connor P. Lesions of the optic radiations mimicking lateral geniculate nucleus visual field defects. J Neurol Neurosurg Psychiatry. 1985;48:982–988, with permission.*)

ominous in character. Especially in younger patients, the causative lesion is likely to be a tumor.

Parietal Lobe Lesions

Lesions of the parietal lobe cause a range of symptoms. Two oculomotor abnormalities are characteristic of parietal lesions, but are very uncommon in tract, temporal lobe, or occipital lesions: (1) Optokinetic nystagmus abnormalities characterized by a diminished slow phase, with rotation of objects toward the side of the lesion (see Chapter 11); and (2) conjugate deviation of the eyes with forced closure of the lids (spastic deviation, Cogan's sign).

Spasticity of conjugate gaze is elicited by asking the patient to forcibly close the lids. If the examiner tries to open them, the eyes are seen to deviate toward the opposite side, in contrast to the normal Bell's phenomenon in which the eyes both deviate upward and outward (see Chapter 11).

Because the parietal cortex is predominantly concerned with sensory modalities, many lesions in this region cause sensory symptoms. *Astereoagnosia* denotes an inability to recognize objects by touch. Thus, the patient is unable to recognize an object placed in the hand opposite the side of the lesion. Vibration sense, two-point discrimination, and position sense may also be lost on the contralateral side of the body.

These patients often show extinction and inattention and may be very difficult to test adequately. The extinction phenomenon may be found by presenting stimuli simultaneously in both hemifields.

Visual symptoms incude metamorphopsia and difficulty with color vision as well as photopsias, hallucinations, and illusions. These latter phenomena tend to occur in the defective portion of the visual field (see Chapter 9). Seizures are also quite frequent in parietal cortex lesions.

Large expansive supratentorial lesions may cause herniation of the hippocampus through the tentorial notch. Third nerve compression results in unilateral mydriasis (a "blown" pupil), and brainstem compression causes decreased consciousness, gaze palsies, internuclear ophthalmoplegia, and nystagmus. If the posterior cerebral arteries are compressed, blindness or hemianopsia may occur.

Disconnection syndromes, disorders of higher visual function, and lesions of the parietal area: These syndromes, such as *alexia*, often involve visual cognitive function. *Alexia* is the loss of comprehension of the written word and is associated with other unusual symptoms of dominant hemisphere lesions—loss of the ability to write (agraphia) and loss of color perception. Prosopagnosia (the inability to recognize familiar faces) also results from lesions in this region. *Alexia with agraphia* is associated with lesions in the region of the angular gyrus and causes an inability to read and write. However, lesions in the region of the splenium of the corpus callosum and dominant anterior occipital lobe cause alexia without agraphia, so the patient cannot read what he or she writes. Visual spatial disorders, especially in lesions of the nondominant hemisphere, include inability to recognize familiar locations or to find one's way through familiar geography (Tables 7–2 to 7–4).

In summary, **lesions of the parietal lobe of the dominant hemisphere disturb language and visual recognition; those of the nondominant hemisphere cause topographic agnosias.**

Large, bilateral parietal lesions may result in **Balint's syndrome,** an extreme lack of awareness of the environment and acquired oculomotor apraxia (see Chapter 12).

The parietal and temporal regions are affected by the common tumors of the central nervous system, including astrocytomas, glioblastomas, and metastases. Because of proximity, temporal lobe tumors more often cause brainstem compression. More acute syndromes occur with vascular accidents, demyelination, and infection.

OCCIPITAL LOBE DISORDERS

The predominant symptom of occipital lesions is a strictly hemianopic defect that tends to be congruous. The one exception is a lesion of the monocular temporal crescent (a lesion involving the anterior portion of the calcarine cortex). Smaller lesions tend to cause the homonymous paracentral scotomas that are pathognomonic of occipital pole disease. Also characteristic is an absence of other symptoms: Optokinetic nystagmus is normal and there is no spasticity of conjugate gaze. The agnosias and spatial disorientation frequent in parietal lesions occur only with anterior lesions that also involve the parietal areas. Hallucinations are relatively rare, although irritative lesions may cause photopsias, which are usually unformed (see Chapter 9). The scintillating

TABLE 7–3. HIGHER VISUAL SYNDROMES ASSOCIATED WITH LESIONS IN THE DISTRIBUTION OF THE POSTERIOR CEREBRAL ARTERIES

Positive phenomena
Hallucinations
Palinopsia
Negative phenomena
Alexia
   Without agraphia
   Hemialexia (unilateral neglect)
Agnosia
   Prosopagnosia
   Visual object agnosia
   Agnosia for environment
Central achromatopsia
Loss of brightness modulation
   Dimness
   Dazzle
Unilateral neglect
Visual field defects
   Cerebral blindness
   Temporal crescent defects
   Homonymous hemianopia
   Homonymous quadrantanopsia
   Altitudinal defects
Absent revisualization (Charcot-Wilbrand syndrome)

From Alexander MP, Cummings JL. Higher-visual functions. In: Lessel S, Van Dalen JTW, eds. Neuro-ophthalmology. Amsterdam: Elsevier, 1984;3.

scotomas of migraine are an exception (see Chapter 8). Again, as in all retrogeniculate lesions, the pupillary responses are normal and there is no optic atrophy.

Bilateral lesions cause *cortical blindness,* which may be associated with denial of the presence of blindness (*Anton's syndrome*). Frequently hemianopia is denied as well. Less often, these patients will also confabulate and hallucinate.

TABLE 7–4. PROPOSED LATERALITY OF INVOLVEMENT OF HIGHER-VISUAL-SYNDROME-ASSOCIATED LESIONS IN THE DISTRIBUTION OF THE POSTERIOR CEREBRAL ARTERIES

Syndromes associated primarily with right-sided lesions
   Visual hallucinations
   Palinopsia
   Topographagnosia
   Absent revisualization
Syndrome associated primarily with left-sided lesions
   Alexia without agraphia
Syndromes requiring bilateral posterior lesions
   Visual object agnosia
   Prosopagnosia
   Central achromatopsia
   Cerebral blindness
   Loss of brightness modulation
Syndrome that may occur with posterior lesions in either hemisphere
   Hemialexia (unilateral neglect)

From Alexander MP, Cummings JL. Higher visual functions. In: Lessel S, Van Dalen JTW, eds. Neuro-ophthalmology. Amsterdam: Elsevier, 1984;3.

TABLE 7–2. EVALUATION OF PARIETO-OCCIPITAL FUNCTION

Name objects by sight and touch
Identify faces
Write a sentence and read it
Read a text and interpret it
Draw a clock
Bisect a line
Imitate actions
Recall a series of numbers and/or designs

Adapted from Mills R. Disorders of the visual system. In: Swanson PD, ed. Signs and Symptoms in Neurology. Philadelphia: Lippincott, 1984:64.

Vascular lesions of the posterior cerebral arteries (PCA) or branches of vertebral basilar system are the most common cause of occipital lobe lesions. The sudden onset of hemianopic defects without other symptoms is pathognomonic of occipital lesions. More proximal PCA occlusions may also involve branches to the temporal lobe and cause memory difficulties, especially recent memory. Hypoxia or transient hypotension may cause bilateral dimming of vision (Chapter 8). Occipital arteriovenous malformations cause occipital epilepsy (usually unformed balls and streaks of light), and occipital apoplexy in which the headache usually precedes the seizure (in contradistinction to migraine).

If the vertebrobasilar arteries are involved, brainstem symptoms frequently result.

Following open heart or bypass surgery, vascular damage to the occipital lobe is very common if looked for. Infarcts result from hypotension and/or emboli and may be associated with hallucinations.

Hallucinations and cortical disorders also occur in transplant patients given cyclosporin therapy, especially if cholesterol is decreased, as it may be after liver transplantation.

Actual infarction of an occipital lobe may present with pain at the medial canthus of the homolateral eye or above and behind the eye. The pain is due to irritation of the overlying tentorium, which receives its nerve supply from the same branches of the trigeminal nerve as the medial canthal region.

Tumors are rarer in this region than in the parietal or temporal lobes. They are more likely to be metastatic than primary. Tentorial meningiomas may compress the occipital lobes. Demyelinating lesions are uncommon.

Because of their proximity to the skull, the occipital lobes are vulnerable to trauma and may be injured in concussive injuries, direct injury by depressed bone fragments, and penetrating injuries. In fact, much of our knowledge of the representation of the visual fields in the calcarine cortex has come by the classical studies of war injuries.

In children with hydrocephalus, blindness may be caused by dilation of the ventricles stretching the surrounding optic pathways. Infants are also susceptible to *Haemophilus influenzae* meningitis, with its predilection to damage the occipital lobes and cause significant visual loss.

Evaluation. The onset and type of symptomatology will frequently give clues as to etiology of the lesions. The diagnosis is further delineated by appropriate imaging studies, especially computed tomography and magnetic resonance imaging. Ultrasonography may occasionally be useful in infants where access can be obtained through the fontanelle. Occasionally, even appropriate imaging studies will not elucidate the diagnosis sufficiently, and brain biopsy may be necessary.

BIBLIOGRAPHY

General

Huber A. *Eye Symptoms in Brain Tumors.* 2nd ed. St. Louis: Mosby, 1971.

Miller N, ed. *Walsh and Hoyt's Clinical Neuroophthalmology.* 4th ed. Baltimore: Williams & Wilkins, 1982;1.

Hemianopias

Boldt HR, et al. Retrochiasmal field defects from multiple sclerosis. *Arch Neurol.* 1963;8:565–575.

Haerer AF. Visual field defects and the prognosis of stroke patients. *Stroke.* 1973;4:163–168.

Smith JL. Homonymous hemianopsia: A review of 100 cases. *Am J Ophthalmol.* 1962;54:616–622.

Trobe JD. Isolated homonymous hemianopia. *Arch Ophthalmol.* 1973;89:377–381.

Keyhole Visual Field Defect

Carter JE, et al. Lesions of the optic radiations mimicking lateral geniculate nucleus visual field defects. *J Neurol Neurosurg Psychiatry.* 1985;48:982–988.

Hoyt WF. Geniculate hemianopias: Incongruous visual field defects from partial involvement of the lateral geniculate nucleus. *Proc Austral Assoc Neurol.* 1975;12:7–16.

Pupil in Optic Tract Lesions

Loewenfeld I. Pupils in optic tract lesions. *J Clin Neuroophthalmol.* 1983;3:221. Letter.

Optokinetic Nystagmus

Kompf D. The significance of optokinetic nystagmus asymmetry in hemispheric lesions. *Neuro-ophthalmol.* 1986; 6:61–64.

Vascular Supply

Margolis MT, Newton TH, Hoyt WF. Cortical branches of the posterior cerebral artery: Anatomic–radiologic correlation. *Neuroradiology.* 1971;2:127–135.

Cortical Blindness

Brindley GS, et al. Cortical blindness and the functions of the non-geniculate fibers of the optic tracts. *J Neurol Neurosurg Psychiatry.* 1969;32:259–264.

Griffith JR, Dodge PR. Transient blindness following head injury in children. *N Engl J Med.* 1968;12:648–651.

CHAPTER 8

TRANSIENT VISUAL LOSS

Temporary reduction of effective blood supply to the visual pathways is the common denominator of transient visual loss. The deprivation must be severe enough to cause loss of function, but not so severe as to cause infarction. The vascular insufficiency may be either arterial or venous; migraine and emboli are two special causes of arterial insufficiency (Table 8–1). In addition, vascular insufficiency needs to be distinguished from seizures and other causes of temporary neurologic dysfunction such as hypoglycemia.

HISTORY

Recalling that the anterior portions of the visual afferent pathway are supplied by the paired carotid arteries and the posterior portions by the single basilar artery, ascertain whether the visual events are uniocular or binocular. Uniocular transient ischemic attacks (TIAs) are due to insufficiency in the internal carotid system; visual cortical TIAs due to insufficiency in the basilar system cause binocular homonymous defects. Anomalies, primitive arteries, and anastomotic blood supplies can occasionally cause variations in this dictum—for example, when the ophthalmic artery is a branch of the external carotid system rather than the internal, or when the posterior cerebral arteries are branches of the carotid system rather than the basilar system. However, these cases are rare and need to be considered only when the symptoms would suggest bizarre vascular origin.

It is important to get a feeling from the *patient's* words for the duration and exact character of the visual loss and of any previous episodes. Frequently patients who have talked to several doctors may wag their heads "yes" to a particular description suggested to them by their interviewers. It can be difficult to elicit an accurate description of what the patient actually experienced. Have the patient describe the episode: Is the entire visual field affected? If not, in what order do the parts disappear? Are the attacks related to specific movements or postures (eg, turning the head, getting out of bed)? How is vision affected—gone, shimmering, disturbed? How long do the attacks last? How does the visual field recover? (Frequently, the patient is so startled at the onset of a TIA that the initial symptoms are not recalled, but the resolution is clearly remembered.)

How often do attacks occur? Is one eye affected, or is it half of the visual field? Did the patient cover one eye? What happened then? Are there any associated symptoms—angina, palpitations, headache, disorientation or confusion, speech problems, diplopia, light-headedness, vertigo, hemiparesis, or hemisensory loss? Are such changes ipsilateral or contralateral to the visual loss? Are there symptoms of temporal arteritis—headache, tender scalp, jaw claudication, arthralgias?

Take a history of prior cardiovascular problems with particular attention paid to histories of rheumatic fever, arrhythmias, vascular surgery, claudication, angina, and dyspnea. A young patient is more likely to have cardiac valvular disease, migraine, or myxoma and an elderly patient more likely to have an atherosclerotic or arteritic lesion. Use of drugs that could conceivably lead to emboli, vasoconstriction, thrombosis, or hypotension should be sought. In particular, ask whether women are taking "the pill," whether antihypertensive or antimigrainous (ergotamine) therapy was recently initiated, or whether the patient is an IV drug abuser. Transient visual loss, both monocular and homonymous, has recently been associated with interleukin-2 therapy.

TABLE 8–1. CAUSES OF TRANSIENT VISUAL LOSS

Cause	Duration	Pattern of Visual Loss	Associated Findings	Etiology
"Classic" Migraine	10–20 min	Binocular, involving homonymous half fields with typical fortification figure that expands toward the peripheral field, often followed by a scotoma. Bilateral homonymous fields may be involved, causing total blackout of vision.	Usually followed by headache, may be associated with nausea, photophobia; patient may have an "aura." Patient usually has excellent recall of precise circumstances in which the attack occurred, but is unable to distinguish between a homonymous field disorder and a uniocular problem.	Vascular spasm or arteriovenous shunting
Ocular Migraine	10–20 min	Much less common; pattern of visual loss may be retinal (quadrantic, altitudinal, or total) or choroidal (concentric constriction). Retinal attacks are distinguished from embolic TIAs by longer duration and association with migraine history or hemicranial headache.	Positive family history.	
Hypotensive attacks, binocular (vertebral–basilar)	Brief, seconds	Gray outs, usually total, rarely altitudinal; patient may describe flickering of field like TV "snow"; may have many attacks without complaining.	Occasional tinnitis, diplopia, vertigo; perioral paraesthesias are rare.	Postural hypotension, autonomic insufficiency; cardiac insufficiency, arrhythmia, compression of vertebral artery
Hypotensive attacks, monocular (orbital–choroidal)	Seconds to minutes	Concentric narrowing of field from periphery toward center, occasionally central acuity may be retained.	Orbital or carotid vascular disease.	Vascular occlusive disease of the orbit or carotid distribution making the orbital circulation susceptible to slight decreases in perfusion that normally would not affect visual function
Embolic TIAs	3–5 min	Quadrantic, altitudinal, or total, corresponding in distribution of retinal arterioles.	Rarely central TIA (contralateral hemiplegia +/– hemihypoesthesia	Embolic, most frequent source ulcerated plaque at carotid bifurcation, also cardiac valves, mural thrombi, and atrial myxomas
Obscuration	Seconds	Gray-out, blur; usually unilateral on each occurrence; but either eye may be affected; sometimes photopsias also occur.	Findings associated with the cause of the papilledema.	Papilledema, orbital venous pressure, venous stasis +/– poor arterial perfusion

Modified from Miller N, ed. Walsh and Hoyt's Clinical Neuro-ophthalmology. *4th ed. Baltimore: Williams & Wilkins, 1982; 1; with permission.*

DIFFERENTIAL DIAGNOSIS OF UNIOCULAR VISUAL LOSS

When the visual loss is truly uniocular, determine the length of the episode. If it is brief, lasting 3 to 10 minutes, the most likely diagnosis is an embolic episode from the ipsilateral carotid circulation. If the visual field defect corresponds to the pattern of distribution of the central retinal artery, or if the TIA is associated with weakness of the contralateral arm, the symptom complex is nearly pathognomonic of an embolus (Table 8–2).

The most common type of embolus is a *cholesterol embolus* (Fig. 8–1), which manifests as a glistening, shiny, slightly irregular object with the vessel and sometimes at a bifurcation. Although the embolus may have broken up and passed on by the time you see the patient, frequently arterial sheathing or narrowing will be present, especially if the patient has a sectoral field defect. These changes should be looked for not only in the part of the retina corresponding to a field defect, but in other areas because embolic events due to cholesterol emboli are frequently multiple.

The finding of an asymptomatic cholesterol plaque in the fundus has the same prognostic and diagnostic significance as the history of an ocular TIA.

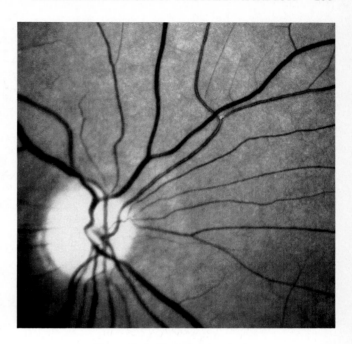

Figure 8–1. Cholesterol embolus.

Fibrin platelet emboli are soft and creamy white in appearance; they mold themselves to the arterial tree like an amorphous plug. These emboli may come from thrombotic changes in ulcerated plaques, mural thrombi in the heart, or abnormalities of the valves. They may occur in conjunction with cholesterol emboli.

Calcific emboli are the rarest. They appear as jagged, bright white spots within the vascular tree. They come almost exclusively from heart valves.

As with patients with retinal artery occlusion, the patient with embolic TIAs is at greatest risk from cardiovascular disease. Although the risk for death from stroke is five times that of the ordinary population, within 5 years more than 50% of the patients with a TIA or cholesterol plaque will die, frequently from cardiac disease.

The **major differential diagnosis** (Fig. 8–2) is that of vascular occlusive disease in which the stenosis of the vessels proximal to the eye is sufficient to critically lower the perfusion pressure when hypotension or cardiac arrhythmias occur. It is this diffuse ischemia that is most often associated with an "ischemic eyeball." These attacks may be either briefer or longer than the attacks associated with embolic events, which are often very stereotyped for each individual.

The signs of an *"ischemic eyeball"* include corneal striae, cells and flare in the anterior chamber, iris atrophy or rubeosis, sluggish pupillary reactions, tensions that may either be high or low, and a venous

TABLE 8–2. RETINAL EMBOLI

Characteristic	Cholesterol (Lipid)	Platelet–Fibrin	Calcium
Appearance	Copper, bright, re-fractile, pulsatile	White, creamy, elongated	Gray-white
Number	Multiple (in two thirds)	Often multiple	Usually single
Location (mostly temporal retina)	Often at bifurcations, disc to periphery	Temporal arcades	On or near disc
Caliber	Appears larger than blood column	Same size or larger than blood column	Same size or larger than blood column
Mobility	Can fragment and move on	Mobile or fixed	Fixed
Retinal ischemia	Rarely	Frequent	Frequent
Source	Ulcerated atherosclerotic lesions of carotid or large vessels (in two thirds)	Platelet aggregations on carotid, large vessels, or heart	Heart (in two thirds)

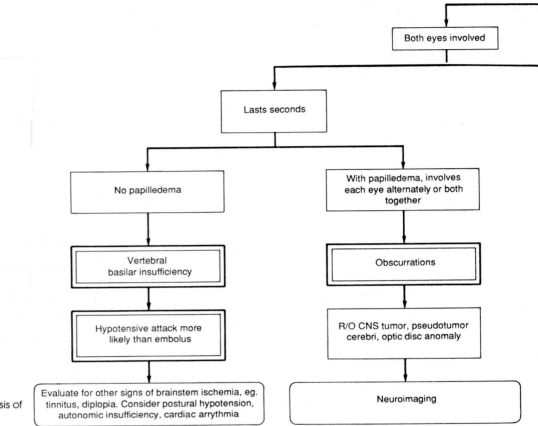

Figure 8–2. Differential diagnosis of transient visual loss.

stasis type of retinopathy that is maximal in the mid-periphery. Not infrequently, the intraocular pressure increases significantly following endarterectomy. Dilated episcleral veins and cataracts may be present. Other causes of the "ischemic eyeball," such as carotid–cavernous fistula and vasculitis, must be ruled out. The ischemic eyeball can progress to neovascular glaucoma and phthisis and eventually need enucleation. It carries a poor prognosis, a five-year mortality of 40%, mostly due to cardiac disease.

Choroidal TIAs. A rare form of uniocular TIA is the choroidal TIA, which occurs in the setting of diffuse orbital or posterior ciliary artery occlusive disease. In this case, the transient episode—rather than being altitudinal, hemianopic, or quadrantic—tends to a concentric narrowing of the field, which may or may not preserve central vision. Given diffuse posterior ciliary occlusive disease, hypotensive episodes are not unlikely to lead to one of these attacks. They may also be seen in the setting of orbital masses that compromise the blood supply. The duration of the attack is variable, from seconds

to minutes. Usually there is either clearly associated hypotension or a history of a systemic vascular disease or arteritis.

EVALUATION OF THE PATIENT WITH TRANSIENT UNIOCULAR VISUAL LOSS

Noninvasive Methods

The **initial diagnostic workup** (Fig. 8–3) consists of a careful fundus exam, measurement of blood pressure, and probably also ophthalmodynamometry. Also evaluate the patient for the "ischemic eyeball" (see Chapter 3). The cervical and facial pulses should be palpated and auscultated and the patient should be examined for Horner's syndrome.

However, as with arteriolarsclerotic retinal vascular disease, carotid artery stenosis is an important marker of generalized atherosclerosis, and is the cardiac vascular disease that poses the greatest threat to the patient. Thus, these patients should be screened for risk factors for atherosclerosis and coronary artery disease, especially hypertension, diabetes,

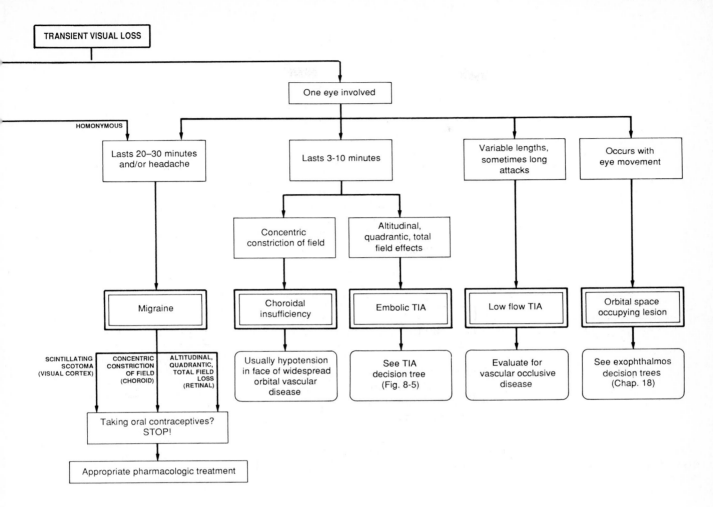

smoking, and hyperlipidemia. Additionally, one should check for arrhythmias and obtain a cardiology consultation as more than one third of patients have sufficiently severe coronary artery disease to warrant revascularization; their mortality from coronary artery disease exceeds that of patients with angina, and the coexisting coronary artery disease increases the operative mortality of carotid endarterectomy. Another rare cause of TIA is a paradoxic embolism through patent foramen ovale. This may be looked for by contrast echography during a valsalva maneuver. This cardiac abnormality is associated with mitral valve prolapse as well.

Because the large majority of ocular TIAs are of embolic origin, attempt to find an embolus in the retinal circulation (Fig. 8–2). However, this results in positive findings much less commonly than one would expect.

In addition to thorough neuro-ophthalmic evaluation, check the patient's blood pressure and auscultate the carotid and vertebral vessels and the heart. On slit-lamp examination, look for dilated episcleral vessels. Then proceed with noninvasive evaluations. Most of these—duplex ultrasound, ophthalmodynamometry, and oculoplethysmography—measure flow and pressure in tributaries of the carotid artery, especially the ophthalmic artery.

Laboratory evaluation. Hematologic evaluation should be done, both to rule out other causes of vascular incompetency and to rule in risk factors for vascular disease. Hematologic tests should include a complete blood count, platelet count, tests of aggregation and adhesiveness of the platelets, erythrocyte sedimentation rate, glucose, fibrinogen, serum protein, cholesterol, triglycerides, and antinuclear antibodies (ANA). In patients with carotid atherosclerosis, the combination of coronary artery disease, elevated low-density lipoproteins (LDL), and increased fibrinogen predicts the progression of carotid stenosis with 88% accuracy. In appropriate circumstances, antithrombin III and proteins C and S should be estimated (see Chapter 3 for other etiologies of embolic and vascular occlusion).

Ophthalmodynamometry (ODM). Ophthalmodynamometry measures the arterial pressure in the ophthalmic artery proximal to the eye by using a

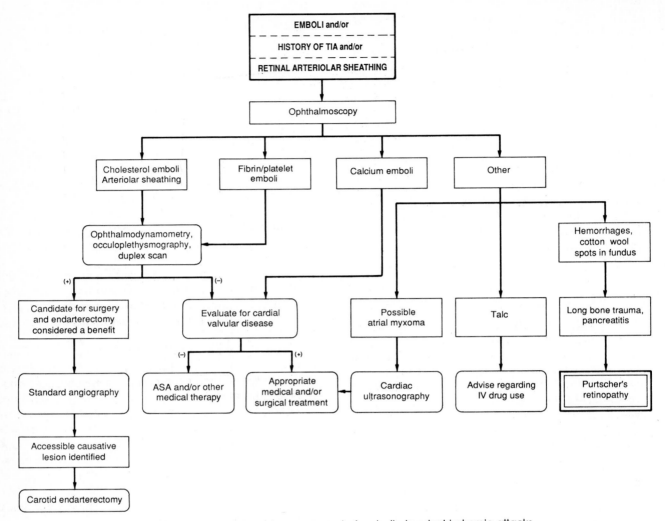

Figure 8–3. Evaluation and management of embolic transient ischemic attacks.

plunger to compress the eyeball and increase intraocular pressure. As with a sphygmomanometer, the point at which the retinal artery begins to pulsate corresponds to diastole and that where it collapses, to systole. There should be no more than a 20% difference in systolic readings between the two eyes and no more than a 15% difference for diastolic. If the readings are low bilaterally, a diastolic reading less than 50% of the brachial diastolic pressure is significant.

Ophthalmodynamometry is performed with topical anesthesia and with either direct or indirect ophthalmoscopy through a dilated pupil. With indirect ophthalmoscopy, two people are preferred, one to do the ophthalmoscopy and the other to exert and record the pressure. The two-person technique, using bracketing to arrive at several estimations of the pressures, is more accurate.

Place the foot plate of the instrument perpendicular to the eye on the temporal bulbar conjuctiva. Observe the major arterioles as they cross the disc margin. Be careful not to measure venous pulsations. Press the instrument against the eye until the vessels pulsate; record the diastolic pressure; then increase pressure until the vessels stop pulsating at the systolic pressure point. If cardiac arrhythmias are present, the measurement can be very difficult because of the fluctuating intensity of the pulsations. Similarly, fluctuating blood pressure can make accurate measurements difficult. You must be sure to have the foot plate of the instrument perpendicular to the globe surface.

The measurements also become inaccurate in the face of very low ophthalmic artery pressures. This test is much more reliable if both systolic and diastolic measurements are made. A simple test, which is cheap and easy to do in the office, ophthalmodynamometry can be very useful in patients whose symptoms are somewhat atypical. In patients with appropriate symptoms, it is about 90% accurate. This is in the same range as most other noninvasive evaluations. It is contraindicated when there is external ocular infection or a dislocated lens, an acute cardiac problem, or history of previous retinal detachment or other surgery that is likely to have thinned and weakened the globe. Ophthalmodynamometry must be carefully done and it is important to gain sufficient experience to be accurate.

Oculopneumoplethysmography (OPG) uses an air-filled suction cup applied to the anesthetized sclera. The negative pressure causes an increase in intraocular pressure to the point that choroidal arterial flow ceases. As the applied vacuum is decreased, the point where pulsation returns is the systolic pressure.

The accuracy of OPG is slightly better than ODM, and when combined with duplex scanning, the detection rate and specificity are excellent.

Both ODM and OPG may miss bilateral lesions and are poor at distinguishing occlusion from very-high-grade stenosis. However, effects of intracranial and orbital occlusion are measured where carotid ultrasonography can only evaluate the accessible portions of the arteries. Transcranial Doppler ultrasonography shows promise, but its accuracy and sensitivity remain to be established. None of the noninvasive tests reliably demonstrates plaque ulceration, although B-scan ultrasound shows intraplaque hemorrhage very well. All these tests are extremely dependent on the skill and experience with which they are performed.

Imaging: Duplex ultrasound of the carotid arteries gives a good picture of the carotid bifurcation via B scan and will document stenosis or plaque formation. Doppler evaluation gives a complimentary assessment by measuring the velocity of flow through the vessels. Although some believe definitive evaluation of arterial lumen is only possible by angiography, recent studies suggest that the sensitivity of duplex scanning is greater than that of arteriography for lesion detection. Furthermore, the accuracy of duplex scanning exceeds that of angiography for detecting intimal surface abnormalities and ulceration. It has also been shown that the inability of duplex scanning to image the great vessels and intracranial vessels, often considered a reason for angiography, does not affect the patient's morbidity. Cardiac echography is also indicated to rule out a cardiac source of emboli (eg, mural thrombosis or an abnormal valve).

Invasive Methods

Angiography: Many still consider it mandatory to perform an angiographic study when a patient is considered for surgical therapy. But many neurovascular surgeons are willing to operate on patients who have been studied by duplex scanning or arterial digital subtraction arteriography (DSA) only. The resolution of digital subtraction angiography is quite good and the complication rate quite low. However, to get the very best quality studies, conventional angiography is necessary. Angiography displays the carotid siphon and intracranial circulation and allows quantification of the degree and location of luminal compromise, but does not demonstrate disease of the arterial wall—interplaque hemorrhage, ulceration, or intraluminal thrombus—as well as B-scan ultrasound.

In centers with experienced angiographers, the rate of any complication is approximately 13%, including a 5% incidence of transient neurologic deficit. The rate of a permanent neurologic deficit is less than 1%.

The rationale to follow in evaluating these patients depends on your philosophy of therapy. If you believe carotid endarterectomy is never indicated, the workup may cease as soon as you have confirmed the diagnosis—for example, a patient with transient visual loss of about 5 minutes in a retinal pattern, no heart disease, a cholesterol retinal embolus, and asymmetric ODM, almost certainly has ipsilateral carotid occlusive disease and should be started on antiplatelet therapy—period.

Patients with less typical presentations must have other causes of TIAs ruled out.

If you have criteria for offering carotid endarterectomy as a choice, the appropriate tests must be done to ascertain whether the patient meets those criteria. If the criteria are met, the patient should be offered surgery; if not, the patient should be followed for progression, usually with duplex scanning.

THERAPY

The primary therapy of patients with TIAs, including amaurosis fugax, is **medical.** Treat associated conditions such as hypertension, arrhythmias, and conditions leading to hyperviscosity and hypercoagulability. Antiplatelet agents, especially aspirin, are the backbones of this treatment. Aspirin (650 mg bid) results in a 25 to 30% decrease in stroke incidence following a TIA. Lower doses (< 500 mg daily) may be equally effective. The addition of dipyramadole or sulfinpyrazone does not confer any additional advantage in stroke prevention; however, as platelet antiaggregants, the drugs could theoretically have a beneficial affect on cardiovascular disease. Ticlopidine produced good results in a recent trial, but is expensive.

Surgical treatment has consisted of carotid endarterectomy and external carotid/internal carotid (EC-IC) artery bypass. The latter is an effort to bypass a totally occluded internal carotid or carotid artery that is occluded in an inaccessible place by anastomosing the superficial temporal artery to a branch on the temporal lobe. Recent studies have shown that this surgical procedure rarely improves prognosis or life expectancy.

Whether there is a group of patients who should be subjected to carotid endarterectomy remains under consideration (Table 8–3). Recent studies indicate that the prognosis, both for morbidity and mortality, in patients who had a TIA is not significantly improved by endarterectomy. This is not surprising, because the major cause of morbidity and mortality is cardiac disease. However, many patients who are quite troubled by their TIAs and in whom one might expect a stroke to ensue, can be made asymptomatic by endarterectomy.

This procedure obviously should not be done for all victims of a TIA or cholesterol embolus. It is still possible, however, that better-controlled studies may show a subgroup of patients who will benefit. Intraluminal balloon angioplasty of accessible lesions is another promising modality.

Patients who are not surgical candidates should be placed on antiplatelet agents. Aspirin 650 mg bid seems the most effective.

Patients who potentially qualify for surgery but who have less than 75% stenosis should be followed with serial duplex scanning and placed on antiplatelet therapy. Progressive stenosis or crescendoes of TIAs favor offering these patients the choice of surgery.

Patients who have greater than 75% stenosis and who are excellent surgical risks should be offered carotid endarterectomy where there are available excellent interventional radiography and neurovascular surgeons (eg, where the risks of angiography and surgery are less than those associated with medical treatment). I leave the choice to perform angiography to the neurovascular surgeon.

LONGER-DURATION (10–20 MINUTES) TIAs

By far the most frequent cause of transient visual loss is migraine; however, the purely ocular migraine that results in unilateral transient visual loss is much rarer than the other varieties of migraine. In ocular migraine, it is hypothesized that arterial spasm involves the arteric artery vasculature. Rarely, spasm leads to infarction and nerve fiber bundle defects (Fig. 8–4); usually it clears within the usual time period and is followed by headache.

More typically, migraine presents with scintillating scotomas in the homonymous portions of the visual field. Almost invariably, the headache follows and may last for hours to more than a day. This "classic migraine" is one of many forms of vascular headache (see Chapter 18).

TABLE 8–3. TREATMENT FOR UNIOCULAR TRANSIENT VISUAL LOSS

Factors Favoring Antiplatelet Therapy
No recent episodes of visual loss
Infrequent episodes of visual loss
No associated CNS TIAs
Poor candidate for surgery
Patient opposed to surgery
Surgical team with risks < natural history
Factors Favoring Endarterectomy
Recent episodes of visual loss
Multiple episodes of visual loss
Associated CNS TIAs
Recurrent visual loss on antiplatelet therapy
Patient in good health, < 70 years old
More than 75% stenosis
Surgical team with results > natural history

Adapted from Beck R. Amaurosis fugax: Controversies in management. Int Ophthalmol Clin. *1986;26:277–284.*

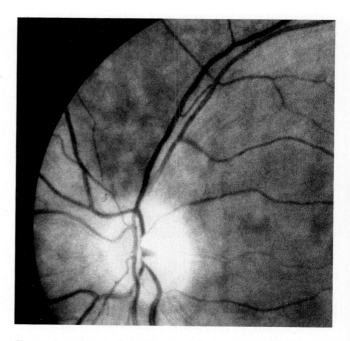

Figure 8–4. Nerve fiber bundle defect caused by retinal migraine.

VERTEBROBASILAR TIAs

A common cause of **binocular** transient visual loss is a vertebrobasilar TIA. These attacks occur predominantly in the elderly, last only a few seconds, and are described as a gray-out or dim-out of vision. They may be associated with spots, "snow," or "flickers." Occasionally, these episodes are related to posture (particularly turning the head, reaching for things on high shelves, or arising from a recumbent position) and/or cardiac arrhythmias. They may be associated with faintness, loss of balance, dizziness, and a generalized sensation of weakness. Obviously, the slit-lamp findings associated with ocular ischemia are not expected to be found here, so the workup should concentrate on the other aspects of vascular disease.

Hypoperfusion is the commonest cause of vertebrobasilar TIAs. Vertebrobasilar thrombosis has a very poor prognosis. Recently, prompt infusion of tissue plasminogen activator has been documented to resolve a thrombotic basilar artery occlusion without hemorrhagic complications. Therapy with thrombolytic agents probably deserves consideration in thrombotic occlusions causing vertebrobasilar TIAs.

TRANSIENT OBSCURATIONS

Obscurations are extremely brief (secondary) episodes of visual dimming that occur in association with well-developed papilledema. The symptoms may affect both eyes simultaneously or either eye alternately; they are related to posture, particularly getting out of bed in the morning. Not infrequently, photopsias occur. There does not seem to be any clear relationship to the underlying disease process, nor does the presence of obscurations signify a worrisome prognosis for the patient.

Although there are relatively few symptoms that would be confused with these very brief episodes of visual loss, Uhthoff's phenomenon, a transient visual episode that occurs associated with demyelinating plaques in the optic nerve, occasionally seems somewhat similar. Presumed interference with optic nerve perfusion by orbital masses, thyroid orbitopathy, and anomalies in the region of the optic nerve head (eg, drusen, staphyloma) also occasionally present with this type of transient visual loss.

BIBLIOGRAPHY

Bernard JT, Ameriso S, et al. Transient focal neurologic deficits complicating interleukin-2 therapy. *Neurology.* 1990;40:154–155.

Bernstein EF, ed. *Amaurosis Fugax.* New York: Springer-Verlag, 1988.

Fisher CM. Observations of the fundus oculi in transient monocular blindness. *Neurology.* 1959;9:333–347.

Gay AJ. Clinical Ophthalmodynamometry, *Int Ophthalmol Clin.* 1967;7:729–744.

Gent M, et al. The Canadian American Ticlopidine Study (CATS) in thromboembolic stroke. *Lancet.*1989;8649: 1211–1220.

Goodson SF, et al. Can carotid duplex scanning supplant arteriography in patients with focal carotid territory symptoms? *J Vasc Surg.* 1987;5:551–557.

Grotta JC. Current medical and surgical therapy for cerebrovascular disease. *N Engl J Med.* 1987;317:1505–1516.

Grotta JC, Yatsu FM, et al. Prediction of carotid stenosis progression by lipid and hematologic measurements. *Neurology.* 1989;39:1325–1331.

Henze T, et al. Lysis of basilar artery occlusion with TPA. *Lancet.* 1987;2:1391.

Hollenhorst RW. Significance of bright plaques in the retinal arterioles. *Trans Am Ophthalmol Soc.* 1961;59:252.

Roederer GO, et al. Is siphon disease important in predicting outcome of carotid endarterectomy? *Arch Surg.* 1983;118:1177–1181.

Savino PJ, Glaser JS, Cassady J. Retinal stroke. Is the patient at risk? *Arch Ophthalmol.* 1977;95:1185–1189.

Sivalingam A, et al. The ocular ischemic syndrome. Mortality and systemic morbidity. *Int Ophthalmol.* 1989;13: 187–191.

CHAPTER 9

PHOTOPSIAS, ENTOPSIAS, ILLUSIONS, AND HALLUCINATIONS

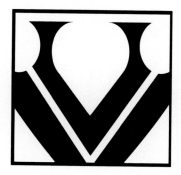

Most visual afferent pathway disorders produce negative effects on visual perception: visual loss and visual field defects. The phenomena considered here are the results of an opposite, positive effect. However, they are equally important signposts in ophthalmic and neuro-ophthalmic disease; frequently, they coexist with retinal and neurologic visual deficits (in fact, they occur in about 50% of these patients). Furthermore, they overlap a number of naturally occurring visual phenomena. Paradoxically, they may not be reported by patients lest their "seeing things" make them seem crazy to others.

Photopsias are bright, unformed light images. **Entopic phenomena** result from optical circumstances that allow perception of structures and particles within one's own eye. **Illusions** are distortions of something actually seen, and **hallucinations** are perceptions of things not present at all.

PHOTOPSIAS

Among the photopsias or sensations of light is a number of normal phenomena, termed **phosphenes,** which generally result from retinal stimulation or retinal/vitreal traction (Table 9–1). **Moore's lightning streaks** are vertical lines in the temporal visual field best seen in dim illumination and with eye movement. Eye movement may also cause **flick phosphenes,** streaks of light occurring in the central field, especially with saccadic (fast) eye movements. Like most phosphenes, they are seen best in the dark-adapted eye. Strong efforts at accommodation may cause peripheral flashes, perhaps from ciliary body traction on the peripheral retina. Following optic neuritis and compressive and ischemic optic neuropathies, photopsias frequently are associated with eye movement. It is not clear whether they are a retinal release phenomenon or result from stimulation of injured neurons in the optic nerve, analogous to electric sensations in the limbs with neck flexion (Lhermitte's sign) found in multiple sclerosis and cervical spinal cord lesions. Similar flashes are occasionally evoked in optic neuropathies by unexpected sounds homolateral to the injured optic nerve.

Another positive phenomenon seen in optic nerve disease is chromatopsia in Leber's optic neuropathy and in tabetic and drug-induced (eg, ethambutol) optic neuropathies. Chromatopsias are also seen in retinal toxicity, as in the "yellow vision" of digitalis toxicity.

TABLE 9–1. PHOTOPSIAS (UNFORMED STREAKS, FLASHES, BALLS OF LIGHT)

Phosphenes
Movement related
    Moore's "lightning" streaks
    Flick phosphenes
    Accommodative phosphenes
Stimulus related
    Direct blow to eye—"seeing stars"
    Haidinger brushes
    Electrical stimulus to eye, visual paths
    Cherenkov radiation
Pathologic
Retinal detachment and/or vitreous traction
Central serous retinopathy, especially after laser
Optic neuropathies—movement or sound induced
Central retinal vein occlusion
CNS—ictal, structural lesions, migraine

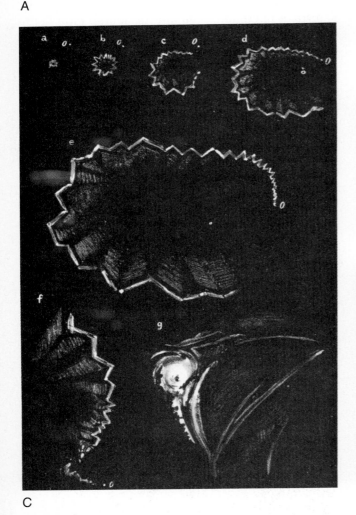

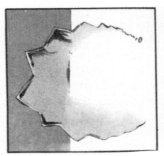

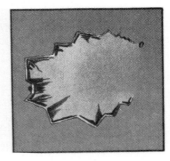

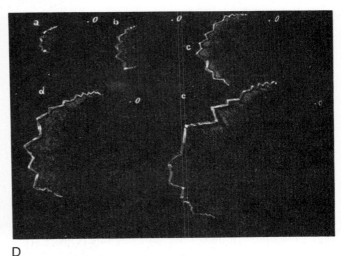

Figure 9–1. A–D Depiction of migrainous scotomas. (*From Gowers WR. Subjective visual sensations.* Trans Ophthal Soc UK. *1895; 15:1–38, with permission.*)

In retinal pathology (central retinal vein occlusion, following photocoagulation, and so forth), similar photic sensations are noted. Central serous retinopathy, in particular, causes a positive scotoma, sometimes colored, that seems to intervene between the patient and the visual target. The scotomas intensify in bright light, forming the basis of the photostress test—an excellent way to distinguish between macular and optic nerve pathology.

In their configuration and variety, the visual auras of classic migraine are examples par excellence of these phenomena (Fig. 9–1). Similar experiences may occur with carotid artery disease, especially incipient occlusion, but usually last only seconds to minutes, in contrast to the 15- to 20-minute duration of the migraine aura.

Other stimuli produce like experiences. A blow to the eye makes us "see stars," as does electrical stimulation of the retina. Electrical stimulation of the visual afferent pathways can also produce geometric shapes: white, black and white, or colored. If two points are stimulated consecutively, there may be an illusion of motion.

Particle-induced visual sensations (PIVS) arise by several mechanisms. The most studied are the result of Cherenkov radiation and occur in dark-adapted eyes subjected to particles accelerated to relativistic velocities. The sensations include large crescent-shaped flashes occupying up to one half the visual field. There are also cloud-like flashes, bright small flashes, streaks, and bands; large flashes with dark centers occur if the particles enter the rear of the eye and exit the cornea. On Apollo space flights PIVs were noted as often as one to two times per minute.

Haidinger brushes are seen if polarized light (especially blue light) shines through a prism into the eye. Yellow brushes are seen on a blue background in the central area (Fig. 9–2). The brushes may be related to the parallel fiber pattern of the outer plexiform layer. They may be used to estimate macular function (eg, in central serous retinopathy). The ability to recognize the brushes is reported to predict improvement in visual acuity after patching in amblyopia or after cataract extraction.

ENTOPSIAS

Entoptic phenomena are visualizations of ocular elements anterior to the rods and cones made obvious by differences in optical density (Table 9–2). The most common of these are the vitreous condensations known as "floaters," which are made apparent by eye movement. They suddenly appear and then float out of view. In time they may settle away from the visual axis and be less noticed. Floaters are benign and occur more often in myopes. However, a shower of floaters may herald an intraocular hemorrhage or inflammation.

Another common entopsia is the *halo* produced by any structure in the eye that acts as a diffraction grating. Any bright light source is seen as a rainbow-like halo. Unlike rainbows and coronas formed by clouds, ocular haloes hide objects between the observer and the light. Physiologic haloes include lenticular haloes, caused by the radial arrangement of lens fibers; and corneal haloes, due to edema of the deeper corneal layers (eg, with increased intraocular pressure).

Awareness of the retinal circulation may occur in *Scherer's phenomenon* (moving bright dots—white blood cells) that track in arcs to the periphery and disappear.

If the eye is illuminated with a diffuse light, especially blue, details of the retinal vessels, the capillary-free area at the fovea, and particulars of retinal pathology (scars, pigment patches) become sensible. Under proper conditions other entopic sensations include awareness of tears and mucous on the cornea, corneal irregularities and edema, the pupil and its movements, lens fibers, star figures, vac-

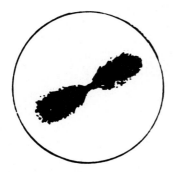

Figure 9–2. Haidinger brushes. Seen in Goldschmidt's apparatus. The brushes appear black on a blue background. (*From Duke-Elder S, ed. System of Ophthalmology. Vol 7 The Foundations of Ophthalmology: Hereditary, Pathology, Diagnosis and Therapeutics. London: H. Kimpton, 1962, with permission.*)

TABLE 9–2. ENTOPSIAS

Tears and mucous on cornea
Corneal irregularities, edema—haloes associated with increased intraocular pressure
Lens—star figure, vacuole, fiber patterns
Vitreous condensations—"floaters"[a]
Scherer's phenomenon—white blood cells in retinal circulation (?)
Light flooding—vessels, retinal details, white blood cells

[a] Most frequent by far.

uoles, and discrete opacities (Fig. 9–3). The perception of these elements may be utilized as a test of retinal sensitivity and function in the face of media opacities (cataract, corneal scars, or edema), but reliability varies as individuals differ greatly in their ability to perceive such phenomena.

ILLUSIONS AND DISTORTIONS

Illusions are misinterpretations of something actually seen (Table 9–3). Relatively common illusions include metamorphopsias, macropsia, and micropsia, seen predominantly with macular lesions (although metamorphopsia may occur with central lesions as well). Sometimes illusions result from treatment of lesions, especially photocoagulation of central serous retinopathy (Fig. 9–4). They may also occur in the absence of structural lesions months to years following drug abuse. Palinopsia (the persistence of something seen after the object has left the field of vision), visual perservation, and illusory visual spread may also be considered illusions. Palinopsia occurs predominantly in right-sided and posterior hemisphere lesions. It has been reported as a side effect of trazodone (Desyryl).

TABLE 9–3. ILLUSIONS

Palinopsia
Illusory visual spread
Visual allesthesia
Cerebral diplopia/polyopia (when monocular most often caused by media changes)
Metamorphopsia
Macropsia
Micropsia

HALLUCINATIONS

A **hallucination** is the perception of an object that is not present (Table 9–4). These percepts may be either formed (recognizable objects, animals, and so forth) or unformed (blobs, geometric shapes, sparkles, shimmers); they may result from a stimulus (ictus, electrode) or as release phenomena. There is considerable overlap between normal states, photopsias, illusions, and hallucinations.

Normal individuals experience afterimages and dreams, as well as hypnogogic and hypnopompic images (images seen when falling asleep and awakening). Formed hallucinations are frequent in children and those skilled at artistic imagery. Specific patterns recur frequently in artistic imagery, retinal and

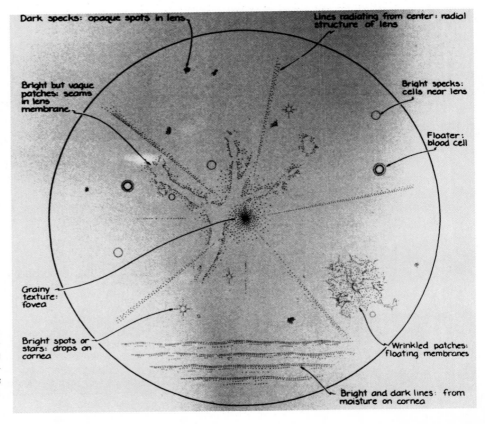

Figure 9–3. Entopsias. A few of the objects that may be seen when a featureless background is viewed through a pinhole. (*From Walker J. "Floaters": Visual artifacts that result from blood cells in front of the retina. Sci Am. 1982; vol. 151, with permission.*)

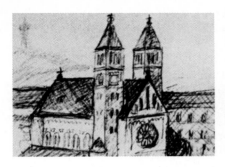
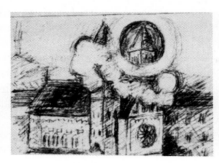
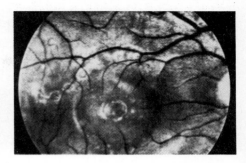

Figure 9–4. Following photocoagulation in central serous retinopathy. The patient's simultaneous drawing of a church as she saw it 2 weeks after photocoagulation with her left eye (left) and right eye (middle) when the fixation point was the roof of the tower. The central scotoma consists of three parts: a circle-like dark gray spot, a surrounding lighter ring, and a dark outer halo. The light flashes, surrounded by colored haloes projected to the lower visual field, are in correspondence with the coagulation spot marked in the fundus picture (right). (*From Kovacs B.* Doc Op. *1977;44:445–53.*)

release phenomena, and hallucinogenic experiences. This common visual thread confounds the distinction between normal and abnormal visual perceptions (Fig. 9–5).

Electrical stimulation or ictal events create visual imagery. In general, images elicited from the eye and occipital areas tend to be unformed—photisms, shadows, colored balls, discs, lights. Multiple stimuli may give an illusion of movement. Stimuli near the temporal lobe tend to elicit formed images that often have an element of unpleasantness and distortion. Their relationship to complete memory processes is unclear. However, any type of hallucination may arise anywhere within the visual system. Visual perception may be entirely normal in between the ictal events that produce the hallucinations.

Hallucinations associated with release phenomena tend to occur within damaged areas of the visual field, but may extend into the normal field and even to the other eye. It is hypothesized that normal central nervous system activity releases impulses that create nonphysiologic perceptions in the defective areas of vision (Table 9–5).

Visual hallucinations associated with seizures, migraine, tumors, and visual field defects contain visual imagery only. In contrast, hallucinations related to psychiatric illness are usually multisen-

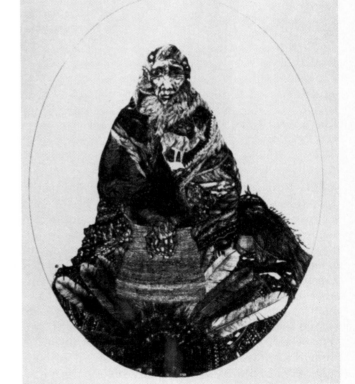

Figure 9–5. Reproduction of the visual hallucination of an artist-migraineur. The complex intricate detail of the hallucination suggests temporal lobe malfunction. (*From Raskin NH, Appenzeller O.* Migraine: Clinical aspects. In: Smith LH Jr, ed. Headache, vol. 14 *in* Major Problems in Internal Medicine. *Philadelphia: Saunders, 1980, with permission.*)

TABLE 9–4. HALLUCINATIONS

Unformed	Ictal, migraine
	Structural lesions—eye, cortex
Formed	Normal phenomena—dreams, afterimages, formed hallucinations in children, hypnogogic and hypnopompic hallucinations
	Irritative—temporal lobe, posterior right hemisphere lesions
	Release—ocular hemorrhage, visual field defects, enucleation, patching, bilateral dense media opacities

TABLE 9–5. FEATURES USEFUL IN DISTINGUISHING ICTAL AND RELEASE HALLUCINATIONS ASSOCIATED WITH HEMISPHERIC LESIONS

Characteristics	Ictal Hallucinations	Release Hallucinations
Duration	Brief (usually seconds to minutes)	Persistent (hours)
Variability	Stereotyped content	May be stereotyped, variable or change slowly over time
Visual field defect	Visual field defect may or may not be present	Visual field defect usually present
Lateralization	May or may not be lateralized	Usually lateralized to side of visual field defect
Environmental influence	Little or no response to environmental influences	Frequently influenced by environmental factors, such as opening, moving or closing eyes
Content	May consist of a visual memory Tend to be unformed with posterior lesions and formed with temporal	Usually novel May be formed regardless of lesion location
Associated findings	Consciousness often altered during or after ictal event; head and eye deviation common during hallucination	No associated ictal behaviors or alteration of consciousness

From Cummings JL, et al. Visual hallucinations: Clinical occurrences and use in differential diagnosis. West J Med. 1987;146:46–51.

sorial—for example, containing auditory and tactile as well as visual imagery.

In ophthalmic and neuro-ophthalmic hallucinatory events, visual deprivation is often a contributory factor. Hallucinations generally occur in defective portions of the visual field. Visual loss or deprivation due to bilateral patching following cataract extraction, bilateral corneal or retinal detachment surgery, enucleation, vitreous hemorrhage, central serous retinopathy, and temporal arteritis all give rise to hallucinations that can be intrusive enough to prevent sleep and make the patient suicidal. Paradoxically, in previously sighted individuals who lose all sight, restoration of vision can cause a similar reaction (Table 9–6).

Within the central nervous system, hallucinations tend to occur while a lesion evolves and to cease as the lesion stabilizes.

Midbrain or peduncular hallucinosis produces a distinctive complex hallucination—that is, like watching a silent movie. These formed hallucinations occur after vertebral angiography, posterior cerebral artery occlusion, hypoxia, and cardiac surgery, as well as with pituitary tumors that extend posteriorly. They are pleasant in contrast to hallucinations of temporal lobe disorders. Because they are not threatening and because they are not unpleasant, they are rarely mentioned as a symptom. They seem to occur with diffuse posterior circulatory lesions involving the posterior occipital regions, medial thalami, midbrain, peduncles, and fornices.

Other phenomena straddle the border between illusion and hallucination. These include palinopsia (visual perservation); illusory visual spread (color extending beyond its normal boundaries); visual allesthesia (displacement of objects from their true location, such as upside-down or to the other visual hemifield); and cerebral polyopia. In contrast, ocular polyopia is nearly always associated with media irregularities, especially corneal opacities and cataracts, which are usually obvious on examination, especially in the retinoscopic reflex.

Hallucinogens and toxic drug reactions result in

TABLE 9–6. CAUSES OF VISUAL HALLUCINATIONS

Ophthalmologic Diseases
  Enucleation
  Cataract formation
  Retinal disease
  Choroidal disorder
  Macular abnormalities
  Glaucoma
Neurologic Disorders
  Optic nerve disorders
  Brain-stem lesions (peduncular hallucinosis)
  Hemispheric lesions
  Epilepsy
  Migraine
  Narcolepsy
Toxic and Metabolic Conditions
  Toxic–metabolic encephalopathies
  Drug and alcohol withdrawal syndromes
  Hallucinogenic agents
Psychiatric Disorders
  Schizophrenia
  Affective disorders
  Conversion reactions
Miscellaneous Conditions
  Dreams
  Hypnagogic hallucinations
  Childhood (imaginary companions)
  Eidetic images
  Sensory deprivation
  Sleep deprivation
  Hypnosis
  Intense emotional experiences

From Cummings JL, et al. Visual hallucinations: Clinical occurrences and use in differential diagnosis. West J Med. 1987;146:46–51.

hallucinations that may overlap the psychiatric state, such as delirium tremens following alcohol withdrawal (Table 9–7). Many of the mydriatic and parasympatholytic drugs (scopolamine, atropine, cyclopentolate) used in ophthalmology have considerable hallucinogenic potential. Toxicity from these drugs is usually associated with confusion, agitation, flush, and tachycardia. In patients receiving cyclosporin for immunosuppression, formed visual hallucinations may occur in association with increasing serum levels of cyclosporin, and appear to be more frequent if serum cholesterol is low.

BIBLIOGRAPHY

Appenzeller O, Raskin NH. Migraine. In: Raskin NH, ed. *Headache.* 2nd. ed. New York: Churchill Livingstone, 1988.

Brindley GE, Lewin W. The sensations produced by electrical stimulation of the visual cortex. *J Physiol London.* 1968;196:479–493.

Chapanis NP, Uematsu S, Konigsmark B, et al. Central phosphenes in man: A report of three cases. *Neuropsychologia.* 1973;11:1–19.

Cogan DG. Visual hallucinations as release phenomena. *Albrecht von Graefes Arch Klin Exp Ophthalmol.* 1973; 188:139–150.

Cohn R. Phantom vision. *Arch Neurol.* 1971;25:468–471.

Gittinger JW, Miller NR, Keltner JL, Burde RM. Sugarplum fairies. Visual hallucinations. *Surv Ophthalmol.* 1982; 27:42–48.

Hoffman DD. The interpretation of visual illusions. *Sci Amer.* 1983;249:154.

Hughes MS, Lessell S. Trazodone-induced palinopsia. *Arch Ophthalmol.* 1990;108:399–400.

Jacobs L, Karpik A, Bozian D, Gothgen S. Auditory-visual synesthesia. Sound-induced photisms. *Arch Neurol.* 1981;38:211–216.

Katirji MB. Visual hallucinations and cyclosporine. *Transplantation.* 1987;43:768.

Kovacs B. Visual phenomena following light coagulation in central serous retinopathy (CSR). *Doc Ophthalmol.* 1977;44:445–453.

Lepore FE. Spontaneous visual phenomena with visual loss: 104 patients with lesions of retinal and neural afferent pathways. *Neurology.* 1990;40:444–447.

Levi L, Miller NR. Visual illusions associated with previous drug abuse. *J Clin Neuro-ophthalmol.* 1990;10:103–110.

McNamara ME, Heros RC, Boller F. Visual hallucinations in blindness: The Charles Bonnet syndrome. *Int J Neurosci.* 1982;17:13–15.

McNulty PJ, Pease VP. Visual sensations induced by Cherenkov radiation. *Science.* 1975;189:453–454.

Murphey F. The scotomata of carotid artery disease as I remember them. Case report. *J Neurosurg.* 1973;39:390–393.

Page NGR, Bolger JP, Sanders MD. Auditory evoked phosphenes in optic nerve disease. *J Neurol Neurosurg Psychiatry.* 1982;45:7–12.

Safran AB, Kline LB, Glaser JS. Positive visual phenomena in optic nerve and chiasm disease: Photopsias and photophobia. In: Glaser JS, ed. *Neuro-ophthalmology.* St. Louis: Mosby, 1980;10:225–231.

Siegel RK. Hallucinations. *Sci Amer.* Oct 1977; vols:131–140.

Weinberger LM, Grant FC. Visual hallucinations and their neuro-ophthalmic correlates. *Arch Ophthalmol.* 1940; 27:166–199.

TABLE 9–7. DRUGS ASSOCIATED WITH VISUAL HALLUCINATIONS

Hallucinogens	Antibiotics
Dimethyltryptamine	Antimalarial agents
Harmine	Cycloserine
Ketamine hydrochloride	Isoniazid
LSD	Podophyllum resin
Mescaline	Procaine penicillin
Nitrous oxide	Sulfonamides
Phencyclidine hydrochloride	Tetracycline
(PCP)	Hormonal Agents
Psilocybin	Levothyroxine sodium
Tetrahydrocannabinol	Steroidal agents
Stimulants	Analgesics and Nonsteroidal
Amphetamine	Antiinflammatory Agents
Cocaine	Indomethacin
Methylphenidate	Nalorphine
Antiparkinsonian Agents	Narcotic agents
Amantadine hydrochloride	Pentazocine
Anticholinergic drugs	Phenacetin
Bromocriptine	Salicylates
Levodopa	Miscellaneous Agents
Lisuride	Baclofen
Mesulergine	Bromide
Pergolide mesylate	Cimetidine
Antidepressants	Clonazepam
Amitriptyline hydrochloride	Cyclosporin
Amoxapine	Diethylpropion hydrochloride
Bupropion hydrochloride	Disulfiram
Doxepin hydrochloride	Ephedrine
Imipramine hydrochloride	Heavy metals
Lithium carbonate	Hexamethylamine
Phenelzine sulfate	Metrizamide
Anticonvulsants	Phenylephrine hydrochloride
Ethosuximide	Promethazine hydrochloride
Phenobarbital	Ranitidine
Phenytoin	Solvents
Primidone	Vincristine
Cardiovascular Agents	Volatile hydrocarbons
Digitalis	
Disopyramide	
Methyldopa	
Propranolol hydrochloride	
Quinidine	
Reserpine	
Timolol	

Adapted from Cummings JL, et al. Visual hallucinations: Clinical occurrences and use in differential diagnosis. West J Med. 1987;146:46–51.

Section II
Eye Movements

CHAPTER 10

SUPRANUCLEAR EYE MOVEMENT SYSTEMS AND THEIR SUBSTRATES

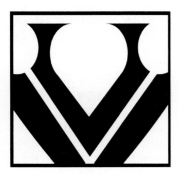

Recent advances in understanding of eye movements are formidable. The last decade produced logorithmic leaps in knowledge through clinical correlations, neuro-imaging, study of normal eye movement physiology and pathologic eye movements, modeling of neural substrates, and incorporation of information theory. Yet an exact understanding of the anatomic and physiologic substrates for eye movements remains elusive. What follows presents a clinical approach to eye movement disorders. The details of control system analysis and parallel processing are difficult to incorporate into this rubric. What used to be thought of as relatively monolithic eye movement subsystems are really groups of subsystems responding to different types of stimuli, processed in parallel, sometimes with parallel efferent pathways as well, until the final common pathway in the brain stem. The optimal facilities for isolation, measurement, and clinical integration of these subsystems are available to few of us. Thus, I have chosen to omit many details of eye movement pathophysiology in favor of a more succinct, pragmatic approach. Consequently, these sections admittedly fall short in providing an up-to-date information-processing oriented approach to eye movements and their disorders. For this aspect of ocular motility, the reader is referred to the excellent book by Leigh and Zee, the other references listed in the bibliography, and the reference lists within those publications.

OVERVIEW

Eye movements serve a number of specific visual functions. Primarily, they direct the fovea to objects of interest, either by aiming the fovea at a stationary target or by pursuing a moving target. At the same time, they maintain proper alignment of the eyes with respect to one another and adjust for movement of the head and body. Normally, all these activities are simultaneous; visual, proprioceptive, and other inputs are continually processed and interrelated to create the visual relationship with our environment.

Eye movements are executed by one or more specific supranuclear eye movement systems, which are functionally and to some degree anatomically separate. The four eye movement systems are the (1) saccadic; (2) smooth pursuit; (3) vergence; and (4) reflex (vestibular, otolithic, and full-field optokinetic nystagmus [OKN]) systems. In addition, the cerebellum influences eye movements—especially the precision of saccadic (fast) eye movements and the ability to adapt to disorders of pursuit.

The *saccadic system* generates fast eye movements that direct the eye to objects of visual interest away from the fovea. *Smooth pursuit* is used to follow slowly and smoothly moving objects and maintain them on the fovea. The third eye movement system, the *vergence system*, turns the eyes toward or away from each other to maintain binocular fixation on objects at various distances. The fourth system, the *reflex system*, encompasses optokinetic, labyrinthine, otolithic, and tonic neck reflexes, which regulate the position of the eyes with respect to the head and body; and includes the vestibulo-ocular reflex (VOR). This system, as its name implies, is primarily reflex in nature.

Pathways for eye movement proceed from their origins in the hemispheres, cerebellum, brain stem, or elsewhere (peripheral receptors) to the premotor areas of the pons (horizontal eye movements) and mesencephalon (vertical eye movements). They converge via parallel distributed networks onto the final common pathway, the ocular motor neurons of cranial nerves III, IV, and VI (Fig. 10–1).

This chapter discusses the general principles that govern the eye movement systems. Each system is considered in isolation from the other eye movement systems to simplify examination and analysis. However, all four eye movement mechanisms normally work simultaneously. Each system has its own stimulus, latency of response, velocity range, and sampling considerations (Table 10–1).

NEURAL CONTROL SIGNALS

For saccades, the premotor innervation includes phasic and tonic components. The *phasic component* (or pulse) is proportional to eye velocity and movement amplitude; the *tonic component* (or step) is proportional to eye position. A neural integrator (in the mathematical sense), as yet unlocalized anatomically, derives the position coding from the eye velocity command. Apparently, one neural integrator operates for all horizontal eye movements (nucleus prepositus hypoglossi?) and another for all vertical eye movements (medial vestibular nucleus or rostral interstitial nucleus of the median longitudinal fasciculus [MLF]?). For horizontal saccades, excitatory burst cells in the ipsilateral paramedian pontine reticular formation (PPRF) generate the saccadic pulse to the agonist abducens nucleus. The motorneurons of the abducens nucleus innervate the ipsilateral lateral rectus, and the interneurons pro-

ceed in the contralateral MLF to the oculomotor nucleus to control the contralateral medial rectus. Inhibitory burst neurons, located in the PPRF, inhibit the contralateral antagonist abducens nucleus and the ipsilateral medial rectus. Omnipause neurons continuously inhibit the excitatory burst cells except during the saccade. The step, derived by the neural integrator, generates the tonic activity, which then holds the eye in its new position (Fig. 10–2). Similar mechanisms generate vertical saccades.

THE SACCADIC SYSTEM (FAST EYE MOVEMENTS)

Saccades are fast eye movements principally mediated by frontal, dorsomedial temporal, and intraparietal cortices and by superior collicular (SC) pathways descending to the paramedian reticular formation in the mesencephalon, pons, and medulla.

The **saccadic system** generates **all** fast eye movements: refixation movements, fast phases of vestibular nystagmus, fast phases of optokinetic nystagmus (OKN) and other true nystagmus, and many abnormal eye movements and microsaccades (probably). Fixation movements place an object of interest on the fovea or move the eyes from one object to another. Thus, when you hear an unusual noise and move your eyes to see what caused it, you make a saccade. You also use a saccade to look up from your desk to see what time it is, or to look from word to word as you read. Hence, saccades are frequently termed voluntary eye movements. However, reflex and involuntary eye movements like fast phases of nystagmus and many abnormal ocular oscillations are also saccades, as are the rapid eye

Figure 10–1. A simplified diagram of premotor networks subserving five eye movement systems. These networks mostly converge at the level of the motoneurone. (Dtn, dorsal terminal nucleus; lgn, lateral geniculate nucleus; ltn, lateral terminal nucleus; min, medial terminal nucleus; not, nucleus of the optic tract; OKR, optokinetic response; pph, nucleus prepositus hypoglossi; rf, reticular formation; sc, superior colliculus; vn, vestibular nuclei; VOR, vestibulo-ocular reflex. *(From Buttner-Ennever J. Anatomy of the ocular motor nuclei. In Kennard C, Rose FC. Physiological Aspects of Clinical Neuro-ophthalmology. Chicago: Year Book, 1988, with permission.)*

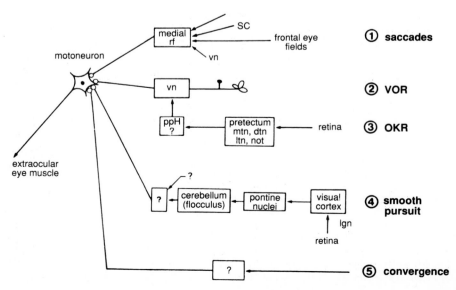

TABLE 10–1. EYE MOVEMENT SYSTEMS

	Saccadic	Pursuit	Vergence	Ocular Motor Reflex System (Vestibular, Otolithic, Neck Reflexes)
Function	Place object of interest on fovea rapidly	Maintain object of regard near fovea, match eye and target	Align visual axes to maintain bifoveal fixation	Maintain eye position with respect to changes in head and body posture
Stimulus	Object of interest in peripheral field	Moving object near fovea	Retinal disparity	Stimulation of semicircular canals, otoliths, neck receptors
Latency (from stimulus to onset of eye movement)	200 msec	125 msec	160 msec	Very short, about 10 msec
Velocity	To 700 degrees/sec	To 100 degrees/sec	Around 20 degrees/sec	To 300 degrees/sec[a]
Feedback	Mostly sampled	Continuous	Continuous	Continuous

[a] Slow phase only. The fast phase is initiated in the pontine reticular formation via the saccadic mechanism and has the same characteristics as that system.
From Gay A, Newman NN, Keltner J, Stroud M. Eye Movement Disorders. *St. Louis: Mosby, 1974.*

movements so characteristic of rapid eye movement (REM) sleep. Conversely, many other types of eye movements may be voluntary.

A tentative division of saccadic labor suggests that cortical areas generate intentional and reflex saccades. For example, the frontal eye fields generate purposeful, nonvisually guided saccades; the parietal–temporal occipital area, visually guided intentional saccades; and the superior colliculi and subcortical paths, spontaneous saccades and the fast phases of nystagmus.

Nearly all fast eye movements are moderated by the cerebellum. In fact, the majority of abnormal ocular oscillations (many erroneously termed "nystag-

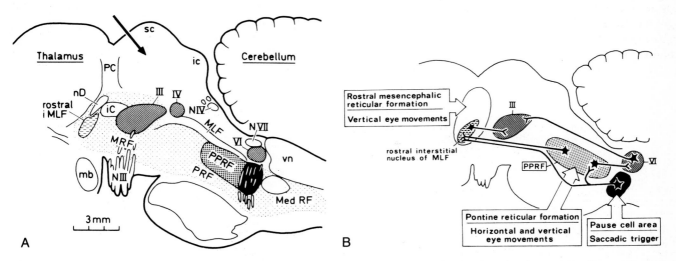

Figure 10–2. A. Schematic sagittal view of the brain-stem reticular formation in the monkey, to demonstrate the anatomical localization of some structures involved in the generation of saccades. Omnipause neurones are located at the level of the abducens rootlets, in caudal PPRF in the black area; the white region just caudal to this in the medullary reticular formation marks the location of the horizontal inhibitory burst units. (III, oculomotor nucleus; IV, trochlear nucleus; VI, abducens nucleus; iC, interstitial nucleus of Cajal; ic, inferior colliculus; iMLF, [rostral] interstitial nucleus of MLF; mb, mammillary body; medRF, medullary reticular formation; MLF, medial longitudinal fasciculus; MRF, mesencephalic reticular formation; MIII, oculomotor nerve; NIV, trochlear nerve; NVII, facial nerve; nD, nucleus Darkschewitsch; PC, posterior commissure; PPRF, paramedian pontine reticular formation; sc, superior colliculus; vn, vestibular nuclei.) **B.** A view of the brain stem showing some of the basic connections involved in the generation of the horizontal and vertical components of saccades. For the sake of simplicity only the oculomotor (III) and abducens nuclei (VI) are drawn. (*From Buttner-Ennever J. Anatomy of the ocular motor nuclei. In: Kennard C, Rose FC. Physiological Aspects of Clinical Neuro-ophthalmology. Chicago: Year Book, 1988, with permission.*)

mus'') are disruptions of the saccadic system (or its cerebellar inputs) or saccadic intrusions into other eye movements.

Characteristics of saccadic eye movements. Saccades are rapid eye movements with a long delay from stimulus to execution. The stimulus for a refixation saccade is an object of interest whose image is distant from the fovea. In laboratory testing, from the onset of the stimulus to the beginning of the recorded saccade, the latent period is about 200 msec. Normal saccades are all very rapid (to 700 degrees/sec), with a velocity that increases proportionally to the size of the saccade.

The saccadic system operates much as a sampled data system, but some stimulus alterations during the latent period do modify the resultant eye movements; thus, the saccadic system seems able to process information continuously. Nevertheless, once a saccade is initiated, the motor output remains very resistant to change. During all saccades, the visual threshold is increased, resulting in decreased visual sensitivity and perception. Movement is preprogrammed and very precise; a slight undershoot or overshoot can be normal.

The electromyogram (EMG) shows an abrupt increase in activity of the agonist (reflecting the neural pulse) and immediate reciprocal inhibition of the antagonist (Fig. 10–3). When the eye movement reaches its target, the tonic electrical pattern appropriate for the new eye position (reflecting the neural step) is adopted and keeps the eye in the target position. This reciprocal, nearly instantaneous change in electrical activity is the same for all saccadic eye movements and correlates with tension curves recorded from the extraocular muscles (Fig. 10–4). During initiation of the saccade, the curves reflect an excess of tension, presumably to overcome the viscoelastic drag of the globe and orbit. The initial burst of electromyographic activity correlates with the initial overshoot of the tension curve.

Anatomic correlates and physiology. Neurons of the frontal cortex (frontal eye fields [FEF]), the dorsomedial temporal regions, and the intraparietal areas and their descending pathways as well as neurons of the superior colliculus (SC) mediate rapid eye movements via at least two parallel pathways. In general, horizontal rapid eye movements are mediated by the contralateral cortex, including the frontal eye fields; in experimental studies using direct electrical stimulation, however, the frontal lobes can produce ipsilateral movements as well.

Vertical conjugate rapid eye movements depend on simultaneous bilateral activity within the cortex in essentially the same cerebral areas that generate horizontal eye movements on unilateral stimulation.

In alert monkeys the frontal lobe neurons discharge during, rather than prior to, saccades. This suggests that the frontal lobes do not initiate rapid eye movements, but instead play an obligatory, poorly understood role, perhaps of a facilitatory nature, while other, probably brainstem, structures act as the saccadic generator. Positron emission tomography (PET) during saccades suggests that saccades are controlled by the contralateral prefrontal cortex. For horizontal saccades the cortical axons descend to the paramedian pontine reticular formation

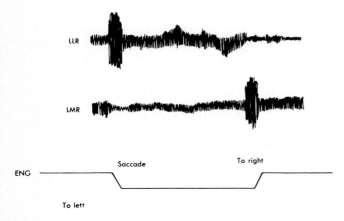

Figure 10–3. EMG pattern of a saccade. Resting activity in primary position. Note burst of activity in agonist LLR and complete reciprocal inhibition of activity in antagonist LMR on gaze left. The reverse occurs on gaze right. (LLR, left lateral rectus; LMR, left medial rectus.) (*From Gay A, Newman NN, Keltner J, Stroud M. Eye Movement Disorders. St. Louis: Mosby, 1974, with permission.*)

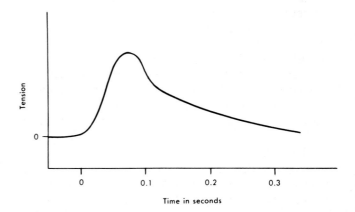

Figure 10–4. Isometric tension of agonist in a saccade. Note the overshoot presumed necessary to overcome the visco-elastic properties of the globe and orbital tissues. Also note the similarity to the EMG pattern. (*From Gay A, Newman NN, Keltner J, Stroud M. Eye Movement Disorders. St. Louis: Mosby, 1974, with permission.*)

(PPRF) after decussating at the level of the ocular motor nuclei. A parallel pathway descends via the superior colliculus. For vertical saccades the paths descend bilaterally to the pretectal area of the midbrain (vertical gaze center). Cortical or SC lesions alone lead to transient defects in saccade generation; lesions of both cortical and SC pathways lead to severe and persistent saccadic deficits.

Processes (such as progressive supranuclear palsy, covered in Chapter 12) that do affect the entire saccadic mechanism are diffuse, widespread disturbances.

Cerebellar and cerebellar pathway lesions. The cerebellum has important roles in the control of saccadic amplitude, repair of saccadic dysmetria, and maintenance of appropriate gaze positions following saccades. The most dramatic alterations of saccadic control, opsoclonus (multidirectional saccades) and flutter (horizontal saccades), are back-to-back saccades without an intersaccadic interval (see Chapters 12 and 14). These occur in lesions of the cerebellar pathways, hypothetically in the omnipause cells that normally inhibit spontaneous saccades misfunction. Saccadic intrusions are less dramatic abnormalities causing disruptive saccades that (like opsoclonus and flutter) move the fovea *away* from its target; however, saccadic intrusions have normal intersaccadic intervals. Saccadic intrusions include square wave jerks, myoclonus, and bobbing (see Chapter 14).

The precise anatomic pathways interconnecting the saccadic ocular motor system with the cerebellum are not defined. Neither is it known at what point the cerebellum exercises control over the ocular motor outflow: It may be close to the final common path (cerebellar efferents connect directly to the ocular motor nuclei; comparable cortical efferents for the cerebral hemispheres remain unidentified), perhaps via connecting loops through the brain-stem PPRF. In any case, the cerebellum continuously modulates head and eye movements. Saccades modulate as a function of head movement, so that head and eye movement add to give the desired excursion; if the head is restrained, the eye movement compensates. This modulation occurs via negative vestibuloocular feedback.

Disorders of saccades per se include slow saccades, prolonged latency of saccades, inaccurate saccades, and inappropriate saccades (see the discussions of disorders of separate eye movements for clinical correlates).

Cerebellar lesions (especially of the flocculus) also cause marked deficits in smooth pursuit, in suppression of inappropriate vestibular nystagmus, and in VOR regulation.

Tests: To evaluate the function of the saccadic system, test the eye movements it generates: refixation movements, fast phases of vestibular nystagmus, and fast phases of OKN. Test both horizontally and vertically. Rapid alternations in fixation will illustrate the lag of an eye with slow saccades. Note the intrusion of inappropriate saccades into fixation or nonsaccadic eye movements. Small-amplitude intrusions (eg, square wave jerks) not visible on observation sometimes are visible when looking at the retina with the magnification of the ophthalmoscope.

Other Considerations

Importance of the macula. The integrity of refixation saccades depends upon the development of the fovea. Thus, while infants are several weeks old before they utilize refixation saccades, they have an intact fast eye movement system at birth, demonstrable as normal fast phases of vestibular or optokinetic nystagmus. As a corollary, congenitally blind subjects do not develop normal refixation saccades. Usually, they develop a meandering, pendular eye movement in the first few months.

Effect of stage of consciousness. Rapid eye movements occur in certain states of consciousness (reticular activating system activity). They are normally present in alert subjects and are selectively depressed in patients with lowered states of consciousness; for example, in coma, under anesthesia, sleep, or following the use of certain drugs. In general, as the state of consciousness decreases, first voluntary and then reflex rapid eye movements are lost. In stuporous patients there may be no spontaneous rapid eye movements, but normal caloric vestibular nystagmus may be elicited; then, as deeper stages of coma intervene, the fast phases of the vestibular response diminish, and a slow tonic deviation is the only response to vestibular stimulation. A similar sequence of eye movement depression is seen as patients progress from light to deeper stages of anesthesia and after taking large doses of sedative drugs such as barbiturates.

Vestibular stimulation or the oculocephalic maneuver can cause tonic deviations in unconscious patients. These maneuvers test the integrity of the nuclear and infranuclear pathways when no voluntary or saccadic eye movements are present.

> For example, you are called to the emergency room to see a patient who was knocked from his motorcycle. He is unconscious. He has no spontaneous eye movements. Because he is unconscious, it is not possible to test OKN. You are reluctant to move his head in the doll's-head maneuver before neuroradiologic evaluation. However, you want to evaluate the function of the cranial nerves. After assuring the integrity of the

tympanic membranes, you perform ice water calorics in each ear separately. (See Chapter 11) for details of the caloric testing procedure and interpretation.) You find that only slow phases are evoked. Both eyes move fully to the right. However, while the right eye moves fully to the left, the left eye barely moves past midline. You have detected a left abduction deficit, probably due to sixth nerve palsy.

When consciousness is severely depressed, even doll's-head and caloric responses are absent. This total absence of eye movement often indicates a metabolic disorder or drug intoxication, especially if the patient is not moribund.

During sleep, rapid eye movements are so characteristic of the stage associated with dreams that this part of the sleep cycle has been named "REM sleep." At least one patient has been described with an abnormal REM, opsoclonus, present always during the alert state but only during the REM stage of sleep.

FOVEAL SMOOTH PURSUIT SYSTEM

The smooth pursuit system is utilized to follow small targets that move smoothly and relatively slowly. It maintains a fixed relationship between eyes and target; the velocity of a pursuit movement is linearly related to the velocity of the target (up to approximately of 40 degrees/sec—much slower than saccadic velocities, which reach 700 degrees/sec). Because smooth pursuit movements directly relate eye position to target position, they are also termed following, or tracking movements. The slow phase of OKN with hand-held tapes or drums is another pursuit movement.

Obviously, because the head usually moves in conjunction with the eye, a mechanism is needed to counteract the contralateral movement generated by the vestibulo-ocular reflex (VOR) (see below: Vestibular-Otolithic System). This VOR cancellation seems to be expressed via the pursuit mechanism.

Characteristics. Pursuit movements are characterized by short latency (125 msec) and, as might be expected, the visual threshold is not altered during pursuit, because eye and target movement must be continuously matched. Consistent with this, the feedback control for the system seems to be continuous. The stimulus for pursuit is slippage of the target off the fovea, detected via errors in eye target position, velocity, and acceleration. When foveal fixation is normal, the pursuit mechanism reaches a maximum velocity of 60 degrees/sec.

When the velocity capabilities of the smooth pursuit mechanism are exceeded, the smooth pur-

suit movement is interrupted by saccades in an attempt to place the target back on the fovea (via catch-up or back-up saccades) so that the pursuit mechanism can begin functioning again. Where central vision is absent (central scotoma), slippage of the target away from the fovea (the stimulus that would normally evoke a saccade) is no longer sensed, and the pursuit system is allowed to operate without interruption from the saccadic mechanism. In other words, in the normal person, once the target has slipped off the fovea, the saccadic system is stimulated, causing an interruption in the normal pursuit movement. However, if there is no parafoveal stimulation, as with a dense central scotoma, target slippage from the fovea does not induce a saccade, and the pursuit mechanism can operate uninterrupted, attaining higher velocities. When the pursuit pathways are damaged or the patient is not alert, saccades may interrupt the pursuit movement earlier, as the pursuing movements do not match the target velocity—so-called "saccadic pursuit."

Electromyographic pattern. During pursuit, the ocular EMG shows a gradual increase of firing (recruitment) in the agonist and a concomitant gradual decrease of firing (inhibition) in the antagonist (Fig. 10–5).

Anatomic correlates. Each cerebral hemisphere participates in smooth pursuit in both directions. The hemispheric substrates for smooth pursuit eye

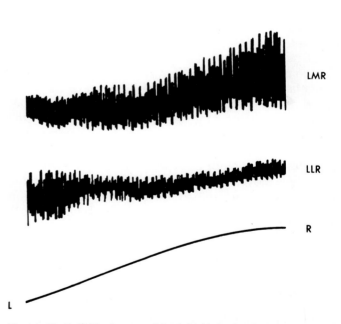

Figure 10–5. EMG of a pursuit to right. Note gradual increase in firing in the agonist LMR and gradual decrease in the antagonist LLR. (LLR, left lateral rectus; LMR, left medial rectus.) (*From Gay A, Newman NN, Keltner J, Stroud M. Eye Movement Disorders. St. Louis: Mosby, 1974, with permission.*)

movements include projections of the motion-sensitive portions of the visual afferent pathways: M-retinal ganglion cells to lateral geniculate nucleus (LGN) magnocellular layers to striate cortex (V_1) to middle temporal and medial superior temporal cortex at the parietal occipital temporal confluence. Axons from this area project (possibly via the posterior limb of the internal capsule) to ipsilateral pontine nuclei (dorsolateral pontine nuclei), which in turn project to the flocculus and posterior vermis of the cerebellum. Possibly, there is a parallel path from the frontal eye fields to the nucleus recticularis tegmenti pontis. Pursuit commands proceed to the medial vestibular nuclei for horizontal pursuit and the "y" group of the vestibular nuclei for vertical pursuit. As-yet-undocumented pathways carry the position signal to the neural integrator and tonic premotor neurons. From there they proceed to the ocular motor nuclei (III, IV, VI) (Fig. 10–6). Lesions of the FEFs and SC also impair pursuit.

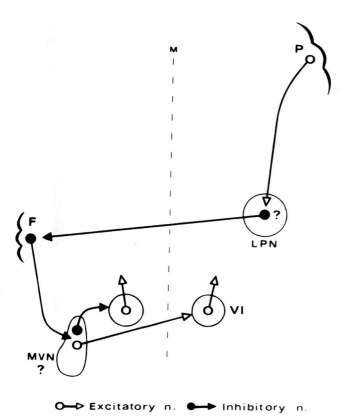

O—▷ Excitatory n.   ●—▶ Inhibitory n.

Figure 10–6. Hypothetical circuitry of foveal smooth pursuit. (F, flocculus; LPN, lateral pontine nuclei; M, midline; MVN, medial vestibular nucleus; P, posterior cerebral cortex; VI, abducens nucleus; ?, the inhibitory nature of the pontofloccular neurone and a relay in the MVN are still uncertain.) (*From Buttner-Ennever J. Anatomy of the ocular motor nuclei. In: Kennard C, Rose FC. Physiological Aspects of Clinical Neuroophthalmology. Chicago: Yearbook, 1988, with permission.*)

The substrates for vertical pursuit proceed to the pretectal area and those for horizontal pursuit to the PPRF.

Tests: Ask the patient to follow a slowly, smoothly moving target. Pursuit is also tested by the slow phase of OKN with hand-held targets and the oculocephalic maneuver (doll's-head maneuver—ask the patient to fix on an object while the head is rotated). Especially in uncooperative patients, this may be a better test than following a target, because it is more automatic and eliminates voluntary effort, but it does contain some nonoptic reflex influence.

VERGENCE SYSTEM

By controlling the visual axes of the eyes, the vergence system keeps the image of a target on appropriate points (corresponding elements) of the two retinas. Vergence is elicited by retinal disparity, when a target falls on noncorresponding retinal elements, or blur. For example, if a target moves toward the eyes, they must turn toward each other (converge) to keep the target on the fovea of each eye (Fig. 10–7). Conversely, as the target moves farther away, the eyes must turn out (diverge). Vergence is thus a disconjugate (nonparallel) movement of the eyes, in contrast to most other eye movements, which are conjugate (parallel). It is basic to stereopsis.

To test for (con)vergence, ask the patient to look from distant to near objects. Lesions of the vergence system cause deficient vergence movements and diplopia.

When the vergence system (fusional vergence) is inadequate to overcome the tendency of the eyes to become misaligned, strabismus results.

Characteristics. The vergence system generates the slowest eye movements of all (about 20 degrees/sec); its latency is about 160 msec.

Anatomic correlates. The anatomic substrates for vergence movements have never been precisely defined. These functions appear to be represented diffusely in the occipitoparietal temporal confluence. The efferent pathway involves the pretectal area, midbrain tegmentum, and paramedian pontine tegmentum. Within the midbrain there appear to be both convergence and divergence burst cells with firing patterns analogous to saccadic burst cells, suggesting that the neural organization of the vergence system in some ways resembles that of the saccadic system despite the significant differences in the resultant eye movement. Recent studies also demonstrate separate cell populations active in vergence and accommodation, despite the tight coupling of these functions in normal visual behavior.

Other considerations. Disease processes rarely

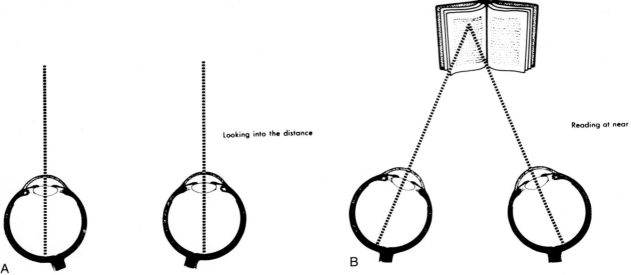

Figure 10–7. Vergence. When looking into the distance, the visual axes are parallel; when reading at near, the visual axes converge. (*From Gay A, Newman NN, Keltner J, Stroud M.* Eye Movement Disorders. *St. Louis: Mosby, 1974, with permission.*)

affect the vergence system alone. Cerebral hemisphere lesions that damage it are usually large and diffuse and will affect pursuit movements and fixation as well. Convergence is most frequently affected by lesions of the pretectal area. Here, disorders of vergence (especially convergence) are frequently associated with pupillary abnormalities, limitation of upward gaze (with or without lid retraction), or convergence–retraction "nystagmus" (Parinaud's syndrome, Chapter 12; sylvian aqueduct syndrome). The near reflex consists of convergence, accommodation, and miosis: spasm of convergence is accompanied by increased hyperopia and miosis. Voluntary nystagmus is thought to be evoked by vergence movements. Divergence palsy is probably early bilateral sixth-nerve palsies.

VESTIBULAR, OTOLITHIC, AND FULL-FIELD OKN REFLEX SYSTEMS

Function. These reflex systems integrate eye movements with head and body movements and stabilize gaze during head and body movements. They include the labyrinthine reflexes mediated by the semicircular canal systems of the inner ears, and reflexes involving the otolith organs of the vestibular system and the neck receptors. These reflex systems produce prompt (minimal latency) but slow eye movements that compensate for head and body movements to maintain a stable retinal image. The vestibular system responds to rotational movements of the head and body (angular acceleration) via the VOR, whereas the otolithic system responds to tilting movements (linear acceleration). Dorsal pontine nuclei appear to record retinal slip. In response to head movement, a smooth eye movement in the opposite direction is generated. It is unclear whether these smooth slow eye movements of the VOR are identical to pursuit movements. In addition, because target, head and body movements can exceed the velocity capabilities of the vestibular system, a velocity storage mechanism mediated by the cerebellar nodulus (for horizontal and possibly vertical eye movements) and, possibly, the interstitial nucleus of Cajal for vertical eye movements, helps to adjust the ocular movements appropriately.

Characteristics. These reflexes are stimulated by head and body rotation. Disruption of the usual balanced sensory input from each semicircular canal system by head rotation is the stimulus for the vestibular reflex system; its balance is disrupted by unilateral increase or decrease in input (eg, head or body rotation, caloric stimulation, or labyrinthine or eighth nerve damage). Latency of response in the vestibular system is very brief. Compensatory eye movements of the vestibular system may reach a velocity of 300 degrees/sec. Head or body tilt activates the otoliths.

Anatomic correlates. The labyrinthine system consists of the semicircular canals and otoliths, the eighth cranial nerves, and the vestibular nuclei and their projections. The pathways serving this system ascend from the vestibular nucleus to the ocular motor nuclei via the MLF and the surrounding pontine reticular formation. The superior and medial vestibular nuclei and Deiters' nucleus are the vestibular nuclei functionally related to the oculomotor nuclei. Their connections are both crossed and uncrossed and appear to be specific, such that vestibular subnuclei and oculomotor subnuclei serving extraocular movements in a specific plane are interconnected (for example, the superior vestibular nucleus and the dorsal ocular motor subnucleus on each side send impulses to the ipsilateral inferior rectus for movements in the vertical plane). The medial vestibular nucleus is the premotor relay for all reflex horizontal slow eye movements: the VOR, the cervico-ocular (tonic neck) reflexes, and full-field OKN.

The slow component is generated entirely within the brain stem. The fast component is also set off within the brain stem. Where this interaction of brain stem and cerebral systems occurs is not known. Lesions of the vestibulocerebellum profoundly affect the VOR, especially adaptive changes.

Tests. These systems can be evaluated by caloric testing, the oculocephalic maneuver, and body and/or head rotation.

Cerebellar pathways. Lesions of the cerebellum and its pathways cause degeneration of the precision of eye movement, particularly the abilities to make accurate saccades and to maintain gaze position or to compensate for eye movement deficits. The cerebellum is particularly important in maintaining the adaptive functions and plastic control of the eye movement systems. Lesions of the vermis and its brain-stem connections cause loss of precision in saccadic movement (ocular dysmetria, ocular flutter, opsoclonus, macrosaccadic oscillations, and intrusions). Oscillations are initiated by saccades; intrusions are sporadic saccadic movements taking the eyes away from the target. Lesions of the vestibulocerebellum (flocculus and nodulus) and its brain-stem connections cause degeneration in the accuracy of smooth pursuit and vestibular movements, inability to maintain eccentric gaze positions, and decreased facility to compensate for disorders of smooth pursuit.

SUPRANUCLEAR "GAZE CENTERS"

Two brain-stem regions are especially important to the supranuclear control of conjugate eye movements (gaze): the paramedian pontine reticular formation and the dorsal mesencephalic or pretectal area.

Pretectal "Gaze Centers"

Pathways for vertical gaze movements are organized in the mesencephalic or pretectal region rostral to the oculomotor nuclei; ascending paths from the cerebellum, vestibular nuclei, paramedian pontine reticular formation, and abducens nuclei converge here. The rostral interstitial nucleus of the MLF (riM-

LF) is critical to vertical saccades and has been attributed to characteristics of the vertical neural integrator. It contains vertical saccadic burst neurons. The saccadic, pursuit, and vestibular systems all feed into this area, and a lesion here may affect all vertical conjugate gaze movements. Upgaze palsy, downgaze palsy, and complete vertical gaze palsy result from bilateral lesions in the region of the posterior commissure. The riMLF projects contralaterally through the posterior commissure so that midline lesions involving these paths sometimes cause bilateral as well as unilateral vertical gaze disorders. The posterior commissure region is especially critical for upgaze; the riMLF region for downgaze. The interstitial nucleus of Cajal (INC) is related to slow eye movements and vertical gaze holding. There seems to be some separation of the upgaze and downgaze pathways. Masses (such as pinealomas that encroach on the center from above and rostrally) and hydrocephalus (in children) eliminate upgaze, but leave downgaze intact until the mass grows larger. In children with hydrocephalus, upgaze palsy may be the first sign of a blocked shunt.

Pontine "Gaze Center"

The **pathways for horizontal gaze movements** terminate near the nucleus of the sixth cranial nerve. In this region the various eye movement mechanisms for horizontal gaze are organized into what has been called the **pontine gaze center** (PGC), a center for conjugate gaze to the same side. This area, the PPRF, is critical for lateral saccades. The PPRF sends the premotor command to the abducens nucleus. Lesions here produce an ipsilateral saccadic paresis, a paresis of ipsilateral conjugate gaze, or both. It is a gaze center in the sense that all horizontal conjugate eye movements are dependent on its proper functioning. Saccades, pursuit, and vestibular nystagmus may all be affected by lesions in this area, selectively or in combination.

Severe lesions cause the eyes to deviate to the contralateral side; the patient cannot bring them back across the midline. Lesser lesions cause a gaze palsy or gaze paretic nystagmus.

BIBLIOGRAPHY

General

Carpenter RHS. *Movements of the Eyes.* London: Pion, 1977.

Fuchs AF, Becker W, eds. *Progress in Oculomotor Research.* Amsterdam: Elsevier, 1981.

Keller EL, Zee DS, eds. *Adaptive Processes in Visual and Oculomotor Systems.* New York: Pergamon, 1986.

Kennard C, Rose FC. *Physiological Aspects of Clinical Neuro-ophthalmology.* Chicago: Year Book, 1988.

Leigh RJ, Zee DS. *The Neurology of Eye Movements.* Philadelphia: Davis, 1983.

Miller N, ed. *Walsh and Hoyt's Clinical Neuro-ophthalmology.* 4th ed. Baltimore: Williams & Wilkins, 1985;2.

Saccades and Saccadic Intrusions

Fox PT, Fox JM, Raichle ME, Burde RM. The role of cerebral cortex in the generation of voluntary saccades: A positron emission tomographic study. *J Neurophysiol.* 1985;54:348–368.

Sharpe JA, Fletcher W. Saccadic intrusions and oscillations. *Can J Neurol Sci.* 1984;11:426–433.

Zee DS. Oculomotor control: The cerebral control of eye movements. In: Lessell S, Van Dalen JTW, eds. *Neuro-Ophthalmology.* New York: Elsevier, 1984:141–156.

Pursuit

Bogousslavsky J, Regli F. Pursuit gaze defects in acute and chronic unilateral parietal occipital lesions. *Eur Neurol.* 1986;25:10–18.

Sharpe JH, Fletcher WA. Disorders of visual fixation. In: Lessell, S, ed. *Neuro-ophthalmology Now.* Chicago: Year Book, 1986;267–284.

Tusa RJ, Zee DS. Cerebral control of smooth pursuit and optokinetic nystagmus. In: Lessell S, Van Dalen JTW, eds. *Current Neuro-ophthalmology.* Chicago: Year Book, 1989;2:115–146.

Cerebellar Control

Ito M. *The Cerebellum and Neural Control.* New York: Raven, 1984.

Vergence

Judge SJ, Cumming BG. Neurons in monkey midbrain with activity related to vergence eye movement and accommodation. *J Neurophysiol.* 1986;55:915–930.

Mays LE, Porter JD, Gamlin PD, Tello CA. Neural control of vergence eye movements: Neurons encoding vergence velocity. *J Neurophysiol.* 1986;56:1007–1021.

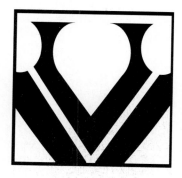

CHAPTER 11

EXAMINATION OF EYE MOVEMENTS

This chapter considers primarily the examination of the supranuclear eye movement mechanisms—those that produce conjugate eye movement disorders without diplopia. For the evaluation of the patient with diplopia or restricted eye movements, see Chapters 13 and 15.

Fixation. Evaluation of fixation is the primary step in the examination of eye movements, because disorders in fixation affect all eye movement systems. To examine fixation, ask the patient to gaze steadily for several seconds, first at a near target (approximatley 15 inches away) and than at a distant target (ideally at least 20 feet away). The patient should be able to maintain steady fixation on both targets for a minimum of 5 seconds, without drifting and without noticeable movement. If fixation is poor, the patient should be asked to hold a thumb approximately 15 inches in front of the face and to look at a mark on the thumbnail. The additional proprioceptive input from the hand and arm often helps to maintain eye position. If the patient still cannot fixate, some questions are raised: Is failure due to lack of effort or cooperation? Is it related to decreased

alertness? Is fixation interrupted by abnormal eye movements? Is there a primary defect of cerebral control of fixation?

Random movements will be observed if the patient is distracted or failing to make adequate effort. If the patient's level of alertness is decreased, the response will vary accordingly. Pathologic disturbances of fixation may be manifest in abnormal ocular motility, such as tonic deviation or nystagmus, opsoclonus, or macro-oscillations. Looking into an eye with an ophthalmoscope can magnify and make obvious abnormal small eye movements.

Smooth pursuit. Test smooth pursuit by asking the patient to follow a target moving slowly (less than 20 degrees/sec) and smoothly across the field of vision. Normally, the subject should do this precisely. Inability to maintain smooth pursuit results in interruption by saccades (Fig. 11–1). Saccadic pursuit is frequently associated with hemispheric lesions; however, its presence cannot be reliably used as a localizing sign, for it occurs with anxiety and fatigue, drug effects (especially barbiturates, diphenylhydantoin, or alcohol), and with lesions of the brain stem and/or cerebellar pathways.

Range of movement. The range of ocular movement and the binocular coordination of motility may be tested while observing the smooth pursuit mechanism. The patient watches a target that is moved slowly and smoothly into the six diagnostic positions of gaze (Fig. 11–2). Ordinarily, both eyes move conjugately into all extremes of gaze (versions). A normally full horizontal movement hides the limbus (the border of the cornea and the sclera) under the medial or lateral canthus. Vertically, upgaze should reach at least 30 degrees. For unknown reasons, upgaze becomes limited as one grows older. If full gaze movements are not elicited, note whether both eyes are equally limited (a problem of conjugate gaze,

Figure 11–1. A. Electronystagmogram (ENG) of normal patient following a pendulum. Note smooth uninterrupted following movements. **B.** ENG of patient with saccadic pursuit to the right. (*From Gay A, Newman NN, Keltner J, Stroud M. Eye Movement Disorders. St. Louis: Mosby, 1974, with permission.*)

Gaze right   Gaze left

A

B

Figure 11–2. Diagnostic positions of gaze (as viewed by the examiner). The indicated muscle is best isolated in the fields designated. (LR - lateral rectus, MR - medial rectus, SR - superior rectus, IR - inferior rectus, IO - inferior oblique, SO superior oblique) (*From Gay A, Newman NN, Keltner J, Stroud M. Eye Movement Disorders. St. Louis: Mosby, 1974, with permission.*)

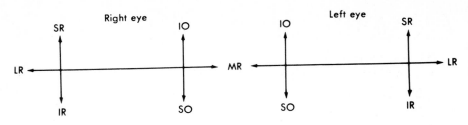

which will be discussed below) or whether one eye alone is limited. If the response is confusing, movement of each eye should be examined separately (ductions).

The **six diagnostic gaze positions** are those that best isolate the action of a single muscle (but not necessarily the most powerful or effective positions of the muscles). With acute paresis of a single muscle, diplopia is maximum in the diagnostic position that represents that muscle (Fig. 11–3). The eye with the lagging or paretic muscle always projects the image further, producing maximal diplopia in the direction of paretic gaze. Once the field of maximal diplopia is determined, the paretic muscle itself may be identified by observing the uniocular movements of the eyes (ductions). For example, if diplopia is greater in looking up and to the right, there are two possible muscles involved: the right superior rectus (RSR) and the left inferior oblique (LIO). If the right eye is limited in movement in this direction, it is the RSR that is paretic (Fig. 11–4). If more than one eye muscle is limited, the eye movement will represent the combined deficit. In long-standing palsies, acquired overaction and contractions confuse the picture.

Diplopia usually indicates a nuclear or infranuclear lesion, especially when it is present in the primary position.

The identification of paretic muscles and the quantification of limitations and restrictions of eye movement by measurement with prisms are usually sufficient for most neuro-ophthalmic evaluations. To follow any limitation objectively, quantification is always necessary. It is also critical for evaluation and treatment planning in strabismus.

When both eyes show equally limited movement in the same direction, usually a *gaze paresis* exists, signifying a supranuclear lesion and involving one or more of the conjugate gaze mechanisms. Because both eyes are equally limited in supranuclear lesions, there is no diplopia and the eyes remain conjugate (tracking together). Exceptions to this rule—cases in which supranuclear lesions are associated with diplopia or disconjugate eye movements—include internuclear ophthalmoplegia (INO) and skew deviation. In such cases, the disconjugate nature of the eye movements may make them difficult to analyze. The evaulation is simplified if the movements are examined one eye at a time.

Full horizontal movements of either eye imply an intact pontine horizontal gaze center; full vertical movements imply intact vertical gaze centers. Thus, in the face of disconjugate eye movements, full gaze movements in either eye signify that the supranuclear gaze mechanisms are intact, and therefore that the lesion is nuclear or infranuclear (with the exception of INO and skew). If a strabismus or paralytic squint is detected, further evaluation is indicated (see Chapters 15 and 17).

Use of gaze positions to determine paretic muscle

Primary positions

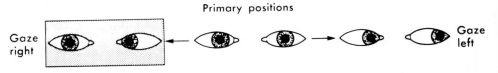

Figure 11–3. Patient with a right lateral rectus muscle weakness. Use of the gaze positions to determine the paretic muscle. (*From Gay A, Newman NN, Keltner J, Stroud M. Eye Movement Disorders. St. Louis: Mosby, 1974, with permission.*)

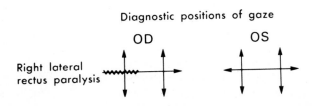

Use of gaze positions to determine paretic muscle

Diagnostic positions of gaze

Maximum diplopia

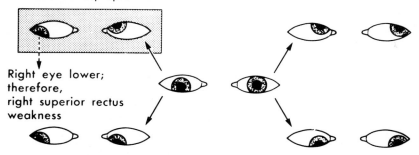

Right eye lower;
therefore,
right superior rectus
weakness

1. In primary position eyes are straight or right
   eye is slightly lower than left eye

2. Maximum defect is on gaze up and to right;
   therefore, weak muscle is either RSR or LIO

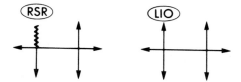

3. Right eye is lower; therefore, right elevator is
   weak; paretic muscle is RSR

Figure 11–4. Patient with right superior rectus muscle weakness. Use of the gaze positions to determine the paretic muscle. (*From Gay A, Newman NN, Keltner J, Stroud M. Eye Movement Disorders. St. Louis: Mosby, 1974, with permission.*)

Saccadic system. After position maintenance, smooth pursuit, and the range of ocular movement have been tested, the saccadic (rapid eye movement, voluntary eye movement) system is evaluated. This eye movement mechanism is tested by having the patient look rapidly and repeatedly from one object to another or from one extreme of gaze to another. Test movements in both horizontal and vertical planes and movements to and from the center and extreme points of gaze. The eyes should swing conjugately and rapidly to the target in one movement, perhaps with a slight correction. Note whether the refixation movements are of normal saccadic velocity or abnormally slow. This qualitative judgment takes some time to master, but it is of diagnostic significance in diseases such as progressive supranuclear palsy (PSP). Close observation of saccadic velocity can be of diagnostic value in INO. Gaze to the side opposite the lesion uses the paretic medial rectus of the adducting eye. Because it cannot make a normally rapid saccade, the adducting eye consequently lags markedly behind the abducting eye.

A slight undershoot on refixation is seen frequently and is a normal finding; a minor overshoot may also be within normal limits. However, large errors in either direction are abnormal. If the at-

tempted saccade is associated with a large overshoot or several oscillations at the end point, the resulting abnormality of eye movement is called ocular dysmetria and is, like limb dysmetria, a symptom of disturbed vestibulo-cerebellar control.

Vergence system. The vergence system controls the degree to which the eyes turn in or out relative to each other. It is tested by having the patient fixate on an object that is slowly brought closer until it touches the tip of the nose; the patient's finger is an appropriate and available target. The eyes should turn inward equally and smoothly. Letters and numbers also provide strong vergence stimuli.

To test convergence is to test a voluntary act that is more sensitive to variations, cooperation, and attention than tests of saccades. Hence, the examiner must ascertain that the patient makes an adequate attempt to converge. This may be done by observing the pupils. Because of the near synkinesis (convergence, miosis, accommodation), pupillary constriction indicates convergence effort even if the eyes do not move. Overaction of the vergence system may contribute to some types of strabismus.

Ocular (Vestibular) reflex system. The vestibular system is tested by observing eye movements while irrigating the external auditory canals with water. Five mL of water may be placed in the external auditory canal, and the patient's head then turned to bring the water in contact with the tympanic membrane. The water is allowed to remain for 40 seconds, and the head is then turned face forward and elevated 30 degrees. Either warm (44°C) or cold (30°C) water may be used.

The normal response to caloric stimulation is jerk nystagmus. With cold calorics, the fast phase is away from the stimulated ear and the slow phase is toward it; the opposite is true when warm water is used. The mnemonic COWS may be used to recall that with Cold calorics, the fast phase is toward the side Opposite the one stimulated; with Warm calorics, the fast phase is toward the Same side. Simultaneous bilateral caloric stimulation evokes vertical movements. With simultaneous cold stimulation, the fast phase is up; with simultaneous warm stimulation, the fast phase is down.

If neither stimulation produces a response, the test should be repeated with ice water (15°C) and the irrigation continued over 1 minute or until a response is elicited. The ice water caloric test represents the maximum single unilateral stimulus available to test the integrity of the oculomotor pathways in the obtunded or unconscious patient.

If a vestibular stimulus produces no response, attempt to reinforce the stimulus by simultaneously turning the patient's head from side to side (oculocephalic or doll's-head maneuver); in trauma patients, attempt this only after you are sure there is no neck injury! Head turning, or the doll's-head maneuver, occasionally is more effective (a greater stimulus), possibly because the vestibular system is stimulated bilaterally. When the saccadic pathways are disrupted, a tonic deviation of the eyes to the side of the stimulus may be the only response to vestibular stimulation with cold water.

Unilateral semicircular canal paresis may be detected clinically by the head-shaking test. Sit the patient upright and fix vision on a distant target. While the patient fixes the target, turn the head rapidly from side to side, starting from a head position about 20 degrees away from the side to which it will be turned. Normally, gaze remains fixed on the target. In patients with total unilateral canal paresis, fixation remains normal when the head turns away from the affected side. When the head turns toward it, compensatory refixation saccades occur in the direction opposite the head motion.

OTHER TESTS OF EYE MOVEMENTS

Additional tests of oculomotor function, evaluating more than a single eye movement mechanism, may be utilized to gain more information.

Optokinetic nystagmus: There are two systems that generate optokinetic nystagmus (OKN). The predominant OKN in humans consists of smooth pursuit of a small target interrupted by a resetting fast phase. The usual stimulus is a repetitive series of targets. The slow phase probably is a slow foveal pursuit movement. Obviously, disordered pursuit or saccades produce abnormal OKN. Beyond this, asymmetric OKN is especially characteristic of lesions deep in the posterior hemisphere, especially the parietal lobe. OKN is normal in lesions restricted to the temporal or occipital lobes, and thus a hemianopia associated with asymmetric OKN strongly suggests a deep parietal lesion. The poorer OKN response occurs on target motion toward the side of the lesion. Brain-stem lesions that disturb eye movements also disturb OKN, but have no associated hemianopia.

The second type of OKN acts to stabilize images on the retina during sustained head rotations, complementing the vestibulo-ocular reflex. This type of nystagmus is less prominent in humans than in lower animals; it is the only system in nonfoveate animals. A full-field rotating stimulus, possibly using the accessory optic pathways, sets OKN in motion. It is usually assessed by measuring optokinetic after nystagmus (OKAN). Because this system is vestigial in humans and necessitates a special testing environment, it will not be considered further here.

Oculocephalic (Doll's-head) maneuver: The oculocephalic maneuver (OCM) consists of briskly turning the patient's head from side to side for horizontal movements or briskly flexing and extending the neck for vertical movements (Fig. 11–5). The conscious patient is asked to fixate on an object straight ahead. In this case, the oculocephalic maneuver tests fixation and the smooth pursuit mechanism, as well as the vestibular ocular reflex (VOR). Normally, the eyes remain fixed on the target while the head moves. In a comatose patient, fixation is not possible and the oculocephalic maneuver is a test of ocular reflexes, primarily the vestibular mechanism. If these reflexes are intact, the eyes deviate in a direction opposite that to which the head is turned. When the deviation is full, nuclear and infranuclear pathways are intact; any gaze paresis must result from a supranuclear lesion of the conjugate gaze pathways. Full vertical movements indicate a normally functioning pretectal area, while full horizontal movements indicate preservation of the pontine conjugate gaze centers. Disconjugate movements resulting from the oculocephalic maneuver signify nuclear or infranuclear disturbances or may indicate the presence of INO or skew (Fig. 11–5).

In the conscious patient, fixation dominates the control of eye movements during the oculocephalic

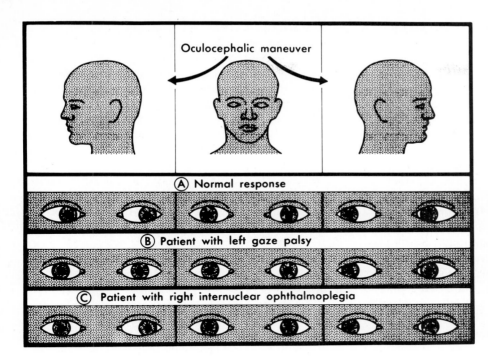

Oculocephalic maneuver

Ⓐ Normal response

Ⓑ Patient with left gaze palsy

Ⓒ Patient with right internuclear ophthalmoplegia

Figure 11–5. Oculocephalic (doll's-head) maneuver. **A.** In a normal patient, as the head turns to the right, the eyes conjugately move to the left; the opposite is true with a head turn to the left. **B.** In a patient with a left gaze palsy, as the head turns to the right, the eyes fail to move to the left, but move normally on left head turn. **C.** In a patient with a right internuclear ophthalmoplegia or right medial rectus palsy, as the head turns to the right, the right eye fails to move to the left; but the right eye moves normally on left head turn. (*From Gay A, Newman NN, Keltner J, Stroud M. Eye Movement Disorders. St. Louis: Mosby, 1974, with permission.*)

maneuver. Therefore, when fixation is defective, the vestibular mechanism is most important in generating eye movements when the head is turned passively. If the vestibular mechanism is also impaired, the tonic neck reflexes become dominant.

Tonic deviation of gaze. To evaluate tonic deviation, ask the patient to close the eyes tightly, as in testing of seventh nerve function. Normally, if the lids are raised forcibly by the examiner while the patient continues the effort to keep them closed, both eyes will deviate or diverge, usually upwards and outwards (Bell's phenomenon). However, Bell's phenomenon is absent in 10 to 15% of normal patients. In many patients with hemispheric lesions, the eyes deviate in parallel toward the side opposite the lesion. This abnormal deviation with the eyes closed is termed *spasticity of conjugate gaze (Cogan's sign).* Alternately, to elicit "spasticity," ask the patient to close the eyes normally for a few seconds, and observe the movement of the eyes as the lids are opened, or observe any deviation of the eyes as the patient blinks rapidly. These tests, which do not involve the examiner struggling with the patient, are more physiologic. Frequently, tonic conjugate gaze is associated with jerky pursuit movements when the patient's eyes follow a target toward the side of the lesion.

Tonic deviation is suggestive of hemispheric pathology, but may occasionally be found with brainstem lesions and rarely in normal patients. Thus, its detection is useful as a confirming piece of evidence, but not in isolation as a localizing sign.

METHOD OF EXAMINATION

All the methods described above are easily applied. Any evaluation of eye movements should include study of fixation, smooth pursuit, saccades, and convergence. The optokinetic responses and tonic deviation of gaze should also be evaluated; they are easily and rapidly tested for, and the results of such testing may reveal unsuspected abnormalities or bring out defective eye movements that are otherwise difficult to detect. For example, adduction lag due to INO may be uncovered by optokinetic testing.

In every case, each eye movement mechanism must be analyzed independently. Although all fast movements are saccadic, there are several types of slow eye movements: smooth pursuit, the slow phase of OKN or of vestibular nystagmus, and convergence. All complex eye movements, such as nystagmus, must be evaluated by consideration of their individual components. It is not adequate to state that the OKN is defective to the right; it must also be noted whether the fast phase or slow phase is defective, or whether both are involved. Absence of any optokinetic response may mean that the patient is not alert or cannot see the targets.

Nystagmus, characterized by rhythmic to-and-fro movements of the eyes, may be encountered in the examination of eye movements. In general, nystagmus is conjugate; occasionally it is disconjugate (such as in the abducting nystagmus that occurs with lesions of the median longitudinal fasciculus [INO]). The most common nystagmus is jerk nystagmus with both fast and slow components; nystagmus may also be pendular (frequently the case in congenital nystagmus) or rotatory (usual with nystagmus of vestibular origin). When nystagmus is present, the examiner must evaluate it carefully, noting the slow and fast phases and any changes in character in each of the diagnostic positions. Nystagmus and other abnormal oscillations are discussed in detail in Chapter 14.

The activity of a specific eye movement mechanism may either augment or mask abnormal eye movements. Thus, attempts at upward saccades generate or augment convergence–retraction "nystagmus" in Parinaud's syndrome. Extreme gaze positions or convergence may mask many kinds of nystagmus. On the other hand, testing for spasticity of conjugate gaze in the face of a vertical gaze paralysis may reveal a paradoxically normal Bell's phenomenon and thus provide important evidence that the disorder is supranuclear.

When eye movement disorders are complex and confusing, examine one eye at a time. As mentioned above, normal horizontal movements in either eye signify a functioning pons; normal vertical movements, a functioning pretectum.

The Bedside Ocular Motor Examination

Examination of each ocular motor subsystem may be performed quickly and without expensive equipment, even at bedside. First, usually as you take the history, observe the patient for abnormal head postures (tilts or turns), head thrusts during refixations, and head tremors; look for lid abnormalities and spontaneous abnormal eye movements.

1. Have the patient fixate first at distance then at near. Instruct the patient to smoothly track a small moving target horizontally and vertically. Look for saccadic intrusions, nystagmus, and limitation of range. Establish the range of motion with versions (both eyes viewing), particularly in the cardinal positions.

2. Test vergence by asking the patient to fixate a target brought in toward the nose. Note pupillary changes during vergence movements.

3. Observe spontaneous saccades and saccades to targets. Note latency, velocity, accuracy, and conjugacy.

4. Test for strabismus using cover tests (see Chapter 15). If the evaluation of either version or cover tests is confusing, test ductions (one eye viewing).

5. Determine the position of the eyes under closed lids (Bell's phenomenon) by noting corrective movements when the patient opens the eyes.

6. Further evaluation may include optokinetic nystagmus testing to bring out pursuit and vestibular testing with small amounts of ice water (less than 1 mL) to elicit caloric nystagmus.

Examination in a well-equipped examination room is more exacting and yields additional information.

Quantitative Eye Movement Recording

Quantitative eye movement data are recorded electrically by electro-oculogram, magnetic search coils, or infrared sensors.

Quantitative eye movement recording allows (1) a permanent record of test results; (2) an accurate quantitative and qualitative comparison between the two eyes of one patient, between different stimulus conditions, and between normal subjects and patients with disorders of eye movement; (3) a graphic comparison of eye movements as well as computerized analysis; (4) comparison of test results from one examination to another; (5) measurementes of various parameters of eye movement, such as waveform, duration, latency, velocity, and acceleration; and (6) recording in the dark.

BIBLIOGRAPHY

Hamalgyi GM, Curthoys IS. A clinical sign of canal paresis. *Arch Neurol.* 1988;45:737–739.

Kjallman L, Frisen L. The cerebral ocular pursuit pathways: A clinicoradiological study of small-field optokinetic nystagmus. *J Clin Neuro-op.* 1986;6:209–214.

Leigh RJ, Zee DS. *The Neurology of Eye Movements.* Philadelphia: Davis, 1983.

Miller N, ed. *Walsh and Hoyt's Clinical Neuro-ophthalmology.* 4th ed. Baltimore: Williams & Wilkins, 1982;3.

CHAPTER 12

DISORDERS OF THE SUPRANUCLEAR EYE MOVEMENT MECHANISMS

Disorders of the ocular motor system are classified in several manners. They are supranuclear, nuclear, or infranuclear. There are also disorders of saccades, pursuit, vergence, and ocular reflexes.

In addition, many eye movement disorders can be attributed to an anatomic location—for example, Parinaud's syndrome (pretectum), internuclear ophthalmoplegia (medial longitudinal fasciculus), or downbeat nystagmus (area of the foramen magnum). Some disease processes involving multiple areas of the central nervous system produce characteristic patterns of eye movement disorders, as occurs in progressive supranuclear palsy and Huntington's chorea.

In this chapter, we consider disorders of the supranuclear eye movement mechanisms. Nuclear and infranuclear disorders, nystagmus, and strabismus are covered in later chapters.

Supranuclear dysfunction results from lesions of the premotor pathways: hemispheric lesions, lesions of the pretectal areas, lesions of the mesencephalic and pontine reticular formations, and lesions of the medial longitudinal fasciculus (MLF), vestibular pathways, cerebellar paths, and areas of the medulla connecting with the ocular motor systems. Most *supranuclear lesions* affect mechanisms for conjugate gaze and, consequently, *are unassociated with diplopia or strabismus*. Exceptions are lesions of the pathways for vergence, lesions of the MLF, and lesions producing skew deviations and seesaw or dissociated nystagmus.

Supranuclear lesions may damage one or more of the ocular motor mechanisms (Fig. 12–1), but by definition at least one substrate remains intact. Thus, adequate testing will *always* demonstrate the integrity of the nuclear and infranuclear pathways; for example, if the lesion involves the pathways for saccades, pursuit or vestibular stimulation may be utilized to move the eyes. Normal, full excursions are not possible with nuclear or infranuclear lesions.

DISORDERS RELATED TO LESIONS OF SPECIFIC EYE MOVEMENT MECHANISMS

Lesions of the Saccadic Mechanisms

A deficit of rapid eye movements to the opposite side is caused by an interruption of the paths for fast eye movements. This is true of lesions anywhere along the parallel descending paths from the frontal eye fields, temporal-parietal-occipital confluence, and superior colliculi to the brain stem where they decussate, somewhere between the third and fourth nerve nuclei. Thus, a right-sided lesion above the decussation will cause a deficit of all fast eye movements to the left: saccades to the left, the fast phase of optokinetic nystagmus (OKN) when it is to the left, and the fast phase of vestibular nystagmus when it is to the left. Acutely, the eyes may show a transient tonic ipsilateral deviation and neglect the opposite hemifield. Because the saccadic pathways are diffusely represented in the cerebral hemispheres and because there are parallel pathways, complete lesions are relatively rare. If recovery is incomplete, contralateral saccades remain slowed both in their initiation and maximum velocity. Somewhat paradoxically, especially acutely, there is an inability to inhibit saccades to novel stimuli in the contralateral visual field.

If the patient is comatose, the tonic deviation

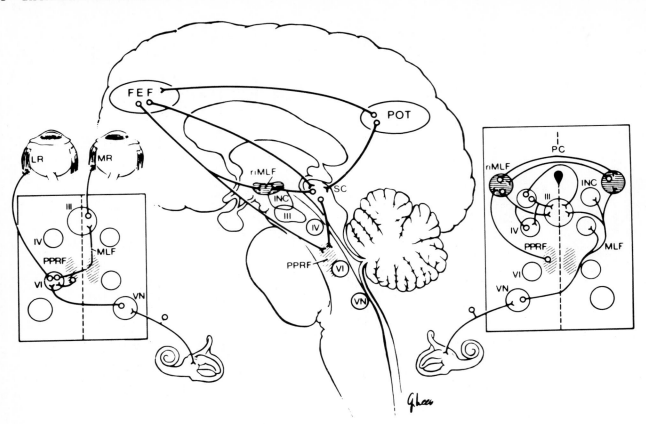

Figure 12–1. Summary of eye movement control. The center figure shows the supranuclear connections from the frontal eye fields (FEF) and the parieto-occipital-temporal junction region (POT) to the superior colliculus (SC), rostral interstitial nucleus of the medial longitudinal fasciculus (riMLF), and the paramedian pontine reticular formation (PPRF). The FEF and SC are involved in the production of saccades, and the POT is thought to be important in the production of pursuit. The schematic drawing on the **left** shows the brain-stem pathways for horizontal gaze. Axons from the cell bodies located in the PPRF travel to the ipsilateral abducens nucleus (VI) where they synapse with abducens motorneurons whose axons travel to the ipsilateral lateral rectus muscle (LR) and with abducens internuclear neurons whose axons cross the midline and travel in the medial longitudinal fasciculus (MLF) to the portion(s) of the oculomotor nucleus (III) concerned with medial rectus (MR) function (in the contralateral eye). The schematic drawing on the **right** shows the brain-stem pathways for vertical gaze. Important structures include the riMLF, PPRF, the interstitial nucleus of Cajal (INC), and the posterior commissure (PC). Note that axons from cell bodies located in the vestibular nuclei (VN) travel directly to the abducens nuclei and, mostly via the MLF, to the oculomotor nuclei. IV, trochlear nucleus. (*From Miller N, ed. Walsh and Hoyt's Clinical Neuro-ophthalmology. 4th ed. Baltimore: Williams & Wilkins, 1983;2; with permission.*)

may last longer; if the opposite descending path has been damaged previously, compensation may be completely lacking, and the tonic deviation may persist.

After the decussation, lesions of these pathways produce the same type of deficit, but the saccadic paresis is ipsilateral to the lesion. Thus, involuntary conjugate ocular deviations toward a normal arm and leg indicate a hemispheric lesion (Fig. 12–2), and toward a paralyzed arm and leg, a pontine lesion (Fig. 12–3). The saccadic pathways are more compactly represented in the brain stem; therefore, total disruption is more common and recovery less frequent. However, in the brain stem other premotor structures usually are affected as well, causing complex combinations of disordered motility.

As recovery occurs, even at the point where saccades seem to be normal, they are much less frequent, either spontaneously or as a response to optokinetic or vestibular stimulation.

Bilateral lesions of these pathways lead to a total absence of saccades (global saccadic paralysis), including lack of the fast phase of OKN and the fast phase of vestibular nystagmus. Metabolic, toxic, and degenerative central nervous system diseases characteristically cause slow saccades. Disorders of the vestibulo-cerebellum and its brainstem connections cause disorders of saccadic accuracy, hypo- and hypermetric saccades, and saccadic intrusions (Table 12–1).

Lesions of the pontine premotor areas in the paramedian pontine reticular formation (PPRF)

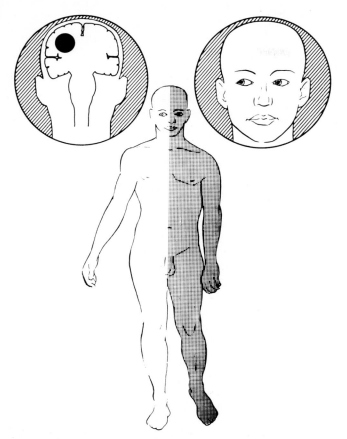

Figure 12–2. Patient with acute right cerebral hemisphere cerebrovascular accident, demonstrating initial deviation of the eyes in the direction of the normal arm and leg away from the paralyzed side (as if to make use of the remaining intact extremities). (*From Newman NM, Keltner JL, Stroud MH, Gay AJ.* Eye Movement Disorders. *St. Louis: Mosby, 1974, with permission.*)

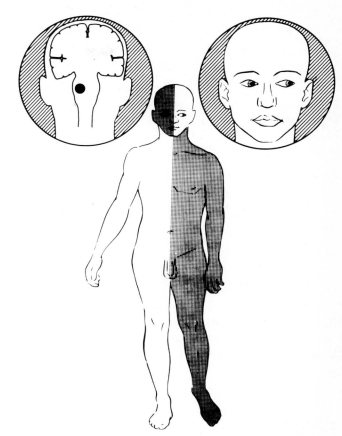

Figure 12–3. Patient with acute cerebrovascular accident of right pons, involving right pontine gaze center. Eyes are deviated toward the paralyzed side and remain deviated in that direction. (*From Newman NM, Keltner JL, Stroud MH, Gay AJ.* Eye Movement Disorders. *St. Louis: Mosby, 1974, with permission.*)

cause abnormalities of horizontal saccades because the pause and omnipause neurons for all saccades reside in this area (nucleus raphe interpositis). Bilateral lesions may also affect vertical saccades. Slow saccades are associated with lesions of the nucleus raphe interpositus.

The seventh nerve, which passes around the sixth-nerve nucleus, is nearly always affected as well, and saccades from the contralateral field are rapid because inhibitory PPRF paths are spared. Often after the conjugate gaze palsy resolves, an ipsilateral sixth-nerve palsy persists, probably due to fascicular involvement. Midbrain lesions involving descending pathways can also produce contralateral conjugate gaze palsies often associated with an ipsilateral pursuit defect, vertical gaze abnormalities, and pupillary abnormalities. In midbrain lesions, vestibular function is always normal.

Ocular motor apraxia is a global lack of voluntary saccades (often with pursuit disorders as well) that emphasizes the functions of the saccadic system. These patients exhibit a near total lack of voluntary saccades, but have occasional random rapid eye movements and more normal reflex eye movements. Normally, small refixation saccades are used to look from one object to another. In the absence of voluntary saccades, patients with ocular motor apraxia cannot refixate easily and are often described as having "spasm of fixation."

Patients with *congenital ocular motor apraxia* develop a characteristic head thrust in order to refixate, the most obvious sign of the disorder. Frequently, the head thrust is the abnormality noted by parents, the reason the child is brought to the doctor's office. The head thrust breaks fixation. As the head is turned, vestibular input (vestibular ocular reflex; VOR) causes the eyes to deviate in the "wrong" direction and actually look away from the

TABLE 12–1. SACCADIC OSCILLATIONS AND INTRUSIONS

Saccadic Oscillations	Saccadic Intrusions
Square wave oscillation	Square wave jerks
Macro square wave jerks	Sporadic macro square wave jerks
—	Saccadic impersistence
Macrosaccadic oscillation	—
Microsaccadic oscillation	
Convergent–retraction pulses	Saccadic pulses
Opsoclonus: flutter, voluntary flutter[a]	Double saccadic pulses
Bobbing	Sporadic bobbing

[a] Convergent–retraction pulses and voluntary flutter are usually referred to as nystagmus but they are not genuine nystagmus, because each is initiated by saccades rather than by the smooth (slow) eye movements that initiate nystagmus.
From Sharpe JH, Fletcher WA. *Disorders of visual fixation*. Neuro-ophthalmology Now. *Chicago: Year Book, 1986.*

target. Therefore, it is necessary to turn the head past the target until the limits of lateral eye deviation are reached and the eyes are artificially forced on to the target by further head turning. Once the target is locked in, the head turns back until the eyes are in primary position (Fig. 12–4). This biphasic movement is very characteristic and distinguishable from other abnormal head movements, such as a head turn to compensate for a paretic muscle or gaze, head movements in motor nystagmus, the head nodding

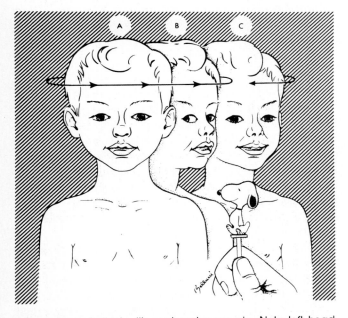

Figure 12–4. Patient with oculomotor apraxia. Note left head thrust, contraversion of the eyes right to fixate target, and realignment of the head to place the eyes in primary position. (*From Newman NM, Keltner JL, Stroud MH, Gay AJ.* Eye Movement Disorders. *St. Louis: Mosby, 1974, with permission.*)

of spasmus nutans (in which the head movements do *not* compensate for the eye movements), and abnormal head movements seen in basal ganglia disorders. In the latter, abnormalities of limb movement analogous to those of eye movement usually occur.

Congenital ocular motor apraxia affects horizontal eye movements predominantly, whereas patients with *acquired ocular motor apraxia* (OMA) have abnormal horizontal and vertical eye movements and much less prominent head thrusts. Acquired OMA occurs in diffuse and large bilateral frontoparietal lesions and in metabolic diseases. It rarely improves over time, whereas congenital OMA improves with age.

Several diffuse central nervous system (CNS) degenerations affect the saccadic mechanism preferentially and early in their course. The prototype of this form of oculomotor disorder is progressive supranuclear palsy. Similar patterns of disturbance have been described in Huntington's chorea and occasionally in lysosomal storage disorders (eg, Tay-Sachs disease, neuronal ceroid lipofuscinoses, and other storage diseases). Some spinocerebellar degenerations show similar slowed saccades.

Progressive supranuclear palsy (PSP) is a degenerative disorder of the CNS, which commony appears in the sixth decade and affects men more frequently than women. It has been confused with Parkinson's disease because of the rigidity (especially nuchal dystonia), bradykinesia, and retropulsion that are frequently a part of the disorder. The oculomotor disorder is distinctive, however, and often is the most striking physical finding, as well as the most disabling part of the illness in its early stages. Nevertheless, these patients have remarkably little insight into their eye movement difficulties and rarely complain of any trouble with their eyes.

The first manifestation of PSP is often an inability to make vertical saccades, particularly downward saccades; the patients bang their shins, eat off only the top part of their plates, and complain of being unable to read because of inability to use their bifocals (they can't look down!). As the disease progresses, vertical pursuit, and then horizontal fast, and finally horizontal pursuit movements become involved as well. When all fast eye movements are affected, the patient is unable to make refixation saccades; optokinetic and vestibular stimuli cause a tonic deviation. When asked to refixate, the patient with PSP makes a slow eye movement. When the patient turns a corner while walking, the vestibular input causes the eyes to swing in the opposite direction, adding to his oculomotor difficulties. These patients also exhibit difficulties with convergence and square wave jerks.

Whipple's disease may cause a similar picture. It also causes a rare but unique movement disorder, oculomasticatory myorhythmia—large-amplitude (±20 degrees), binocular, asymmetric pendular vergence oscillations at ±1 Hz. Oculomasticatory myorhythmia occurs in the setting of vertical ophthalmoparesis and is synchronous with smooth, rhythmic contractions of masticatory musculature. It is worthwhile to keep this rare entity in mind, as it is treatable with antibiotics. *Parkinson's disease* also produces distinctive aberrations in saccadic behavior, primarily a delay in initiation of saccades, a tendency for hypometric saccades (undershoots), and decreased saccadic velocity. Multiple saccades are used to complete a given movement. Patients with Parkinson's disease also exhibit defective velocity gain of pursuit movement.

Lesions of the Pursuit Mechanism

Lesions of the pursuit pathways in the hemispheres cause saccadic pursuit in which the abnormally slow smooth pursuit movement (due to a decrease in ipsilateral gain) is interrupted by catch-up saccades. The major deficit is in ipsilateral pursuit, although maximal velocity pursuit seems to depend on bilaterally intact hemispheres. In contrast to rapid recovery of saccadic function in hemispheric lesions, the pursuit defects endure. Pathologic conditions involving the cerebellar pathways, decreasing alertness, or sedation also produce saccadic pursuit, as can anticipation of the target in a nervous patient and inattention. However, these latter factors affect pursuit bilaterally. Thus, when pursuit movements are entirely normal in one direction and abnormal in the opposite direction, a lesion of the pursuit pathways themselves is probable.

Eye movements such as OKN, which depend on the smooth coordination of saccades and pursuit, can be interrupted when either saccadic or pursuit mechanisms are damaged.

Lesions of the vergence system cause diplopia. Because the primary differential diagnosis is between cranial nerve lesions and strabismus, they will be considered in more detail in Chapters 15 and 17.

DISORDERS RELATED TO LESIONS OF SPECIFIC ANATOMIC AREAS (TABLE 12–2)

Parietal lobe: Cortical lesions of the parietal lobe produce no characteristic defect of eye movement mechanisms. In contrast, deep or massive parietal lesions produce a disturbance of optokinetic nystagmus (OKN), impairment of ipsilateral pursuit, and, sometimes, abortive corrective saccades to the side opposite the lesion.

TABLE 12–2. EYE MOVEMENT FINDINGS THAT MAY BE LOCALIZING

Clinical Manifestations	*Anatomic Lesion*
Seesaw nystagmus	Posterior diencephalon/pretectum (interstitial nucleus of Cajal?)
Convergence–retraction "nystagmus"	Dorsal midbrain
Upgaze palsy	Posterior commissure
Downgaze palsy	Rostral mesencephalon (rostral interstitial nucleus of the median longitudinal fasciculus?)
Internuclear ophthalmoplegia (INO)	Median longitudinal fasciculus (MLF)
1½ syndrome (INO plus ipsilateral gaze palsy)	MLF plus PPRF or sixth-nerve nucleus
Paralytic pontine exotropia	Acute plus PPRF or sixth-nerve nucleus
Horizontal gaze palsy (VOR intact) with slow saccades in contralateral field of gaze	PPRF
Horizontal gaze palsy with rapid saccades in contralateral field of gaze	
Horizontal gaze palsy, complete	Sixth-nerve nucleus
Skew deviation	Brain stem, usually on side of higher eye
Upbeat nystagmus	Central tegmentum of pons, medulla
Bobbing	Central pontine lesions
Brun's nystagmus	Cerebellar pontine angle masses
Lateropulsion	Dorsolateral medulla
Downbeat nystagmus	Cervico–medullary junction

Severe abnormalities of the true OKN (full field, surround stimuli) occur with deep parietotemporal lesions. More moderate OKN defects occur nonselectively in hemispheric lesions, as do pursuit OKN defects (small target (drum, tape) stimuli).

Spasticity of conjugate gaze is a tonic horizontal or diagonally upward deviation of the eyes under closed lids. The deviation is to the side contralateral to the lesion.

As the efferent ocular motor pathways leave the cerebral hemispheres, the pathways for saccades and pursuit become more closely associated. Those concerned with vertical movements proceed to the pretectal center for vertical gaze and those concerned with horizontal movements decussate and proceed to the pontine gaze center. Thus, most lesions of the brain stem produce deficits in both saccadic and pursuit mechanisms. Consequently, simultaneous defects in both horizontal saccades and pursuit, without evidence of widespread neurologic damage, indicate damage in the pons. Similarly, defects in vertical saccades and pursuit indicate damage in the pretectal area.

Accommodation and convergence insufficiency with a left parietotemporal lesion following a middle cerebral artery occlusion has been described. Aside from saccadic pursuit movements, other eye movements and the pupillary light reaction were normal, providing clinical evidence for an anatomical localization of these functions in the hemisphere.

Pretectal Area (Center for Vertical Gaze)

Lesions in the area of the sylvian aqueduct are associated with Parinaud's syndrome (dorsal midbrain syndrome, Koerber-Salus-Elschnig syndrome): paresis of vertical gaze (especially upgaze) and convergence, associated with pupillary abnormalities. The most common pupillary abnormality is light–near dissociation (a depressed light response and nearly normal near response). (Parinaud actually described a lack of pupillary reaction on convergence and a *retained* light reflex.) Retraction of the lids on attempted upgaze (Collier's sign) and convergence–retraction "nystagmus" are associated signs.

This constellation of signs demonstrates that the pathways for vertical saccades and vertical pursuit have become associated, and that the substrates for convergence and pupillary reactions lie in the same vicinity. However, they may all be affected differentially, and the differential effects are frequently seen with the extension of a pineal tumor into the pretectal region (a relatively common etiology of the rare Parinaud's syndrome). With slow expansion of the tumor, an acquired myopia and vertical diplopia are early signs of tectal involvement as compression from above increases. Upgaze becomes limited before downgaze, probably due to posterior commisure lesions, and saccades are limited before pursuit movements. Lesions median and dorsal to the red nuclei (rostral, interstitial nucleus of the MLF?) are responsible for downgaze paresis. The clinical progression of lesions in this area implies that components for downgaze run ventrocaudal to those for upgaze. Horizontal movements remain intact until there is massive involvement of brain-stem structures.

The phenomenon of convergence–retraction "nystagmus" is one of the most striking and characteristic signs of pretectal damage. Any attempt at upgaze brings on bilateral movements of retraction, convergence, or both. The movement that predominates depends on the innervation delivered to the extraocular muscles. Inappropriate simultaneous ac-

tivity in normally antagonistic muscles produces co-contraction of the muscles and hence retraction of the globe.

Other aberrations of ocular motor function are attributed to lesions in the midbrain area. Frequently, tonic downward and convergent deviation of the eyes occurs with thalamic hemorrhage.

In **pseudoabducens palsy,** an apparent abducens palsy ipsilateral to a lesion in the pretectal areas, ipsilateral abduction is defective for all modalities except caloric stimulation.

In contrast, a monocular paresis of adduction in the ipsilateral eye, paresis of contralateral saccades in the opposite eye, and conjugate paresis of ipsilateral smooth pursuit, occur in midbrain tegmentum lesions, suggesting that the mesencephalic reticular formation subserves contralateral saccades and ipsilateral pursuit.

A uniocular acquired impairment of upgaze, **double elevator palsy,** is attributed to a unilateral lesion in the pretectum (path from the rostral interstitial nucleus of the MLF to the oculomotor nucleus?), presumably secondary to a vascular lesion. There is sudden unilateral onset of limited upgaze, which is constant for all horizontal positions. The eye usually will not elevate further by Bell's phenomenon. Pupillary and convergence abnormalities are frequently associated. Their presence supports localization of the responsible lesion to the dorsal midbrain. Double elevator palsy must be differentiated from skew deviation (where the misalignment is present in all gaze directions on versions but where upward ductions are full) and the more common mechanical limitations of upgaze (eg, thyroid orbitopathy, blow-out fracture, and inferior rectus fibrosis), which are diagnosed by positive forced ductions.

Seesaw nystagmus (Chapter 14) is a rare disorder that gets its descriptive name because one eye rises while the other falls; simultaneously the eyes show a conjugate rotatory nystagmus, with the upgoing eye intorting and the downgoing eye extorting.

The majority of described patients had masses or trauma involving the chiasm or anterior third ventricle, frequently causing a bitemporal hemianopsia as well. However, other patients have had lesions more caudal in the brain stem, and unassociated with field defects (especially in the region of the interstitial nucleus of Cajal, a possible coordinating center for vertical and torsional eye movements).

Paramedian Pontine Reticular Formation (PPRF)

Although the efferent premotor paths for eye movements are closely associated in the brain stem, they still may be differentially affected by disease processes. The pursuit pathways either are located in a different area at this level or are more diffuse; therefore, defective pursuit movements alone do not occur with pontine lesions.

Pontine Gaze Center

Although not a discrete anatomic entity, the neurons that function as the pontine center for horizontal conjugate gaze project directly to the ipsilateral sixth-nerve nucleus and to the contralateral third-nerve nucleus by way of the medial longitudinal fasciculus (MLF). Lesions of the abducens nucleus produce a complete paralysis of ipsilateral horizontal conjugate gaze, involving saccades, pursuit, and vestibular nystagmus, an ipsilateral gaze palsy. Central isolated sixth-nerve palsies result from lesions of the sixth-nerve fasciculus and spare the sixth-nerve nucleus. Some lesions (especially lesions of the PPRF area) also cause an ipsilateral gaze palsy, but may spare the pursuit or vestibular mechanism. In contrast to the transient deviations that follow hemispheric lesions, deficits due to lesions of the pontine gaze center persist for a long period. Other abnormal eye movements, most associated with pontine lesions and lesions of vestibulo-cerebellar function, are considered in Chapter 14, as are ocular bobbing, upbeat nystagmus, and downbeat nystagmus.

Medial Longitudinal Fasciculus (Internuclear Ophthalmoplegia)

Lesions of the medial longitudinal fasciculus (MLF; Table 12–3) between the third and sixth nerve nuclei produce the clinical picture termed internuclear ophthalmoplegia (INO). The typical MLF syndrome

TABLE 12–3. CAUSES OF INTERNUCLEAR OPHTHALMOPLEGIA

Multiple sclerosis (commonly bilateral); postirradiation demyelination
Brainstem infarction (commonly unilateral)
Brainstem and fourth ventricular tumor
Arnold-Chiari malformation and associated syringobulbia
Infection: viral or other forms of encephalitis
Wernicke's encephalopathy
Mass effect (eg, subdural hematoma)
Metabolic disorders (eg, hepatic encephalopathy and maple syrup urine disease)
Drug intoxications (eg, from phenothiazines and tricyclic antidepressants)
Head trauma
Degenerative conditions: progressive supranuclear palsy
Syphilis
Pseudo-internuclear ophthalmoplegia of myasthenia gravis and Fisher syndrome

From Leigh RJ, Zee DS. The Neurology of Eye Movements. Philadelphia: Davis, 1983.

consists of an apparent medial rectus paresis in the eye on the side of the lesion, nystagmus of the abducting eye on lateral gaze to the side opposite the lesion, and normal medial rectus activity on convergence. The anterior INO of Cogan, in which convergence is also absent, probably is found only in larger lesions, possibly with third-nerve nucleus involvement.

The MLF syndrome is a typical supranuclear disorder, because the apparently paretic muscle is able to produce normal convergence and there is no diplopia (no heterotropia) in the primary position. A

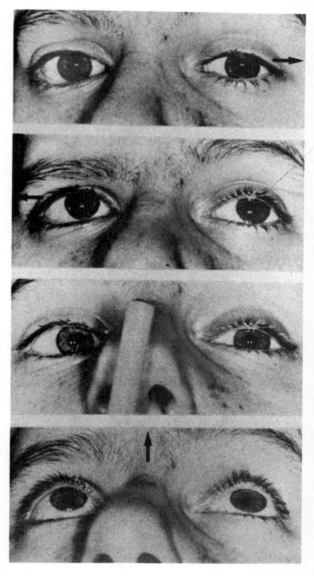

Figure 12–5. One-and-a-half syndrome in a 19-year-old patient with a brainstem glioma. (*From Sanders EACM: Syndromes of the medial longitudinal fasciculus. In: Sanders EACM, et al, eds. Eye Movement Disorders. Hingham, MA: Kluwer, 1987;11; with permission.*)

MLF lesion produces disconjugate eye movements and diplopia on lateral gaze, because impulses to the lateral rectus travel normally, whereas those to the medial rectus are interrupted. In mild degrees of INO, the abducting nystagmus may be made more obvious by eliciting asymmetric convergence or by producing fast movements in the direction of the abducting nystagmus. That is, when there is a right MLF lesion, the abducting nystagmus in the left eye on left lateral gaze is augmented by optokinetic or vestibular nystagmus with fast phases to the left.

Combined PPRF and MLF lesions cause striking motility disorders. If the PPRF and MLF are damaged, there is an ipsilateral gaze palsy and medial rectus palsy. As a result, the ipsilateral eye can make no horizontal movements and the contralateral eye can abduct only—the "one-and-a-half syndrome" (Fig. 12–5). Acutely, the deviation due to the gaze palsy may cause the contralateral eye to be exotropic (the ipsilateral eye can't follow because of its internuclear medial rectus paresis), causing a paralytic pontine exotropia (PPEX; Fig. 12–6). **Skew deviation** occurs frequently with lesions of the MLF, especially when unilateral, but may occur in many brain-stem lesions. Usually the higher eye is on the side of the lesion. A skew deviation is thought to represent an interruption of otolithic inputs.

Cerebellum

The detailed cerebellar control of eye movements is not well understood. However, the cerebellum is important in the precise control of eye movements and of saccades in particular. It probably integrates eye movements, as it does limb movements, in order to provide smooth, effective control of movement and compensation for ocular motor abnormalities. Information flowing into the cerebellum is integrated and organized. The resulting output is either directly to the spinal cord or to the cerebral cortex via the thalamic nuclei. With reference to the ocular motor system, it is of interest that the cerebellum has **direct** input to the ocular motor nuclei; some of its outflow fibers travel to these nuclei without synapse.

In contrast, direct fibers from the cerebral cortex to the ocular motor nuclei have never been found, and the exact number of synapses between the cerebral cortex and the ocular motor nuclei remains unknown. Certainly, a direct connection of the cerebellum with the ocular motor nuclei would be of great value for precise ongoing control of eye movement. In current thinking, the cerebellum provides continuous ongoing correction of eye movements, "incessantly subject to revision by the continuous feedback of information to the cerebellum with the further integration in its output and so on continuously throughout all postures and movements." (Eccles)

The cerebellum and its projections include premotor areas in which afferent information (visual, vestibular) projects to the neurons involved in eye movement. The cerebellum adaptively regulates eye movement with respect to the environment and re-

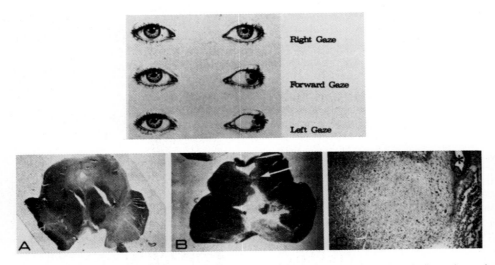

Figure 12–6. *Top.* Oculomotor findings. Right eye is completely immobile in the horizontal plane. Left eye is moderately exotropic during forward gaze, adduction to the midline is achieved; with attempted left gaze, further abduction occurs. *Bottom.* Histopathologic findings. **A.** Cross section at level of mesencephalon. Midline third-nerve nuclei, ventrally exiting nerves are intact. (Slits in tissue are processing artifacts.) (2.5 ×). **B.** Cross section at level of upper pons. Destruction of median tegmentum (arrow) to right of midline (ie, in region of MLF and PPRF) as well as necrosis of the basis pontis is present. The left PPRF and MLF are intact (2.5 ×). **C.** Magnified view of **B.** Asterisk represents midline. The left PPRF and MLF are intact. Ischemic necrosis of the right MLF and PPRF is seen (10 ×). *(From Newman NM, Day SH, Aguilar MJL. Paralytic pontine exotropia: A case report with clinicopathologic confirmation. In Kommerell G, ed. Disorders of Ocular Motility. Neurophysiological and Clinical Aspects. Munich, Germany: JF Bergman, 1978, with permission.)*

pairs abnormal eye movement production. It controls saccadic amplitude and repairs saccadic dysmetria via the vermis and fastigial nuclei; it also works to stabilize the retinal image (via the flocculus, which appears to act as part of the neural integrator) and repairs mismatches of eye, head, and target movement via the VOR (nodulus).

Cerebellar pathway lesions result in a spectacular group of oculomotor disorders: dysmetria, flutter, opsoclonus, and other abnormal oscillations. Most are conjugate disturbances and predominantly disturbances of fast eye movements (see Chapter 14).

Two other disorders of eye movement involving cerebellar pathways have been described. One group of patients with cerebellar degenerations has no normal pursuit movements, only saccadic pursuit. Families with heredofamiliar spinocerebellar degeneration show a spectrum of slowed eye movements, including slowed or absent saccades and pursuit. Many intrinsic "pure" cerebellar degenerations are associated with several less common types of nystagmus and other abnormal eye movements of unexplained mechanism (Table 12–4).

Medulla

Three forms of unusual eye movements are frequently correlated with medullary lesions: (1) *downbeat nystagmus*; (2) *dissociated nystagmus*, in which one eye moves vertically and the other horizontally; and (3) *periodic alternating nystagmus*. These abnormal eye movements are of infrequent occurrence and are very difficult to explain by what is known of ocular motor pathways and control mechanisms. Spontaneous nystagmus to the contralateral side and lateropulsion of saccades occur in Wallenberg's lateral medullary syndrome.

TABLE 12–4. OCULAR MOTOR ABNORMALITIES IN "PURE" CEREBELLAR DEGENERATIONS

1. Inaccurate (dysmetric) saccades; normal velocities and latencies
2. Fixation abnormalities: square wave jerks (saccadic intrusions) and increased slow drift
3. Impaired smooth pursuit with head still or moving (VOR cancellation); impaired OKN; impaired fixation suppression of caloric-induced nystagmus
4. Postsaccadic drift (glissades)
5. Gaze-evoked nystagmus (occasionally centripetal nystagmus)
6. Rebound nystagmus
7. Downbeat nystagmus
8. Positional nystagmus
9. Increased VOR gain
10. Alternating hyperdeviation on lateral gaze (skew)

From Leigh RJ, Zee DS. The Neurology of Eye Movements. Philadelphia: Davis, 1983.

TABLE 12–5. SOME DRUGS AND TOXINS THAT AFFECT EYE MOVEMENTS

Drug or Toxin	Reported Effects
Diazepam	Reduces saccadic peak velocity. Impairs smooth pursuit and gaze holding. Decreases VOR amplitude.
Tricyclic antidepressants	Internuclear ophthalmoplegia. Total gaze paresis.
Phenytoin	Impaired smooth pursuit and gaze holding. Downbeat nystagmus, periodic alternating nystagmus. Total gaze paresis.
Phenobarbital and other barbiturates	Impaired smooth pursuit and gaze holding. Impaired vergence. Total gaze paresis. Decreased accommodative convergence–accommodation ratio.
Carbamazepine	Ophthalmoplegia, oculogyric crises, downbeat nystagmus.
Phenothiazines	Oculogyric crises. Internuclear ophthalmoplegia.
Methadone	Saccadic hypometria. Impairs smooth pursuit.
Alcohol and marijuana	Impaired smooth pursuit and gaze holding. Alcohol may cause positionally induced nystagmus.
Chloral hydrate	Impaired smooth pursuit.
Amphetamine	Increased accommodative convergence–accommodation ratio.
Chlordecone, lithium, and thallium	Opsoclonus.
Botulinum toxin	Ophthalmoparesis.

From Leigh RJ, Zee DS. The Neurology of Eye Movements. Philadelphia: Davis, 1983.

Table 12–5 lists some of the drugs and toxins that may affect eye movements.

BIBLIOGRAPHY

General

Leigh RJ, Zee DS. *The Neurology of Eye Movements.* Philadelphia: Davis, 1983.

Miller N, ed. *Walsh and Hoyt's Clinical Neuro-ophthalmology.* 4th ed. Baltimore: Williams & Wilkins, 1983;2.

Hemisphere

Thurston SE, Leigh RJ, Crawford T, et al. Two distinct deficits of visual tracking caused by unilateral lesions of cerebral cortex in humans. *Ann Neurol.* 1988;23:266–273.

Pretectum/Midbrain

Jampel RS, Fells P. Monocular elevator paresis caused by a CNS lesion. *Arch Ophthalmol.* 1968;80:45–57.

Kanter DS, et al. See-saw nystagmus and brain stem infarction: MRI findings. *Neuro-ophthalmol.* 1987;7:279–283.

Masden JC, Rosenberg M. Midbrain diencephalic horizontal gaze paresis. *J Clin Neuro-ophthalmol.* 1987;7:227–234.

Wilkins RH, Brady IA. Parinaud's syndrome. *Arch Neurol.* 1972;26:91–93.

Zakon DH, Sharpe JA. Midbrain paresis of horizontal gaze. *Ann Neurol.* 1984;16:495–504.

Pons

Hanson MR, et al. Selective saccadic palsy caused by pontine lesions: Clinical, physiologic and pathologic correlations. *Ann Neurol.* 1986;20:209–217.

Cerebellum

Eccles JC et al. Mode of operation of the cerebellum in the dynamic control of movement. *Brain Res.* 1972;40:73–80.

OKN

Kompf D. The significance of optokinetic nystagmus asymmetry in hemispheric lesions. *Neuro-ophthalmol.* 1986;6:61–64.

Convergence

Ohtsuka K, Maekawa H, Takeda M, et al. Accommodation and convergence insufficiency with left middle cerebral artery occlusion. *Am J Ophthalmol.* 1988;106:60–64.

Oculomotor Nuclei

Warwick RJ. Representation of the extraocular muscles in the ocular motor nuclei of the monkey. *J Comp Neurol.* 1953;98:480.

CHAPTER 13

NUCLEAR AND INFRANUCLEAR CONTROL OF EYE MOVEMENTS

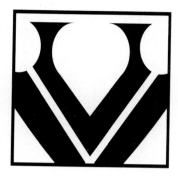

The globes are moved in their orbits by the six extraocular muscles; for each globe there are four rectus muscles (the medial rectus, superior rectus, inferior rectus, and lateral rectus) and two oblique muscles (the inferior and superior obliques).

Lesions in the brain stem, cranial nerves, extraocular muscles, or orbit cause nuclear and infranuclear disorders, disorders associated with disconjugate (nonparallel) eye movements, diplopia, and (usually) deviation of the eyes in the primary position.

For additional information about how to examine the patient with limitation of eye movements, see Chapter 15.

THE OCULAR MOTOR NERVES

Cranial nerves III, IV, and VI are the motor nerves of the eye and arise from the oculomotor, trochlear, and abducens nuclei, respectively. The nuclei lie in the brain stem from the dorsal midbrain region to the pontomedullary junction supplying the extraocular muscles and levator palpebrae. Additionally, the oculomotor (third) nerve carries the parasympathetic fibers to the smooth muscles of the eye (pupillary sphincter and ciliary muscle). The sympathetic fibers to the pupillary dilator muscle join the sixth (briefly) and then fifth nerve in the cavernous sinus, and then run in the nasociliary branch of the fifth nerve through the long ciliary nerves to the dilator pupillae.

Paralysis of the ocular motor nerves causes deficits of ocular motility in the fields of action of the muscles innervated. Recent paralyses demonstrate primary and secondary deviations. The *primary deviation* is measured with the nonparetic eye fixing, and *secondary deviation* with the paretic eye fixing. Obviously, when looking into the paretic field of gaze, the secondary deviation will be greater than the primary deviation. Long-standing paralyses (especially long-standing fourth nerve palsies) may be more difficult to diagnose because of spread of comitance with time.

THIRD NERVE DISORDERS

Clinical Presentation. The third nerve supplies the superior rectus, inferior rectus, medial rectus, inferior oblique, and levator palpebrae muscles; ciliary body; and pupillary sphincter. Lesions cause ptosis; inability to rotate the eye up, down, or in; inability to accommodate; and a dilated pupil. Total palsy can be associated with up to 3 mm of proptosis. The most frequent causes are diabetes and other microvascular (usually pupil-sparing) lesions; trauma; aneurysm; uncal herniation with supratentorial masses; infection; inflammation; and neoplastic disease of the interpeduncular region, cavernous sinus, and orbit.

Anatomy: The *third nerve nuclei* are located below the aqueduct of Sylvius in the periaqueductal gray matter of the rostral mesencephalon at the level of the superior colliculi. They are V-shaped with the medial longitudinal fasciculi forming their ventral and lateral boundaries.

The organization of the third nerve nucleus in the schema of Warwick divides the paired nuclei into subnuclei, each of which innervates a single extraocular muscle: the ventral subnucleus supplies the medial rectus (MR) muscle, the dorsal subnucleus supplies the inferior rectus (IR) muscle, and the intermediate cell column supplies the inferior oblique (IO) muscle. All these provide *uncrossed* innervation. The medial subnucleus supplies the superior rectus with *crossed* innervation. The single medial superior nuclei provide *bilateral* innervation: the caudal central nucleus supplies both levator palpebrae, and the parasympathetic subnucleus of Edinger and Westphal supplies the ciliary body and pupil, bilaterally (Fig. 13–1, Table 13–1). More recent studies with neuro-anatomical tracers give the medial rectus a multifocal representation and separate the large and small neurons—the latter lie around the border of the classical nucleus with MR and IR neurons dorsomedial and SR and IO motor neurons in the midline (Fig. 13–2).

The roots of the third nerve pass ventrally through the brain stem through the medial longitudinal fasciculus, red nucleus, substantia nigra, and anterior midbrain; exiting the brain stem through the medial portion of the peduncle, and emerging in the interpeduncular fossa.

Results of lesions in this brainstem region produce *Benedikt's syndrome* (homolateral third nerve

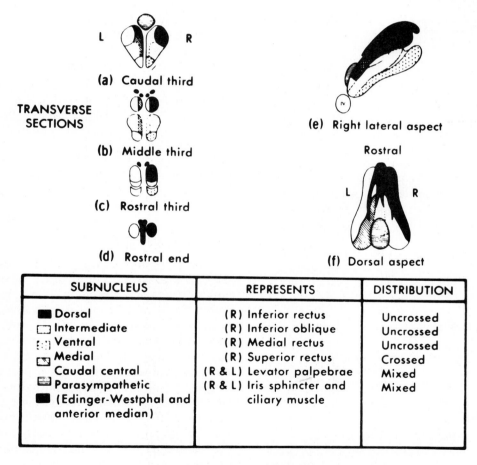

SUBNUCLEUS	REPRESENTS	DISTRIBUTION
■ Dorsal	(R) Inferior rectus	Uncrossed
▢ Intermediate	(R) Inferior oblique	Uncrossed
⸬ Ventral	(R) Medial rectus	Uncrossed
◫ Medial	(R) Superior rectus	Crossed
Caudal central	(R & L) Levator palpebrae	Mixed
▤ Parasympathetic	(R & L) Iris sphincter and	Mixed
■ (Edinger-Westphal and anterior median)	ciliary muscle	

CLINICAL CORRELATES

Physical Findings

1. Unilateral third nerve palsy, with contralateral superior rectus palsy
2. Bilateral total third nerve palsies, with spared levators   Lesion **must be** nuclear
3. Unilateral total third nerve palsy, with normal contralateral superior rectus
4. Unilateral internal ophthalmoplegia   Lesion **cannot be** nuclear
5. Unilateral ptosis

Figure 13–1. Subnuclei of the oculomotor nucleus. (*From Gay A, Newman NN, Keltner J, Stroud M. Eye Movement Disorders. St. Louis: Mosby, 1974, with permission.*)

TABLE 13–1. CLINICAL CORRELATIONS OF OCULOMOTOR NERVE PALSY

Lesions	Physical Findings[a]
Must be nuclear[b]	Unilateral third nerve palsy with contralateral superior rectus palsy Bilateral third nerve palsies with spared levators and/or spared parasympathetic functions
Cannot be nuclear	Unilateral third nerve palsy with normal contralateral superior rectus Unilateral internal ophthalmoplegia Unilateral ptosis

[a] All superior muscles—SR, SO, levator—are cross innervated.
[b] Ptosis and pupillary involvement must be either bilateral or absent.

palsy with contralateral tremor due to red nucleus involvement; Fig. 13–3) and *Weber's syndrome* (homolateral third-nerve and contralateral hemiplegia).

The interpeduncular portion of the third nerve courses forward and laterally between the posterior

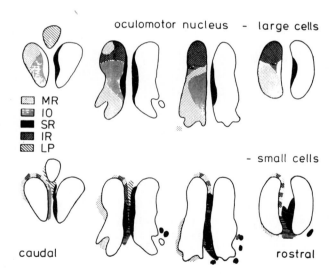

Figure 13–2. Drawing of four levels of the monkey oculomotor nucleus showing the organization of the motoneurone pools of the five muscles (MR, IO, SR, IR, and LP). In the upper drawing the organization of the large motoneurones (cell diameter > 22 μm) is plotted. The lower drawings show the localization of the small motoneurones (cell diameter < 22 μm). The small motoneurones lie around the perimeter of the classical oculomotor nucleus, and are not intermingled with the large motoneurones. (Extraocular eye muscles. IO, inferior oblique; IR, inferior rectus; LP, levator palpebrae; LR, lateral rectus; MR, medial rectus; SO, superior oblique; SR, superior rectus.) (*From Buttner-Enever JA. Anatomy of the ocular motor nuclei. In: Kennard C, Rose FC, eds. Physiological Aspects of Clinical Neuro-Ophthalmology. Chicago: Year Book, 1988, with permission.*)

cerebral artery and superior cerebellar artery and then parallel to the posterior communicating artery (Fig. 13–4). Pupillary fibers initially lie superiorly and medially and are especially vulnerable here.

In this region the third nerve is involved especially by compressive and vascular lesions (posterior communicating, posterior cerebral, superior cerebellar, and basilar arteries such as aneurysms or dolichoectatic vessels) as well as uncal herniation occurring with supratentorial mass lesions. *Pain in the face and headache* are important and characteristic associated symptoms of a posterior communicating aneurysm, *the most common cause of acute third nerve palsy involving the pupil* (due to compression or intraneural hemorrhage). The third nerve is frequently involved in this region by processes involving the meninges (meningitis, infections and granuloma, tuberculosis, syphilis, carcinomatous meningitis, and so forth). This type of involvement frequently causes *bilateral paralysis* (Table 13–2).

Cavernous sinus. The third nerve enters the cavernous sinus lateral to posterior clinoid process, close to the uncus of the temporal lobe. It runs forward in the lateral wall of the sinus (superior to the fourth nerve and first and second divisions of the fifth nerve; Fig. 13–5) lateral to the carotid artery. It then divides into a superior ramus supplying the superior rectus and elevator muscles, and an inferior ramus supplying the inferior rectus, medial rectus, and inferior oblique muscles and short ciliary branches to the ciliary ganglion (pupillomotor and accommodative fibers).

Results and etiology of lesions. Lesions of the third nerve in the cavernous sinus and orbit (Tables 13–2 and 13–3) are rarely isolated, except for microvascular third nerve palsies. Involvement of sympathetic fibers in the cavernous sinus may cause an associated Horner's syndrome causing the pupil to be less dilated than expected (test with hydroxyamphetamine). Aneurysms of the intracavernous carotid tend not to rupture because of investment by the walls of the sinus; they may grow very large, expanding the superior orbital fissure and compressing the optic nerve or pituitary gland. Thrombosis of the cavernous sinus is usually associated with orbital and ocular venous congestion, exophthalmos, and sepsis.

Primary aberrant regeneration of the third nerve is frequently seen with slowly evolving lesions of the cavernous sinus, especially aneurysms and meningiomas. The slow compression allows regeneration of third nerve fibers. However, the regeneration is disorderly such that most axons terminate on muscles other than those for which they are intended. This leads to abnormal coordination of ocular, lid, and pupil movements—the pseudo-Von-

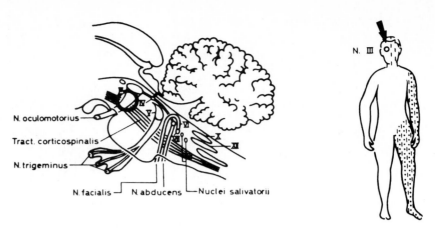

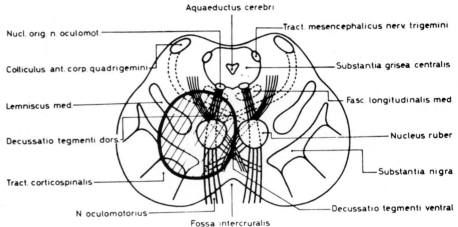

Figure 13–3. Benedikt's syndrome (lower syndrome of the red nucleus, midbrain syndrome, syndrome of the tegmentum of the midbrain). Vertical strokes indicate sensory deficiency; dots, extrapyramidal deficiency. (*From Sachsenweger R. Clinical localization of oculomotor disturbance. In: Vinken PJ, Bruyn GW. Handbook of Clinical Neurology. Amsterdam: North Holland, 1969;2:347, with permission.*)

Graefe phenomenon or lid elevation on downgaze, pupillary constriction on adduction, and so forth. **Secondary aberrant degeneration** occurs after ischemia or trauma.

Pupil-sparing third nerve palsies classically have been attributed to the interpeduncular and cavernous portions of the third nerve. They are caused by vascular occlusion, especially in diabetes mellitus (less often in temporal arteritis, hypertension, and periarteritis). **Pain** is a frequent complaint and may precede the palsy by a few days. Recent reports suggest many isolated third-nerve palsies with or without pupillary sparing originate in the brain stem, either in the tegmentum or fascicles of the third nerve. Histopathology demonstrates central softening of the third nerve by microinfarcts that spare the more peripheral pupillary fibers.

Superior orbital fissure and orbit. The third nerve enters the orbit most medially and inferiorly of the motor nerves of the eye; the superior and inferior divisions may be affected separately, although isolated superior and inferior division third-nerve palsies also result from midbrain lesions. In the orbit, isolated third nerve palsies are rare due to the mul-titude of structures in the orbital apex; aberrant regeneration does not occur. Concomitant optic nerve involvement indicates anterior cavernous sinus or orbital involvement of the third nerve. Tumors frequently affect the orbital third nerve (meningioma, nasopharyngeal carcinoma, metastatic carcinoma; also sphenoid sinus mucocele). Idiopathic orbital inflammatory disease (orbital pseudotumor) and the Tolosa-Hunt syndrome (frequently associated with severe pain) are of inflammatory origin. The differential diagnosis of third nerve palsies in the orbit also includes thyroid orbitopathy, orbital fibrosis syndromes, muscle entrapment, myasthenia gravis, and botulism. These latter processes all usually spare the pupil.

Other causes of third nerve palsy include ophthalmoplegic migraine and cyclic oculomotor palsy. *Ophthalmoplegic migraine* occurs most frequently in youngsters. Its etiology is uncertain; it is repetitive. Ophthalmoplegic migraine is a fairly comfortable diagnosis in the setting of migraine. Where no history of migraine exists, computed tomography (CT) or magnetic resonance imaging (MRI) are probably indicated. However, controversy exists as to

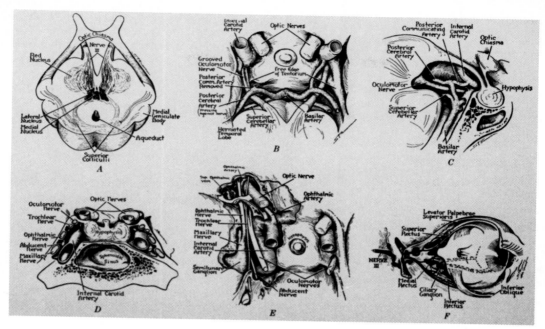

Figure 13–4. The position of the third nerve is shown as it leaves the midbrain and passes between the posterior cerebral and superior cerebellar arteries. On the left the posterior communicating artery has been removed. It had seemingly produced grooving of the third nerve. This diagram makes it obvious that an aneurysm on any of the vessels in the circle can press on one or the other third nerve. On the left of the diagram an effort has been made to show that herniation of the temporal lobe would produce pressure on the third nerve. (*From Walsh FB, Hoyt WF. The ocular motor system. In:* Clinical Neuro-Ophthalmology. *3rd ed. Baltimore: Williams & Wilkins, 1969;1; with permission.*)

when to proceed to angiography if the history is negative.

Cyclic oculomotor palsy is an oculomotor paresis with ptosis, mydriasis, and decreased accommodation; it occurs approximately every 2 minutes. The lid elevates, the globe adducts, the pupil constricts, and accommodation increases for a 10- to 30-second period, and then returns to the paretic state. It is

TABLE 13–2. ETIOLOGY OF THIRD NERVE LESIONS[a]

Undetermined	23%
Trauma[b]	16%
Neoplasia	12%
Vascular	21%
Aneurysmal	14%
Other[c]	15%

[a] The problem with compendia of cases such as this is that the clinical picture—associated signs and symptoms—is not considered. For example, no differentiation is made between a supratentorial mass causing uncal herniation, intrinsic third nerve tumor, orbital tumor, or pituitary tumor as "neoplastic" causes of third nerve palsy; and so little help is provided in clinical decision making.
[b] If trauma is minor, investigate for another cause (eg, tumor).
[c] Congenital third nerve palsies are frequently followed by aberrant regeneration.
From Rush JA, Younge BR. Paralysis of cranial nerves III, IV, and VI. Cause and prognosis in 1000 cases. Arch Ophthalmol. *1981;99:76–79.*

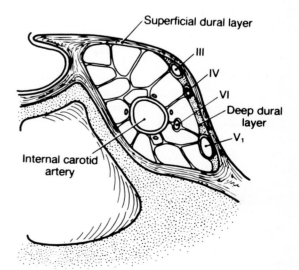

Figure 13–5. Diagram of the cavernous sinus as described by Umansky and Nathan showing the location of the oculomotor (III), trochlear (IV), ophthalmic (V) nerves and abducens nerve (VI). (*From Miller N, ed.* Walsh and Hoyt's Clinical Neuroophthalmology. *4th ed. Baltimore: Williams & Wilkins, 1982;1; with permission.*)

TABLE 13–3. ETIOLOGY OF OCULOMOTOR NERVE PALSY

Location	Etiology
Nuclear	Congenital hypoplasia
	Infarction
Fascicular	Vascular disease and tumor
Subarachnoid	Aneurysm (typically, posterior communicating artery; rarely, basilar artery)
	Meningitis (infectious, syphilitic, and neoplastic)
	Infarction (associated with diabetes)
	Tumor
	Neurosurgical complication
At the Tentorial Edge	Uncal herniation
	Pseudotumor cerebri
	Trauma
Cavernous Sinus and Superior Orbital Fissure	Aneurysm
	Carotid–cavernous fistula
	Thrombosis
	Tumor (pituitary adenoma, meningioma, nasopharyngeal and other metastases)
	Pituitary infarction (apoplexy)
	Nerve infarction (associated with diabetes or hypertension)
	Sphenoidal sinusitis
	Herpes zoster
	Tolosa-Hunt syndrome
Orbit	Trauma
Localization Uncertain	Infectious mononucleosis and other viral infections
	Following immunization
	Migraine

From Leigh RJ, Zee DS. Peripheral ocular motor palsies and strabismus. In: The Neurology of Eye Movements. *Philadelphia: Davis, 1983:171.*

almost always unilateral and is a lifelong problem. Over time the lid movement and adduction may decrease, but the pupil abnormality remains obvious.

Evaluation. Table 13–4 summarizes the evaluation of isolated third-nerve palsies.

Prognosis. In vascular third-nerve palsies the prognosis is good; usually recovery occurs in 2 to 3 months. In compression of the third nerve, the outcome depends on the degree and duration of the lesion.

Treatment. First, treat any underlying condition appropriately. Then allow a minimum of 6 months of stable deficit before considering surgery for strabismus or ptosis. Complex movement disorders due to multiple extraocular muscle involvement can be very difficult to correct surgically (especially aberrant regeneration). In these cases, marked improvement in function is rare; stability in primary position and a small field of binocular single vision is all that can be hoped for. Even with multiple operations, cosmesis is usually poor. Symptomatic diplopia may be treated by patching, opaquing one lens of glasses, or an opaque contact lens. Small deviations may be helped by prisms. If the dilated pupil causes a cosmetic problem, a weak Pilocarpine solution to constrict the pupil sometimes helps.

FOURTH NERVE DISORDERS

Clinical Presentation. The fourth nerve supplies the superior oblique muscle. It is the cranial nerve with the longest course and the one most frequently involved by trauma. A superior oblique palsy results in extorsion of the affected eye and weakness of depression; acutely, the deficit is maximum on looking down and in. Consequently, patients have great difficulty reading and going down stairs. They may have a compensatory head tilt to the opposite side. To test for a fourth-nerve palsy in the face of a third-nerve palsy, look for loss of intorsion (shown by movement of conjunctival blood vessels) on gaze down and to opposite side (Fig. 13–6). *Fourth nerve palsies are the most common cause of acquired vertical strabismus.* With time, the deviation may decrease and the inferior oblique overaction predominate. Congenital fourth nerve palsies are frequently accompanied by large (25 to 45 diopter) vertical phorias; diplopia may be absent. Bilateral fourth nerve palsies are not uncommon and must be ruled out in every vertical strabismus. They can be very difficult to identify (use the head tilt test and double Maddox rod). Often there is little inferior oblique overaction and symptoms are primarily referable to esotropia and excyclotropia in downgaze (see Chapter 15).

The **fourth nerve nuclei** are paired nuclei below the aqueduct of Sylvius in the periaqueductal gray matter of the mesencephalon at the level of the inferior colliculi; they are bounded by the median longitudinal fasciculus (MLF) laterally and ventrally and are continuous with the third nerve nuclei.

Brain-stem lesions. Isolated fourth nerve palsies from brain-stem lesions are rare; nevertheless, isolated bilateral fourth nerve palsies may be nuclear because the nuclei are very close to each other. When a superior oblique palsy is detected, it is the contralateral brain stem that is affected because the fourth nerve decussates. Vascular occlusion and trauma are the most common causes of fourth-nerve palsy in this location.

The trochlear nerves themselves course dorsally and laterally around the central gray, *decussating completely* in the roof of the mesencephalon to emerge from the brain stem just behind the inferior

TABLE 13–4. EVALUATION OF ISOLATED THIRD NERVE PALSIES

Findings	Clinical Setting	Look For	Tests
1. Pupil only	Comatose patient	Expanding supratentorial mass	MRI, CT
	Alert patient	Adie's syndrome, pharmacologically dilated pupil	Pharmacologic testing
2. Total third nerve palsy	Pain, meningeal signs	Aneurysm	MRI, CT, angiogram, lumbar puncture
Bilateral palsy		Intrapeduncular involvement	MRI, CT, angiogram, lumbar puncture
3. Pupil-sparing third nerve palsy[a]	Pain	Diabetes mellitus, other vascular causes	Fasting blood sugar, erythrocyte sedimentation rate vasculitis w/u, if neg. and no improvement, CT, angiogram, MRI for local midbrain infarct
4. Smaller-than-expected pupil	any	Cavernous sinus lesion	MRI, CT, test for Horner's syndrome with hydroxyamphetamine
5. Aberrant regeneration	insidious onset following trauma	Cavernous sinus meningioma/aneurysm	MRI, CT
		History of trauma or congenital third nerve palsy	
6. Isolated internal ophthalmoplegia	Botulism following viral infection		History, culture
7. Paralysis of accommodation without pupillary involvement	ill patient	Diphtheria	History, culture

[a] Observe closely (especially in young patients) first week; an aneurysm may occasionally seem to spare the pupil early on (but usually sparing is only relative if *carefully* studied). Rule out orbital disease, myasthenia gravis, thyroid disease.

colliculi. The fourth nerves are unique in exiting the brain stem dorsally and in decussating completely; they then pass anteriorly around the brain stem parallel to the posterior cerebral artery and pierce the dura to enter the cavernous sinus just posterior to the posterior clinoid. The fourth nerves presumably are compressed against the tentorium in head trauma (especially frontal); alternatively, trauma injures the nerves in the anterior medullary velum where they decussate, causing bilateral fourth nerve palsies. The fourth nerve may also be injured in neurosurgical procedures that split the tentorium. The paramesencephalic fourth nerve is presumably the portion of the nerve involved in vascular lesions. Like the third nerve, the fourth nerve is susceptible to meningitis and other meningeal processes in this region.

Cavernous sinus. The fourth nerve runs in the lateral wall of the cavernous sinus, inferior to the third nerve, superior orbital fissure, and superior oblique. In this area, isolated fourth nerve palsies are rarely recognized. The fourth nerve is liable to the same cavernous sinus problems as the third nerve (tumor, aneurysm, thrombosis).

Orbit. The nerve passes superonasally in the orbit, where it is frequently injured by procedures on the sinuses along with fractures of the supraorbital rim.

Other causes. *Brown's syndrome* consists of limited elevation of the adducted eye secondary to restricted movement of the superior oblique tendon through the trochlea. It is often congenital and may be acquired in inflammatory, systemic, and orbital diseases. It is important to differentiate from acquired fourth nerve palsy with implying central nervous system pathology. *Superior oblique myokymia* manifests as a rapid fine twitch of the superior oblique. It is idiopathic. The movements are of small amplitude and hard to observe. Look at torsion of conjunctival vessels with the slit-lamp or for torsion of retinal vessels with the ophthalmoscope. This unusual disorder frequently responds to Tegretol and rarely is associated with myokymia elsewhere.

Evaluation of isolated fourth nerve palsies. Because the majority of nonvascular fourth nerve palsies is caused by trauma or tumor, appropriate neuroradiologic evaluation is necessary. As with other cranial nerve palsies, if the fourth nerve palsy is truly isolated (without other signs or symptoms), especially in an older patient likely to have vascular disease, you can wait expectantly for resolution in 1

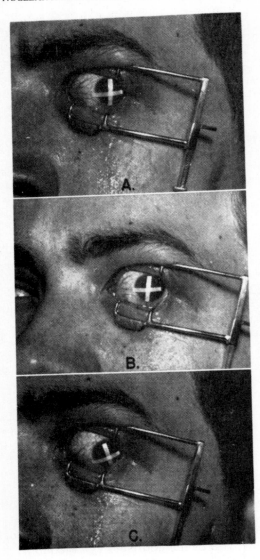

Figure 13–6. Intorsion of the eye due to the action of the superior oblique muscle in the presence of a third nerve paralysis. (*From Cogan DG.* Neurology of the Ocular Muscles. *2nd ed. Springfield, IL: Thomas, 1956, with permission.*)

to 3 months. If there is no improvement, or if the palsy worsens or other signs appear, the patient should be further evaluated (Tables 13–5 and 13–6).

Differential diagnosis. *Skew deviation* is a vertical imbalance of the eyes that occurs in brain-stem lesions. It may be constant (eg, one eye always higher) or alternating (higher eye depends on direction of horizontal gaze). If the skew is isolated, rule out torsion due to fourth nerve palsy with a negative head tilt test. However, like most brain-stem disorders, a skew deviation is not often isolated; it is usually constant in up- and downgaze unilke fourth-nerve or double-elevator palsies.

Double-elevator palsy causes inability to elevate

TABLE 13–5. ETIOLOGY OF FOURTH-NERVE LESIONS

Undetermined	36%
Head trauma	32%
Neoplasm	4%
Vascular	17%
Aneurysm	2%
Other	8%

From Younge BR, Sutula F. Analysis of trochlear nerve palsies: Diagnosis, etiology, and treatment. Mayo Clinic Proc. *1977;52:11–66.*

the eye in either abduction or adduction. It is probably due to a paranuclear or premotor third-nerve lesion.

Prognosis. The prognosis is good in ischemia, mild to moderate closed head trauma, and compression of brief duration. In severe head trauma and transection by surgical procedures, prognosis is usually poor.

Treatment. For diplopia, patch one eye, and opaque the patient's glasses or use an opaque contact lens for symptomatic relief. Prisms may be used for small deviations. Prior to surgery, allow a minimum of 6 months of stable deviation. The procedures to consider are inferior oblique weakening; weakening of the contralateral inferior rectus, ipsilateral supe-

TABLE 13–6. ETIOLOGY OF TROCHLEAR NERVE PALSY

Location	Etiology
Nuclear and Fascicular	Aplasia
	Mesencephalic hemorrhage or infarction
	Trauma
	Demyelination
	Neurosurgical complication
Subarachnoid	Trauma
	Tumor (pinealoma, tentorial meningioma, trochlear schwannoma, ependymoma, metastases)
	Neurosurgical complication
	Mastoiditis
	Meningitis (infectious and neoplastic)
Cavernous Sinus and Superior Orbital Fissure	Tumor, thrombosis, aneurysm, Tolosa-Hunt syndrome[a]
	Herpes zoster
Orbit	Ethmoidectomy
	Ethmoiditis
	Trauma
Localization Uncertain	Infarction (associated with diabetes or hypertension)

[a] More commonly accompanied by other ocular motor nerve palsies
From Leigh RJ, Zee DS. Peripheral ocular motor palsies and strabismus. The Neurology of Eye Movements. *Philadelphia: Davis, 1983:169.*

rior rectus, or both; superior oblique tucking; and advancing the superior oblique tendon.

SIXTH NERVE DISORDERS

Clinical presentation: The sixth nerve supplies the lateral rectus muscle. Sixth-nerve palsies cause double vision on gaze to the side of the lesion. The affected eye is turned in and abducts poorly. The patient may adopt a head turn to the side of the weak muscle (eyes turned to normal side). Primary and secondary deviations are most obvious in recent sixth nerve paresis. The sixth nerve has the longest course at the base of the brain, and is therefore susceptible to trauma, meningitis, tumor, and increased intracranial pressure.

Like the third and fourth nerve nuclei, the **sixth nerve nuclei** are paired structures; they lie in the floor of the fourth ventricle, at the pontomedullary junction, just anterior to the vestibular nuclei. The seventh nerve fibers circumnavigate the nuclei. The center for conjugate horizontal gaze is close to and nearly always affected at the same time as the sixth nerve nucleus, so that lesions of the sixth nerve nucleus lead to gaze palsies, **not** sixth nerve palsies. The medial longitudinal fasciculi are medial to the nuclei and separate them. *Wernicke's encephalopathy* frequently involves the sixth nerve and also causes gaze palsies and nystagmus. *Möbius syndrome* is the occurrence of congenital bilateral sixth nerve and facial nerve deficits (Fig. 13–7) because the nerves, nuclei, or both do not develop. It is usually bilateral and often there is an associated gaze palsy with abnormal adduction and convergence. In *Duane's syndrome* (see below), there is aplasia of the oculomotor nucleus and nerve.

Roots. The sixth nerve fibers run ventrally through the tegmentum of the pons, emerging lateral to the pyramids, level with the posterior border of the pons. *Foville's syndrome* (syndrome of the dorsal pons) consists of a sixth nerve palsy, ipsilateral facial weakness, facial anesthesia, Horner's syndrome, and deafness (Fig. 13–8). *Millard-Gubler syndrome* (syndrome of the ventral pons) (Fig. 13–9) is a contralateral hemiplegia or a sixth nerve palsy. *Raymond's syndrome* includes a sixth-nerve palsy and contralateral hemiplegia (Fig. 13–10).

The sixth nerve runs forward and laterally in the pontine cistern along the clivus through Dorello's canal (petroclinoid ligament) bending forward at the petrous tip of the temporal bone to enter the cavernous sinus below and medial to the fifth nerve (Fig. 13–11). It is very susceptible here to trauma, purulent meningitis, increased intracranial pressure, and displacement following lumbar puncture (sixth nerve palsy and papilledema do not have localizing

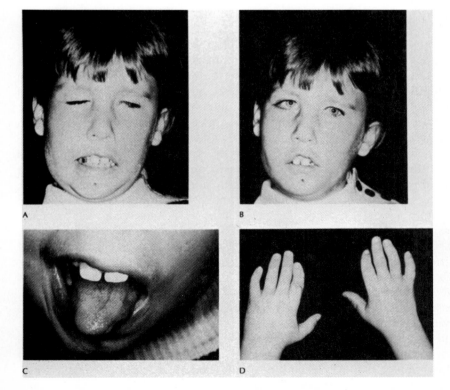

Figure 13–7. A. Child born with bilateral facial paralysis due to Möbius syndrome. Note asymmetric involvement with left eye more involved than right and normal lower face. **B.** Attempting to look right or left. No eye movement indicates involvement of the sixth cranial nerve. Head tilt to left is the result of efforts to compensate for eye muscle imbalance. **C.** Partial atrophy of left side of tongue indicates involvement of twelfth cranial nerve. **D.** Anomalous fingers. (*From May M, ed. The Facial Nerve. New York: Thieme, 1986, with permission.*)

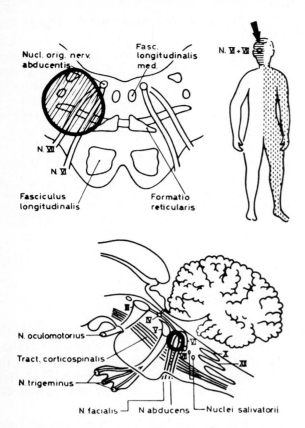

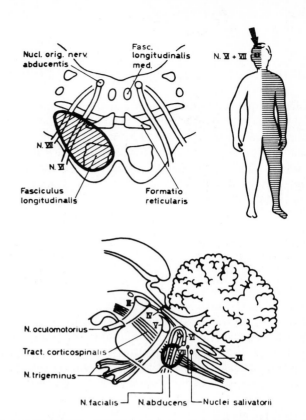

Figure 13–8. Foville's syndrome (hemiplegia abducento–facialis alternans, dorsocaudal syndrome of the pontine tegmentum). Striped bars and vertical strokes indicate motor deficiency. (*From Sachsenweger R. Clinical localization of oculomotor disturbance. In: Vinken PJ, Bruyn GW. Handbook of Clinical Neurology. Amsterdam: North Holland, 1969;2; with permission.*)

Figure 13–9. Millard-Gubler syndrome (hemiplegia alternans inferior, ventrocaudal syndrome of the pontine tegmentum). Striped bars indicate motor deficiency. (*From Sachsenweger R. Clinical localization of oculomotor disturbance. In: Vinken PJ, Bruyn GW. Handbook of Clinical Neurology. Amsterdam: North Holland, 1969;2; with permission.*)

value, and are often bilateral). Congenital absence of the sixth nerve with innervation of the lateral rectus by the third nerve is *Duane's syndrome*. The consequent co-contraction of the lateral and medial recti causes retraction of eye on lateral gaze; diplopia is rare. *Gradenigo's syndrome* occurs after middle ear infection and includes diplopia and ipsilateral facial pain with deafness. It is due to osteitis of petrous tip and/or petrosal vein thrombosis. In **cerebellopontine angle syndrome,** acoustic neuromas, meningiomas, and cholesteotomas often affect the sixth nerve along with the fifth, seventh, and eighth nerves.

Cavernous sinus. The sixth nerves pierce the dura and enter the cavernous sinus at the level of the dorsum sella. Unlike the other ocular motor nerves (III and IV), the sixth nerve runs through the cavernous sinus itself rather than in the lateral wall. Hence it is more vulnerable to expansile processes (internal carotid artery aneurysm, pituitary tumor, sphenoid mucocele) and vascular poblems (carotid–cavernous thrombosis, carotid–cavernous fistula, and dural arteriovenous fistula). In the cavernous sinus the sixth

nerve is joined briefly by some sympathetic fibers from the carotid plexus that supply the pupil and lid. With the third and fourth nerves, the sixth nerve enters the orbit through the superior orbital fissure and in the orbit innervates the lateral rectus muscle.

Benign sixth nerve palsy occurs in children (to age 15), frequently after viral illness, and may be recurrent but always recovers. Occasionally, it evolves into a comitant esotropia with full ductions. It is a truly *isolated* sixth nerve palsy. **Divergence palsy,** uncrossed comitant diplopia at distance and single binocular vision at near, is usually sudden in onset. The pupils are not miotic as they are in convergence spasm. It is probably a manifestation of early bilateral sixth nerve palsies. (Tables 13–7 to 13–9).

Evaluation. Truly isolated sixth nerve palsies can be watched like third- and fourth-nerve palsies, especially in children (benign postviral sixth-nerve palsy).

Prognosis. Because many sixth nerve palsies are not due to direct injury (sixth nerve palsy with increased intracranial pressure, after lumbar puncture,

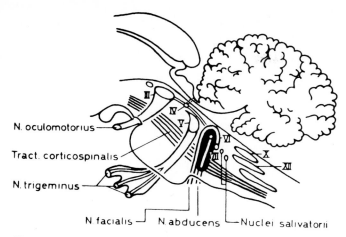

Figure 13–10. Raymond's syndrome (hemiplegia alternans abducens). (*From Sachsenweger R. Clinical localization of oculomotor disturbance. In: Vinken PJ, Bruyn GW. Handbook of Clinical Neurology. Amsterdam: North Holland, 1969;2; with permission.*)

TABLE 13–7. CAUSES OF PARALYSIS OF THE SIXTH CRANIAL NERVE (N = 49)

Cause	No. (%)
Undetermined	124 (29.6)
Head trauma	70 (16.7)
Neoplasm	61 (14.6)
Vascular[a]	74 (17.7)
Aneurysm[b]	15 (3.6)
Other	75 (17.9)
Total	419 (100.0)

[a] Twenty-four patients had diabetes mellitus, 22 had hypertension, 9 had atherosclerosis, and 19 had more than one condition.
[b] Includes 11 cases of subarachnoid hemorrhage.
From Rush JA, Younge BR. Paralysis of cranial nerves III, IV, and VI. Cause and prognosis in 1,000 cases. Arch Ophthalmol. 1981;99:76–79.

and so forth) or benign sixth nerve palsy (in children), prognosis can be very good. This is also true with ischemic lesions and compressive lesions of mild degree and short duration. Sixth nerve palsies due to severe head trauma and long-standing compression have a poorer prognosis.

Treatment. Early on, patch or use an opaque glass or contact lens to eliminate diplopia. In children alternate patch to avoid amblyopia. Oculinum can be used to prevent contracture of the medial rec-

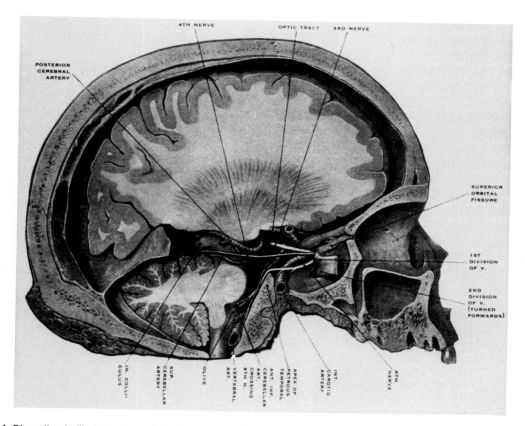

Figure 13–11. Dissection to illustrate the bend in the course of the sixth cranial nerve. (*From Woolf S. Anatomy of the Eye and Orbit. 6th ed. Revised by Last EJ. London: Lewis, 1968, with permission.*)

TABLE 13–8. ETIOLOGY OF ABDUCENS NERVE PALSY

Location	Etiology
Nuclear (characterized by horizontal gaze palsy)	Möbius syndrome
	Other congenital or hereditary gaze palsies
	Duane syndrome (some cases)
	Infarction
	Tumor (particularly pontine glioma and cerebellar tumors)
	Wernicke-Korsakoff syndrome
Fascicular (nucleus to exit from brain stem)	Infarction
	Demyelination
	Tumor
Subarachnoid	Compression by arteriosclerotic or anomalous vessels or berry aneurysm (usually of anterior inferior cerebellar artery or basilar artery)
	Subarachnoid hemorrhage
	Trauma
	Meningitis (infective and neoplastic)
	Clivus tumor
	Neurosurgical complication
	Postinfectious
Petrous	Infection of mastoid or tip of petrous bone
	Thrombosis of inferior petrosal sinus
	Trauma (fracture of petrous bone)
	Persistent trigeminal artery
	Trigeminal schwannoma
	Downward displacement of brain stem by supratentorial mass (eg, tumor, pseudotumor)
	Following lumbar puncture, myelography, spinal or epidural anesthesia
	Aneurysm
Cavernous Sinus and Superior Orbital Fissure	Aneurysm
	Thrombosis
	Carotid–cavernous fistula
	Dural arteriovenous malformation
	Tumor (pituitary adenoma, nasopharyngeal carcinoma, meningioma)
	Tolosa-Hunt syndrome
	Herpes zoster
Orbital	Tumor
Localization Uncertain	Infarction (often associated with diabetes or hypertension)
	Migraine

From Leigh RJ, Zee DS. Peripheral ocular motor palsies and strabismus. The Neurology of Eye Movements. *Philadelphia: Davis, 1983:167.*

tus. The best results are obtained if the fixing eye is not the eye injected. After 6 months of stable deviation, consider surgery.

Prisms are less successful in treating sixth-nerve palsies than third- and fourth-nerve palsies.

MULTIPLE OCULOMOTOR NERVE PALSIES

Lesions causing palsies of more than one ocular motor nerve most frequently are compressive, infiltrative, or traumatic (Table 13–10). Toxic motor nerve

TABLE 13–9. CAUSES OF PARALYSIS OF CRANIAL NERVES III, IV, OR VI

	CN III (%)	CN IV (%)	CN VI (%)
Undetermined	23	36	30
Head trauma	16	32	17
Neoplasm	12	4	15
Vascular	21	19	18
Aneurysm	14	2	4
Other	14	8	18

From Rush JA, Younge BR. Paralysis of cranial nerves III, IV, and VI. Cause and prognosis in 1,000 cases. *Arch Ophthalmol. 1981;99:76–79.*

TABLE 13-10. ETIOLOGY OF MULTIPLE OCULAR MOTOR NERVE PALSIES

Location	Etiology
Brain Stem	Tumor
	Infarction
	Motor neuron disease
	Leigh's disease
Subarachnoid	Meningitis (infectious and neoplastic)
	Trauma
	Clivus tumor
	Aneurysm
Cavernous Sinus and Superior Orbital Fissure	Aneurysm
	Tumor (meningioma, pituitary adenoma with apoplexy; metastases, particularly nasopharyngeal carcinoma)
	Thrombosis
	Tolosa-Hunt syndrome
	Neurosurgical complication
	Herpes zoster
	Infarction (associated with diabetes)
	Carotid–cavernous fistula
	Mucormycosis and other fungal infections
Orbital	Trauma
	Tumor
Localization Uncertain	Toxins
	Postinflammatory neuropathy (Guillain-Barré syndromes)
	Arteritis
	Behçet's disease

From Leigh RJ, Zee DS. Peripheral ocular motor palsies and strabismus. In: The Neurology of Eye Movements. Philadelphia: Davis, 1983:174.

palsies have no distinguishing characteristics. A good history is critical for suspecting the diagnosis.

Tumors may affect the nerves or their roots or nuclei anywhere along the pathway. Discrete masses compress contiguous nerves (sixth, seventh and, less frequently, fourth and fifth), especially in the cavernous sinus and orbital apex. Any combination may occur. In the orbital apex, the optic nerve is often involved. Intrinsic brain-stem tumors and large infarcts may involve any of the ocular motor nerves and roots, frequently in combination with supranuclear and infranuclear defects of ocular motility as well.

Pituitary tumors cause ophthalmoplegia by compression of the ocular motor nerves (especially in the cavernous sinus). They also may be associated with enlargement of the extraocular muscles, giving a radiologic picture indistinguishable from thyroid orbitopathy (see below). Growth-hormone-secreting tumors are especially prone to do this.

Severe **head trauma** affects the ocular motor

nerves in sphenoid fractures (orbital apex), temporal bone fractures (sixth and seventh nerves), and uncal herniation (the third nerve).

Multiple, bilateral, and sometimes fluctuating palsies may be associated with increased intracranial pressure and processes at the base of the brain: meningeal infection, inflammation, carcinomatosis, and nasopharyngeal tumor spreading into the intracranial cavity, and giant ICA aneurysm.

The **differential diagnosis of multiple cranial nerve palsies** includes orbital and cavernous sinus processes (especially aneurysm, pituitary tumor, meningioma, and rarely multiple myeloma and actinomycosis); thyroid, pseudotumor (myositis), orbital apex, and Tolosa-Hunt syndromes; muscle entrapment; neurologic disorders (myasthenia gravis; rarely, the Lambert-Eaton syndrome) and myopathies; chronic progressive external ophthalmoplegia (PEO, ophthalmoplegia plus); the Miller-Fisher syndrome; botulism and diphtheria (Table 13–11); and metabolic abnormalities (Wernicke's and Leigh's syndromes). Rare disorders affecting multiple cranial nerves include trichinosis, amyloid, and arteritis (especially temporal arteritis) and tumor infiltration of the muscles.

Apart from the multiple of central nervous system (CNS) diseases causing specific cranial nerve palsies (discussed above) there is one striking symptom complex, the *Miller-Fisher syndrome*, thought to be a postviral neuropathy and variant of the Guillain-Barré syndrome (GBS) in which *ophthalmoplegia* as well as *ataxia and areflexia* dominate the clinical picture. The pupil may be involved occasionally. It may also occur following vaccination and specific viral infection (such as Epstein-Barr virus or Herpes zoster). This disorder is poorly understood, but has autoimmune features and seems to cause symptoms by demyelination. The signs and symptoms may suggest either intrinsic CNS or cranial nerve involvement. These tend to remit sponta-

TABLE 13-11. RARE TOXIC CAUSES OF MULTIPLE OCULAR MOTOR PALSIES

Botulism
Ophthalmoplegia with pupil involvement and accommodative paresis, symmetrical
Evaluation: History, postingestion or wound, identify toxin in food
Therapy: Antitoxin

Diphtheria
Accommodative paresis, with spared pupil, occasional ophthalmoplegia after malaise, headache, sore throat, and palatal paralysis
Therapy: Antitoxin, prior to symptoms will prevent neurologic complications

neously in 5 to 6 weeks, but may affect progressively descending parts of the CNS, becoming a threat to medullary centers. Steroids and plasmapheresis may be effective in therapy. These cases seem to merge with the descending neuropathy of GBS, which shares a characteristic autoimmunologic–cytologic dissociation in the cerebrospinal fluid. Conversely, the GBS rarely ascends to cause ophthalmoplegia.

Carotid–cavernous fistulas also involve cranial nerves in the cavernous sinus and the petrous apex and may be associated with enlarged extraocular muscles and ophthalmoplegia.

NEUROMUSCULAR JUNCTION PROBLEMS

Myasthenia gravis (MG) is a neuromuscular disorder characterized by fatigability, abnormally rapid exhaustion, and loss of strength in muscles under voluntary control—particularly facial, bulbar, and ocular muscles.

MG is caused by postsynaptic neuromuscular junction dysfunction characterized by a reduction in the number of acetylcholine receptors (30% of normal ACh receptors) and mediated by an autoimmune disorder (IgG is formed against postsynaptic protein; Fig. 13–12).

Myasthenia gravis affects 1 in 20,000 to 30,000 people, with a ratio of females to males of 3:2. The peak incidence in women is in the third decade, and in men in the sixth decade. In contrast, ocular MG preferentially affects men over 40.

Generalized myasthenia gravis is characterized by excessive fatigability of muscle function, made worse by muscle activity, and improves with rest ("variability and fatigability"). The symptoms are often more severe at the end of the day; weakness often begins in muscles innervated by cranial nerves causing **ptosis,** oculomotor palsies, weakness of the orbicularis, face, swallowing, phonation, and respiration. Limb muscles are also involved, especially proximally. Ocular symptoms are the initial symptoms in 70% of patients (50% of patients first consults an ophthalmologist), are present during the course of the illness in 90%, and are the sole symptoms in 21% of patients.

Ocular myasthenia. Approximately 80% of patients ultimately will exhibit generalized myasthenia. Most exhibit generalized signs of myasthenia within 3 years of the first ocular symptoms.

Ocular MG typically presents with ptosis and diplopia. Less usual are gaze palsy, muscle palsy, an apparent internuclear ophthalmoplegia, vertical nystagmus, or "progressive external ophthalmoplegia." All may be variable, switching from side to side and eye to eye.

Differential diagnosis. Myasthenia gravis must be differentiated from other ocular motor problems. Amyotrophic lateral sclerosis (ALS) rarely causes ptosis or ocular motor signs and fasciculations are prominent (they are **not** present in MG). Multiple sclerosis may be ruled out with visual evoked potential and MRI studies. In myotonia dystrophica there is a positive family history, myotonia, and myotonic cataract. It is worse in the morning and may get **worse** with Tensilon. In progressive external ophthalmoplegia there is usually a positive family history (50%), symmetry of symptoms, and no variation. In botulism there is a decrease in accommodation and the pupillary light reaction but on occasion a positive Tensilon response may be present (as in many other neurogenic and myopathic processes).

Consider myasthenia in all pupil-sparing disturbances of ocular motility with or without ptosis (although rare pupillary abnormalities have been detected in MG). Ocular myopathies can be confused with cases of myasthenia gravis when the myasthenic motility disorder is relatively stable. Stable myasthenia gravis is also confused with cranial-nerve palsies or double-elevator palsy. In contrast, thyroid orbitopathy usually is associated with other signs and symptoms, lid lag or retraction, and characteristic findings on ultrasound, CT, or MRI scanning. However, the incidence of myasthenia is increased in thyroid orbitopathy. The pattern of extraocular muscle enlargement on ultrasound, CT, or MRI differentiates myasthenia gravis from uncommon cases of orbital myositis that present without the characteristic inflammation and pain. Diphtheria never is associated with ptosis; paresis of accommo-

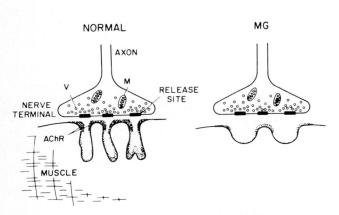

Figure 13–12. Diagrams of normal and myasthenic neuromuscular junctions. The MG junction shows reduced numbers of AChRs (stippling); sparse, shallow postsynaptic folds; a widened synaptic space; and a normal nerve terminal. (*From Drachman DB, ed. Myasthenia gravis: Immunobiology of a receptor disorder. TINS. 1983;6:447, with permission.*)

dation is the most frequent sign of diphtheria but is nearly never seen in myasthenia gravis.

In myasthenics, beware of induced or increased weakness (which can be life threatening) with antibiotics and other drugs (Table 13–12).

Any unexplained ocular palsy or ptosis deserves a Tensilon test!

The **Lambert-Eaton** myasthenic syndrome (LES) is an autoimmune disorder associated with carcinomas (50%), especially small-cell carcinoma of the lung; and immunologic disorders. It is characterized by impaired presynaptic release of acetylcholine. The autoantibodies interfere with the neurotransmitter release by diminishing the function of voltage operated calcium channels.

LES is symptomatically similar to MG, with muscle weakness, hyporeflexia, and autonomic dysfunction. Ocular signs are rare, but diplopia is a frequent complaint. It has a pathognomonic electromyogram (EMG) that is just the opposite of the EMG in MG; there is a posttetanic increase in potentials. LES autoantibodies detected by quantitative radioimmunoassay distinguish this disease from myasthenia and other neurological disorders. Both the motor and autonomic defects of the syndrome can be effectively treated with 3,4 diaminopyridine.

Diagnostic evaluation. Carefully evaluate ocular motility. Look for lid twitches (a characteristic excessive "popping" and lifting of the lid that occurs as the lid is elevated), orbicularis weakness and other facial weakness ("myasthenic snarl"); and check for increase of ptosis, and/or nystagmus, squint, and so forth, with prolonged effort at upgaze. Be alert for motility abnormalities that change from examiner to examiner. In bilateral myasthenic ptosis, if the lid with the greater ptosis is elevated, the other lid will fall (myasthenic "curtaining"). This "enhanced" ptosis is a helpful diagnostic sign. In MG, the pupil is spared.

Pharmacologic evaluation. Perform a *Tensilon test*—establish a reliable baseline; an objective end point is absolutely necessary as the criterion against which the reaction to Tensilon will be measured. In small, hard-to-measure deviations a Hess or Lancaster screen can be very helpful. Carefully quantitate the ptosis or squint. For an adult use 10 mg (1 cc) of Tensilon in a tuberculin syringe. Give a placebo, a saline injection, if you suspect a fictitious weakness, followed by a 0.2 cc in a test dose. This is important as some myasthenics are exquisitely sensitive and excess Tensilon may produce worsening of symptoms. If no reaction occurs in 1 minute, give the remainder. Some physicians pretreat with 0.4 mg of atropine IV to prevent the muscarinic side effects; I just have the atropine handy, but do use a three-way stopcock on a butterfly infusion set to facilitate quick access of atropine and flushing the Tensilon into the vein.

A positive test is a definite return toward normal of the baseline signs.

Tensilon tonography also may be used if the usual test is equivocal or if no measurable signs are present. A positive response is a 2 mm Hg increase in intraocular pressure, 10 seconds after injection.

False positives do occur in cases of myositis, myopathy, and even cranial neuropathy and tumors. False negatives are rare. Very rarely a true myasthenic will get worse, especially if overdosed. Neostigmine may also be used and is especially helpful in infants or children who will not sit still for careful measurements during an injection. Give IM; use (weight [kg] × 1.5 mg)/70, plus 0.4 mg atropine. Check the abnormal signs after 30 minutes.

One can be certain that a sufficient dose was absorbed if there are muscarinic side effects: diaphoresis, salivation, lacrimation, fasciculations, and increased bowel activity. These will go away in less than 1 minute as will any improvement in symptoms. Asthma or cardiac arrhythmias are relative contraindications to Tensilon testing. It is wise to warn the patient of the transient side effects.

Laboratory evaluation. CT and MRI scans for thymoma should be performed; 15 to 20% of patients with MG has a thymoma (10% are malignant). Conversely, 40 to 50% of patients with a thymoma has MG. An EMG of extraocular muscles with Tensilon may be done and will show jitter, as in peripheral EMGs. Anti-ACh-receptor antibodies are present in about 80% of myasthenics.

Associated disorders. Malignancies occur in 7.5% of MG patients, autoimmune disease in 5%, and thyroid disease in 13%.

Treatment. Four general approaches to treatment are currently utilized for MG: (1) enhancement of neuromuscular transmission by anticholinesterase agents (Prostigmin, Mestinon); (2) immunosuppres-

TABLE 13–12. DRUGS THAT MAY INDUCE OR EXACERBATE MYASTHENIC WEAKNESS (CAN BE LIFE THREATENING)

Aminoglycosides	Kanamycin
Ampicillin	Librium
Bacitracin	Neomycin
Chloroquine	Penicillamine
Chlorpromazine	Polymycin
Clindomycine	Procainamide
Colistin	Quinidine
Curare	Quinine
Diazepam-like drugs	Streptomycin
Dihydrostreptomycin	Succinyl choline
Imcomysin	Tetracycline
Inhalation narcotics	Valium

sion with steroids and cytotoxic drugs, (azothio-prine, cyclosporine); (3) "maximal" thymectomy, which over the years has gained increasing acceptance; and (4) plasmapheresis, which can induce short-term improvement in severe exacerbations.

In my experience, steroids have been especially effective in children with ocular myasthenia. Frequently, the steroids may be tapered or even stopped after several months. This is a relief, as the long-term effects of the immunosuppressive agents have not been fully determined.

Selective elimination of the autoimmune response is very encouraging. Generally, immunosuppressive agents improve more than 90% of patients, but are a lifelong treatment with well-known risks. However, recent studies suggest that even a limited period of treatment with cyclosporin can induce long-lasting or permanent tolerance. In addition, production of anti-idiotypes (anti-antibodies) against the antibodies to the ACh receptor have been produced and may provide an effective treatment. Even more excitingly, the exact molecular structure of the mammalian muscle ACh receptor has been determined. This knowledge will be invaluable in developing a specific treatment of MG.

Unfortunately, the ocular symptoms (especially the diplopia)—perhaps because very little muscle weakness (eg, a degree of weakness that might not produce symptomatic limb weakness) may result in ptosis or diplopia—often do not respond as well to anticholinergic agents as do the systemic symptoms.

OPHTHALMOPLEGIAS

The ophthalmoplegias as defined here are a dissimilar group of hereditary, local, and systemic disease processes, having in common the limitation of ocular motility by a process that affects neither the specific muscles and nerves nor is a space-occupying lesion. Because these disease processes have little in common aside from causing ophthalmoplegia, I have found it easiest to group them by the age of onset (Table 13–13).

Congenital ophthalmoplegias: Included in this group of disorders are the orbital fibrosis syndromes, where abnormal fibrotic bands within the orbits restrict eye movement and even replace extraocular muscles. Also included are disorders of the muscles that present at birth, including the congenital myopathies (central core disease, nemaline myopathy, and so forth) and muscular dystrophies that involve the extraocular muscles. Ocular motility may also be affected in congenital myotonia and congenital MG, especially in children of myasthenic mothers. Con-

TABLE 13–13. OPHTHALMOPLEGIAS

Congenital

Orbital fibrosis syndromes
Congenital myopathies (central core, nemaline, etc)
Muscular dystrophies
Myotonia
Congenital myasthenia gravis
Bassen-Kornsweig syndrome (vitamin E deficiency due to malabsorption), ophthalmoplegia, retinitis pigmentosa, ataxia, areflexia, acanthosis of red blood cells

Onset in Late Childhood, Second Decade

Myotonic dystrophy, autosomal dominant; myotonia, hatchet facies, wasting of hand muscles, ptosis, weakness, orbital occlusion, relatively mild ophthalmoplegia, Christmas tree cataract, low intraocular pressure, increased VEP latency. Less frequently: corneal changes, chorioretinopathy

Onset Second to Third Decade

Chronic Progressive External Ophthalmoplegia: Mitochondrial cytopathy
Ophthalmoplegia is presenting feature in two thirds; pupil spared, diplopia rare
Kearns-Sayre variant—retinitis pigmentosa, frequently complete heart block

Onset Third to Fourth Decade

Oculopharyngeal dystrophy—dysphagia and ptosis; autosomal dominant

Rare

Familial periodic paralysis
Chondrodystrophic myotonic (Schwartz-Jampel syndrome) dwarfism; long-bone abnormalities; blepharospasm, myotonia
Familial static ophthalmoplegia

genital or neonatal ophthalmoplegia is part of the Bassen-Kornzweig syndrome (abetalipoproteinemia, in which malabsorption of vitamins A and E results in manifestations of ophthalmoplegia, retinitis pigmentosa, ataxia, areflexia, and acanthosis of the red blood cells.

Onset in late childhood, second decade: Only one relatively frequent cause of ophthalmoplegia has its onset in late childhood: myotonic dystrophy. This autosomal dominant dystrophy can be recognized by generalized myotonia—difficulty in muscular relaxation that is more profound in cold and that infrequently involves the eye muscles. Those with the disorder may be recognized by their "hatchet facies" and wasting of the hand muscles. These patients also suffer premature frontal balding and men from testicular atrophy. The ocular signs include a predominant ptosis, relatively mild ophthalmoplegia, Christmas tree cataracts, and less often corneal changes and a diffuse chorioretinopathy. Myotonic dystrophy is one of the rare disorders to cause low intraocular pressure (usually ≤ 10). An association with disorders of the cardiac conduction system should be evaluated by serial electrocardiograms.

Onset in second or third decade: Again, only one cause of ophthalmoplegia commonly presents in the second or third decades, the group of mitochondrial cytopathies, recognized as chronic progressive external ophthalmoplegia "plus." The plus is often a pigmentary retinopathy and, in the Kearns-Sayre variant, heart block (Table 13–14). Cerebellar dysfunction and increased cerebrospinal fluid protein also are found commonly.

These ophthalmoplegias are associated with a multitude of other clinical and laboratory abnormalities, usually are only slowly progressive, and are rarely associated with diplopia. Ptosis is prominent. The limitation of ocular motility may be profound. The ophthalmoplegia does not vary and is unassociated with fatigue, in contrast to myasthenia gravis. The disorder is associated with deletions of mitochondrial DNA.

Onset in third or fourth decade: Oculopharyngeal dystrophy usually presents in the third and fourth decades with ptosis and dysphagia. It is autosomal dominant and has a large concentration in families of French-Canadian origin.

Rare disorders: Familial periodic paralysis, familial static ophthalmoplegia, and the Schwartz-Jampel syndrome (dwarfism, long bone abnormalities, blepharospasm, and myotonia) are less common causes of ophthalmoplegia.

TABLE 13–14. CLINICAL FEATURES OF THE KEARNS-SAYRE SYNDROME

CPEO[a]
Retinal pigmentary degeneration
Heart block[a]
Small stature
Hearing loss (vestibular disturbance)
Cerebellar ataxia
Pendular nystagmus
Corticospinal tract signs
Impaired intellect
Cranial muscle weakness (face, palate, neck)
Peripheral neuropathy
"Myopathy" affecting skeletal muscles (ragged-red fibers)
Corneal clouding
Scrotal tongue
Spinal fluid abnormalities (elevated protein)
Slowed electroencephalogram
Endocrine abnormalities (steriod, calcium, glucose metabolism)
Elevated serum glutamic oxaloacetic transaminase, creatinine phosphokinase, lactic dehydrogenase, altered lactate-pyruvate metabolism

[a] For diagnosis of Kearns-Sayre syndrome, these features should be present before 20 years of age.

Traditional teaching has held that where the ptosis or ophthalmoplegia is progressive, it should not be treated by surgical procedures. Because many of these processes are very slowly progressive, the more disabling and cosmetically disfiguring aspects of the disease may be approached surgically as long as the patient understands the result may not be permanent. However, where the ophthalmoplegia is not associated with diplopia, as in many of these disorders, any realignment of the extraocular muscles should be approached with great caution and only with the expectation of significant function or cosmetic benefit. Ptosis surgery should also be done with caution because of the danger of exposure if the Bell's phenomenon is poor, as it usually is. Special attention should also be paid to the increased sensitivity of many of these patients to anesthetic inducation agents, curare, and nondepolarizing muscle relaxants.

Especially where downgaze is limited, the use of prisms to read can be very helpful in these patients.

ORBITAL INFLAMMATORY DISEASE

Thyroid orbitopathy. Thyroid orbitopathy (Graves' disease, thyroid eye disease, and so forth) causes an inflammatory involvement of orbital structures, especially the extraocular muscles mediated by an autoimmune reaction with antigens common to the thyroid and the extraocular muscles. It is *the most common cause of exophthalmos,* unilateral or bilateral. The end result is enlargement and ultimately fibrosis of the extraocular muscles, leading to proptosis, diplopia, ophthalmoplegia, lid retraction, and lid lag. The restrictive myopathy also may cause an increase in intraocular pressure, especially on upgaze, sometimes leading to erroneous diagnosis of "glaucoma" (see Chapter 18). Severe involvement may lead to corneal exposure or optic neuropathy.

Diagnosis is made by finding limitation of eye movement, especially in upgaze with positive **forced ductions,** proptosis, lid lag, lid retraction, and laboratory evidence of thyroid dysfunction. However, occasional patients do not have abnormal thyroid tests despite clinical thyroid orbitopathy and confirmatory imaging studies. Even with "fast" thyrotropin-releasing hormone and antibody determination, up to 20% may be "euthyroid."

Ultrasound, CT, and MRI show enlarged extraocular muscles, usually multiple and in both orbits. Ultrasound is probably the most sensitive in experienced hands. The tendinous muscle insertions usually remain normal in contrast to their involvement in idiopathic orbital inflammatory disease.

"Newman's hypothesis:" Orbital involvement

appears to occur with changes in thyroid status, whether it is from normal to hyper, hyper to normal (especially following treatment of hyperthyroidism), or normal to hypothyroid.

Differential diagnosis. Usually lid lag and retraction differentiate thyroid orbitopathy from orbital pseudotumor (usually unilateral with more severe inflammatory signs) and from neuropathic and myopathic disease (negative forced ductions and rare proptosis). A small number of patients has both myasthenia and thyroid orbitopathy.

Trichinosis is associated with chemosis, **lid edema,** ophthalmoplegia, pain on movement, and eosinophilia. A history of ingestion of pork that may have been inadequately cooked is helpful.

Treatment. The treatment of mild to moderate symptoms is symptomatic: tears as needed and a moisturizing ointment at bedtime to prevent drying. Elevate the head of the bed and use protective shields and moist chambers.

Severe symptoms, especially eye-threatening corneal exposure and optic neuropathy, may necessitate orbital decompression, high-dose steroid treatment, or radiation. For optic-nerve symptoms,

medial and posterior decompression of the orbital apex is needed.

Cosmetic surgery should be undertaken only after the disease is quiescent for a 3-month minimum with normalized thyroid function. Procedures include orbital decompression, lid surgery, and extraocular muscle surgery.

Occasionally a patient doing poorly on synthroid therapy after thyroid ablation will be much less symptomatic on Cytomel.

Idiopathic orbital inflammatory disease (Orbital pseudotumor), Tolosa-Hunt syndrome, Orbital apex syndrome/painful ophthalmoplegia. These poorly understood inflammatory disease(s) of the orbit may preferentially affect the extraocular muscles (orbital myositis), superior orbital fissure, or cavernous sinus. Involvement in the apex or cavernous sinus may also involve the optic nerve. Any combination of muscle palsies may occur. Orbital inflammatory disease is primarily a disease of middle age, which may show an elevated erythrocyte sedimentation rate (ESR), especially in the bilateral cases, which are more likely to have a systemic cause (periarteritis nodosa, Wegener's syndrome). Symp-

TABLE 13–15. PAINFUL OPHTHALMOPLEGIAS

Etiology	Ophthalmoplegia	Age	Other
Orbit infection	Any combination of palsies possible	Child	Sinus disease
Orbit inflammation	Any combination of palsies possible	Any	Inflammation
Orbital apex syndrome	Any combination of palsies possible	Any	Optic nerve
Superior orbital fissure syndrome	Any combination of palsies possible	Middle	Decreased V_1 sensation
Tolosa-Hunt syndrome	Any combination of palsies possible	Middle	Steriod sensitive
Vascular third, fourth, sixth nerve lesions			
Microvascular	**Pupil sparing,** III most often	Older	Headache, diabetes
Aneurysm	III, **with pupil affected**	Young, middle	Severe headache
Ophthalmoplegic migraine	Recurrent III	Child	History: family history, migraine, aberrant regeneration
Raeder's syndrome	Uncommon	Older	Horner's syndrome, V
Pituitary tumor	VI first, III, IV	Middle	Headache
Pituitary apoplexy	Any III, IV, VI	Middle	Decreased visual acuity, **headache**
Parasellar mass			
Aneurysm	Any	Middle	Aberrant regeneration or (rarely) neuromyotonia
Invasive pituitary adenoma	VI first		
Nasopharyngeal carcinoma, basal tumors (chordoma)	VI first	Older	Multiple cranial nerves, pain
Sphenoid sinus mucocele	VI		
Gradenigo's syndrome	VI	Child	Middle ear infection, otitis media
Temporal arteritis	Due to orbital vascular occlusion; cranial nerves less commonly involved	Elderly	Tender scalp, jaw claudication, polymyalgia rheumatica, increased erythrocyte sedimentation rate, steroid response

TABLE 13–16. DIFFERENTIAL DIAGNOSIS OF PTOSIS

Pseudoptosis	Protective—secondary to ocular irritations, foreign body (double evert eyelid to check)
	Orbital malformations
	Enophthalmos
	Vertical muscle imbalance (watch lid on cover testing!)
	Apraxia of lid opening (Huntington's chorea)
	Blepharospasm
	Malingering
	Contralateral lid retraction
	Contralateral exophthalmos
Congenital Ptosis (no lid fold)	Isolated
	Associated with other lid and eye anomalies (epicanthal folds, blepharophimosis, etc)
	Bilateral familial
	Associated with superior rectus weakness
	Congenital Horner's syndrome
	Syndromes: Marcus-Gunn, jaw winking
Neurogenic Ptosis	Third nerve palsy—including cyclic third nerve, ophthalmoplegic migraine, misdirection of third nerve
	Myasthenia gravis
	Myotonic dystrophy, progressive external ophthalmoplegia, and other myopathies and ophthalmoplegias
	Horner's syndrome (1- to 3-mm ptosis only) and miosis
	Ptosis "pseudoparalytica" is really blepharospasm
	Marin Amat syndrome
Orbit	Masses and inflammation—especially lid tumor, lacrimal gland tumor, orbit and lid infection (even with a chalazion!)
	Trauma—including orbit and ocular surgery, especially strabismus, cataract, retinal detachment, levator disinsertion
	Thyroid orbitopathy—both true ptosis and pseudoptosis with contralateral lid retraction
Senile	Ptotic lid with good levator function

toms include pain, diplopia, chemosis, and exophthalmos. Usually, there is a prompt response to steroids, which some suggest as a diagnostic trial (see Chapters 18 and 19).

Differential diagnosis includes neoplasm, infection, trauma, aneurysm, and diabetic ophthalmoplegia (Table 13–15; see also Chapter 18).

Evaluation includes ultrasound, CT, or MRI; occasionally contiguous involvement of intracranial or sinus and cavernous sinus structures is found on CT or MRI; an ESR and ANA should be obtained.

Therapy: Steroids! The response is usually so good that lack of response should make you question the diagnosis.

ORBITAL TUMORS

Occasionally orbital tumors may present as a primary limitation of ocular motility. This is especially true of rhabdomyosarcoma in infants. Appropriate neuro-imaging evaluation usually makes the differential diagnosis from a neurogenic lesion, if not a specific diagnosis (see Chapter 18).

PTOSIS

We have already considered neurogenic ptosis with third nerve palsy, myasthenia gravis, ophthalmople-

gia, and myopathy. Orbital disease is covered in Chapter 18 and as part of the pathognomonic triad of Horner's syndrome with other disorders of the pupil (see Chapter 16). Most other ptoses are not easily confused with neurogenic ptosis, but you should keep in mind a clear differential diagnosis (see Table 13–16).

In third nerve palsies, ptosis is often the first sign of damage; its improvement, the first sign of recovery. It is often the first sign of myasthenia gravis. In nuclear third nerve palsies, ptosis is always bilateral if present.

Treatment: The treatment of nonmyaesthenic ptosis is usually surgical, although corticosteroid drops and neosynephrine drops can elevate the lid a millimeter or two. There are two major approaches to the correction of ptosis: resection of conjunctiva and Müller's muscles and resection of the levator. These are usually adequate where there is some residual levator function. Less commonly, when levator function is minimal or associated with abnormal synkinesis (Marcus Gunn jaw winking, Marin Amat syndromes; see Chapters 17 and 18), a suspension of the lid is necessary.

In children, surgery should usually be delayed until accurate measurements of levator function can be made, unless unilateral ptosis causes amblyopia.

BIBLIOGRAPHY

General

Buttner-Ennever JA. Anatomy of the ocular motor nuclei. In: Kennard C, Rose FC, eds. *Physiological Aspects of Clinical Neuro-Ophthalmology.* Chicago: Year Book, 1988.

Kerr FWL, Holowell OW. Location of pupillomotor and accommodation fibers in the oculomotor nerve: Experimental observations on paralytic mydriasis. *J Neurol Neurosurg Psychiatry.* 1964;27:473–481.

Leigh RJ, Zee DS. Peripheral ocular motor palsies and strabismus. In: *The Neurology of Eye Movements.* Philadelphia: Davis, 1983.

Rush JA, Younge BR. Paralysis of cranial nerves III, IV and VI. Cause and prognosis in 1,000 cases. *Arch Ophthalmol.* 1981;99:76–79.

Sachsenweger R. Clinical localization of oculomotor disturbance. In: Vinken PJ, Bruyn GW. *Handbook of Clinical Neurology.* Amsterdam: North Holland, 1969.

Warwick B. Representation of the extra-ocular muscles in the oculomotor nuclei of the monkey. *J Comp Neurol.* 1953;98:449–504.

Myasthenia Gravis and Lambert-Eaton Syndrome

Cogan DG. Myasthenia Gravis: A review of the disease and a description of lid twitch as a characteristic sign. *Arch Ophthalmol.* 1965;74:217.

Cruciger M, et al. Clinical and subclinical oculomotor findings in the Lambert-Eaton syndrome. *J Clin Neuroophthalmol.* 1983;3:18–22.

Drachman DB, ed. Myasthenia Gravis: Biology and clinical aspects. *Ann NY Acad Sci.* 1981;377.

Glaser JE, et al. The edrophonium tonogram test in myasthenia gravis. *Arch Ophthalmol.* 1966;76:368–373.

Grob D, ed. Myasthenia gravis: Pathology and management. *Ann NY Acad Sci.* 1981;377.

Hedges TR Jr. Ophthalmoplegia of myasthenia and bronchial neoplasm. *Arch Ophthalmol.* 1963;70:333–334.

McEvoy K, Windebank A, et al. 3,4-diaminopyridine in the treatment of Lambert-Eaton myasthenic syndrome. *N Engl J Med.* 1989;321:1567–1571.

Noda M et al. Cloning and sequence analysis of cells with DNA and human genomic DNA encoding alpha subunit precursor of muscle acetylcholine receptor. *Nature.* 1983;305:818–823.

Sher E, Gotti C, et al. Specificity of calcium channel autoantibodies in Lambert-Eaton myasthenic syndrome. *Lancet.* 1989;1:640–643.

Wray SH, Pavan-Langston D. A re-evaluation of edrophonium chloride (Tensilon) in myasthenia gravis. *Neurology.* 1971;21:586–593.

Ophthalmoplegia Plus

Berenberg PA, et al. Lumping or splitting? Ophthalmoplegia plus or Kearns-Sayre syndrome. *Ann Neurol.* 1977;1:37–54.

Third-Nerve Disorders

Asbury AK, Aldredge H, Hershberg R, et al. Oculomotor palsy in diabetes mellitus. A clinicopathological study. *Brain.* 1970;93:555–566.

Collard M, Saint-Val C, et al. Paralysie isolée du nerf moteur oculaire commun par infarctus de ses fibres fasciculaires. *Rev Neurol (Paris).* 1990;146:128–132.

Eyster EF, Hoyt WF, Wilson CB. Oculomotor palsy from minor head trauma. An initial sign of basal intracranial tumor. *JAMA.* 1972;220:1083.

Hopf HC, Gutmann L. Diabetic third nerve palsy: Evidence for a mesencephalic lesion. *Neurology.* 1990;40:1041–1045.

Lowenfeld IE, Thompson HS. Oculomotor paresis with cyclic spasms. A critical review of the literature and a new case. *Surv Ophthalmol.* 1975;20:81–124.

Schatz NJ, Savino PJ, Corbett JJ. Primary aberrant oculomotor regeneration—A sign of intracavernous meningioma. *Arch Neurol.* 1977;34:29–32.

Weber RB, Daroff RB, Mackey EA. Pathology of oculomotor nerve palsy in diabetics. *Neurology.* 1970;20:835–838.

Fourth Nerve Disorders

Hoyt WF, Keane JR. Superior oblique myokymia. *Arch Ophthalmol.* 1970;84:461–467.

Younge BR, Sutula F. Analysis of trochlear nerve palsies—Diagnosis, etiology and treatment. *Mayo Clin Proc.* 1977;52:11–66.

Sixth Nerve Disorders in Children

Knox DL, Clark DB, Schuster FF. Benign VI nerve palsies in children. *Pediatrics.* 1967;40:560–564.

CHAPTER 14

NYSTAGMUS AND OTHER OCULAR OSCILLATIONS

Nystagmus is a rhythmic biphasic oscillation of the eyes. Usually, both eyes move together (conjugately) and the two phases of nystagmus are equal in amplitude. In true nystagmus the initial deviation is a slow eye movement; the corrective or return phase may be fast (jerk nystagmus) or slow (pendular nystagmus). Commonly, however, the term "nystagmus" has been used to describe a multitude of ocular movements. These other types of eye movements (such as opsoclonus and convergence–retraction "nystagmus"), even if they are nystagmoid in appearance, are best classed as *other ocular oscillations* when they do not result from slow eye movement abnormalities. In fact, most of them are **fast** eye movements.

Nystagmus has many forms and many causes (Table 14–1). Some nystagmus is considered physiologic (end point nystagmus); some is the result of visual pathology (visual deprivation nystagmus) or associated with strabismus (latent nystagmus); some nystagmus may be disconjugate (abducting nystagmus in internuclear ophthalmoplegia) or dissociated (seesaw nystagmus). Nystagmus may be named by its gross appearance on examination (upbeat nystagmus), its presumed anatomical substrate (vestibular nystagmus), its general configuration (jerk nystagmus), analysis of eye-movement recordings (decreasing-velocity exponential nystagmus), the patient's age at onset (congenital nystagmus), or how it is elicited (positional nystagmus). All jerk nystagmus is named by the direction of the fast phase.

ANATOMICAL SUBSTRATES

Because all nystagmus and all ocular oscillations have eye movement in common, their analysis must rest upon a thorough knowledge of the underlying anatomic substrates and appropriate methods for their examination (see Chapters 10 and 13).

Supranuclear inputs to the oculomotor nuclei. Major central nervous system systems significant to the generation of nystagmus and related ocular oscillations converge upon the oculomotor nuclei. These systems include the visual afferent systems, eye movement subsystems, cerebellar pathways, vestibular apparatus, and proprioceptive inputs. Nystagmus results from an imbalance either within these inputs to the oculomotor system, between one input and another, or in the oculomotor output itself. If nystagmus has been noted during the examination of ocular motility, it should be described accurately. Is it conjugate? If not, is it disconjugate (involving one eye exclusively or significantly more than the other), or dissociated, (with each eye moving in a somewhat different direction)? Nystagmus is most frequently of the jerk variety, with both fast and slow components, but may also be pendular or rotary. The examiner should note the direction of slow and fast phases, any changes with different gaze or head positions, the amplitude of the nystagmus, and whether or not it is affected by vergence.

The easiest way to describe all this information is graphically (Fig. 14–1). If the nystagmus is of the jerk variety, the fast phase is indicated by a single arrow pointing in the direction of the fast phase. Pendular nystagmus can be indicated by arrows of equal magnitude pointing in different directions. If the amplitude is indicated by the length of the arrows, the frequency can be indicated by the number of "feathers."

As pointed out above, it is important to go

TABLE 14–1. CLASSIFICATION OF NYSTAGMUS

I. Jerk nystagmus
  A. Induced
    1. Optokinetic
    2. Vestibular
    3. Drug-induced
  B. Gaze evoked
    1. Physiologic end-point
    2. Common gaze evoked
    3. Gaze paretic
    4. Muscle paretic, myasthenia gravis
    5. Brun's nystagmus
    6. Internuclear ophthalmoplegia (INO)
    7. Rebound
  C. Primary position
    1. Downbeat
    2. Upbeat
    3. Periodic alternating (PAN)

II. Pendular nystagmus
  A. Convergence and convergence evoked
  B. Seesaw
  C. Circular/elliptic/oblique
  D. Dissociated

III. Nystagmus of infancy
  A. Motor imbalance nystagmus
    1. Congenital
    2. Nystagmus associated with strabismus
      a. manifest latent/latent
  B. Visual deprivation
  C. Spasmus nutans

IV. Other ocular oscillations (mostly abnormalities of fast eye movements)
  A. Convergence–retraction
  B. Ocular bobbing
  C. Ocular flutter, opsoclonus
  D. Ocular dysmetria
  E. Square wave jerks and macro square wave jerks
  F. Macro saccadic oscillations
  G. Ocular myoclonus
  H. Voluntary "nystagmus"
  I. Superior oblique myokymia

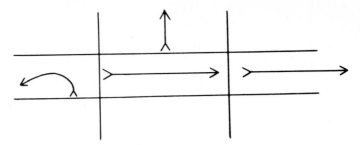

Figure 14–1. Nystagmus is observed and recorded in the five positions of gaze: primary, upward, down, left, and right. Direction of arrow indicates fast phase, curve of arrow indicates rotary nystagmus, length of arrow indicates amplitude or excursion of beat. (*From Gay AJ, Newman NM, Kiltner J. Eye Movement Disorders. St. Louis: Mosby, 1974, with permission.*)

coils). In order to accurately ascertain whether or not the movements are disconjugate, each eye must be recorded separately, allowing accurate measurement of velocity and precise characterization of wave forms. Thus, jerk nystagmus has been characterized by the form of the slow phase: linear, decreasing velocity exponential, or increasing velocity exponential. When eye movement recording is combined with careful examination of the eye movement subsystems, a more complete description of eye movement abnormalities, including nystagmus, is obtained. For example, upbeat nystagmus may be seen to result from defective pursuit, while the slow phase of vestibular nystagmus remains intact.

CLASSIFICATION OF NYSTAGMUS

Although the recent advances in eye movement physiology have produced a great deal of information about nystagmus, there is still not complete classification of nystagmus that satisfies both the needs of the clinician and the control system engineer. The classification used here (Table 14–1) is a pragmatic one. It is necessarily incomplete and only touches briefly on the mechanistic and control system attributes of nystagmus. (For those interested in pursuing those aspects further, the chapter bibliography provides a guide.)

Jerk Nystagmus

Most acquired forms of nystagmus have definite slow and fast phases; hence, the appellation *jerk nystagmus*. The slow phase is the abnormal deviation and the fast phase a corrective return. The nystagmus is named for the direction of the fast phase, which often beats in the direction of defective gaze and is increased in amplitude by attempts to gaze further in this direction.

through all the steps of eye movement analysis. For example, attempts at upward saccades may be the only manner in which the characteristic convergence-retraction "nystagmus" of Parinaud's syndrome can be elicited. On the other hand, a very fine congenital nystagmus may be masked if the patient is only examined with near targets as convergence may block or dampen nystagmus, especially nystagmus of congenital origin.

This chapter deals almost exclusively with nystagmus that can be observed in the office or at the bedside. Accurate evaluation of eye movements and abnormal eye movements, in particular, can be made only by quantitative oculography (EOG with DC recording, infrared goggles or magnetic scleral search

Induced Nystagmus

Optokinetic nystagmus. Optokinetic nystagmus (OKN) is elicited by repetitive visual stimuli moving through the visual field. To small targets, the slow phase is a pursuit movement with the eyes following the moving target. The fast phase is a saccadic movement in the opposite direction. Presumably, the slow phase is mediated by the pursuit pathways and the fast phase by the saccadic paths. Apart from lesions of these pathways and the brain-stem areas that act as the integrators and final common pathways for eye movements, deep parietal lesions cause a deficit in OKN when movement of the tape is toward the side of the lesion. Thus, with a left parietal lesion, movement of the tape from right to left will demonstrate a decreased optokinetic response. Any hemianopsia present is incidental, occurring only because the optic radiations are adjacent to the ocular motor paths in the parietal lobe. Thus, although homonymous hemianopsias are frequently present when the optokinetic response is defective, patients with complete hemianopsia may have normal OKN and patients without hemianopsia can have abnormal OKN. Conversely, when the optokinetic response is normal in the presence of a homonymous hemianopic defect, the lesion is rarely in the parietal lobe.

The optokinetic response overrides many voluntary eye movements and vestibular nystagmus. Thus, it can be used to estimate visual acuity in infants, as it is present within a few months of birth; it may be useful in establishing the presence of vision in patients who are hysteric or malingering. By varying the size of the targets presented, a rough estimate of visual acuity may be obtained. Because OKN tests both saccadic and pursuit systems, it is an extremely useful part of the examination of ocular motility.

In congenital nystagmus, OKN may be abnormal or absent.

Vestibular jerk nystagmus. Normally, both vestibular nuclei send balanced impulses to the gaze centers. The gaze centers send the impulses to the ipsilateral lateral rectus via the sixth-nerve nucleus and to the contralateral medial rectus through the medial longitudinal fasciculus and reticular formation. Any alteration in the inputs from the vestibular system—whether within the ear, the cerebellar pontine angle, or intramedullary portions of the pathway—will result in a jerk nystagmus with a slow phase to the side opposite the lesion. Thus, the vestibular system is often tested by caloric stimulation. Positional testing and the differentiation of central and peripheral vestibular nystagmus are discussed in Chapter 17 (see also Chapter 11).

Vestibular nystagmus may be induced by caloric stimulation or rotation, often has a rotary compo-

nent, and is accompanied by oscillopsia and vertigo.

Oscillopsia is a symptom and not a type of eye movement. It is the subjective illusion of bidirectional environmental movement. It occurs most frequently with disorders of the vestibular system, cerebellum, or brain-stem areas. *Vertigo* is the sensation of unidirectional movement of self or environment that occurs with nystagmus of large amplitude, usually with decreased vestibulo-ocular reflex (VOR) gain, causing slippage of the image over the retina (see Chapter 10). Since vision is suppressed during fast phases, the sensation of vertigo is due to the experience of environmental motion during the slow phase of nystagmus, with the environment appearing to move in the direction opposite to the slow phase. Vertigo indicates vestibular dysfunction and is more persistent and more pronounced in end-organ than in central disorders.

Drug-induced nystagmus. The most common etiology of nystagmus seen in clinical practice is drug intake. The most common drugs producing nystagmus are alcohol, phenytoin, barbiturates, or other central nervous system depressants. Many illicit drugs cause nystagmus.

This nystagmus is usually a horizontal jerk gaze-evoked nystagmus. It may be associated with vertical upgaze nystagmus or, rarely, downgaze nystagmus. With increasing intoxication, especially with barbiturates, there is a degeneration of slow smooth pursuit movements, resulting in saccadic pursuit (cogwheeling).

Even higher levels of intoxication with barbiturates or phenytoin will eliminate saccadic eye movements so that patients in a light barbiturate coma will show only tonic conjugate responses to caloric irrigation. More profound intoxication will cause an absence of caloric responses. Thus, a patient with absent caloric responses and an intact pupillary light reflex probably is in metabolic coma related to barbiturate overdose.

Additionally, in any given patient, one can roughly quantitate the degree of Dilantin toxicity with the degree of nystagmus.

Gaze-evoked Nystagmus

The most common form of nystagmus seen clinically is gaze-evoked nystagmus; it is a jerk nystagmus not present in primary position, which occurs when the patient attempts to maintain an eccentric position of gaze.

Unsustained End-point Nystagmus. This is the most frequently encountered gaze-evoked nystagmus. It is of fine amplitude and intermediate frequency, although the rhythm and amplitude may be variable. The fast phase of end-point nystagmus is in the direction of gaze. Not infrequently, horizontal end-point nystagmus may be dissociated, usually with the larger amplitude nystagmus in the abducting eye. Usually, it is a physiologic nystagmus and diminishes in fixation at distance.

Where there is uncertainty whether nystagmus is physiologic or gaze paretic (see below), eye movement recording can be used to differentiate between the linear slow phases of physiologic nystagmus and the descending velocity slow phase of gaze paretic nystagmus.

Common gaze-evoked nystagmus. Gaze-evoked nystagmus that is not induced by drugs usually occurs in the presence of brain-stem or cerebellar pathway dysfunction. This nystagmus is fairly rapid and increases in amplitude with increasing eccentricity of gaze. Frequently, when there is bilateral horizontal gaze-evoked nystagmus there is also an associated gaze-evoked nystagmus on upgaze, but rarely a downbeating nystagmus on downgaze.

Gaze paretic nystagmus. Patients who have lesions in the ocular motor areas of the hemispheres or brain stem show a gaze paretic nystagmus when the deficit is subtotal. These patients seem unable to hold gaze, resulting in the eyes drifting slowly back towards primary position, the nystagmus occurring when a corrective saccade returns the eye to the eccentric position of gaze. This nystagmus is a relatively low-frequency nystagmus with a decreasing velocity slow phase, postulated to be due to a leaky neural integrator and inappropriate step.

Muscle paretic nystagmus. A special type of paretic nystagmus occurs when a muscle is paretic whether on a neurogenic basis, because of muscular contraction associated with long-standing strabismus or thyroid orbitopathy or as a result of eye muscle surgery or orbital trauma. In this case the nystagmus occurs when the eye with the paretic muscle moves into that muscle's field of action. When medial rectus muscles are paretic, muscle paretic nystagmus in the yoke lateral rectus may mimic an intranuclear ophthalmoplegia (see below). This may occur following large medial rectus recessions, with medial blowout fractures entrapping the medial rectus or with medial rectus involvement in thyroid ophthalmopathy. This same type of nystagmus also occurs with myasthenia gravis. Thus, it is important to elicit a complete history from your patient, including history of orbital injury or previous strabismus surgery. Patients having a muscle paretic type of nystagmus, no other evidence of central nervous system disease, and no history of strabismus or orbital trauma or other orbital disease should have a Tensilon test.

Brun's nystagmus. Brun's nystagmus is a combination of gaze paretic nystagmus and vestibular nystagmus that is characteristic of cerebellopontine angle tumors. It is a horizontal jerk nystagmus with large-amplitude gaze paretic nystagmus when gaze is directed toward the side of the lesion. When gaze is directed to the side opposite the lesion, there is a small-amplitude vestibular nystagmus. With eyes closed, the nystagmus beats in the direction opposite the side of the lesion. Brun's nystagmus occurs when the cerebellar pontine angle lesion is large enough to cause both a vestibular lesion and brainstem compression.

Internuclear ophthalmoplegia (INO). Lesions of the medial longitudinal fasciculus between the third- and sixth nerve nuclei produce internuclear ophthalmoplegia (INO). This is an apparent medial rectus paresis ipsilateral to the lesion associated with nystagmus of the abducting eye on lateral gaze to the side opposite the lesion (ocular motor purists do not consider the abducting saccades true nystagmus because the slow phases are normal). In the most common type of internuclear ophthalmoplegia there is normal medial rectus activity on convergence. In an anterior internuclear ophthalmoplegia (presumably due to rostral lesions involving the third-nerve nucleus or its fibers), convergence may be absent. Skew deviation (with the ipsilateral eye higher) is common in unilateral INO. Bilateral INO frequently is associated with impaired upgaze and upbeating nystagmus.

The medial longitudinal fasciculus syndrome is a typical supranuclear disorder since the "paretic" medial rectus is able to produce normal convergence and there is no diplopia or exotropia in primary position.

When the internuclear ophthalmoplegia is subtle or even subclinical, the abducting nystagmus may be elicited or magnified by asking the patient to converge (asymmetric convergence) on a target brought toward the abducting eye, or stimulating or producing repetitive fast phases in the direction of the abducting nystagmus with either optokinetic or caloric stimulation.

The medial longitudinal fasciculus syndrome is characteristic of a pontine lesion and is frequently seen in multiple sclerosis in younger patients or ischemic lesions in elderly patients.

Rebound nystagmus. Rebound nystagmus is a horizontal jerk nystagmus that appears to fatigue and then change direction when lateral gaze is sustained or with refixation to primary position. It is a manifestation of cerebellar pathway disease and is similar to periodic alternating nystagmus as it changes direction (see below).

After sustained lateral gaze, when the eyes return to primary position the fast phase reverses direction. For example, jerk nystagmus with fast phases to the right on right gaze, becomes jerk nystagmus with fast phases left when gaze returns to primary position.

Primary Position Nystagmus.

Downbeat nystagmus is a vertical jerk nystagmus of large excursion and low frequency; downbeat nystagmus is present in primary position and thus differs from gaze-evoked downbeat nystagmus, which occurs only with gaze away from primary position. It has a slow phase that beats upward and fast corrective phases in the downward direction. It is usually associated with structural lesions in the region of foramen magnum such as the Chiari-I malformation, with cerebellar lesions and degenerations. It has also been reported in numerous other disorders including multiple sclerosis (MS), syringomyelia, brainstem infarction and encephalitis, Wernicke's syndrome, hydrocephalus, and magnesium and thiamine deficiency; as a toxic response to alcohol, phentoin, carbamazepine, and lithium; and as a congenital eye movement disorder. Contrary to gaze-evoked nystagmus, the nystagmus is not maximum in the extreme position of gaze. In fact, downbeat nystagmus is frequently of greater amplitude when the eyes are positioned laterally and slightly downward.

Upbeat nystagmus: Upbeat nystagmus, again, as differentiated from gaze-evoked upbeat nystagmus, is a vertical nystagmus present in primary position with the fast phases upward. One form of upbeat nystagmus is of large amplitude increasing in intensity with increased upward gaze. Another type is of smaller amplitude and decreases in intensity with increased upward gaze. Both types of upbeat nystagmus are usually seen with pontomedullary lesions, disorders of the cerebellar pathways, or Wernicke's encephalopathy. In infants, upbeat nystagmus may be associated with retinal disease and not brain-stem pathology.

Periodic alternating nystagmus: This dramatic nystagmus is a spontaneous horizontal jerk nystagmus that periodically changes direction. Typically the nystagmus will beat in one direction for 60 to 90 seconds, begin to slow down and decrease in amplitude, reach a neutral phase in which no nystagmus may be detected or in which there are only small apparently pendular oscillations, and then begin to beat in the opposite direction for a similar period of time. Periodic alternating nystagmus has many etiologies, but is frequently associated with lesions in the region of the foramen magnum or vestibulocerebellar pathway. Because at any given moment it may appear to be a rather ordinary jerk or pendular nystagmus, the alternating pendular nature will be-

come evident only if the eyes are observed over a period of several minutes. Sometimes, noting the patient alternately turn the head to minimize the nystagmus suggests this disorder. Its presence is suggested when each notation in the patient's chart seems to describe a different nystagmus!

Pendular Nystagmus

Convergence and convergence-evoked nystagmus: Convergence nystagmus is a disconjugate, acquired convergent nystagmus. Sometimes it is present spontaneously and other times it is evoked by convergence efforts.

Convergence-evoked nystagmus is evoked when an effort is made to converge. Both congenital and acquired cases have been reported to cause or modify most other types of nystagmus.

Seesaw nystagmus: Seesaw nystagmus is a dramatic disconjugate nystagmus. One eye rises and intorts, while the opposite eye falls and extorts. It is usually associated with disorders of the diencephalon/rostral mesencephalon, thalamus, or both, and many cases occur when chiasmal lesions produce a bitemporal hemianopia. Congenital cases have also been reported. Lesions of the interstitial nucleus of Cajal are implicated.

Circular/elliptic/oblique nystagmus: These forms of pendular nystagmus are also very dramatic in appearance because the globes move around the orbit in a path caused by simultaneous horizontal and vertical pendular nystagmus. When the oscillations are out of phase, the eyeball appears to roam around the orbit. Oblique nystagmus may also have a jerk component. All of these types of nystagmus may be disconjugate and either congenital or acquired. They occur in diffuse neurologic disease, MS, Pelizaeus Merzbacher disease, large brain-stem infarcts, and profound visual loss. In fact, the combination of elliptical pendular and upbeat nystagmus may be characteristic of Pelizaeus Merzbacher disease.

Dissociated nystagmus: Dissociated nystagmus refers to nystagmus with each eye moving differently.

Nystagmus of Infancy

These types of nystagmus usually begin at birth (congenital nystagmus) or in the first year of life.

Obviously, all types of nystagmus discussed above may occur in infants as well as adults with lesions of the same underlying pathways. The types of nystagmus described below are those that do not appear to be related to known disease processes affecting the oculomotor system or its supranuclear inputs.

Motor Imbalance Nystagmus

Congenital nystagmus. Congenital nystagmus is a binocular and conjugate nystagmus present at birth or very soon thereafter. It is noted in the first few weeks of life and may be hereditary. Several different patterns of congenital nystagmus waveform have been described. Perhaps the most common kinds are a nystagmus that tends to be relatively small amplitude and pendular near primary gaze and nystagmus with a null point with jerk nystagmus of increasing amplitude developing with gaze away from these points. The null point (a point of minimum eye movement) is characteristic of congenital nystagmus, as is a lack of response to optokinetic stimulation or "inverted" OKN response. Congenital nystagmus is usually horizontal, and remains horizontal in upgaze. This characteristic distinguishes congenital nystagmus from acquired horizontal nystagmus, which is associated with vertical nystagmus on upgaze.

As mentioned, convergence may dampen several forms of nystagmus, especially congenital nystagmus. This partially explains why the patient with congenital nystagmus has poor distance visual acuity when the eyes are moving substantially, but perfectly normal visual acuity at near when convergence is brought into play. In fact, patients with congenital nystagmus are often found to read at a very close distance in order to make best use of this effect.

On the other hand, efforts to fixate accurately frequently increase the severity of the nystagmus.

With congenital nystagmus, there may be an associated head nodding or "head nystagmus," which is the result of the same disordered motor outflow and not a compensatory head movement as has been thought previously.

The hereditary congenital nystagmus may be X-linked, recessive or dominant, as well as occurring sporadically. In about 50% of patients spontaneous improvement occurs as the patient grows older.

It is not unusual for the families of patients and even the patients themselves to be entirely unaware of the presence of the nystagmus. Thus, these patients at times are admitted to neurosurgical services for evaluation of presumed brain-stem disease. Awareness of the characteristics of congenital nystagmus will prevent this in most cases. In cases that remain doubtful, eye movement recordings may be helpful in clearly identifying several of the distinct waveforms typical of congenital nystagmus and rarely found in any other kind of nystagmus.

These patients may adopt a head turn in order to keep their eyes near the null point and thus maximize visual acuity. When the head turn is excessive, or the nystagmus seems to significantly interfere with the child's development, treatment may be considered. Phenobarbital and other medications that appear to work by their effect on the reticular formation can occasionally have a dramatic effect. Prisms may displace the null point, or surgery may place the eyes in a position that changes the null point to minimize the head turn.

Nystagmus associated with strabismus. *Manifest latent/Latent nystagmus:* Latent nystagmus is a congenital nystagmus that appears or is made more apparent when one eye is covered. The eyes move conjugately with the fast phase directed toward the uncovered or fixing eye. Strabismus (usually esotropia) is present in 95% of patients with latent nystagmus, and conversely about 20% of patients with strabismus will have latent nystagmus. Dissociated vertical deviation commonly is seen in a triad with esotropia and latent nystagmus. This nystagmus may be hereditary, but the mode of inheritance is unclear. Latent nystagmus may also be a component of a congenital nystagmus. Conversely, patients with latent nystagmus and strabismus may be thought to have congenital nystagmus because the latent nystagmus is made manifest by the monocular viewing associated with strabismus (ie, manifest latent).

It is important when testing visual acuity in these patients that the nonfixing eye is not covered, thus inducing the nystagmus in the fixing eye and decreasing its visual acuity. The nonfixing eye may be blurred with plus lenses or a pencil held in front of fixation.

Visual deprivation nystagmus. This type of nystagmus is associated with loss of central vision. It is unknown whether visual deprivation and congenital nystagmus are associated or whether the visual loss is causative. In a study by Gelbart and Hoyt of 152 infants with congenital nystagmus from a university pediatric ophthalmology practice, 119 had "sensory nystagmus" and 13 "pure motor nystagmus." Frequently this type of nystagmus is indistinguishable from congenital nystagmus in appearance, being pendular in the primary position and becoming a jerk nystagmus on gaze to either side. With acquired visual loss, nystagmus can be circular or elliptical. The nystagmus seems to vary proportionately with the degree of visual loss, such that with profound visual loss the oscillations can be so irregular that the eyes appear to drift aimlessly.

This nystagmus appears at 3 to 4 months of age, even if the visual deficit is congenital, distinguishing it from congenital motor nystagmus, which may be present at birth (but rarely noted then). The abnormal eye movements may be the first indication that a baby cannot see. Visual loss later in life rarely results in similar eye movements. As with congenital nystagmus, head oscillations are frequently present.

When the nystagmus is the result of congenital blindness or severe visual loss, the eye movements are often wandering in character, slow, and large in amplitude. Causes of visual deprivation nystagmus include optic nerve hypoplasia, Leber's congenital amaurosis, congenital cone dystrophy, congenital optic atrophy, ocular albinism, and achromatopsia (total color blindness). Miner's nystagmus, described almost exclusively in Great Britain, has been related to lack of light in the coal mines. In the few recent cases, suspicion exists that some cases of miner's nystagmus may really be voluntary "nystagmus" (see below) or a congenital nystagmus reported for reasons of secondary gain.

Spasmus nutans is a generally self-limited syndrome of infancy. It usually develops between the sixth and twelfth months of life and disappears spontaneously by the third or fourth year. It is a clinical triad: head nodding (87%), nystagmus (80%), and head turning (38%). The nystagmus is frequently monocular or predominantly monocular and may be pendular, jerk, rotary, horizontal, or vertical. It is a very fine and rapid nystagmus (3 to 10 Hz). The etiology is unclear. It may be unassociated with any recognizable central nervous system deficit or with nonspecific cerebral deficits. A recent note by Bray suggests an association with the fetal alcohol syndrome.

A similar nystagmus occurs (without the other triad features) in infants with optochiasmatic gliomas and one case has been reported in Leigh's disease. Optic atrophy is often present in those patients with gliomas and spasmus-nutans-like eye movements. Thus, do careful ophthalmoscopy in all patients thought to have spasmus nutans, especially if the nystagmus develops before 6 months of age.

Other Ocular Oscillations

Nearly all of the following oscillations are fast eye movement abnormalities.

Convergence–retraction "nystagmus". Convergence–retraction "nystagmus" is a frequent component of the dorsal midbrain syndrome (Parinaud's syndrome, sylvian aqueduct syndrome, Koerber-Salus-Elschnig syndrome). Attempted upgaze, especially at fast, upward movements, results in jerky bilateral eye movements of retraction, convergence, or both. The movement that predominates depends on which ocular muscles are maximally innervated. Co-contraction of normally antagonistic extraocular muscles causes retraction of the globe. These are saccadic movements and thus are not a true nystagmus in the limited definition adopted here.

Clinically, this dramatic eye movement is seen with compression of the upper midbrain by pineal-

omas, vascular accidents, neoplasia, infection, or demyelination in the pretectal area. In youngsters, obstructed shunts cause the dorsal midbrain syndrome before other signs of decompensation or papilledema develop. Thus, any child shunted for hydrocephalus should be observed carefully for this phenomenon.

Ocular bobbing. Massive lesions of the pons may be associated with a distinctive ocular motor phenomenon, ocular bobbing, rapid downward movements of the eyes with a very slow return to primary position. Generally conjugate, the movements may be disconjugate or even uniocular. Other oculomotor function may be present, but commonly bobbing represents the only possible ocular motor response to attempts at voluntary gaze, doll's-head maneuver, or caloric stimulation. Because bobbing is associated with massive destruction of the pontine tegmentum, it usually has a poor prognosis.

Ocular flutter, opsoclonus. These ocular movements are a saccadic decompensation of eye movements. Ocular flutter is a series of small saccades with a normal intersaccadic interval and occurring with efforts at fixation. Opsoclonus (saccadomania) is chaotic, repetitive saccadic movements in all directions, preventing fixation. These movements are back-to-back saccades without the normal intersaccadic interval. Opsoclonus has also been termed "dancing eyes" and "lightning eye movements." Some success in suppressing any associated oscillopsia has been reported with baclofen, haloperidol, and amitryptyline therapy.

In an adult or an older child, opsoclonus is commonly associated with a postinfectious encephalopathy and accompanied by ataxia and other cerebellar signs. Prognosis is excellent. In younger children, opsoclonus has been described in association with neuroblastoma. It often ceases after removal of the tumor or is a sign of regressing tumor. Thus, any young child with opsoclonus should be evaluated for neuroblastoma. Opsoclonus has also been described as a remote effect of tumor in adults, most frequently with carcinomas of the breast or lung, sometimes associated with histopathologic changes in the dentate nucleus.

Ocular dysmetria. Ocular dysmetria is a loss of control of saccadic accuracy, a calibration problem with saccades that overshoot and undershoot. Commonly in the vestibulo-cerebellar pathway, pathology causes a mismatch in the pulse and step.

Square wave jerks and macro square wave jerks. These are pairs of saccades that cause deviation from fixation, and after a short latency, a return to fixation. They are involuntary and their name derives from the characteristic appearance on eye movement tracings. Square wave jerks are of small amplitude (a few degrees) and occur normally as well with cerebellar disease. Macro square wave jerks are almost always pathologic and more frequently occur in bursts.

Macro-saccadic oscillations. Macro-saccadic oscillations are bursts of to-and-fro saccades similar to those seen in square wave jerks in that they have normal intersaccadic latencies. However, macro-saccadic oscillations differ from macro square wave jerks because their amplitudes gradually increase and then decrease and because they straddle fixation, rather than consisting of movements away from and back toward fixation. Like macro square wave jerks, they are frequently associated with cerebellar pathway disease.

Ocular myoclonus (ocular myorythmia). Ocular myoclonus is possibly a true nystagmus with a continuous, rhythmic oscillation, frequently vertical and frequently dissociated. It can only be termed myoclonus when it is associated with similar movements of the brachial musculature, most frequently the palate, but also (in order of descending frequency) the pharynx, larynx, face, mouth, eyes, tongue, diaphragm, extremities, and intercostal muscles. The frequency is quite rapid, varying from 200 to 400 beats per minute. Thus, in any patient who is suspected of having an acquired pendular nystagmus, particularly if it is rapid and dissociated, myoclonic movements of the palate and other brachial musculature should be sought for. Myoclonic movements occur with lesions of the myoclonic triangle (the Guillain-Mollaret triangle: the red nucleus, the ipsilateral inferior olive, and the contralateral dentate nucleus) and are associated with pseudohypertrophy of the inferior olive. It is interesting that the myoclonus may not have its onset until several months after the insult that caused the damage.

Voluntary "nystagmus". Voluntary nystagmus is a series of rapid, low-amplitude saccadic, convergent movements that are back to back and brought on at will. They are of high frequency, of approximately 90 to 400 beats a minute. Because of the effort necessary, they can be sustained for only a few seconds. The oscillations are almost always horizontal.

Superior oblique myokymia. A uniocular, torsional, high-frequency microtremor that evokes oscillopsia, superior oblique myokymia occurs spontaneously in otherwise healthy individuals. At times, the movement is difficult to observe; it is best seen by noting torsional movements of small perilimbal vessels, use of the slit-lamp, or ophthalmoscopic magnification.

The tremor may be self-limiting, but when persistent and troublesome, frequently responds to Tegretol. Superior oblique tenotomy is sometimes curative.

TABLE 14–2. NYSTAGMUS AND EYE MOVEMENTS WITH LOCALIZING VALUE

Type of Eye Movement	Location
Seesaw nystagmus	Posterior diencephalon/pretectum (interstitial nucleus of Cajal)
Convergence–retraction "nystagmus"	Dorsal midbrain
Abducting nystagmus in internuclear ophthalmoplegia	Pons (medial longitudinal fasciculus)
Brun's nystagmus	Cerebellopontine angle
Vestibular nystagmus	Pontomedullary junction and vestibular paths
Ocular bobbing	Central pons
Ocular myoclonus	Myoclonic triangle
Upbeat nystagmus	Medulla, central tegmentum of pons, cerebellar pathways
Contralateral nystagmus, lateropulsion of saccades	Dorsolateral medulla (Wallenberg's syndrome)
Downbeat nystagmus	Foramen magnum and cerebellum
Periodic alternating nystagmus (PAN)	Foramen magnum and cerebellum
Rebound nystagmus	Cerebellar pathways, brain stem
Ocular flutter, dysmetria	Cerebellar pathways, brain stem
Opsoclonus	Cerebellar pathways, brain stem
Square wave jerks, microsaccadic oscillations	Cerebellar pathways, brain stem
Square wave jerks, macrosaccadic oscillations	Cerebellar pathways, brain stem

Some of the eye movements described above are typically associated with lesions in specific areas or in specific pathways within the central nervous system. These correlations are listed in Table 14–2.

TREATMENT OF NYSTAGMUS

Most nystagmus is difficult to treat. In general, first address any amenable underlying process. Those forms of nystagmus, mostly congenital, that have a constant null point may be helped by prisms or surgical procedures that realign the eyes so that the null point comes closer to primary position and sometimes becomes larger so the eyes are stable for a larger percentage of time. Biofeedback has also been reported to be helpful in congenital nystagmus. Prisms induce vergence movements, which will dampen some types of horizontal and downbeat nystagmus. In addition, downbeat nystagmus associated with the Arnold-Chiari malformation often responds to cervical decompression.

TABLE 14–3. DRUG TREATMENT OF NYSTAGMUS

Type of Nystagmus	Drug Reported to Help
Periodic alternating	Baclofen
Seesaw	Baclofen
	Baclofen plus clonazepam
	ETOH
	Carisoprodol
Downbeat congenital	Clonazepam
	Baclofen
	5-Hydroxy-tryptophan
	Barbiturates
	Scopolamine
Vestibular	Innovar
	Scopolamine
	Promethazine
Elliptical	Isoniazid
Opsoclonus	
Infections	ACTH, corticosteroids
Paraneoplastic	High-dose thiamine
Multiple carboxylase deficiency	Biotin
Miscellaneous	Propanolol
Ocular myoclonus	Clonazepam
Myasthenic	Prostigmin and similar agents
Oculopalatal myoclonus	Scopolamine
	Tegretol
	5-hydroxy-tryptophan and carbidopa
Nystagmus in Wernicke's syndrome, Leigh's disease	High-dose thiamine
	Magnesium, zinc
Superior oblique myokymia	Tegretol

Modified from Carlow T. Medical treatment of nystagmus and ocular motor disorders. In: International Ophthalmology Clinics. Boston: Little, Brown, 1986.

Medical treatment is occasionally helpful. Some drugs are used expectantly and others based on neurotransmitters known to function in the ocular motor system. Specific excitatory transmitters include glutamate and aspartate and specific inhibitory neurotransmitters include gamma-aminobutyric acide (GABA), glycine, and acetylcholine. Two of the most effective drugs probably act to alter the activity of these neurotransmitters. Clonazepam is a gabanergic augmenter and baclofen, a glutamate inhibitor. Other drugs known to act on brain-stem transmission include barbiturates and scopolamine (Table 14–3).

Optical retinal image stabilization using a high plus spectacle lens and minus contact lens may improve visual function in some patients with nystagmus and good vision.

BIBLIOGRAPHY

Bray PF. Can maternal alcoholism cause spasmus nutans in offspring? *N Engl J Med.* 1990;322:554. Letter.

Carlow T. Medical treatment of nystagmus and ocular motor disorders. In: Carlow, T, ed. *International Ophthalmology Clinics.* Boston: Little, Brown, 1986.

Daroff RB, Troost BT. Nystagmus and related ocular oscillations. In: Duane TD, ed. *Clinical Ophthalmology.* Hagerstown, MD: Harper & Row, 1982;2.

Dell'Osso LF. Nystagmus and other ocular motor oscillations. In: Lessel S, van Dalen JTW. *Neuroophthalmology.* Amsterdam: Excerpta Medica, 1980;1.

Dell'Osso LF. Nystagmus and other ocular motor oscillations. In: Lessel S, van Dalen JTW. *Neuroophthalmology.* Amsterdam: Excerpta Medica, 1982;2.

Dell'Osso LF. Nystagmus and other ocular motor oscillations. In: Lessel S, van Dalen JTW. *Neuroophthalmology.* Amsterdam: Excerpta Medica, 1989;3.

Gelbart SS, Hoyt CJ. Congenital nystagmus: A clinical perspective in infancy. In: Smith JL, Katz R. *Neuroophthalmology Enters the 90s.* Florida: Dutton, 1988.

Miller N, ed. Disorders of ocular motor system. *Walsh and Hoyt's Clinical Neuro-ophthalmology.* 4th ed. Baltimore, MD: Williams & Wilkins, 1985;3.

Rushton D, Cox N. A new optical treatment for oscillopsia. *J Neurol Neurosurg Physiol.* 1987;50:411.

Traccis S, Rosati G, et al. Successful treatment of acquired pendular elliptical nystagmus in multiple sclerosis with isoniazid and base-out prisms. *Neurology.* 1990;40:492–494.

CHAPTER 15
STRABISMUS

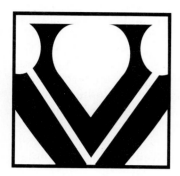

Normally, the eyes are aligned, directing the visual axes and foveas to the same point in space. Misalignment of the visual axes is called **strabismus** (or squint). Strabismus may be

1. Comitant (the more typical strabismus, usually of childhood onset). The deviation is stable in nonextreme directions of gaze.
2. Incomitant (the deviation varies in different gaze positions), related to either cranial nerve palsies (paralytic) or mechanical limitation of eye movement (restrictive). The deviation varies in different gaze positions.

Fusional mechanisms work continually to maintain alignment of the eyes, frequently compensating for small squints.

When strabismus exists, it is named by the direction of deviation: if the eyes turn in, *eso*deviation; if the eyes turn out, *exo*deviation; if one eye is up, *hyper*deviation; if one eye is down, there is a *hypo*deviation; if one is torted, a *cyclo*deviation.

Most normal eye movements are conjugate; the eyes move in parallel. When the visual axes of the two eyes point in different directions, each eye views a separate target, producing diplopia, except with suppression. Consequently, diplopia may not be present in comitant strabismus with suppression, whereas diplopia is a major symptom of acute paralytic and mechanical strabismus or decompensated comitant strabismus. In children, suppression occurs rapidly and may prevent the complaint of diplopia. Rarely, monocular diplopia (Table 15–1) occurs as a result of aberrations in the ocular media or, more rarely, central nervous system (CNS) lesions (especially right parietal lesions). Strabismic (binocular) diplopia can be differentiated from monocular diplopia simply by covering one eye. If the diplopia is no longer present, it is binocular in origin. In monocular diplopia due to media abberations one image often is brighter than the other and the diplopia is usually eliminated by viewing through a pinhole.

Comitant strabismus is usually of infantile or childhood onset, although sometimes a decompensated phoria (see below) will present later. If the measured fusional reserves are large, the deviation is nearly always of childhood origin. In young children (less than 6 years old) with a constant or very frequent deviation, the deviating eye is "suppressed," so the second image is not seen. With time, amblyopia may result. In adults, diplopia is the rule.

When constant (or present with both eyes uncovered), a strabismus is termed *tropia* (manifest deviation). If the tendency for the eyes to deviate is usually controlled by fusion, the brain's facility to maintain alignment of the eyes (eg, present only when one eye is covered to break fusion), the strabismus is called a *phoria* (latent deviation).

When an adult notes sudden diplopia, it is critical to differentiate between comitant strabismus and neurogenic strabismus. In adults with a decompensated phoria, there may be a long history of intermittent diplopia. A phoria may decompensate to a tropia with a decrease in consciousness (fatigue, sedatives, CNS depression); trauma (even minor); the onset of a new neurogenic paresis; illness or stress.

When present, history of such intermittent diplopia helps to differentiate comitant strabismus from paralytic strabismus. The limited motility in paralytic squint is an important differentiating sign. Acute comitant strabismus shows minimal or no limitation of eye movement, although muscle contraction may lead to restriction later on; paralytic strabismus always results in a motility deficit. However, caution is advised in interpretation of the history; old comitant horizontal strabismus frequently decompensates with addition of a neuro-

TABLE 15–1. CAUSES OF MONOCULAR DIPLOPIA

Location	Cause
Cornea	Oil droplet in precorneal tear film
	Epithelial irregularity
	Corneal dystrophy
	Corneal astigmatism
	Keratoconus
Iris	Polycoria
	Iridodialysis
Lens	Subluxation, decentered intraocular lens
	Multi-refractile cataract
Aqueous Humor/Vitreous Body	Foreign body (eg, air bubbles, glass, parasites)
Retina	Giant retinal tear with folded over retina
	Macular cyst
	Subretinal choroidal neovascular membrane
Neurologic	Occipital lobe lesions
	Dissociative lesions between frontal eye fields and occipital associative areas
	Tonic conjugate gaze deviation
	Anomalous retinal correspondence
	Superior oblique myokymia?
	Palinopsia

Modified from LePore FE, Yarian DL. Monocular diplopia of retinal origin. J Clin Neuro-ophthalmol. 1986;6:181–183.

genic vertical strabismus. When the new vertical paralysis is minor relative to the old horizontal deviation, it may be overlooked. In addition, any strabismus that varies in extent and over time, especially if worse later in the day or with fatigue or exercise, suggests myasthenia gravis.

Usually the term strabismus or squint refers to comitant strabismus. Reference to a paralytic strabismus or restrictive strabismus is by the appropriate causative agent and a description of the motility limitation—for example, a third nerve palsy with exotropia and hypertropia; or a blow-out fracture with a left hypertropia.

TYPES OF DEVIATION

Esotropia. The most common kind of esotropia, "infantile" esotropia, usually develops prior to 6 months of age. It is usually a large esotropia (more than 30 prism diopters), which worsens as a child grows older. Frequently the eyes turn in so far that the infant adapts a pattern of cross fixation (the right eye is used for looking to the left and the left eye is used for looking to the right). This "cross fixation" may be mistaken for a bilateral sixth nerve palsy, which is ruled out if the infant makes normally rapid abducting saccades or exhibits a full range of lateral eye movement. If the child doesn't follow laterally voluntarily, use an optokinetic stimulus or spin the child to elicit eye movements. If there is still a question about normal abduction, patch one eye for several minutes to hours. Usually, the other eye will begin to move normally unless there is a true sixth nerve palsy. Because the eyes are turned so far, contraction of the medial rectus often occurs and abducting saccades may be slowed. Overacting oblique muscles, dissociated vertical deviation (DVD), and latent or manifest–latent nystagmus frequently are associated with infantile esotropia. In older children, spasm of the near reflex must be ruled out. Usually the accompanying miosis gives this disorder away (see Chapters 10 and 20 for more details).

Treatment of congenital esotropia. The treatment of congenital esotropia usually is surgical, although oculinum treatment also is used (see below). Controversy persists as to the optimal age to perform the surgery. Some believe that the earlier the surgery is performed and the eyes aligned, the better chance to develop normal or more normal binocular behavior. However, a good binocular result is rare and many experts believe that operation at a later age allows more accurate evaluation of the patient, more accurate surgery, and a better end result.

A child with congenital esotropia rarely develops totally normal binocular vision. Thus, the goal for treatment is to maintain good vision in both eyes (obviate the possibility of amblyopia) and obtain stable alignment with good cosmetic appearance. Because the best results are obtained if both eyes have good vision, any amblyopia should be treated prior to surgery. Prevention of amblyopia must be continued after surgery.

Accommodative esotropia. Accommodative esotropia has a later onset, at an average of about 2 years, but may start earlier. About half the infants with congenital esotropia will develop an accommodative component. Children with pure accommodative esotropia usually have a hyperopic refractive error and a variable esotropia, depending on the degree of accommodation being utilized at a given moment. There is frequently a family history. When the child can cooperate for evaluation of the accommodative convergence/accommodation (AC/A) ratio, a high AC/A is found.

Many of these children are treated effectively by eliminating the accommodative effort that leads to the esotropia. This may be done by correcting their hyperopia, using bifocals to prevent excess convergence at near, miotic therapy to decrease the amount of convergence with near effort, or both.

With time, congenital and accommodative esotropias may both show overaction of the obliques causing "A&V" syndromes (syndromes in which the deviation is different in upgaze as opposed to downgaze). Latent nystagmus and other aberrations such as dissociated vertical deviation may be present.

Rare occurrences must all be considered and ruled out. These include Möbius and esotropic Duane's syndromes (see Chapter 13); missing and fibrotic muscles; cyclic esotropia (a rare periodic esotropia with a 24- to 48-hour periodicity, onset in early childhood, and poorly understood etiology); and migrainous ophthalmoplegia with esotropia.

Exotropia. After esotropia, this is the next most frequent type of comitant strabismus. An exophoria exists if the deviation is completely contr~lled by fusion. An intermittent exotropia occurs when the deviation can be intermittently controlled; however, if the deviation is constant, an exotropia exists. Comitant exotropia frequently starts out as an intermittent exotropia of childhood and often becomes progressive with time. These children frequently close one eye in bright light. Diplopia and amblyopia are rare.

Special types of exotropia include convergence insufficiency, where the deviation is greater at near than at distance and a low AC/A is present. Divergence excess is the reverse, where the deviation is greater at distance with a high AC/A.

Treatment. Asymptomatic patients need no treatment. In those who deviate a small percentage of the time, prisms or stimulation of convergence by excess minus lens correction may be helpful. If there is a significant symptomatic or cosmetic problem, the surgery for exodeviations is extremely successful.

Vertical deviations. Isolated comitant vertical deviations unassociated with horizontal deviations are relatively rare. The majority of vertical squints are restrictive and acquired. Thus, if you initially suspect a comitant vertical deviation, look carefully for superior oblique palsies and vertical rectus palsies (especially after trauma and blowout fractures), myasthenia, thyroid orbitopathy, or neurogenic pareses. Small deviations can be treated with prisms. Larger deviations necessitate surgery.

A special type of vertical deviation is the *dissociated vertical deviation (DVD)* frequently associated with infantile esotropias. DVD is usually bilateral and often symmetrical. Under occlusion or with inattention, one eye will drift upward. It may be noticed by a parent when the child is not concentrating or by the physician as each eye alternately moves upward when doing a cross-cover test. Ther-

apy is rarely necessary and is not especially satisfactory, although large superior rectus recessions do minimize DVD.

THE EVALUATION OF STRABISMUS

History. As always, a complete history is the first step in the evaluation of the patient. When evaluating strabismus, childbirth and childhood history are more important than in many other types of neuro-ophthalmic disorders. Comitant strabismus usually has its onset in childhood; thus, try to establish a history consistent with early onset. Many esotropias have their onset in the first months of life and those associated with an excess of accommodation in the preschool years. Exotropia may present at any time, but frequently has its onset in later childhood. If the patient does not recall which eye turned in or out in childhood, sometimes the mother or grandmother can be very helpful, as can family photographs or school photographs. If there was a compensated phoria during childhood, there may be a history of intermittent eye-turning during periods of fatigue, illness, or stress, or of squinting or closing one eye, especially out of doors or in sunlight with exotropia. A history of wearing glasses, especially a strong correction for hyperopia or a bifocal in childhood (indicative of an accommodative esotropia), as well as history of a head tilt or turn, should be sought. In children, abnormal head positions should be considered to indicate an ocular problem until proven otherwise. They are indicative not only of strabismus, but also congenital nystagmus with a null point eccentric from the primary position. If your patient has a head tilt or turn, patching one eye of the patient can be a diagnostic test; if it eliminates the head tilt, a strabismic etiology is probable. Accommodative strabismus is frequently associated with developmental delay and congenital neurologic difficulties, both structural and nonstructural.

Questions about general neurologic problems can highlight a possible paralytic strabismus. Family history is important, as strabismus is frequently familial, as are congenital nystagmus and hereditary myopathies. Ask about other family members with eyes that turn, strong glasses, "lazy" eyes, or eye muscle surgery. Transitory myasthenia may be present in a neonate who is the child of a myasthenic mother.

A drug history is also critical, as antibiotics may cause neural toxicity, and ingestion of large amounts of vitamin A may cause a pseudotumor syndrome with sixth nerve palsies. Additionally, patients taking sedative drugs for seizure disorders may manifest a strabismus that is latent when the patient is not on drugs or taking a smaller dose.

In summary, nonparalytic *strabismic deviations* are comitant, usually not accompanied by diplopia, and usually have normal eye-movement kinetics. Of course, prior surgery or muscle contraction may alter the usual findings.

On the other hand, *paralytic squint* usually causes incomitant eye movements and diplopia (although young children suppress readily and quickly), maximal in the field of action of the paretic muscle or muscles. Primary and secondary deviations are found, and because the neural impulse is not transmitted normally to the muscle, saccades will be slow. In addition, a paresis in the field of action of muscles innervated by single or multiple cranial nerves should be obvious. Although strabismus is common in children, paralytic third nerve palsies are rare; thus, a history of trauma or migraine (ophthalmoplegic migraine, Chapter 19) should be sought in any child with a third nerve palsy. Conversely, in children, sixth nerve palsies often follow viral illnesses (benign sixth nerve palsy) or may even be the first sign of hydrocephalus.

Myopathic disorders, muscular dystrophies, and myasthenia gravis usually are associated with diplopia if they are asymmetric and occur in an adult. However, when they occur in children, diplopia may not be reported. The limited movement should be obvious, however. When the abnormal movements do not correspond to a cranial nerve distribution or show much variation, look for an etiology other than strabismus.

EXAMINATION OF THE PATIENT WITH STRABISMUS

First, best corrected visual acuity is obtained at distance and near. In children too young to test objectively, observation of visual behavior and visual fixation patterns must suffice. Optokinetic nystagmus, preferential looking tests, and visual evoked potentials are other means to estimate acuity. When visual acuity in one eye is decreased without any obvious other findings to explain it, amblyopia must be considered and tested for. A 10-diopter vertical prism placed in front of the eye in question is often useful, with lack of movement indicating dense amblyopia. Amblyopia, the most frequent cause of visual loss in children, is more likely to be associated with strabismus. In adults, newly discovered visual loss is more frequently neurologic. However, a structural abnormality within the eye—such as a congenital cataract, optic nerve hypoplasia, or other cause of visual loss—can cause the strabismus. In these cases, abnormalities of color vision or an afferent pupillary defect may be present.

Anisometropia can also cause strabismus. Some refractive errors occur more often in specific types of strabismus. Hyperopes frequently are esotropic, especially if there is a high accommodative ratio; myopes often are exotropic.

On the external examination, a broad base of the nose and epicanthal folds often contributes to pseudostrabismus, as does macular ectopia; obvious craniofacial abnormality may distort the orbit and cause true strabismus or pseudostrabismus. Ptosis or a large pupil suggests a third nerve palsy. Pseudoptosis often accompanies hypotropia.

Note abnormal head postures used to compensate for strabismus as well as abnormal head or eye movements.

Stereoscopic vision. It is especially important to test stereopsis with tests designed for that purpose, such as Titmus, TNO, Randot (see Chapter 2). The four-diopter prism test and the neutral density filter test, if positive, both suggest amblyopia. In contrast, an afferent pupillary defect suggests organic visual loss and is extraordinarily rare in strabismic amblyopia. In fact, if an afferent pupillary defect is present, look hard for hypoplastic optic nerves or other neurologic problems.

The General Evaluation of Eye Movements

The *examination of children* necessitates special attention and techniques. First, control fixation and accommodation. Toys, especially those with moving parts or the latest in toy fashion, and interesting noises, can be especially helpful. Slow eye movements are present within a few days of birth and fixation is well established by 4 to 6 weeks. However, good and purposeful pursuit and saccadic movements are usually not made until approximately 3 months. At this point, if visual acuity is poor, typical wandering eye movements may appear.

Visual acuity cards and projection slides with pictures work well for older children, as does the so-called "illiterate" E. In the latter test, the children point their fingers in the direction that the "fingers" of the E point. Even if the child is too young for you to get his or her attention and cooperation by any of these means, optokinetic nystagmus (OKN) and preferential looking tests may be used both to elicit eye movements and to test visual acuity. The acuity will approximate the angle subtended by the stripes on the OKN stimulus. Visual evoked potential (VEP) testing can also be used to give an objective, but only approximate, estimate of visual acuity. Testing of vestibular nystagmus with spinning or by rotating the child at arm's length can also elicit nystagmus and test the range of eye movements.

Examine eye movements thoroughly if the history or the findings suggest strabismus or amblyopia. For the evaluation of strabismus, the fixation target should approximate normal visual situations; for example, numbers and letters, not just a light. Binocular excursions of the eyes are termed *versions*. The movements of each eye tested separately are called *ductions*. The cover and uncover tests (see the following sections) in the cardinal positions of gaze are used to measure any deviation.

Cover test. Using a target visible to the patient, cover and then uncover the eye that appears to fixate by a paddle, first with the patient fixing at distance and then at near.

When a tropia (a constant deviation) is present and the occluder is placed in front of the fixing eye, the other (deviated) eye moves to take up fixation. If the covered eye is not the fixating eye, no movement occurs, and the test is repeated on the other eye. If no movement occurs when either eye is covered, there is no manifest strabismus.

Cover–uncover test: Watch the covered eye as the cover is removed to identify a latent strabismus.

Alternate (Cross-cover) test: Cover each eye sequentially. If there is no movement, there is no tropia. The occluder then is moved from eye to eye (cross-cover test). This is done so that the eyes are not allowed to fixate together, and thus fusion is interrupted. If, after a normal cover test, movement occurs with the cross-cover test, a latent strabismus or phoria exists.

All these tests give a qualitative estimate of ocular deviation. The deviation can be quantified in several ways.

Prism cover test. A prism bends light, and thus prisms of various strengths are used to quantify ocular deviations. A prism is placed in front of the deviating eye so that it points in the direction of the deviation (eg, if there is a right hypertropia, the prism is placed in front of the right eye pointing upward, or base down). The cross-cover test is then repeated and the strength of the prism increased until there is no movement of the eyes. The strength of the prism equals the ocular deviation in prism diopters (prism diopters equal twice the measurement in degrees; for example, a 10-degree deviation is equivalent to a 20-prism diopter deviation).

The position of the light reflex on the cornea can also be used to estimate the magnitude of strabismus; this is known as the *Hirschberg test*. When the reflection on the deviating eye is located halfway between the center of the cornea and the limbus (the border between the sclera and the cornea) the deviation is about 45 prism diopters (22.5 degrees). If the reflex falls at the limbus, the deviation is 90 prism diopters or 45 degrees (each millimeter of decentration corresponds to 7 degrees of deviation).

Another estimate of strabismus based on the corneal reflex, the *Krimsky test,* is performed by increasing prism strength in the same way as for the prism cover tests. In this case, the prism is increased until

the corneal light reflex is centered in both eyes. The strength of the prism then equals the ocular deviation in prism diopters. Neither the Hirschberg nor the Krimsky tests are as accurate as the prism cover test; however, they are more quickly performed, and frequently are the only tests that can be performed in small children or uncooperative patients. These techniques are used predominantly to evaluate comitant squints.

For diagnosis of *vertical* deviations, especially those involving the superior oblique (eg, a fourth nerve palsy), check versions and then do a forced head tilt. First, observe and measure the deviations in lateral gaze. Note the position of the greatest tropia. Second, notice whether the deviation is greater on upgaze or downgaze on the side with the greatest tropia. Third, measure the deviation with the head tilted to the right and then to the left (Bielschowsky head-tilt test). The head-tilt test is especially effective for superior oblique palsies of long standing with spread of comitance (see Chapter 11 for more details).

These evaluations define the strabismus and frequently differentiate between comitant strabismus (the deviation is the same in all fields of gaze) and paralytic or restrictive strabismus (the deviation differs by field of gaze).

In situations where the results are confusing or where the history suggests double vision but your tests have been unable to elicit it, there are two diplopia tests that are especially effective because the images are made dissimilar.

Diplopia Testing

The red glass test tests diplopia by covering one eye with a red glass. The patient (looking at a light) indicates the relative positions of the red and white images in the cardinal gaze positions. In paralytic or mechanical strabismus, the maximum image separation occurs in the direction of action of the affected muscle(s). The patient is asked which image, the red or the white, disappears when an eye is covered. If the image on the same side as the covered eye disappears, the diplopia is uncrossed, and there is an esotropia. If the images are crossed, there is an exotropia. Similarly, the higher image belongs to the hypotropic eye.

The **Maddox rod test** is a similar test that creates an even more dissimilar image. With fusion eliminated, a larger deviation is produced. The Maddox rod may be either red or white and consists of small glass rods oriented parallel to each other. When a light is viewed through a Maddox rod, the patient sees a line perpendicular to the orientation of the glass rods (Fig. 15–1). With both eyes viewing the light, the areas of maximal separation are noted be-

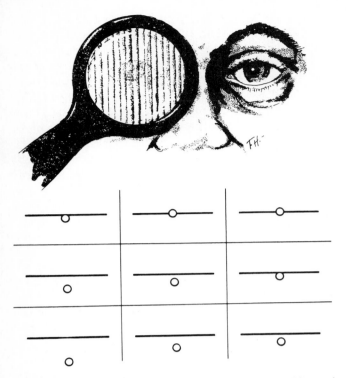

Figure 15–1. The Maddox rod test. Because the Maddox rod breaks fusional vergence, it tests for both phorias and tropias. This patient has a left superior oblique weakness. The separation of images is greatest when the patient looks down and to the right. (*From Leigh RJ, Zee DS. The Neurology of Eye Movements. Philadelphia: Davis, 1983, with permission.*)

tween the image of the light and the line in the cardinal positions of gaze. Because the Maddox rod completely eliminates the ability for fusional compensation, the small phorias present in the majority of people are elicited. These deviations are usually comitant and of small magnitude and should be ig-

nored. Conversely, a large magnitude phoria in an asymptomatic patient signifies a phoria normally kept in check by fusion and suggests a comitant strabismus of long standing.

The *double Maddox rod test* is especially useful for measuring cyclovertical deviations. In this case, a red Maddox rod is used in front of one eye and a white one in front of the other. Vertical and horizontal separations and cyclotortion of each eye can be quantitated. However, Maddox rod testing does not separate a phoria from a tropia.

Testing with the Hess Screen

The *Hess screen* quantifies and documents limitation of eye movement. It is reliable, accurate, and inexpensive and makes little demand on the patient. The findings are readily interpreted and, most importantly, facilitate objective comparisons at different stages of illness.

Method: The patient is seated in front of the Hess grid (Fig. 15–2) marked on a white surface. The head is fixed and the eyes put at the same level as the central point of the grid. Wearing red-green dissociating spectacles, the patient is asked to point with a green light rod to red spots marked on the grid by the examiner. The red-covered eye sees the red spots on the grid and the green-covered eye the green mark of the pointer. The patient points to each spot on the grid, first with the red glass over the right eye and the green glass over the left, and then with the glasses reversed. The positions at which the mark on the pointer appears to coincide with the dots on the grid are recorded on a chart. In mild degrees of paralysis the patient is asked to indicate the peripheral grid dots to magnify any abnormality.

If the fields are displaced equally for both eyes but show no distortion, the diagnosis is concom-

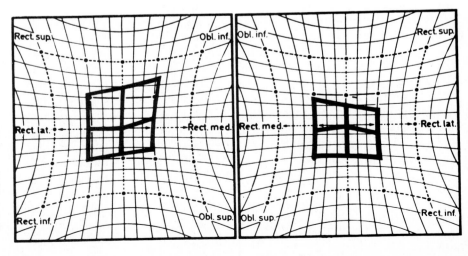

Figure 15–2. Hess chart showing paresis of right superior rectus, overaction of left inferior oblique, inhibitional palsy of left superior oblique. (Left: green glass over left eye. Right: green glass over right eye.) (*From Sachsenweger R. Clinical localization of oculomotor disturbance. In: Vinken PJ, Bruyn GW. Handbook of Clinical Neurology. Amsterdam: North Holland, 1969;2; with permission.*)

itant strabismus, not muscle palsy. In contrast, muscle paresis or overaction produces field distortion—field shrinkage signifies underaction and field enlargement overaction. The paralysed eye is the one whose field is diminished when it is covered with the green glass. The muscle corresponding to the most internally displaced point of a shrunken field is paralysed, and its name can be read off the edge of the chart. Overaction of the ipsilateral antagonist and of the contralateral synergist leads to displacement of the points peripherally in the direction of action of the overacting muscle, and consequent enlargement of the field at this point.

The method does not differentiate muscle paralysis from contracture or mechanical restriction. In multiple palsies the findings can be equivocal while minimal aberrations from the normal may be difficult to determine. Where the condition is not pronounced, patching both eyes for about an hour before the test is sometimes helpful.

Several other points should be made. When the movement of each eye alone (ductions) is tested, a minimal weakness may not be obvious. However, testing the movements of both eyes together (versions) may make a minimal weakness more obvious. One reason is the occurrence of primary and secondary deviations (Fig. 15–3).

Primary deviation is the deviation with the normal eye fixing. *Secondary deviation* is the deviation with the paretic eye fixing. In the field of gaze of the paretic muscle, the deviation will be much larger when the paretic eye fixes, as more effort is utilized to move that eye by the paretic muscle. By Hering's law, the corresponding muscle of the normal eye receives equal innervation; thus, the normal eye will move further and the separation between the images will be larger. The primary and secondary deviations are charcteristic of paretic strabismus and especially strabismus of recent onset. Discrepancies in estimating and measuring strabismus can sometimes be attributed to the different deviations that exist depending on which eye is fixing. So remember primary and secondary deviation when you get variable results.

Spread of comitance also accounts for changes in the primary and secondary deviations over time. In chronic paresis, the antagonist of the paretic muscle may contract or the innervation pattern may be altered, such that the deviation is less obvious. In this case, the deviation becomes more equal in all directions of gaze; "comitance" has spread.

Several other tests should be briefly mentioned. If the patient appears to have an accommodative esotropia, the *AC/A ratio* (accommodative convergence/accommodation) should be determined. The

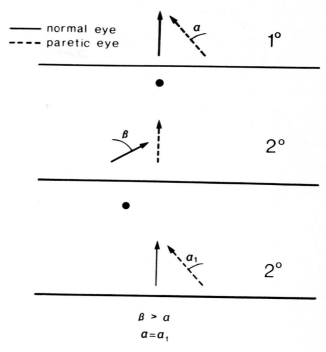

Figure 15–3. The principle of primary and secondary deviations. **Top.** When the normal eye fixes on a target directly ahead, the paretic eye deviates from the primary position by a certain amount (alpha). This is called the primary deviation. **Middle.** When a paretic eye fixes on a target in primary position, the normal eye also deviates from primary position by a certain amount (beta), but this secondary deviation of the normal eye when the paretic eye is fixing is greater than the amount of deviation of the paretic eye when the normal eye is fixing (beta > alpha). **Bottom.** Although the accepted explanation of primary and secondary deviation is based on Hering's law of equal innervation to yoke muscles, Leigh and Zee have suggested that the secondary deviation is greater than the primary deviation in paretic strabismus because when the paretic eye is fixing in primary position, it is forced further into its field of limitation. If the paretic eye were fixing on an object in the opposite direction, the deviation of the eye from primary position (alpha 1) would be the same as if the normal eye were fixing on an object straight ahead (alpha = alpha 1). (*From Miller N, ed.* Walsh and Hoyt's Clinical Neuro-ophthalmology. *4th ed. Baltimore: Williams & Wilkins, 1982;1; with permission.*)

easiest way to do this is to measure the esotropia while the patient (with refractive error fully corrected) views a distant reading target. If a −1.00 sphere is then placed over each eye, 1 diopter of accommodation is stimulated. Then the deviation is remeasured. For example, if the deviation changes from 10 to 15 diopters of esotropia, the AC/A ratio is 5 (5-diopter change in convergence/each diopter of lens-induced accommodation; the normal AC ratio is approximately 3.5). This "gradient method" is thought by many to give the most reliable estimate of the AC/A (see the chapter bibliography for other methods and discussion). When this ratio is high, part or all of an esotropia may be treated by decreasing accommodation and its associated convergence with an appropriate hyperopic correction or the use of drops such as phospholine iodide.

Measurement of Vergence

It is often useful to determine the *amplitude of vergence*. As mentioned above, high vergence amplitudes are characteristic of comitant or long-standing strabismus. Noting low vergence amplitudes may explain intermittent diplopia or aesthenopia in the face of an otherwise normal examination.

Vergence amplitude is measured by placing increasing prisms in front of one eye and noting when diplopia occurs. This may be done for convergence, divergence, and cyclovergence. At distance there are normally 15 to 20 diopters of convergence and 6 to 8 of divergence; at near, convergence is 25 to 30 diopters and divergence 12 to 14 diopters. Marked discrepancies at distance and near may also indicate convergence or divergence paralysis; however, the "normal" values for vergence amplitude show considerable interperson variability.

At this point, the history and the examination should yield a fairly good idea of the etiology of the motility limitation and quantify the degree of limitation.

Forced Duction Tests

Whenever an obvious limitation of eye movement is not clearly explained by a cranial nerve palsy, a forced duction test should be done to rule out a restriction. The forced duction test is done after anesthetizing the conjunctiva with a topical anesthetic. Ask the patient to look in the direction of the paretic muscle and push on the opposite side of the globe with a Q-tip in an attempt to move the eye into the paretic field of gaze. If the eye moves easily, then there is obviously no restriction. If it will not move, a restrictive force is demonstrated. But be sure to watch the other eye to be sure the patient is not deliberately working against you!

Sometimes this method does not obtain sufficient traction on the globe for an adequate test. In these cases, the insertion of the antagonist muscle should be anesthetized by holding a Q-tip dipped into a 4% Xylocaine solution over the insertion for several minutes. The insertion is then grasped with toothed forceps, and again an effort is made to move the eye into the paretic direction (Fig. 15–4). Any limitation can usually be felt. Additionally, note the amount of pull on the forceps as the patient is asked to look in the direction of the "paretic" muscle (*force-generation test*). If normal force (pull) is generated, the limitation of gaze is due to restriction rather than

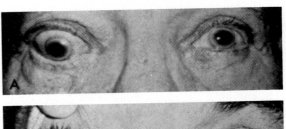
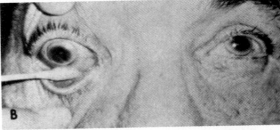
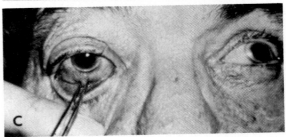
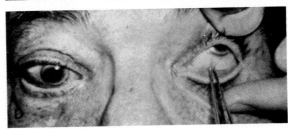

Figure 15–4. Forced duction test. **A.** Inability of patient to elevate right eye on upward gaze. **B.** Using cocaine 10%, insertion of right inferior rectus is anesthetized. **C.** Insertion of inferior rectus is grasped with toothed forces (Elschnig) and, with patient looking upward, attempt is made to manually rotate right globe upward. **D.** For comparison, left globe is manually rotated upward following cocainization. (*From Glaser J. Neuro-ophthalmology examination. In: Duane TT, ed.* Clinical Ophthalmology. *Hagerstown, MD: Harper & Row, 1976;2; with permission.*)

paresis. In addition, with restriction, when saccades are made into the field of restriction, it will be noted that in contrast to a paresis the eye moves with normal rapidity until the restriction comes into play, at which point it will be abruptly tethered. Comitant strabismus usually shows normal saccades.

Mechanical limitation of eye movements. For many types of restrictive limitation of eye movements, the history suggests the likely diagnosis: blowout fracture, previous eye muscle surgery, thyroid disease, orbital mass, congenital fibrosis syndromes. However, restriction may be mimicked by abnormal innervation causing cocontraction of the antagonist (eg, Duane's syndrome or aberrant regeneration of the third nerve, see Chapter 3). Duane's syndrome and Brown's tendon sheath syndrome should be looked for. The fibrosis syndromes frequently are familial, are among the few causes of true restriction in an otherwise normal child, and are the most frequent cause of a double-elevator palsy in a child. Duane's and Brown's syndromes follow typical patterns and are explained more fully in Chapter 13. *Thyroid orbitopathy* is probably the most common cause for acquired, nonparetic, unusual eye movement limitation in adults. When the classic pictures of thyroid orbitopathy or orbital inflammation present, the diagnosis is easy; but remember, both may present subtly until the diagnosis is established and are always important considerations.

In *blowout fractures,* the globe usually is tethered in the inferior portion of the orbit, with either the muscle itself, or more frequently its suspensory ligaments, being caught in a trap-door fracture of the maxilla. Because most blowout fractures do not injure the muscle, you can afford to wait 6 weeks or so for the condition to resolve spontaneously; it usually will. Again, forced ductions will be positive but force generation normal. Whenever restriction exists, intraocular pressure may be elevated when measured with effort to look in the direction of restriction.

If the condition does not resolve after 3 months of stability, surgery to repair the entrapment and to correct any remaining vertical deviation is indicated.

Tensilon testing for myasthenia is described in the section on cranial nerve palsies and myopathies of Chapter 13.

Two other unusual causes of limited eye movement are Möbius syndrome and double-elevator palsy. These are explained in Chapter 13 and should not be confused with the syndromes considered above, as they are not restrictive. However, congenital double-elevator palsies are often caused by inferior rectus fibrosis.

AMBLYOPIA

Amblyopia is decreased visual acuity without obvious organic basis. It occurs in approximately 2% of the population and may be related to strabismus, unequal refractive error in the two eyes (anisometropia), or congenital degradation of the visual image (cataract, vitreous hemorrhage, or corneal opacity). The deviating or poorly seeing eye is suppressed. The physiologic basis appears to be a neurogenic change, an assumption of the weaker eye's neural connections in the visual cortex by those of the dominant eye.

There must be at least a two-line difference in acuity between the two eyes to make the diagnosis of amblyopia. In an eye that doesn't have any obvious aberration in the media to account for the loss of vision, there are several other associated phenomena that help in establishing amblyopia as the diagnosis.

Amblyopic eyes usually show *"crowding"* when tested on an acuity chart. This refers to the unexplained phenomenon of being able to read smaller letters and lines of acuity if tested one letter at a time as opposed to viewing the whole line of letters.

When tested with a *neutral density filter,* the visual acuity of an amblyopic eye will not decrease significantly. Additionally, if a *four-diopter prism* is placed in front of the eye while fixing distant targets with both eyes, the amblyopic eye will not move. In infants and young children, inability to fix and follow targets, or crying and fussing if one eye is occluded, may indicate amblyopia.

It is important to make an effort to prevent or treat amblyopia before a child reaches 5 to 6 years of age, after which attempts to rectify the situation are rarely successful. Children with a media opacity, congenital ptosis, or other lesions obstructing the visual axis should be treated as early as is feasible. Refractive errors should be corrected and, in children, the good eye patched in order to force the amblyopic eye to perform. Do everything possible to eliminate amblyopia prior to any eye muscle surgery to give the patient the best chance to fuse. However, be careful to allow the patched eye to be used intermittently so it does not develop amblyopia! A disturbing recent report suggests that patching may cause a decrement in visual acuity and contrast sensitivity in a "normal" eye.

Orthoptics or **visual training** helps overcome weakness of vergence and decrease the frequency of diplopia. Following surgery, orthoptic training may

TABLE 15–2. INDICATIONS FOR BOTULINUM INJECTION

Unique	Acute nerve palsy
	Acute Graves' disease with diplopia
	Other contraindications to surgery
	Surgical enhancement
Excellent	Small: < 20 prism diopters
Good	Moderate: 20 to 40 prism diopters
Poor	Large: > 40 prism diopter deviation
Relative Contraindications	Complete paralysis
	Severe restriction
Special Situations	Surgical enhancement
	Postoperative rescue

From Magoon E. The use of botulinum toxin injection as an alternative to strabismus surgery. Contemp Ophthalmol Forum. 1987;5–9.

improve an imperfect result, but rarely is it adequate as the only therapy for large deviations.

In general, small deviations may be helped by changes in corrective lenses, prisms, and exercises. *Oculinum injection* should be considered in paralytic strabismus where there is contraction of the antagonist or in comitant strabismus if surgery is indicated and refused. The best results are with small (<20-degree) deviations as primary therapy, following strabismus surgery with a less than perfect result, and in accommodative esotropias (Table 15–2). For best results, the nonfixing eye should be the one treated.

BIBLIOGRAPHY

Burde RM. The extraocular muscles: Anatomy, physiology, and pharmacology. In: Moses RA, ed. *Adler's Physiology of the Eye.* 7th ed. St. Louis: Mosby, 1981.

Parks MM. Ocular motility and strabismus. In: Duane T, ed. *Clinical Ophthalmology.* Hagerstown, MD: Harper & Row, 1975;1.

Rogers GL et al. The contrast sensitivity function and childhood amblyopia. *Am J Ophthalmol.* 1987;104:64–68.

Von Noorden GK. Burian's binocular vision and ocular motility. 2nd ed. St. Louis: Mosby, 1980.

Section III
The Pupil, Other Cranial Nerves, and the Orbit

CHAPTER 16
THE PUPIL

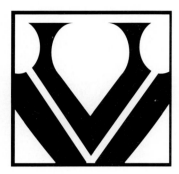

The pupil is our window on the world, a diaphragm through which light rays enter the eye. As very few light rays exit, the pupil appears dark. The size of the diaphragm is determined by the dilator and sphincter muscles of the pupil, controlled by sympathetic and parasympathetic innervation, respectively.

Innervation

The **sympathetic pathways** (Fig. 16–1) originate in the hypothalamus and descend through the mesencephalon and pons to the spinal cord. Here they synapse in the ciliospinal center of Budge (C8–T2). The second-order neuron exits the spinal cord and runs in the sympathetic chain to the superior cervical ganglion, passing over the apex of the lung and close to the brachial plexus. After a second synapse in the superior cervical ganglion, the third-order neuron joins the carotid plexus, accompanying the internal carotid artery (ICA), except for the sudomotor and vasoconstrictor fibers, which accompany the branches of the external carotid artery (ECA) to the face. The fibers from the ICA plexus leave the artery in the cavernous sinus to accompany the fifth and sixth nerves, passing through the superior orbital fissure (SOF) to enter the orbit. Ultimately they pass with the nasociliary nerve to the long ciliary nerves that supply the pupil dilator and with other orbital nerves to Müller's muscles in the lids.

The **parasympathetic pathway** fibers that subserve the light reflex (Fig. 16–2) are activated in the retina and run in the optic nerve, chiasm, and tract, leaving the latter prior to the lateral geniculate body (LGB) to enter the brain stem via the brachium conjunctivum. They synapse in the pretectum and are distributed bilaterally to the Edinger-Westphal (EW) nucleus of the third nerve. The efferent pupillary fibers run with the third nerve and enter the orbit with its inferior ramus to synapse in the ciliary gan-glion lateral to the optic nerve in midorbit. The postsynaptic parasympathetic fibers run in the short ciliary nerves to the pupillary sphincter and ciliary body. Some recent research suggests there may be fibers that pass directly to the ciliary body.

Determinants of Pupillary Size

The size of the pupil is determined by the amount of light impinging on the retina, the physical status of the iris, the near reaction, state of vergence (convergence or divergence of the eyes), state of alertness, and the tonus of the parasympathetic and sympathetic nervous systems.

Pharmacology

Pharmacologic agents that act on the autonomic nervous system will alter the size of the pupil. Parasympathetic drugs constrict the pupil (causing miosis, and therefore are called *miotics*); sympathomimetic drugs dilate the pupils (causing mydriasis, and therefore are called *mydriatics*). Similarly, drugs that inhibit sympathetic activity will cause miosis and those that inhibit parasympathetic activity will cause mydriasis (Tables 16–1, 16–2). Sympathomimetic drugs are used to dilate the pupil for examination of the fundus and for cycloplegia (paralysis of accommodation; Table 16–3). Although frequently used to reverse diagnostic mydriasis and its discomforts, pilocarpine acts slowly, often causes headache, and may precipitate an attack of angle closure in predisposed eyes because it reduces the depth of the anterior chamber. Dapiprazole 0.5%, an alpha-adrenergic blocker, reduces diagnostic mydriasis by nearly 50% in 1 hour without adverse effects except mild conjunctival injection.

Processes that stimulate the sympathetic system (altertness, alarm, interest) cause pupillary dilation;

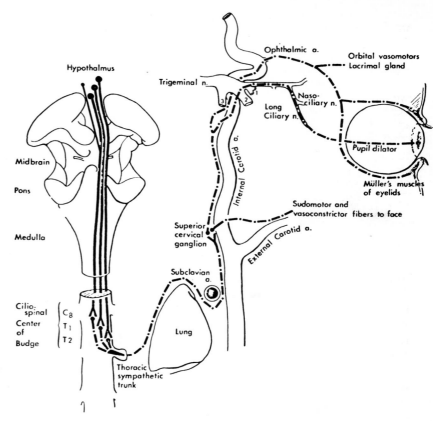

Figure 16–1. Ocular sympathetic pathways. Hypothalamic sympathic fibers comprise a polysynaptic (?) system as they descend to the ciliospinal center. This intra-axial tract is functionally considered the "first-order neuron." The second-order neuron takes a circuitous course through the posterosuperior aspect of the chest and ascends in the neck in relationship to the carotid system. Third-order neurons originate in the superior cervical ganglion and are distributed to the face with branches of the external carotid artery and to the orbit via the ophthalmic artery and ophthalmic division (1) of the trigeminal nerve. (*From Basic and Clinical Science Course 1986–1987, Section 5, Neuro-ophthalmology. San Francisco: American Academy of Ophthalmology, with permission.*)

processes that stimulate the parasympathetic system (sleep) cause miosis.

Pupillary Reactions

The normal pupil. The normal pupil ranges from 2.5 to 7 mm in diameter with less than 1 mm difference between the two pupils. (An anisocoria of up to this amount is present in 25% of the population; the larger pupil may alternate from eye to eye on repeated inspection.) With age, the pupils change from miotic in the newborn to a relatively large size throughout childhood and most of adulthood, be-

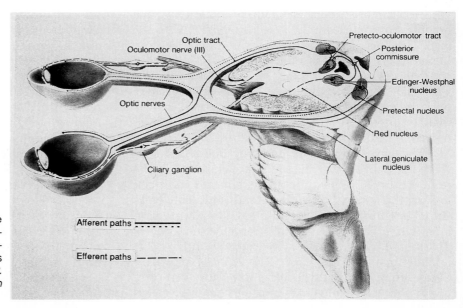

Figure 16–2. Diagram of the path of the pupillary light reflex. (*From Pupil: Embryology, anatomy, innervation and reflex movements. In: Miller N, ed. Walsh and Hoyt's Clinical Neuro-ophthalmology. 4th ed. vol. 2. Baltimore: Williams & Wilkins, 1983;1; with permission.*)

TABLE 16–1. COMMON *OCULAR* PHARMACOLOGIC AGENTS AFFECTING PUPIL SIZE[a]

Mydriatics
Sympathomimetics: phenylephrine, epinephrine, cocaine, OH-amphetamine (paredrine)
Parasympatholytics: atropine, hyoscine, Cyclogyl (anticholinergics)
Steroids

Miotics
Parasympathomimetics (cholinergic, anticholinesterase agents): pilocarpine, carbachol, mecholyl

[a] Partial list.

coming miotic again in the aged. Blue eyes have larger pupils than more darkly pigmented eyes.

Input to the Edinger-Westphal subnucleus of the third nerve complex is crossed and innervation of the pupillary sphincters is bilateral. Thus, *the pupils normally are equal in size,* even with visual afferent pathway (VAP) lesions. Therefore, when the light reaction is tested, the pupils react equally to light-stimulation of either or both retinas. The reaction of the stimulated eye is termed the **direct light reaction;** the reaction of the unstimulated eye is termed the **consensual light reaction.** Normally, pupil reactions to near and to convergence are also equal. **Unequal pupils (anisocoria) result from lesions of the efferent pupillary fibers or the iris itself.**

The Near Reflex. **The near reflex** (near triad, near synkinesis) can be elicited experimentally from dif-

TABLE 16–2. COMMON *SYSTEMIC* PHARMACOLOGIC AGENTS AFFECTING THE PUPIL/ACCOMMODATION[a]

Mydriasis/Decreased Acommodation/Increased Hyperopia	Miosis/Increased Accommodation/Increased Myopia
Amphetamine	Blockers—guanethidine, reserpine, etc.
Amyl nitrite (large doses)	
Anticholinergics	Caffeine
Antihistamines	Chloral hydrate
Artane	Clonidine
Benedryl	Chlorpromazine
Cogentin	Guanethedine
Fenfluramine	Hexamethonium
Glutethamide	Histamine
Jimson weed	MAO inhibitors
L-dopa (dopamine)	Morphine
LSD	Nicotine
Marijuana	Opiates
Oleander	Parasympathomimetics
Parasympatholytics	Sympatholytics—eg, ergotamine, hydralyzine, reserpine
Sympathomimetics	
Tricyclic antidepressants	

[a] Partial list.

fuse cortical inputs that project to the EW nucleus. It consists of concurrent accommodation, convergence, and miosis. Thus, supranuclear lesions (cortex to EW nucleus) can affect the near triad (miosis, accommodation, convergence), but are uncommon; supranuclear lesions usually occur with diffuse disease of the hemispheres or brain stem including multiple sclerosis, upper brain-stem vascular lesions, and tumors. Occasionally *spasm of the near reflex* results from the pathologies mentioned above, but most commonly it is a functional problem. The synkinetic nature of the near reflex makes this functional problem easy to detect; diplopia or esotropia because of excessive convergence is associated with miosis and increased accommodation. Occasionally, convergence may be asymmetric, simulating an acquired sixth nerve palsy. Here again, blurred vision at distance and miosis can be important in establishing the correct diagnosis.

EXAMINATION OF THE PUPILS

Examination of the pupils (Table 16–4) begins with careful attention in a normally lighted room. First, the state of the pupils is noted in room light with the patient looking in the distance. It is important to control convergence and accommodation which affect the pupillary reaction. The pupils should be equal in size and reaction. Some normal pupils appear to be restless, showing nearly constant small variations in pupil size, called *hippus.* When marked, this movement can make pupillary evaluation difficult.

Note any clues suggestive of a pupillary abnormality (eg, a history of trauma or a central nervous system lesion), signs associated with pupillary changes (eg, ptosis occurs with Horner's syndrome), or evidence of other cranial nerve palsies.

Then look at the pupils in very dim light. Normally both pupils should dilate equally and briskly. However, in dim light, some differences in pupil size are exaggerated, often making an equivocally smaller (Horner's) pupil into an obvious anisocoria. In contrast, in bright light, physiologic anisocoria will decrease and anisocoria due to an Adie's pupil will increase. The extent as well as the *quality of the pupillary reactions* must be noted as well (eg, the "tonic" dilation of the Adies' pupil).

Next, *pupillary reactions to a light stimulus* are noted. To do this, a penlight is shone into each pupil alternatively and the reaction noted. Again, both pupils should react equally and briskly, as *no lesion of the VAP alone causes anisocoria.*

In each condition, the pupillary size is recorded. The reactions are noted on a scale of 0 to 4 +, where 4 + is normal (Fig. 16–3).

TABLE 16–3. CYCLOPLEGIA AND MYDRIASIS

Cycloplegia

Drug	Procedure of Instillation	Time of Max. Effect	Duration of Max. Effect	Patient Able to Read After	Accommodation Normal After
Scopolamine	2 Drops 30 min apart	40 min after second drop	90 min	3 days	8 days
Cyclopentolate HCl (Cyclogyl)	2 Drops 5 min apart	25 min after second drop	50 min	3 hr	18 hr
Atropine sulfate	Tid for 3 days	32 hr after first drop	8–24 hr	3–4 days	10–14 days
Tropicamine (Mydriacyl)	2 drops 5 min apart	20 min after second drop	15 min	45 min	4 hr
Homatropine	6–8 drops 10–15 min apart	40 min	50 min	6 hr	36 hr

Mydriasis

	Latency (min)	Rate of Dilation (mm/min)	Time to Maximum Dilation (min)	Time to ½ Recovery Without 1% Pilocarpine	Time to ½ Recovery With 1% Pilocarpine	Time to 9/10 Recovery Without 1% Pilocarpine	Time to 9/10 Recovery With 1% Pilocarpine
Mydriacyl 0.5%	7	0.3	40	3 hr	1.5 hr	7 hr	3.5 hr
Homatropine 2%	14	0.2	70	7 hr	5.5 hr	20 hr	20+ hr
Paredrine 1%	21	0.15	65	3 hr	14 min	7 hr	18 min
Neosynephrine 10%	21	0.14	70	3 hr	16 min	5 hr	22 min

If the direct reaction in an eye is less than its consensual reaction (eg, reaction when the other eye is stimulated), an afferent pupillary defect (**APD or Marcus Gunn pupil**) is present. For example, when the light alternates to the involved eye, the pupils dilate, and when moved to the unaffected eye, the pupils constrict. This apparently paradoxical dilation of the eye is one of the most important signs in neuro-ophthalmology (Fig. 16–4).

Even when the pupil of the suspect eye is dilated (trauma, third nerve palsy, or by drops), watching the reaction of the mobile pupil (because the pupils normally react identically) will expose an afferent pupillary defect; when the light shines in the good eye, its pupil constricts; when it shines in the eye with the affected optic nerve, the good eye's pupil dilates.

The extent to which the afferent pupillary defect is abnormal may be quantified by the use of neutral density filters. Place the filter(s) over the normal eye and continue the "swinging flashlight test." When the pupillary reactions become equal, the amount of neutral density filter used equals the degree of afferent pupillary defect. Pupillary reactions may also be quantitated by pupillography and pupil cycle time (timing of pupil oscillation induced by placing a light beam at the pupillary margin); however, these methods are more complex, time consuming, and difficult to interpret, and have not yet been proven to have a significant advantage over clinical observation.

Light–Near dissociation. Normally, the pupillary reactions to both light and near should be brisk and equal in each eye. To test the pupillary response to near, have the patient look at a target placed about 6 inches in front of the eyes. If the reflex is equivocal, use the patient's own finger as a target. (The added proprioceptive input helps; even patients with acquired blindness can look at their own finger.) It is sometimes useful to bring the target from a small distance (±10 inches) to 6 inches so that convergence is examined simultaneously. However, if any ambiguity remains, a quick refixation from distance (20 feet) to near (6 inches) will accentuate any problem with the near reflex.

TABLE 16–4. EXAMINATION OF THE PUPIL

Room light
Dim light
Bright light
Convergence/near
Swinging flashlight test (APD)

Light Conditions

Size		Room	Dim	Bright	Near	APD
	R					
	L					

Figure 16–3. Schema for recording pupillary reactions: 0–4+.

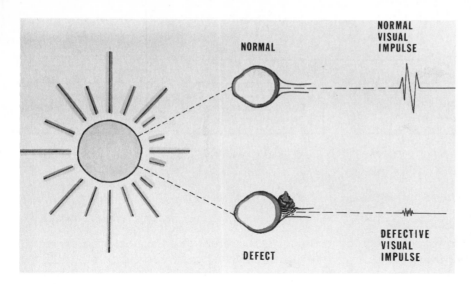

Figure 16–4. Diagram demonstrating the origin of an afferent pupillary defect. In this case a mass compresses the optic nerve and causes a decreased visual impulse on the effected side. (*From Newman NM, Arsham G, Creech J.* Self-Instructional Materials in Ophthalmology—Neuro-ophthalmology. *Washington, DC: National Audio-Visual Center, 1975, with permission.*)

Three major pupillary abnormalities are associated with light–near dissociation (poor light reaction with retained near reflex): the Argyll-Robinson (AR) pupil of tertiary central nervous system (CNS) syphilis, light–near dissociation with mildly dilated pupils in pretectal lesions, and Adie's "tonic" pupils.

Slit-lamp Examination

The magnification offered by the slit-lamp is very helpful in the diagnosis of pupillary abnormalities. You can see in detail the wormian movements of an Adie's pupil, sphincter ruptures, hyphemas, and lens changes following trauma; increased pressure, narrow angles, and inflammation in acute angle closure glaucoma; corneal changes, anterior chamber inflammation, rubeosis of the iris, lens changes, and abnormal intraocular pressure in the ischemia of carotid or orbital arterial occlusive disease (see Chapter 8); subtle abnormalities related to congenital defects, colobomas, pupillary membranes, and adhesion of the iris to lens or cornea; and postoperative defects.

In a pupil with light–near dissociation, slit-lamp observation of wormian movement (segmental constriction) of the pupillary sphincter is pathognomonic of an Adie's pupil.

Pharmacologic Examination of Pupillary Abnormalities

Pharmacologic testing is an important aid in the diagnosis of pupillary abnormalities. It is especially helpful in confirming suspicions of Horner's syndrome and Adie's pupil when the clinical findings are very subtle or equivocal. (Tables 16–5, 16–6)

The differential diagnosis of abnormal pupils is diagrammed in figure 16–5, 16–6, and 16–7 and their anatomic localization discussed below.

ANATOMIC LOCALIZATION OF ABNORMAL PUPILLARY REACTIONS

Pupillary Abnormalities with VAP Lesions

When the visual afferent pathways are damaged prior to the decussation of the visual fibers in the chiasm,

TABLE 16–5. PHARMACOLOGIC TESTING OF SMALL PUPILS

Drug	Pupil Reaction	Diagnosis
Cocaine 10%	Dilates	Normal
	Impaired dilation	Horner's syndrome
Hydroxyamphet-amine (Pare-drine) 1% (2 drops)	Dilates	Normal or preganglionic Horner's syndrome
	Fails to dilate	Postganglionic Horner's
Mydriatics	Poor dilation	AR pupil
	Dilates	Normal

TABLE 16–6. PHARMACOLOGIC TESTING OF LARGE PUPILS[a]

Drug	Pupil Reaction	Diagnosis
Pilocarpine 0.1% (2 drops)	Constricts	Adie's pupil
	No reaction	Normal
Pilocarpine .5% (2 drops)	Constricts	Not pharmacologically dilated
	Fails to constrict	Pharmacologic dilation

[a] Perform pharmacologic tests on different days. Use no topical anesthetic (eg, for applanation tension) and omit corneal testing so corneal epithelial integrity is maintained.

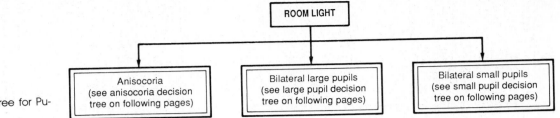

Figure 16–5. Decision Tree for Pupillary abnormalities.

the direct light reaction of the affected eye is decreased, while its consensual reaction remains normal (Fig. 16–8). This **afferent pupillary defect (Marcus Gunn pupil)** is an important hallmark of optic nerve damage. Very large and dense retinal le-

sions, especially those affecting the macula, can cause a small afferent pupillary defect. However, in retinal lesions causing an afferent pupillary defect, vision is severely affected (usually less than 20/200) and the lesion is obvious on examination. Media

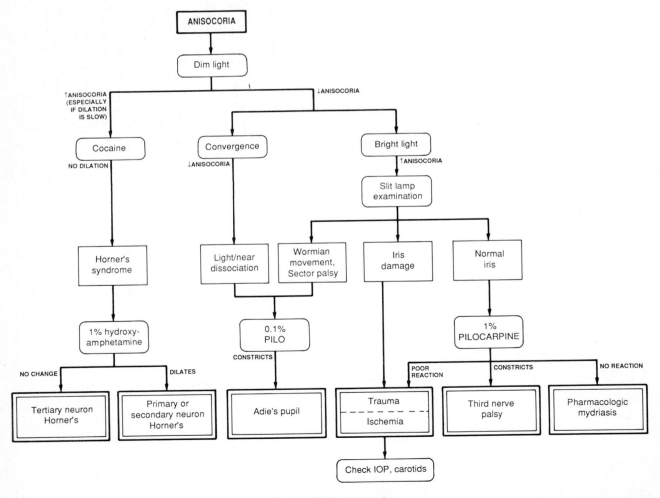

Figure 16–6. Anisocoria.

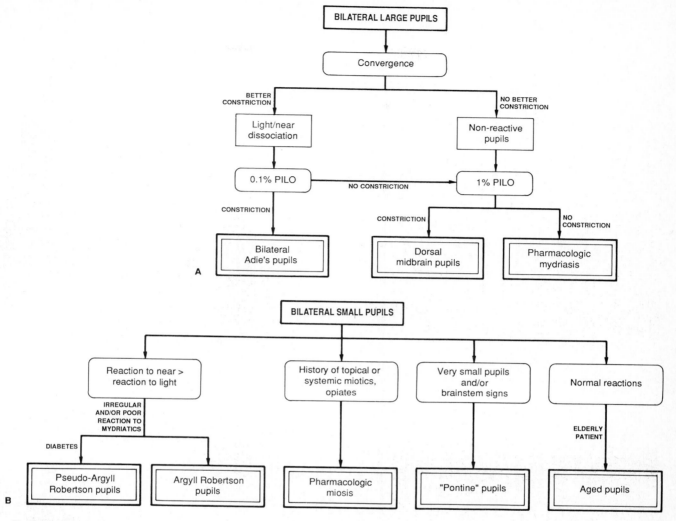

Figure 16–7. **A.** Decision tree–differential diagnosis of bilateral large pupils. **B.** Decision tree–Differential diagnosis of bilateral small pupils.

opacities (corneal scar, cataract, vitreous hemorrhage) almost never cause an afferent pupillary defect unless there is associated optic nerve damage. In optic nerve lesions, a significant afferent pupillary defect may be present with relatively good visual acuity, even with 20/20 or 20/15 vision (especially following optic neuritis). Thus, *an eye with an afferent pupillary defect can be presumed to have an optic nerve lesion unless another very obvious cause is present* (associated loss of color vision and a visual field defect should be looked for). On the other hand, significant unilateral visual loss should not be attributed to optic nerve pathology unless the afferent pupillary defect, loss of color vision, and associated visual field defects are present.

Lesions of the VAP affecting the chiasm and postchiasmal pathways affect decussated fibers and thus almost always affect the reactions of both pupils equally.

Behr's pupil: A rare exception exists when the pupil contralateral to an *isolated* optic tract lesion shows a weaker light reaction than the pupil ipsilateral to the lesion. Behr's pupil is rarely documented clinically, but can be found if carefully tested for. It is caused by the asymmetric decussation of fibers in the chiasm (53% of the fibers cross). Therefore, as these fibers correspond to the nasal retina, the eye with the temporal visual field defect (the eye *contralateral* to the lesion) will show an afferent pupillary defect but have normal acuity (because the lesion is postchiasmal). The associated anisocoria described by Behr probably does not exist in pure tract lesions. When seen it represents an ipsilateral associated Horner's syndrome.

TABLE 16–7. EVALUATION OF PUPILS BY REACTIONS

Flowchart:

- **Pupils equal in ambient light?**
  - **NO → Anisocoria**
    - **One pupil dilated?**
      - **NO → In constricted pupil**
      - **YES → In dilated pupil**
  - **YES → Both large (> 6 mm.)?**
    - **YES →** (both-large scenarios)
    - **NO → Both normal size?**
      - **YES →** (both-normal-size scenarios)
      - **NO → Both small (< 2 mm.)**

	In constricted pupil		In dilated pupil		Both large (> 6 mm.)			Both normal size		Both small (< 2 mm.)		
Direct Light Reaction	Poor	Normal	Poor	Normal	Both Eyes Normal	Both Eyes Poor	Both Eyes Poor	Normal	One Eye Poor	Both Eyes Poor	Both Eyes Poor	Both Eyes Normal
Near Reaction	Normal	Normal	Equally Poor	Normal	Both Eyes Normal	Both Eyes Normal	Both Eyes Poor	Normal	Normal	Both Eyes Normal	Both Eyes Poor	Both Eyes Normal
Diagnostic Considerations		ptosis?, ↓ sweating? Possible Horner's syndrome.	Adie's pupil? (Check deep tendon reflexes.)								Drug history? (e.g. glaucoma meds) or senile miosis.	Patient obtunded? Any other evidence of pontine lesion.
Diagnosis	Argyll-Robertson Pupil		Drug effect or efferent lesion.	Congenital anisocoria likely. (Compare old pictures.)	Congenitally large pupils.	Bilateral afferent defect or bilateral Adie's. (If V.A. ↓, afferent defect likely.)	Drug effect or bilateral efferent lesion.	Normal	Unilateral afferent defect likely.	Argyll-Robertson likely.		

TABLE 16–8. EVALUATION OF SPECIFIC PUPIL ABNORMALITIES

Syndrome	Appearance		Size	Light Reaction	Near Reaction	Comments and Special Tests
Left Tonic pupil (Adie's tonic pupil)		Dark	Large except when old, then small	Vermiform, trace or segmental. Best seen under slit-lamp	Strong, slow and tonic	Pilocarpine 0.12% reveals denervation supersensitivity. Adie's syndrome = tonic pupil + areflexia
		Light				
		Near				
		pilo 0.1%				
Left Horner's syndrome		Dark	Small	Normal	Normal	Ptosis, upside down ptosis, anhidrosis & early hypotony with conjuctival injection
		Light				
1st/2nd neuron Horner's		Cocaine 10%				Cocaine 10% test is positive in 1st, 2nd, 3rd-neuron damage.
3rd neuron Horner's		Paredrine 1%				Paredrine 1% fails to dilate 3rd neuron Horner's syndrome
Argyll-Robertson pupils		Dark	Small	Trace or absent	Brisk	VDRL FTA-AbS Pupils may be irregular. (FBS for diabetic pseudo AR pupils)
		Light				
		Near				

Wernicke's pupil. Pupillary hemiakinesia or Wernicke's pupil is a difference in the light reaction depending on whether the nasal or temporal retina is stimulated (Fig. 16–9). Theoretically, stimulating the blind hemiretina in a tract lesion would give less pupillary reaction than stimulation of the seeing hemiretina. However, even with sophisticated testing (pupillography), light scatter and other variables make this sign nearly impossible to detect. Because of this and the fact that suprageniculate lesions can cause a similar phenomenon, this sign has negligible clinical value.

Brain-stem lesions (Light–Near dissociation). More easily detected are immediately prenuclear lesions of the dorsal midbrain affecting the parasympathetic outflow. These lesions differentially affect the descending fibers subserving the light reaction and those subserving the near synkinesis, causing light–near dissociation. In these cases, the pupillary reaction to light is preferentially affected, so that on examination there is poor light reaction, but normal constriction to a near stimulus. This occurs because the pupillary fibers for accommodation approach the Edinger-Westphal nucleus separately from the pupillary light fibers descending from the brachium conjunctivum and posterior commissure superiorly.

The two most important pupillary abnormalities of this region are the small irregular *Argyll-Robertson* pupils (where the lesion is thought to be in the region of the posterior commissure) and the larger pupils of Parinaud's syndrome. (Fig. 16–7)

In *Parinaud's syndrome* (dorsal midbrain syndrome, Koerber-Salus-Elschnig syndrome, sylvian aqueduct syndrome) the pupils are usually normal or slightly larger than normal in size and the light–near dissociation is often accompanied by limitation of upgaze, lid retraction on attempted upgaze (Collier's sign), and convergence–retraction "nystagmus." When the dorsal midbrain syndrome is caused by downward expansion of a pineal tumor or slow

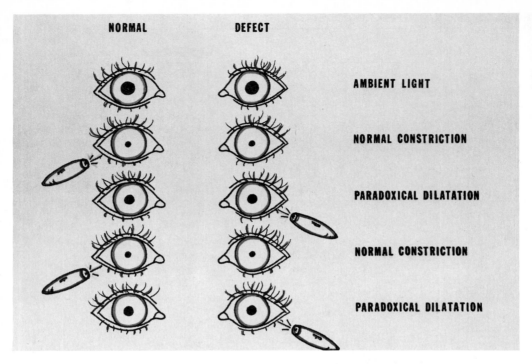

NORMAL   DEFECT

AMBIENT LIGHT

NORMAL CONSTRICTION

PARADOXICAL DILATATION

NORMAL CONSTRICTION

PARADOXICAL DILATATION

Figure 16–8. Diagram of a positive test for an afferent pupillary defect. (*From Newman NM, Arsham G, Creech J. Self-Instructional Materials in Ophthalmology—Neuro-ophthalmology. Washington, DC: National Audio-Visual Center, 1975, with permission.*)

dilation of the sylvian aqueduct in obstructive hydrocephalus, loss of upward saccades and an acquired myopia are early signs followed by light–near dissociation. Vascular lesions, demyelinating lesions, or abruptly increased intracranial pressure (eg, blocked shunt) tend to cause all the signs to appear simultaneously.

Argyll-Robertson pupils (Fig. 16–10) are *small*, usually bilateral, irregular, and dilate poorly even with mydriatics; they are a sign of tertiary CNS syphilis. The light reaction is minimal and the near reaction normal.

Although Argyll-Robertson (AR) pupils are pathognomonic of CNS lues, other disorders cause **pseudo-Argyll-Robertson pupils:** diabetes, systemic amyloid (may cause polygonal pupils!), and myotonic dystrophy. These pupils are small, irregular, and bilateral, but usually show asymmetrical involvement. In contrast to true Argyll-Robertson pupils, pseudo-Argyll-Robertson pupils generally **do not** show light–near dissociation and **do** dilate to atropine and other anticholinergics.

In fact, the classic AR pupil is not the only pupillary abnormality of tertiary syphilis. Eighty-five percent of patients with tertiary syphilis shows pupillary irregularity. Less than 50% of these abnormal pupils are true AR pupils. Most are not constricted. The alterations in size, shape, and reactivity include an Adie's-like pupil (however, this "tonic" pupil of

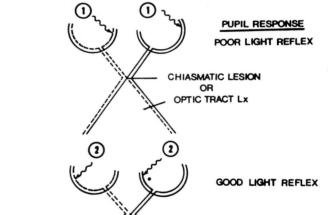

WERNICKE'S HEMIANOPIC PUPILLARY REFLEX

PUPIL RESPONSE
POOR LIGHT REFLEX

CHIASMATIC LESION
OR
OPTIC TRACT Lx

GOOD LIGHT REFLEX

Figure 16–9. Wernicke's hemianopic pupillary reflex. In lesions of the optic tract or of the optic chiasm, there is a differential response of the pupil (miosis) when the nasal versus the temporal half of the retina is stimulated with light. In the diagram, with a lesion on the right, light is directed (1) toward the side of the lesion and the pupillary response is a weak miosis. But light directed (2) away from the side of the lesion evokes a better miosis reaction. However, in most clinical situations the light stimulus is not discrete enough and there is internal scatter with a loss of the hemianopic pupillary reflex. (*From Zinn KM. The Pupil. Springfield, IL: Thomas, 1972, with permission.*)

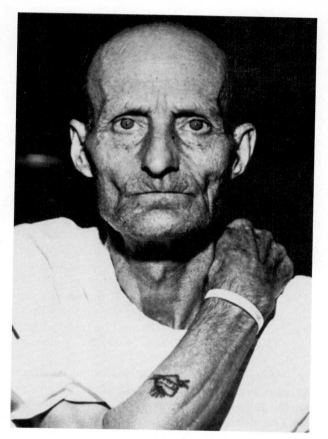

Figure 16–10. Argyll-Robertson pupils in a tabetic merchant seaman. Even in the semidarkness that preceded the photographer's flash, the pupils are so small as to be hidden behind the corneal reflection. (*From disorders of pupillary function, accommodation, and lacrimation. In: Miller N, ed. Walsh and Hoyt's Clinical Neuro-ophthalmology. 4th ed. Baltimore: Williams & Wilkins, 1985,1; with permission.*)

syphilis will react briskly to near stimuli and is nearly always bilateral). Thus, FTA-Abs testing is indicated with many bilateral pupillary abnormalities.

Other causes of miotic pupils include (1) eyedrops, especially glaucoma medications; (2) opiates; (3) ocular inflammation; and (4) pontine lesions. Appropriate serologic testing is mandatory.

Measurable bilateral pupillary abnormalities are less common in lesions of other portions of the central nervous system. Diffuse lesions of the hypothalamus and pons (especially in coma) associated with bilateral miosis occur most frequently with large tumors and vascular lesions.

In **nuclear lesions of the third nerve** that involve the EW nucleus there is bilateral internal ophthalmoplegia, loss of accommodation, and mydriasis (see Chapter 13). **Infranuclear lesions** cause unilateral pupil abnormalities on the side of the affected third nerve (Table 16–9).

TABLE 16–9. CAUSES OF DILATED PUPILS

Damage to Dorsal Midbrain (Pretectal and Edinger-Westphal Nuclei and Connections)
Isolated pupil defect is rare; light–near dissociation may occur
  Ischemia, tumor, demyelination, infection Ictal (?) migraine (sympathetic hyperactivity?)
Damage to the Preganglionic Oculomotor Nerve (From Interpeduncular Fossa to Ciliary Ganglion)
Isolated pupil defect extremely rare (including internal carotid–posterior communicating artery aneurysm)
Except basal meningitis (eg, tuberculosis), uncal herniation (early), basilar aneurysm (rare)
Damage to the Ciliary Ganglia and Postganglionic Short Ciliary Nerves
Usually causes "tonic pupil"; may have light–near dissociation
  Idiopathic (Adie's) tonic pupil
  Local tonic pupil
    Viral infection (eg, herpes zoster)
    Orbital trauma, tumor, surgery
    Retrobulbar anesthesia
    Choroidal trauma, tumor
    Blunt trauma to the globe (ciliary plexus damage)
    Temporal arteritis (18)
    Episodic unilateral mydriasis (springing pupil)
    Panretinal photocoagulation
    Rheumatoid arteritis with episcleritis
  Neuropathic tonic pupil
    Syphilis
    Diabetes
    Amyloidosis
    Sarcoidosis
    Familial and acute dysautonomias
    Guillain-Barré syndrome
Damage to the Iris
Iritis and posterior synechiae
Angle-closure glaucoma (iris sphincter ischemia)
Blunt injury to the globe with sphincter tear (traumatic iridoplegia)
Ipsilateral internal carotid artery occlusion (including Takayasu's disease), iris ischemia, and atrophy
Corneal transplantation (Urrets-Zavalia syndrome)
Pharmacologic Blockade by Atropinic Substances
Accidental mydriatic drops (eg, hand contamination in medical personnel)
Deliberate (factitious) mydriasis
Jimson weed ("cornpickers pupil") and other plant materials
Perfumes and cosmetics
Scopolamine patches
Nutmeg intoxication (?)

Modified from Rubinfeld RS, Currie JN. Accidental mydriasis from blue nightshade "lipstick." J Clin Neuro-Ophthalmol. 1987;7:34–37.

ANISOCORIA (Fig. 16–6)

Efferent Pathway Lesions (Unilateral Large Pupil)

Third Nerve Lesions. Because the pupillary fibers run superficially in the superomedial portion of the third nerve, compressive lesions of that nerve in the intrapeduncular space or cavernous sinus can cause a dilated pupil without other signs of a third nerve palsy. This occurs with posterior communicating artery aneurysms, internal carotid aneurysms, and uncal herniation with supratentorial mass lesions. In contrast, when the third nerve is involved without involving the pupil, the cause is usually ischemic.

Local Abnormalities of the Pupil (Eye and Orbit)

An **Adie's "tonic" pupil** usually is a large pupil with better near than light reaction. The light reaction is slow or "tonic," as is redilation. Adie's pupils result from damage to the ciliary ganglion and/or postganglionic parasympathetic fibers. Following the injury the nerve fibers regenerate; and because the large majority (93%) of postganglionic fibers originally innervated the ciliary body, fibers originally involved in accommodation now subserve the pupil. Thus, the pupil reacts poorly to light, but well to accommodation. At slit-lamp examination, the typical Adie's pupil shows segmental constriction (wormian movement) to light stimulation. An **acute** Adie's pupil (prior to regeneration and less common) is dilated, nonreactive, and shows little wormian movement and less obvious cholinergic supersensitivity.

The pupillary sphincter is partially denervated and supersensitive to cholinergic agents. Thus the **pharmacologic test for an Adie's pupil** is instillation of 1/8% pilocarpine, to which a normal pupil is not sensitive but to which the Adie's pupil constricts; however, large pupils usually constrict more to dilute pilocarpine. Accommodation is also frequently subnormal, resulting in blurred near vision.

Adie's syndrome refers to the frequently familial occurrence of Adie's pupils and areflexia, which affects women more often than men. Other apparent causes of an Adie's pupil are viral illnesses and local trauma. In the case of unilateral Adie's pupils of unclear etiology, the second pupil will become involved in about two thirds of cases. With time, the original Adie's pupil may become smaller and ultimately be the smaller of the two pupils.

Episodic unilateral pupillary dilation frequently associated with headache and visual blur may be a migraine variant and typically occurs in young subjects, mostly women. It results (presumably) from involvement of basal arteries. A history of migraine is helpful in making this diagnosis.

Local disturbances of pupillary function also cause a dilated pupil. **Pharmacologic mydriasis** results in a fixed, widely dilated pupil reactive to neither light nor near stimuli. Pupils dilated from other causes rarely exceed 6 mm, but the pharmacologically dilated pupil is frequently 8 mm. Sometimes a history of mydriatic drug use is present or suspected (eg, the patient's child was given dilating drops for a strabismus exam). More often the use of the drug is accidental or factitious. Less often, environmental factors such as jimson weed or oleander can dilate a pupil.

Detecting the pharmacologically dilated pupil: The pharmacologically dilated pupil can be detected by installing a drop of 1% pilocarpine. A pupil dilated by third nerve compression will constrict, but the pharmacologically dilated pupil will not, because the mydriatic agents block the postganglionic cholinergic receptors and are not displaced by pilocarpine.

In contrast, a dilated pupil due to local trauma usually demonstrates sphincter ruptures and irregularity of the pupillary ruff, especially if examined at the slit-lamp. Iatrogenic trauma—such as sphincterotomies, iridectomies, and iridotomies—should also be looked for. These pupils may not respond normally to 1% pilocarpine but usually do react partially.

Sphincter trauma can also result from ischemia. Thus, a dilated pupil can be seen in vascular occlusion (carotid, orbit) or local vascular compromise (eg, narrow angle glaucoma).

Congenital pupillary anomalies are usually obvious at slit-lamp examination and do not pose neuro-ophthalmologic dilemmas. Aniridia may appear as a dilated pupil because iris stroma is absent and only the stump of the ciliary muscle is visible. These patients frequently have poor visual acuity and nystagmus as well as other ocular problems such as glaucoma or cataract. Systemic anomalies also occur (eg, Wilm's tumor) in sporadic cases of aniridia.

A less extensive anomaly is the **iris coloboma,** a full-thickness defect that usually occurs inferonasally and may be associated with colobomas of the ciliary body, optic nerve, choroid, retina. Colobomas are caused by failure of closure of the fetal fissure, frequent in chromosomal abnormalities and other dysgenetic syndromes.

Other peripheral disturbances of pupillary function include frequent involvement in botulinum toxin poisoning. Pupillary abnormality is rare in diphtheria; accommodation is affected primarily. Infiltration of the iris in familial amyloid polyneuropathy can cause a polygonal pupil with an abnormal pupillary light reflex.

UNILATERAL SMALL PUPIL

Horner's syndrome involves ptosis, miosis, anhidrosis, apparent enophthalmos, and narrowing of the palpebral fissure (Fig. 16–11). The loss of sympathetic stimulus causes decreased pupil dilation (loss of dilator stimulus), ptosis, and apparent enophthalmos (loss of stimulus to Müller's muscles); anhidro-

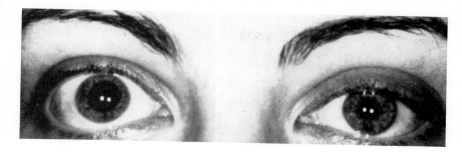

Figure 16–11. Left Horner's syndrome.

sis (loss of sudomotor stimulus); conjunctival vascular engorgement (loss of vasoconstrictor stimulus); and decreased accommodation (increased myopia).

The sympathetic outflow may be damaged by dorsal brain-stem lesions that also cause ipsilateral cranial nerve palsies, hemiparesis, and Horner's syndrome.

Infarcts cause the majority of brain-stem syndromes, including the lateral medullary syndrome (Wallenberg's syndrome)—vertigo, lateropulsion of body and eye movements, hemianesthesia, facial pain, and ipsilateral Horner's syndrome. Problems peculiar to the craniocervical junction may also cause Horner's syndrome; these include Arnold-Chiari and Dandy-Walker malformations, the Shy-Drager syndrome, and disorders that affect the spinal cord in the neck (eg, syringomyelia and compression of the cervical cord). Central lesions may be bilateral or unilateral (most vascular lesions) and cause anisocoria.

These brain-stem and cord areas are so compactly organized neurologically that the accompanying signs and symptoms usually provide good localization of the lesion—cranial nerve palsies in intracranial lesions and their lack in cervical lesions. Once the sympathetic outflow exits the spinal cord, hemianalgesia and hemiparesis are no longer associated; a new constellation of signs and symptoms occurs. In its somewhat tortuous path to the superior cervical ganglion, the second order neuron passes the apex of the lung and is contiguous with the brachial plexus.

Congenital Horner's syndrome secondary to birth trauma frequently has a lightly pigmented iris (heterochromia) on the affected side because there is less sympathetic stimulus to melanin formation. **Tumors in the lung apex** or adjacent lymphatics frequently damage the sympathetic outflow and are the lesions that make the recognition of a Horner's syndrome worrisome. Horner's syndromes due to apical and supraclavicular tumors nearly always are identifiable as second-order neuron lesions and associated with *arm and hand pain*. When unassociated with pain, Horner's lesions in this region may result

from compression (''fiddler's Horner's''), iatrogenic procedures (Swan-Ganz catheter, hyperalimentation lines), or medianoscopy, or be self-inflicted by IV drug abusers.

An isolated Horner's syndrome is more likely to be vascular in nature and the lesion situated higher in the neck, presumably caused by involvement of the carotid sympathetic plexus by arteriosclerotic disease of the carotid artery (rarely by a dissection or aneurysm), and is nearly always a third neuron lesion. If the lesion occurs below the carotid bifurcation, facial sweating is impaired because the sudomotor and vasoconstrictor fibers branch off here to follow the branches of the external carotid artery (ECA) to the face.

Other third neuron lesions occur with involvement of the carotid plexus at the base of the brain (nasopharyngeal tumor), petrous apex (otitis media), and in the cavernous sinus.

In the **region of the cavernous sinus,** the Horner's pupil may be associated with a third-nerve (or other cranial nerve) palsy and cause the pupil to appear less dilated than with a third-nerve palsy alone. More rarely, the sympathetic fibers that temporarily join the sixth nerve in the cavernous sinus may be affected along with that nerve, causing an ipsilateral sixth-nerve palsy and Horner's syndrome. In all lesions occurring superior to the carotid bifurcation, sweating is intact.

Lesions in this area also cause **Raeder's syndrome** (the paratrigeminal syndrome): Horner's syndrome, fifth-nerve palsy, and facial pain. Especially when associated with other cranial nerve palsies, this combination of signs and symptoms frequently occurs with tumors (as in several of Raeder's original patients). Patients with **cluster headache (severe** headache at or behind the eye) frequently occurring during the night for a period of weeks to months and associated with tearing, also have injection of the conjunctiva, nasal stuffiness, and commonly a Horner's pupil (see Chapter 19).

Pharmacologic testing: Cocaine testing is the classic test and effectively detects Horner's syndrome. Hydroxy-amphetamine testing localizes the lesion to the tertiary neurone.

A reversible Horner's syndrome has been described in Lyme disease (by Glauser and associates). Although the patient described had a first- or second-order neuron lesion, Lyme borreliosis now must be included in the differential diagnosis of Horner's syndromes of questionable etiology.

BIBLIOGRAPHY

General

Miller N, ed. *Walsh and Hoyt's Clinical Neuro-ophthalmology.* 4th ed. Baltimore: Williams & Wilkins, 1985;1:385–556.

Toxic

Grant WM. *Toxicology of the Eye.* 3rd ed. Springfield, IL: Thomas, 1986.

Rubinfeld RS, Currie JN. Accidental mydriasis from blue nightshade "lipstick." *J Clin Neuro-Ophthalmol.* 1987; 7:34–37.

Afferent Pupillary Defects

Fineberg E, Thompson HS. Quantification of the afferent pupillary defect. In: Smith JL, ed. *Neuro-ophthalmology Focus 1980.* New York: Masson, 1979.

Adie's Pupil

Fletcher WA, Sharpe JA. Tonic pupils in neurosyphilis. *Neurology.* 1986;36:188–192.

Argyll-Robertson Pupil

Englestein ES, et al. Dilated tonic pupils in neurosyphilis. *J Neurol Neurosurg Psychiatry.* 1986;49:1455–1457.

Finelli P. Pupil shape in syphilis: Case report. *Military Med.* 1977;144:342–343.

Behr's Pupil

Cox TA, Drewes CP: Contraction anisocoria resulting from half-field illumination. *Am J Ophthalmol.* 1984;97:527–582.

Newman SA, Miller NR. The optic tract syndrome: Neuroophthalmologic considerations. *Arch Ophthalmol.* 1983;101:1241–1250.

Horner's Syndrome

Glauser TA, Brennan PJ, Galetta SL. Reversible Horner's syndrome and Lyme disease. *J Clin Neuro-ophthalmol.* 1989;9:225–228.

Hawkins KA, Brichstein AA, Guthrie TC. Percutaneous heroin injection causing Horner's syndrome. *JAMA.* 1977;237:1963–1964.

Maloney WF, Younge BR, Moyer NJ. Evaluation of the causes and accuracy of pharmacologic localization in Horner's syndrome. *Am J Ophthalmol.* 1980;90:394–402.

Teich SA, Halprin SL, Tay S. Horner's syndrome secondary to Swan-Ganz catheterization. *Am J Med.* 1985;78:168–170.

Spasm of Near Reflex

Dagi LR, Chrousos GA, Cogan DC. Spasm of the near reflex associated with organic disease. *Am J Ophthalmol.* 1987; 103:582–585.

Pharmacology

Allison RW, Gerber DS, et al. Reversal of mydriasis by dapiprazole. *Ann Ophthalmol.* 1990;22:131–138.

CHAPTER 17

THE OTHER CRANIAL NERVES

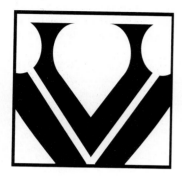

The cranial nerves with frequent neuro-ophthalmic manifestations (II through VI), and the oculomotor aspects of vestibular (cranial nerve III) function have been presented in other chapters. This chapter reviews the first and seventh cranial nerves, the auditory portions of the eighth cranial nerve and "dizziness." Examine these nerves in detail when symptoms, history, or other findings suggest their possible involvement. Detection of abnormal functioning may help localize the lesion or make the diagnosis.

Chapter 13 also considered the common etiologies for multiple cranial nerve palsies. Multiple, especially fluctuating, cranial nerve palsies are characteristic of meningeal disease: infection, carcinomatous or invasive processes (eg, nasopharyngeal tumor). Headache and leg weakness often are associated, whereas, in contrast, intrinsic brain-stem lesions usually show early long-tract signs and cranial nerve palsies only later (Table 17–1). Carcinomatosis is often associated with elevated carcinoembryonic antigen (CEA) in the cerebrospinal fluid.

THE OLFACTORY NERVE: CRANIAL NERVE I

The peripheral receptors of the first cranial nerve lie in the roof of the nasal cavity (Fig. 17–1). They give rise to the unmyelinated olfactory nerves that penetrate the cribriform plate to reach the olfactory bulb. From there their fibers course posteriorly to form the olfactory tract, which passes near the anterior perforated substance, and then in the medial and lateral olfactory striae to the olfactory cortex of the temporal lobe (the pyriform lobe) and to the septal area of the hemisphere.

Evaluation. To test the sense of smell, use aromatic substances such as oil of cloves or coffee to stimulate one nostril at a time (with the other occluded).

Disorders. Disorders of olfaction occur predominantly with peripheral lesions that affect the olfactory receptors, nerves, or tract, causing anosmia. Central disturbances of the olfactory pathways do not disturb the sense of smell. In the anterior fossa bilateral involvement of the peripheral olfactory apparatus is much more frequent than unilateral involvement because the two olfactory tracts run parallel to and very close to each other. Patients with disorders of olfaction often incorrectly complain of a loss of taste, since taste and smell are closely associated in everyday experience.

The most common cause of disturbed olfaction is the common cold, whether or not associated with sinus disease. Trauma frequently causes fractures across the cribriform plate, which may tear the olfactory nerves. In fact, bilateral periorbital ecchymosis, cerebrospinal fluid rhinorrhea, and anosmia form a triad pathognomonic of a fracture across the anterior cranial fossa.

Unilateral anosmia, especially if it develops gradually, is an important sign of subfrontal tumors, especially meningiomas of the olfactory groove. These tumors may also present with optic atrophy in one eye and contralateral papilledema, the Foster-Kennedy syndrome (see Chapter 4).

Although central lesions very rarely cause olfactory symptoms, lesions of the temporal lobe cause olfactory hallucinations and uncinate fits. Albinism is associated with congenital anosmia.

THE FACIAL NERVE: THE SEVENTH CRANIAL NERVE

The seventh cranial nerve innervates the muscles of facial expression (Fig. 17–2). It also sends secretory

TABLE 17–1. SYMPTOMS AND SIGNS OF LEPTOMENINGEAL CARCINOMATOSIS

Symptom	Frequency (%)	Sign	Cranial Nerve	Frequency (%)
		Cerebral		
Headache	66	Mental status changes	—	62
Mental status changes	33	Seizures	—	11
Gait ataxia	27	Generalized (60%)	—	6
Nausea and vomiting	22	Focal (40%)	—	4
Loss of consciousness	4	Papilledema	—	11
Language disorders	4	Diabetes insipidus	—	4
Dizziness	4	Hemiparesis	—	2
		Cranial Nerve		
Diplopia	36	Oculomotor paresis	(III, IV, VI)	36
Hearing loss	14	Facial weakness	(VII)	30
Visual loss	10	Hearing loss	(VIII)	18
Facial numbness	10	Optic neuropathy	(II)	10
Decreased taste	6	Trigeminal neuropathy	(V)	10
Tinnitus	4	Hypoglossal neuropathy	(XII)	10
Dysphagia	4	Decreased gag reflex	(IX, X)	6
		Spinal		
Weakness	46	Reflex asymmetry	—	86
Paresthesias	42	Weakness	—	73
Pain (back/neck)	31	Sensory loss	—	32
Radicular pain	26	+ Straight leg raising	—	15
Autonomic dysfunction	16	Decreased rectal tone	—	14
		Nuchal rigidity	—	9

Adapted from Wasserstrom WR, Glass JP, Posner JB. Diagnosis and treatment of leptomeningeal metastasis from solid tumors: Experience with 90 patients. Cancer. 1982;49:760.

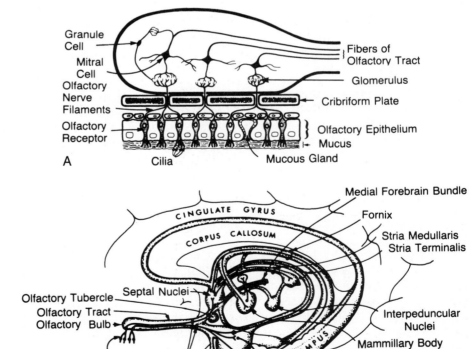

Figure 17–1. A. Anatomy of the olfactory nerves and the olfactory bulb. **B.** Central connections of the olfactory pathways. (*From Rengachary SS. Cranial nerve examination. In: Wilkins RH, Rengachary SS, eds. Neurosurgery. New York: McGraw-Hill, 1985;1; with permission.*)

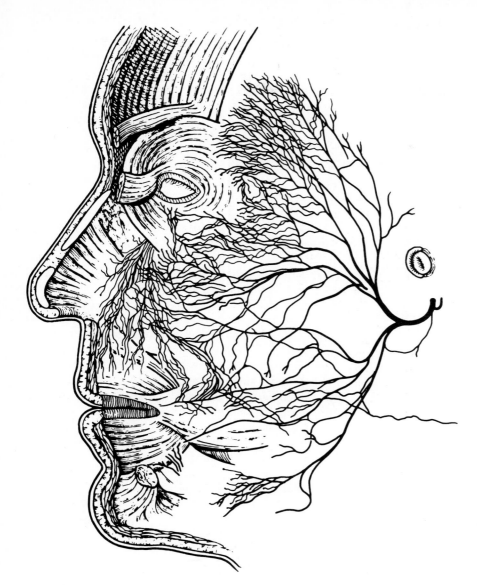

Figure 17–2. Extracranial facial nerve distribution. (*From May M, ed.* The Facial Nerve. *New York: Thieme, 1986, with permission.*)

and sensory fibers to the salivary gland, lacrimal gland, and mucosa of the nose and pharynx. It receives sensory fibers from the external ear and taste fibers from the anterior two thirds of the tongue.

The nucleus lies in the roof of the pons in proximity to the sixth-nerve nucleus. Fibers leave the nucleus and loop around the sixth-nerve nucleus in the facial genu. They then turn ventrally and laterally to emerge at the pontomedullary junction. The facial nerve traverses the subarachnoid space and enters the internal acoustic meatus, passing to the facial canal and exiting the skull via the stylomastoid foramen (Fig. 17–3). It then passes through the substance of the parotid to the muscles and glands of the face.

Examination. Significant disorders of the facial nerve are usually obvious. Asymmetry of the face is one clue. Absence of wrinkles on the forehead, a wide palpebral fissure, incomplete blinking, flattening of the nasolabial fold, or drooping of the corner of the mouth are associated with facial paresis. To test for more minor degrees of weakness, ask the patient to close both eyes tightly (the Bell's phenomenon, upward and outward deviation of the eyes, is tested at the same time). Also look for spasticity of gaze (see Chapter 11). The eyes should close symmetrically and the lashes should be buried. Ask the patient to wrinkle the forehead, smile, frown, or whistle to demonstate other motor nerve functions.

Test taste by putting a small spot of salt, sugar, or vinegar on the anterior two thirds of the tongue

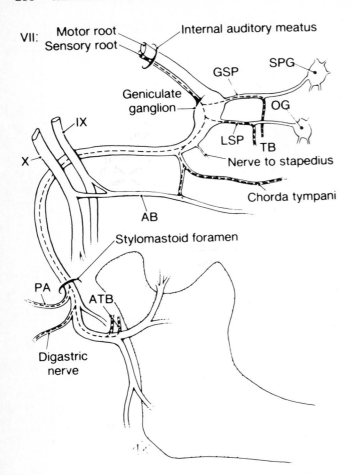

Figure 17-3. Diagrammatic representation of the facial nerve, showing the geniculate ganglion, sensory root, and peripheral divisions. The sensory system is represented by a dashed line. (AB, anastomosis between the facial nerve and auricular branches of the glossopharyngeal (IX) and vagus (X) nerves; ATB, facial nerve branches that anastomose with the auricular temporal branch of the trigeminal nerve (not pictured); GSP, greater superficial petrosal nerve; LSP, lesser superficial petrosal nerve; OG, otic ganglion; PA, posterior auricular nerve; SPG, sphenopalatine ganglion; TB, tympanic branches. (*From Miller N, ed. Facial pain and neuralgia. In:* Walsh and Hoyt's Clinical Neuro-ophthalmology. *4th ed. Baltimore: Williams & Wilkins, 1982;1; with permission.*)

and asking the patient to identify the taste by circling a written list of the sensations: "sweet," "salty," "sour."

The localization of lesions causing facial nerve dysfunction is described in Figure 17-4 and their evaluation in Table 17-2.

Disorders of the facial nerve: Upper motor neuron facial paralysis usually results from a lesion of the corticobulbar pathway and preserves function of the muscles of the forehead, which are bilaterally innervated (Fig. 17-5A, C). Lower motor neuron palsies cause weakness of the entire ipsilateral half of the face (Fig. 17-5B).

Lesions of Neuro-ophthalmic Significance

Bell's palsy. The most common cause of peripheral seventh-nerve palsy (Table 17-3) is Bell's palsy (Fig. 17-6). It is usually unilateral, lasts for hours to days, and may be associated with diabetes mellitus, multiple sclerosis, pregnancy, and Lyme disease. Seventy to eighty percent of the patients experiences a complete recovery, which usually starts before the third week. Another 10% has only partial recovery; and the rest regains little, if any, facial function. If no recovery has started 2 months after the onset of the palsy, not much improvement can be expected. In many peripheral palsies, there may be an associated dry eye (test by the Schirmer test) or, paradoxically, increased tearing caused by irritation associated with the dry eye, paralytic ectropion, and exposure keratitis. When associated with corneal hypesthesia, the resulting keratitis can be very difficult to control. Frequent instillation of artificial tears or 0.1% sodium hyaluronate during the day, and a lubricating ointment before sleeping, will help with most cases. In addition, taping the eyes shut at night and wearing side shields on glasses during the day may aid in slightly more severe cases. Difficult cases will need a lid suture, tarsorrhaphy, medial canthoplasty, punctal occlusion, or a combination.

The efficacy of steroid treatment or surgical decompression of the seventh nerve has not been proven to improve the prognosis in Bell's palsy.

As in third-nerve palsies, aberrant regeneration may occur, causing (1) the crocodile tear syndrome, when misdirected fibers going to the lacrimal gland cause tearing at inappropriate times, especially during eating; or (2) the Marin Amat syndrome, where the misdirected fibers course to the orbicularis oculi and cause eye closure when the mouth is opened widely.

The Marin Amat syndrome is the reverse of the Marcus Gunn phenomenon (see Chapter 19). In this case, with jaw opening, the eye closes. Proprioceptive impulses for facial stretch distributed to the orbicularis oculi are postulated to cause this synkinesis due to aberrant regeneration of seventh-nerve fibers.

Facial Spasm

There are two types of **facial myokymia** (Table 17-4). One is a very common and benign twitching of the lid margins, involving the lower lid more than the upper. This is self-limited and lasts days to months. It is not known to be associated with any pathologic lesions but may be more frequent with fatigue, bright light, ocular irritation, or stress.

The second, rarer myokymia is a spontaneous wave of undulating contraction that spreads across and usually involves facial musculature, frequently

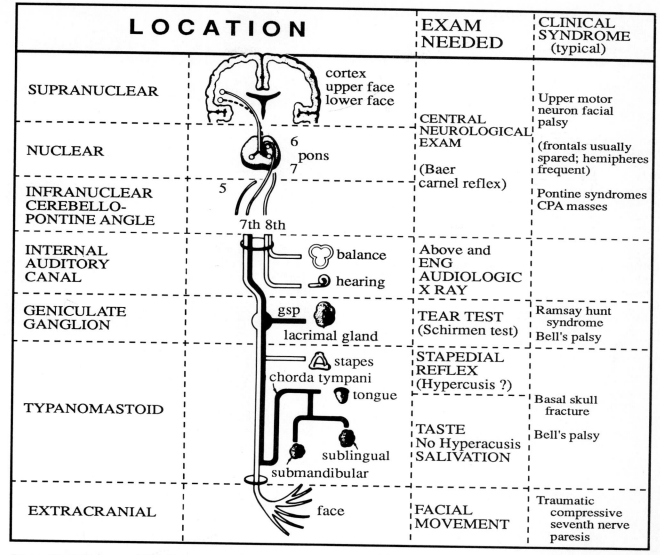

LOCATION		EXAM NEEDED	CLINICAL SYNDROME (typical)
SUPRANUCLEAR	cortex upper face lower face	CENTRAL NEUROLOGICAL EXAM (Baer carnel reflex)	Upper motor neuron facial palsy
NUCLEAR	6 pons 7		(frontals usually spared; hemiferes frequent)
INFRANUCLEAR CEREBELLO-PONTINE ANGLE	5 7th 8th		Pontine syndromes CPA masses
INTERNAL AUDITORY CANAL	balance hearing	Above and ENG AUDIOLOGIC X RAY	
GENICULATE GANGLION	gsp lacrimal gland	TEAR TEST (Schirmen test)	Ramsay hunt syndrome Bell's palsy
TYPANOMASTOID	stapes chorda tympani tongue sublingual submandibular	STAPEDIAL REFLEX (Hypercusis ?) TASTE No Hyperacusis SALIVATION	Basal skull fracture Bell's palsy
EXTRACRANIAL	face	FACIAL MOVEMENT	Traumatic compressive seventh nerve paresis

Figure 17–4. Diagram of facial nerve anatomy. (*From May M, ed.* The Facial Nerve. *New York: Thieme, 1986, with permission.*)

including the platysma. Over time, **spastic paretic facial contracture** occurs. This is pathognomonic of true facial myokymia in contrast to the benign movements described above, which are not associated with atrophy, weakness, or contracture. Facial myokymia occurs with lesions rostral to the facial nucleus, in the pons and cerebellar pontine angle. It is often associated with slow-growing lesions that have been present for lengthy periods of time, such as cholesteatomas, dermoids, and meningiomas, as well as pontine gliomas. Multiple sclerosis may also cause myokymia. In the latter case, the findings may remit spontaneously.

Essential blepharospasm is an intermittent paroxysmal involuntary contraction of the orbicularis oculi causing the lids to close (Fig. 17–7). It is bilat-

eral, idiopathic, and worsens with stress, bright light, or movement. Otherwise, the spasms occur spontaneously. Elderly women are affected predominantly. Although many authors have considered this to be a psychiatric disorder, this etiology has never been substantiated. More recently it has been considered a facial dystonia, like other dystonias associated with supranuclear (basal ganglia?) dysfunction. Many, often relatively extreme, surgeries have been suggested to cure the very troubling symptoms of this disorder, because when it is severe, eye closure does not allow the patients to continue their normal daily activities. Some are functionally blind.

The blepharospasm is often associated with other dystonias, such as orolingual, mandibular, and cervical dystonias; in the latter case it is termed

TABLE 17–2. DIAGNOSTIC EVALUATION OF FACIAL PALSY

History[a]
Physical examination[a]
Topognostic tests
   Hearing[a] and balance tests
   Schirmer test[a]
   Stapes reflex[a]
   Submandibular flow test
   Taste test[a]
Electrical tests
   Maximal stimulation test (MST)
   Evoked electromyography (EEMG)[a]
   Electromyography (EMG)
Radiographic studies
   Plain views of mastoid and internal auditory canal
   Pluridirectional tomography of temporal bone
   Computerized tomography of brain stem, cerebellopontien
      angle, temporal bone, skull base; contrast sialography of
      parotid
   Chest radiographic survey to detect sarcoidosis, lymphoma,
      carcinoma
Surgical exploration
Special laboratory tests
   Lumbar puncture (cerebral spinal fluid) to detect meningitis,
      encephalitis, Guillain-Barré syndrome, multiple sclerosis,
      meningeal carcinomatosis
   Complete white blood cell count and differential infectious
      mononucleosis, leukemia
   Mono spot test to detect infectious mononucleosis
   Heterophil titer to detect infectious mononucleosis
   Fluorescent treponemal antibody titer to detect syphilis
   Erythrocyte sedimentation rate to detect sarcoidosis, collagen
      vascular disorders
   Urine and fecal examinations
      Acute porphyria—elevated porphyrins and urinary porpho-
         bilinogen
      Botulism—*botulinum* toxin in stool specimen
      Sarcoidosis—urinary calcium
   Serum cryoglobulins and immune complexes to detect Lyme
      disease
   Serum globulin level to detect sarcoidosis
   Serum and urine calcium determinations to detect sarcoidosis
   Serum angiotensin-converting enzyme level to detect sarcoi-
      dosis
   Serum antinuclear antibody test (ANA), and rheumatoid fac-
      tor (RF) to detect collagen vascular disorders (periarteritis
      nodosa)
   Serum antibody test for Lyme disease
   Bone marrow examination to detect leukemia, lymphoma
   Glucose tolerance test to detect diabetes mellitus

[a] Performed routinely; the rest of the studies are ordered based on suspicion raised by history and physical examination or abnormalities noted in the routine tests.
From May M, ed. The Facial Nerve. *New York: Thieme, 1986:185.*

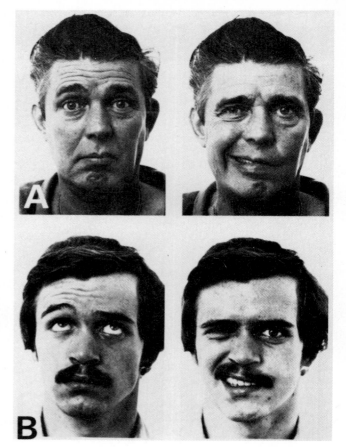

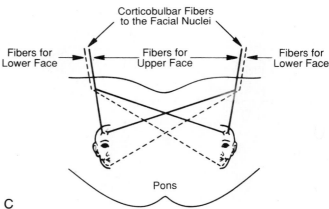

Figure 17–5. A. Upper motor neuron type of facial palsy showing paralysis mainly of the left lower face. **B.** Lower motor neuron type of facial palsy showing paralysis of the entire left half of the face. **C.** Anatomy of the facial nuclei in the pons and their supranuclear control. The facial nuclei in the pons are figuratively respresented by one half of the face. Upper parts of the facial nuclei receive bilateral cortical control, whereas the lower parts receive control only from the contralateral side. (*From Rengachary SS. Cranial nerve examination. In: Wilkins RH, Rengachary SS, eds.* Neurosurgery. *New York: McGraw-Hill, 1985;1; with permission.*)

Meige's syndrome (cranial–cervical dystonia). This is the most common form of dystonia and affects 80% of these patients. Blepharospasm without the associated findings is "essential blepharospasm."

    Blepharospasm, which is always bilateral, must be differentiated from unilateral processes (hemifacial spasm, synkinetic movements of muscles inner-vated by the seventh nerve, the Marin Amat syndrome, misdirection following seventh-nerve palsy, pathologic myokymia, and focal seizures in-

TABLE 17–3. CAUSES OF FACIAL NERVE DISORDERS IN 1575 PATIENTS SEEN OVER 20 YEARS (1963–1983) BY ONE CLINICIAN

Cause[a]	Patients
Bell's palsy	895 (57%)
Herpes zoster cephalicus	117 (7%)
Trauma	268 (17%)
Tumor	91 (6%)
Infection	70 (4%)
Birth (congenital and acquired)	48 (3%)
Hemifacial spasm	28 (2%)
Central nervous system (axial) disease	18 (1%)
Other	30 (2%)
Questionable	10 (1%)
Total	1575 (100%)

[a] Lyme disease is a not infrequently diagnosed cause today.
From May M, ed. The Facial Nerve. *New York: Thieme, 1986;183.*

TABLE 17–4. FACIAL SPASM

	Presumed Locale of Lesion	Unilateral	Bilateral
Myokymia			
Benign	Peripheral (?)	+	Rarely
Pathologic	Brain stem	+	
Essential Blepharospasm/ Meige's syndrome	Supranuclear		+ +
Hemifacial spasm	Infranuclear	+	Rarely
Synkinetic movements	Infranuclear	+	–
Habit spasm (tic)	Supranuclear	+	+
Reflex blepharospasm	Local irritation eye or lids	–	+
Focal seizures	Supranuclear	+	–

volving muscles innervated by the seventh nerve) and bilateral processes (habit spasm or tics and reflex blepharospasm caused by ocular irritation or primary or referred orbital pain).

Treatment: Because the mechanism of the spasm remains obscure, therapy is symptomatic. Pharmacotherapy has been largely disappointing and ineffective. The most effective pharmacologic agents are Clonazepam, Lorazepam, and Baclofen (see Table 17–5). Relatively massive kinds of surgery can provide effective relief, but the nerves often regenerate. Currently, the optimal treatment is pharmacologic denervation by injections of Oculinum (botulinum toxin), which are safe and effective (90%) but have the drawback of needing to be repeated approximately every 3 months.

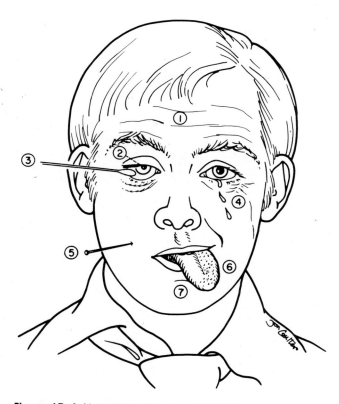

Figure 17–6. Neurologic signs in patients diagnosed as having Bell's palsy. **1.** Intact forehead. **2.** Miosis. **3.** Loss of corneal sensation. **4.** Tearing on uninvolved side only. **5.** Loss of sensation. **6.** Deviation of tongue. **7.** Loss of taste papillae. (*From May M, ed. The Facial Nerve. New York: Thieme, 1986, with permission.*)

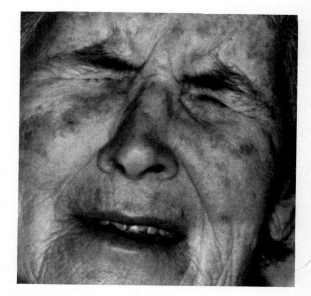

Figure 17–7. Essential blepharospasm. Uncontrolled spasm of the orbicularis muscle produces functional blindness. (*From Doxanas MT, Anderson RL. Clinical Orbital Anatomy. Baltimore: Williams & Wilkins, 1984, with permission.*)

TABLE 17–5. PHARMACOLOGIC AGENTS USED IN TREATMENT OF BLEPHAROSPASM

Anticholinergics	Trihexiphenidyl, trihexethyl-chloride, benztropine mesy-late, orphenadrine citrate, amantadine, ethopropazine
Cholinomimetics	Deanol, choline, lecithin
Dopamine-blocking agents	**Haloperidol,** pimozide, phe-nothiazines
Monamine-depleting agents	**Tetrabenazine,** reserpine
Dopaminergic agonists	Lisuride, levodopa/carbidopa, amantadine
Benzodiazapines	**Clonazepem, lorazepam,** chlordiazepoxide, diaz-epam
Gamma-aminobutyric acid agonists	**Baclofen,** valproate
Tricyclic compounds	Imipramine, chlomipramine
Monoamine oxidase inhibitors	Tranylcypromine, pargyline
Catacholamine-synthesis inhibitor	Alpha-methyltryosine
Anticonvulsants	Barbiturates, phentoin, car-bamazepine
Other	Lithium, methsergide, dexam-phetamine, tryptophan, 5-hydroxy-tryptophan, cyproheptadine

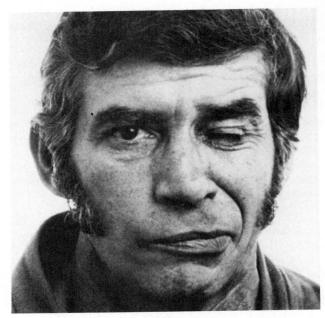

Figure 17–8. Left hemifacial spasm. (*From Rengachary SS. Cranial nerve examination. In: Wilkins RH, Rengachary SS, eds. Neurosurgery. New York: McGraw-Hill, 1985;1; with permission.*)

Hemifacial spasm is another spasmodic disorder of the facial musculature, which involves one half of the face and consists of involuntary spasmodic contraction (Fig. 17–8). It may start with spasms in the ocular region that spread to involve the rest of the facial musculature. It is usually caused by cross-compression of the facial nerve at its exit from the pons, in analogy to the etiology of tic doloureaux (Table 17–6). Hemifacial spasm also is effectively treated with Oculinum injections.

DISORDERS OF CRANIAL NERVE VIII

Evaluation of the "Dizzy" Patient

It is important to distinguish **true vertigo** associated with a false sensation of spinning, either of the individual or of the environment, from other sensations of unsteadiness, light-headedness, and disequilibrium. True vertigo is almost always a symptom of vestibular end-organ disease. Other symptoms of disequilibrium may be related to vestibular nerve disease, central nervous system disease, or vascular insufficiency—especially of the brain stem and cerebellar or vestibular pathways.

As always, take a careful history. Particular at-

tention should be paid to the type of subjective sensation. How long does it last? Is it constant, intermittent, recurrent? Are there provocative factors, especially specific postures of the head or body, that bring on the symptoms? Are there associated symptoms—tinnitus or autonomic disorders, sweating, nausea, vomiting? Is there a history of past trauma, especially head injury or whiplash? Is there an aura that precedes the vertiginous sensation? The use and abuse of drugs and withdrawal from them can cause feelings of unsteadiness. Although hangover is an experience with which many people can identify, even relatively minor doses of tranquilizers or sedatives can cause significant central changes. In

TABLE 17–6. CAUSES OF HEMIFACIAL SPASM IDENTIFIED INTRAOPERATIVELY IN 229 PATIENTS

Cause	No. Patients
Arterial compression	210
Mixed compression	10
Venous compression	4
Tumor	3
Aneurysm	1
Arteriovenous malformation	1
Total	229

From May M, ed. The Facial Nerve. New York: Thieme, 1986:504.

fact, because of these central effects, formal electro-nystagmographic testing should not be performed within 48 hours of ingestion of these medications (sedatives, tranquilizers, ETOH, and so forth). Nystagmus is the only objective correlate of vertigo.

Note other neurologic symptoms, especially those involving the other cranial nerves or ocular motor systems; involvement of the fifth, sixth, and seventh nerves in association with eighth-nerve difficulties is almost pathognomic of a cerebellar pontine angle (CPA) tumor. CPA tumors and brain-stem disorders may also be associated with cerebellar and pyramidal signs. In addition, carefully assess the patient's psychologic status. Diffuse complaints of disorientation and unsteadiness are frequently associated with depression, stress, or malingering.

True vertigo is the illusion of rotation of either the environment or the patient (Table 17–7). **Postural vertigo** is frequently associated with benign paroxysmal positional vertigo (BBPV). In this case, testing for vertigo and its associated nystagmus with the head hanging in different positions often will establish the diagnosis. This vertigo tends to adapt with time.

Benign paroxysmal positional vertigo is the commonest cause of acute vertigo. It is caused by a disorder of the posterior semicircular canal (degenerated otoconia falling on the cupula) and is precipitated by rapid head turns.

Vestibular neuronitis usually has a sudden onset and lasts for many days. It may or may not be associated with a decrease in hearing and is nonrecurring.

Peripheral disorders are much more likely to cause symptoms of vertigo than central disorders; this vertigo is provoked by specific movements and shows conjugate nystagmus with horizontal and rotary components.

Central disorders often show adaptation and demonstrate brain-stem signs. Thus, if the history is negative in the face of moderate to severe objective signs, the lesions either may be bilateral or adaptation has occurred.

Patients with acute labyrinthine lesions lie with the affected ear to the pillow to decrease the vertigo.

Dizziness is frequently associated with disturbance of the brain-stem vascular supply occurring in orthostatic hypotension, Stokes-Adams attacks, carotid sinus syncope, anemia, and hypoglycemia. Neurologic causes include tumor, vascular occlusion, multiple sclerosis, epilepsy, and migraine. Table 17–8 summarizes the differential diagnosis.

On examination, particular attention should be given to abnormalities of eye movement. Subclinical eye movement difficulties, small deviations, diplopia, and secondary effects of eye movement limitation like past pointing can cause disorientation. However, complaints of disorientation are uncommon in patients with visual afferent pathway problems. A positive Pulfrich phenomenon is often present in unilateral optic nerve disease and may explain the disorientation experienced by such patients. Ataxia and other cerebellar signs are also important signposts of an organic basis for disequilibrium.

One test peculiar to the vestibular system should be familiar to you, the **head-hanging maneuver.** In this case, the patient is seated at the edge of a table or a reclining chair and rapidly dropped into the supine position and the head either turned to one side or the patient dropped back to the supine position. The head is made to hang below the level of the shoulders and may either be turned laterally before moving the body downward or as the body is moved (Fig. 17–9). After a latency of approximately 10 seconds, this maneuver will almost always elicit the nystagmus of benign paroxysmal positional vertigo (BPPV). Then, if the head is maintained in the same position, the nystagmus will decrease over the next 30 seconds. Turning the head to the opposite side, repeating the maneuver to the opposite side, or sitting the patient up after the appropriate latency will cause nystagmus to occur in the opposite direction. A positive test, one with the appropriate delay and nystagmus in a decrescendo pattern, is almost pathognomonic for BPPV.

TABLE 17–7. SYMPTOMS COMMONLY ASSOCIATED WITH VERTIGO CAUSED BY LESIONS AT DIFFERENT NEUROANATOMIC SITES

Labyrinth	Brain stem
Hearing loss	Diplopia
Tinnitus	Visual hallucinations (un-
Pressure	formed)
Pain	Dysarthria
Internal auditory canal	Drop attacks
Hearing loss	Extremity weakness and
Tinnitus	numbness
Facial weakness	Cerebellum
Cerebellopontine angle	Imbalance
Hearing loss	Incoordination
Tinnitus	Temporal lobe
Facial weakness and	Absence spells
numbness	Visual hallucinations
Extremity incoordination	(formed)
	Visual illusions
	Olfactory or gustatory hallu-
	cinations

From Baloh RW. Neurotology. In: Wilkins RH, Rengachary SS, eds. Neurosurgery. New York: McGraw-Hill, 1985;1:115.

TABLE 17—8. DIFFERENTIAL DIAGNOSIS OF "DIZZINESS"

Etiology	Onset	Course	Severity	Deafness
End Organ (*True Vertigo*)				
Viral labyrinthitis	Sudden	4–5 days	+	+
Vestibular neuronitis	Sudden	1–2 weeks	+ + +	—
Middle ear infection	Sudden	Nonrecurring, lasts days	+ + +	—
Benign paroxysmal positional vertigo (BPPV)	Sudden with change in head position only	Lasts months, subsides rapidly (<30 sec) if head still	+ + +	+
Ménière's disease	Sudden	Recurrent attacks, subsides over hours/days	+ + +	Hearing loss progressive with each attack
Trauma	Sudden	Hours/weeks	+	+/−
Ischemic internal auditory artery occlusion	Sudden	Days/weeks, with gradual improvement	+ +	+ +
Eighth nerve Tumor	Insidious	Slowly progressive	Varies	Decrease in hearing, tinnitus, occipital headache
CNS Ischemia				
Vertebral basilar insufficiency, ischemia	Sudden, episodic	Minutes	varies	—
Multiple sclerosis	Varies	Intermittent with exacerbations	varies	Occasionally
Brain-stem compression or tumor	Gradual	Progressive	Mild	Slowly progressive hearing loss
Migraine	Varies	Minutes	—	+/−
Systemic				
Myxedema, Wernicke's syndrome, epilepsy (rare) Drugs: sedatives, tranquilizers, anticonvulsants Ocular, cerebellar disease—disequilibrium, not true vertigo				

Total unilateral loss of horizontal semicircular canal function is tested by rapidly turning the patient's head to the side while the patient fixes a distant target. Patients with unilateral canal paresis make compensatory refixation saccades when their head turns to the side of the canal paresis.

If following the history and examination the diagnosis still is unclear, the remainder of the workup includes neuro-imaging and neuro-otologic evaluation. Magnetic resonance imaging is especially useful in detecting parenchymal tumors, demyelinating lesions, and basilar artery thrombosis. Computed tomography (because of its ability to perform thin sections) is probably still most accurate for the detection

Nausea/ Vomiting	Associated Symptoms	Other	Nystagmus	Therapy
+	Otherwise healthy	Viral illness? Otherwise healthy patients		Symptomatic
+ +	—	Worse in certain positions	Horizontal with rotary component	Symptomatic (Dramamine, antivert)
+ + +	+	"Stuffy" ear	Uncommon	Antibiotics
+ +	—	Middle age; diagnose with head-hanging test; benign	+ + with change of head position, subsides spontaneously and faster with exercise, adaptation (?)	Appropriate exercises
+ + +,	Fluctuating tinnitus may precede vertigo	Fullness in ear	May be bilateral	Vestibular neurectomy if intractable
+	Vary with extent and location of trauma	Past pointing	+	As indicated
+	Ataxia, abnormal labyrinthine function (caloric testing); usually recovers	—	Increased with head movement	—
0	V, VI, VII cerebellar ataxia, VII myokymia occipital headache	Rarely true vertigo, but "dizziness" often	Horiz., increased with gaze to side of lesion	Removal of tumor
+ +	Other brain-stem signs: ataxia, diplopia, pry. signs	May be related to head position, age >50	+/−	Symptomatic
Rate	Other CNS symptoms	+/−	+ +	Antimetabolites
Other cr.nn, pyr. symptoms	Depends on location	+ +		
Other brain-stem symptoms	History and family history	Rare	Migraine treatment, abortive or prophylatic	

of small intracanalicular vestibular neurinomas. Audiometric testing can distinguish between cochlear and retrocochlear causes of decreased hearing, and is especially important if a cerebellopontine angle tumor is under consideration. Any vestibular imbalance or associated nystagmus can be documented by caloric testing and electro-nystagmography. Brain-stem auditory evoked potentials can frequently localize the lesion and are especially sensitive to demyelinating processes.

Myxedema is associated with symptoms of light-headedness and, in mysterious cases, where one suspects real disease but has not made a diagnosis to this point, thyroid evaluation is suggested.

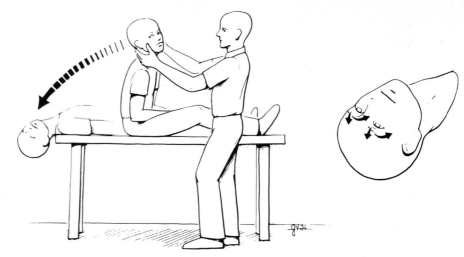

Figure 17–9. Left. The right head-hanging maneuver as described by Dix and Halpike. **Right.** Direction of rotatory nystagmus in right head-hanging position. (*From Mohr DN. The syndrome of paroxysmal positional vertigo: A review. West J Med. 1986;145: 646, with permission.*)

BIBLIOGRAPHY

General

Rengachary SS. Cranial Nerve Examination. In: Wilkins RH, Rengachary SS, eds. *Neurosurgery.* New York: McGraw-Hill, 1985;1.

Carcinomatosis Meningitis

Klee GS. Elevation of CEA in CSF among patients with meningeal carcinomatosis. *Mayo Clin Proc.* 1986;61: 9–13.

Facial Nerve

May M, ed. *The Facial Nerve.* New York: Thieme, 1986.

Blepharospasm

Elston JS, Marsden CD, Grandas F, Quinn NP. The significance of ophthalmologic symptoms in idiopathic blepharospasm. *Eye.* 1988;2:435–439.

Jankovich J. Blepharospasm. In: *Current Therapy in Neurologic Disease,* 2nd ed. Philadelphia: Decker, 1987.

Eighth Nerve

Baloh RW. Neurotology. In: Wilkins RH, Rengachary SS, eds. *Neurosurgery.* New York: McGraw-Hill, 1985;1.

Drachman DA, Hart CW. An approach to the dizzy patient. *Neurology.* 1972;22:323–334.

Mohr DN. The syndrome of paroxysmal positional vertigo: A review. *West J Med.* 1986;145:645–650.

Canal Paresis

Halmagyi GM, Curthoys IS. A clinical sign of canal paresis. *Arch Neurol.* 1988;45:737–739.

Hemifacial Spasm

Digre K, Corbett JJ. Hemifacial spasm: Differential diagnosis, mechanism and treatment. *Adv Neurol.* 1988;49: 151–176.

Jankovic J, Tolosa E, eds. *Facial Dyskinesias.* New York: Raven, 1988.

CHAPTER 18

ORBIT

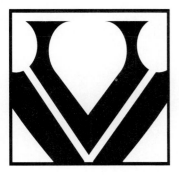

ANATOMY

The bony orbit is a pyramidal or pear-shaped cavity—narrow posteriorly at the apex and widest anteriorly, just behind the orbital opening. Its walls are formed by seven bones—the frontal, sphenoid, maxillary, zygomatic, palatine, ethmoid, and lacrimal bones (Fig. 18–1)—enclosing a volume of approximately 30 cc. The medial walls of the orbit are nearly parallel to the sagittal plane of the cranium; the lateral walls diverge at nearly a 90-degree angle to one another. The orbit is virtually surrounded by the paranasal sinuses except temporally (Fig. 18–2).

The **medial wall** is formed from the lamina papyracea of the ethmoid bone with anterior contributions by the lacrimal bone and frontal process of the maxilla and a posterior contribution from the lesser wing of the sphenoid. The bone of the medial wall is extremely thin as it separates the ethmoid air cells from the orbit. The anterior and posterior ethmoidal arteries and their accompanying veins and nerves pass from the orbit to the ethmoidal air cells through foramina in the medial orbital wall which mark the extent of the anterior cranial fossa. Surgical approaches along the medial wall must carefully consider these structures and the thinness of the lamina papyracea. A deep groove in the lacrimal bone anteriorly houses the lacrimal sac from which the nasolacrimal duct communicates with the inferior meatus of the nose.

The **roof of the orbit** is formed almost entirely by the triangular orbital plate of the frontal bone. Medially it separates the orbit from the frontal sinus; the lateral portions support the frontal lobe of the brain. There are no major vessels or nerves that pierce the orbital roof, simplifying surgical access over this route. Posteriorly, a small portion of the roof is formed from the lesser wing of the sphenoid. The

trochlea, the pulley for the superior oblique tendon, rests medially about 5 mm posterior to the orbital rim; the fossa of the lacrimal gland forms a shallow depression anterolaterally which houses the orbital portion of the lacrimal gland.

The **lateral wall of the orbit** is formed posteriorly by the greater wing of the sphenoid and anteriorly by the zygoma. It lies at approximately 45 degrees to the sagittal plane and medial wall of the orbit. It is the thickest orbital wall.

The **floor of the orbit** is formed primarily from the orbital plate of the maxilla. Posteriorly a small section of the palatine bone and anteriorly part of the zygoma form parts of the floor. The inferior orbital fissure runs forward and laterally from the apex of the orbit, separating the floor from the lateral wall. The palatine and maxillary bones lie medially; the zygoma and the greater wing of the sphenoid lie laterally. Through the fissure the orbit is in contiguity with the pterygoid (sphenopalatine) fossa. The maxillary (V_2) branch of the trigeminal nerve runs through the *inferior orbital groove* in the orbital floor and into the *inferior orbital fissure* before joining with branches from the sphenopalatine fossa to enter the cavernous sinus. Within the inferior orbital fissure there are usually anastomoses between the orbital vasculature originating from the ophthalmic artery, an internal carotid artery branch, and extraorbital vasculature such as the infraorbital branch of the maxillary artery, from the external carotid artery. There are also profuse venous interconnections.

The **superior orbital fissure** separates the lesser and greater wings of the sphenoid bone and lies just inferior and lateral to the optic canal. Structures that pass through the superior orbital fissure include the third, fourth, and sixth cranial nerves and the branches of the ophthalmic (V_1) division of the trigeminal nerve, as well as the superior ophthalmic

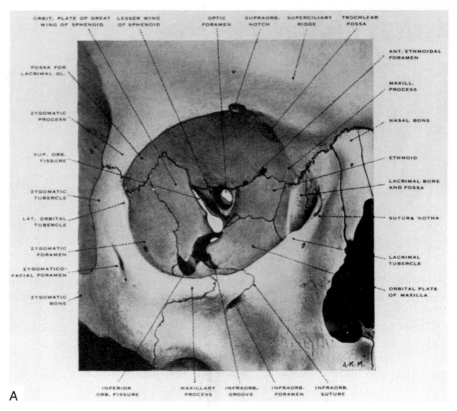

A

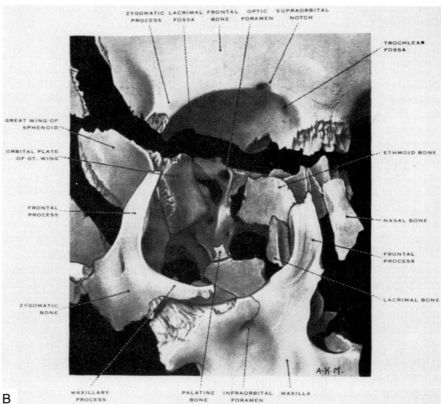

B

Figure 18–1. A. The right orbit viewed along its axis. **B.** The bones of the right orbit in situ but separated. (*From Woolf S. The bony orbit and paranasal sinuses. In:* Anatomy of the Eye and Orbit. *6th ed. Revised by EJ Last. London: Lewis, 1968, with permission.*)

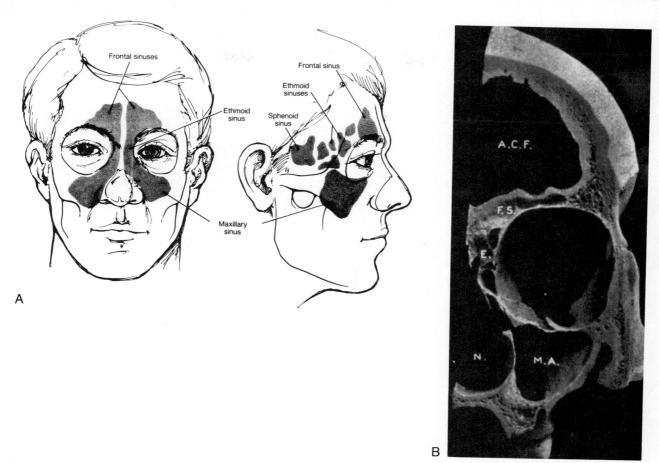

Figure 18–2. **A.** Relationship of the orbits to the paranasal sinuses. **B.** Frontal section of the left half of the skull just behind orbital margin and passing through largest part of cavity (greatest orbital height = 37.5 mm); seen from in front, natural size. (**A.** *From Doxanas MT, Anderson RL. Osteology. In:* Clinical Orbital Anatomy. *Baltimore: Williams & Wilkins, 1984, with permission.* **B.** *From Woolf S. The bony orbit and paranasal sinuses. In:* Anatomy of the Eye and Orbit. *6th ed. Revised by EJ Last. London: Lewis, 1969, with permission.*)

vein. The inferior ophthalmic vein may pass through either the superior or inferior orbital fissure or join the superior orbital vein on its way to the cavernous sinus.

The orbital rim is relatively thick compared to the bones that form the walls of the orbit.

The orbit is lined by periorbita. Anteriorly, it is continuous with the periosteum of the facial bones at the orbital rim; posteriorly, it is continuous with the dura of the intracranial cavity. The optic canal, which exits the orbital apex medially, like the stem of the orbital pear, bridges the orbit and the intracranial cavity, surrounds the optic nerve and the ophthalmic artery, and is separated from the superior orbital fissure by the optic strut.

Orbital Contents. The **four recti muscles** and the superior oblique arise from the tendinous annulus of Zinn, a fibrous ring contiguous with the periorbita

and surrounding the optic canal and medial portion of the superior orbital fissure. The muscles fuse with the sclera in tendinous insertions approximately 6 mm behind the limbus of the globe. The *superior oblique*, the longest of the extraocular muscles, runs forward in the superonasal portion of the orbit, becomes tendinous, passes through the trochlea, and turns obliquely downward, passing beneath the superior rectus muscle to attach to the sclera in the upper temporal quadrant of the eye posterior to the equator. The *inferior oblique* muscle arises from the periorbita at the lacrimal crest of the maxilla just behind the nasal orbital rim and runs superiorly and posteriorly, inferior to the inferior rectus muscle, to attach to the globe inferiorly and temporally but above the level of the lateral rectus in the region of the macula (Fig. 18–3). The *levator palpebrae* arises from the annulus of Zinn and runs anteriorly above the superior rectus in the roof of the orbit. It ends in

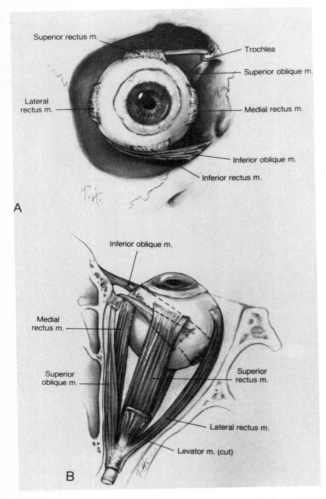

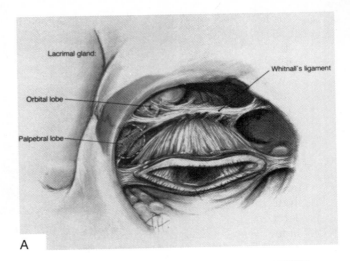

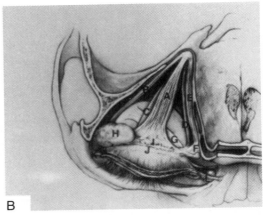

Figure 18–3. The extraocular muscles, orientation in the orbit. **A.** Frontal view. **B.** View from above. (*From Doxanas MT, Anderson RL. Extraocular muscles. In:* Clinical Orbital Anatomy. *Baltimore: Williams & Wilkins, 1984, with permission.*)

Figure 18–4. Superior view of the orbit. *Top.* Schematic diagram. (A, levator muscle; B, lateral rectus muscle; C, superior rectus muscle; D, medial rectus muscle; E, superior oblique muscle; F, trochlea; G, superior oblique tendon; H, lacrimal gland; I, Whitnall's ligament; J, levator aponeurosis; K, lateral canthal tendon; L, medial canthal tendon.) **B.** The lacrimal gland. The levator aponeurosis divides the lacrimal gland into an orbital and palpebral lobe, with the palpebral lobe laying beneath the levator aponeurosis. Whitnall's ligament provides support for the lacrimal gland. *Bottom.* Histologically, the fibers of the levator aponeurosis split the lacrimal gland into its two components. (OL, orbital lobe of lacrimal gland; PL, palpebral lobe of lacrimal gland; LA, levator aponeurosis; B, main excretory duct of lacrimal gland.) (H&E, ×50.) (*From Doxanas MT, Anderson RL. Eyebrows, eyelids and anterior orbit. In:* Clinical Orbital Anatomy. *Baltimore: Williams & Wilkins, 1984, with permission.*)

a broad triangular aponeurotic insertion that fans out to insert on the breadth of the tarsus of the upper lid and on the orbital rim. The tendon continues medially and laterally as tendinous insertions that join the tendon of the superior oblique and the capsule of the orbital lobe of the lacrimal gland, respectively (Fig. 18–4).

Many masses in the superior orbit are of an infiltrating or inflammatory nature (invasive lacrimal gland tumors, "pseudotumor," mucocele) and may involve the levator. Beware of the patient with a preoperative ptosis as the levator fibers may be intimately involved in the mass. In these cases, excisional surgery may extirpate significant portions of the levator as well as tumor, causing a postoperative ptosis that is exceedingly difficult to repair.

Connective tissue condensations encase the globe as Tenon's capsule, continuous posteriorly around the optic nerve with the perineural sheaths, which are in turn continuations of the meninges. Anteriorly, the reflections of Tenon's capsule surround the tendons and muscles of the globe with sleeve-like extensions, also forming a broad circumferential band, the intermuscular septum, and a large inferior suspensory ligament of the globe, Lockwood's ligament. Throughout the orbit, the connective tissue structures form complex and variable compartments (Fig. 18–5).

At the anterior margins of the orbit, the periorbita is thickened, giving attachment to the orbital septum which fuses with the levator aponeurosis in the upper lid and the tarsal plate in the lower lid, forming an incomplete partition across the orbital opening.

The nerves of the orbit. (Fig. 18–6) The ocular motor nerves are described in Chapter 19. Only a brief description is given here.

The **ocular motor nerves** all enter the orbit through the superior orbital fissure (Table 18–1). The trochlear nerve enters the superior oblique muscle superolaterally in its posterior quarter. The oculo-

motor nerve divides into two divisions, either in the cavernous sinus or the superior orbit. The superior division supplies the superior rectus and levator muscles entering the posterior thirds of both muscles on their undersurfaces. The inferior ramus supplies the medial rectus on its medial surface and the posterior third of the inferior rectus similarly. Another branch carries the parasympathetic fibers to the ciliary ganglion before entering the inferior oblique muscle posteriorly, approximately halfway along the length of the muscle. The abducens nerve supplies the lateral rectus muscle at approximately its posterior third and enters the muscle from its medial surface.

The **sensory nerves of the orbit** are branches of

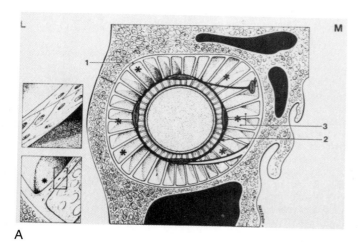

A

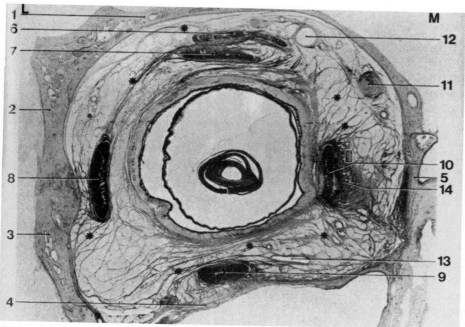

B

Figure 18–5. A. Schematic arrangement of the fibrous septa. Asterisks indicate the areas where smooth muscle tissue was found. (1, periorbit; 2, common muscle sheath at eyeball level; 3, fibrous septa. L, lateral; M, medial.) **B.** Frontally sectioned histologic section (60u) of an adult right orbit, at a level in the orbit 3.2 mm anteriorly from the hind surface of the eye. (Asterisks, connective tissue septa; 1, frontal bone; 2, greater wing of the sphenoid; 3, zygomatic bone; 4, maxilla; 5, ethmoid; 6, superior levator palpebral muscle; 7, superior rectus muscle; 8, lateral rectus muscle; 9, inferior rectus muscle; 10, medial rectus muscle; 11, superior oblique muscle; 12, superior ophthalmic vein; 13, branches of the inferior ophthalmic vein; 14, medial check ligament; M, medial; L, lateral.) (Acidic fuchsin–picrin acid/von Gieson, ×2.5.) (*From Koorneef L. Human orbital connective tissue.* Arch Ophthalmol. *1977;95:1269–1273, with permission.*)

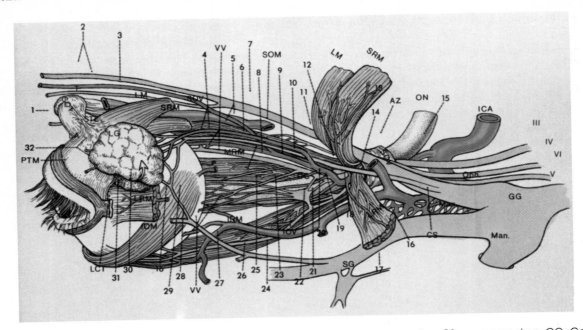

Figure 18–6. Nerves of the orbit and orbital contents. Annulus of Zinn. CG, ciliary ganglion; CS, cavernous sinus; GG, Gasserian ganglion; ICA, internal carotid artery; IOM, inferior oblique muscle; IOV, inferior ophthalmic vein; IRM, inferior rectus muscle; LA, levator aponeurosis; LCT, lateral canthal tendon; LG, lacrimal gland; LM, levator muscle; LRM, lateral rectus ophthalmic nerve; Man, mandibular nerve; Max, maxillary nerve; MRM, medial rectus muscle; ON, optic nerve; Oph, ophthalmic nerve; PTM, pretarsal muscle; SG, sphenopalatine ganglion; SOM, superior oblique muscle; SOT, superior oblique tendon; SOV, superior ophthalmic vein; SRM, superior rectus muscle; STL, superior transverse ligament; T, trochlea; VV, vortex veins; 1, intratrochlear nerve; 2, supraorbital nerve and artery; 3, supratrochlear nerve; 4, anterior ethmoid nerve and artery; 5, lacrimal nerve and artery; 6, posterior ethmoid artery; 7, frontal nerve; 8, long ciliary nerves; 9, branch of oculomotor nerve (III) to medial rectus muscle; 10, nasociliary nerve; 11, trochlear nerve (IV); 12, ophthalmic (orbital) artery; 13, superior ramus of oculomotor nerve (III); 14, abducens nerve (VI); 15, ophthalmic artery, origin; 16, anterior ciliary artery; 17, vidian nerve; 18, inferior ramus of oculomotor nerve (III); 19, central retinal artery; 20, sensory branches from ciliary ganglion to nasociliary nerve; 21, motor (parasympathetic) nerve to ciliary ganglion from nerve to inferior oblique muscle; 22, branch of oculomotor nerve (III) to inferior rectus muscle; 23, short ciliary nerves; 24, zygomatic nerve; 25, posterior ciliary arteries; 26, zygomaticofacial nerve; 27, nerve to inferior oblique muscle; 28, zygomaticotemporal nerve; 29, lacrimal secretory nerve; 30, lacrimal gland-palpebral lobe; 31, lateral horn of levator aponeurosis; 32, lacrimal artery and nerve, terminal branches. (*From Stewart WB. Ophthalmic Plastic and Reconstructive Surgery. 4th ed. Rochester, MN: Academy Manual Program/American Academy of Ophthalmology, 1984, with permission.*)

the trigeminal nerve. The first division, the ophthalmic division (V_1), divides into three orbital branches: the nasociliary, frontal, and lacrimal branches. The frontal nerve runs forward and below the roof of the orbit and superior to the levator, dividing into the supraorbital and supratrochlear nerves to the tissues of the supraorbital area. The lacrimal nerve supplies sensory fibers to the lacrimal gland, skin of the lid, and superolateral orbital tissues. It anastomoses prior to entering the orbital portion of the lacrimal gland with the lacrimal secretory branch of the zygomaticotemporal nerve, a branch of the maxillary nerve (V_2).

The nasociliary branch gives rise to the long ciliary nerves, the anterior and posterior ethmoidal nerves, and the infratrochlear nerve which supplies sensation to the side and tip of the nose.

The **ciliary ganglion** is primarily a parasympathetic way station but also transmits sympathetic and sensory fibers to the globe. Recent studies suggest that some parasympathetic fibers also either pass through the ganglion without synapsing or reach the globe without transmitting the ciliary ganglion. It lies approximately 10 mm from the apex (20 mm from the globe) of the orbit, lateral and sometimes slightly inferior to the optic nerve. It may be injured in lateral approaches to the optic nerve and in retinal and extraocular muscle surgery, resulting in an Adie's-like pupil (see Chapter 16).

From the ciliary ganglion, **short ciliary nerves** carry fibers to the globe, bridging the sclera circumferentially around the optic nerve.

The **maxillary nerve** (V_2) enters the orbit from the sphenopalatine ganglion, having picked up lacrimal secretory fibers, and runs into the inferior orbital fissure. Here the zygomatic nerve branches off, divides into the zygomaticotemporal branch mentioned above, and anastomoses with the lacrimal

TABLE 18–1. CONTENTS OF ORBITAL FISSURES AND CANALS

	Location	Contents
Optic canal	Lesser wing of sphenoid	Optic nerve, meninges, ophthalmic artery, and sympathetic fibers
Superior orbital fissure	Lesser and greater wing of sphenoid	Nerves 　Motor: (oculomotor—III (superior and inferior divisions), IV (trochlear), and VI (abducens) 　Sensory: V_1 (trigeminal—ophthalmic division) frontal lacrimal, nasociliary branches Sympathetic fibers Vessels 　Superior ophthalmic vein 　Anastomosis of recurrent lacrimal and middle meningeal arteries
Inferior orbital fissure	Greater wing of sphenoid, palatine, zygomatic, and maxillary bones	Nerves 　Sensory: V_2 (trigeminal—maxillary division) infraorbital and zygomatic branches 　Parasympathetic 　Branches from pterygopalatine ganglion Vessels: inferior ophthalmic vein and branches to pterygoid plexus
Anterior ethmoid canal	Frontal and ethmoid	Nerve: Anterior ethmoid becomes dorsal nasal Vessel: Anterior ethmoid artery
Posterior ethmoid canal	Frontal and ethmoid	Nerve: Posterior ethmoid Vessel: Posterior ethmoid
Nasolacrimal fossa	Lacrimal and maxillary bones	Nasolacrimal sac and duct

From Rootman J. Anatomy of the orbit. In: Rootman J, ed. Diseases of the Orbit: A Multidisciplinary Approach. New York: Lippincott, 1988:8.

nerve before entering the lacrimal gland. The zygomaticofacial nerves exit the orbit through the zygoma to provide sensation to the lateral and inferior periorbital area. The maxillary nerve continues in the infraorbital groove, anterior to the inferior orbital fissure, and as the infraorbital nerve pierces the infraorbital foramen of the maxillary bone and supplies sensation to the cheek and upper lip. It is frequently damaged in trauma or neoplastic invasion of the orbital floor.

Arising from the sympathetic plexus surrounding the internal carotid artery, the **sympathetic nerves** enter the orbit with the ophthalmic artery. They are thought to follow the various branches of the ophthalmic artery to their target tissues in the orbit.

As was mentioned above, the **orbital portion of the optic nerve** is approximately 30 mm in length and takes an S-shaped course to the orbital apex and optic canal.

The **blood supply to the orbit** comes almost exclusively from the ophthalmic artery, which branches from the internal carotid artery and passes into the orbit with the optic nerve through the optic canal. It supplies muscular branches to the muscles of the orbit; supplies the globe via the short posterior ciliary arteries, anterior ciliary arteries, and central retinal artery; and feeds the pial plexus which nourishes the optic nerve. There are extensive anastomoses with external carotid artery (ECA) branches.

The **venous drainage of the orbit and the eye** forms two major channels, the superior and inferior ophthalmic veins. The superior ophthalmic vein originates in the region of the trochlea and exits the orbit through the superior orbital fissure, having been joined by the superior vortex veins and veins from the superior portion of the orbit. The inferior ophthalmic vein may join the superior ophthalmic vein in the orbital apex or may enter the cavernous sinus independently.

The **lacrimal gland** lies in the superior lateral portion of the orbit. The orbital lobe sits in the lacrimal fossa whereas the palpebral lobe resides subconjunctively, being separated from the orbital lobe by the levator aponeurosis. Thus, the ducts from the orbital lobe of the gland must pass through the palpebral lobe, joining with its ducts to pierce the conjunctiva.

All the orbital contents are cushioned in the orbital fat.

The **eyelids** protectively slide over the front surface of the eyeball. They are structured on the framework of the tarsi and orbital septum, covered by very thin skin and lined by conjuctiva. The tarsal plates (tarsi) are formed by very dense connective tissue, anchored laterally by the ribbonlike lateral palpebral ligament to the orbital tubercle of the zygoma. Medially, the tarsi are connected with a limb of the Y-shaped medial palpebral ligament, which passes in front of the lacrimal sac to the frontal process of the maxilla with deep fibers merging with the lacrimal fascia. The subcutaneous tissue of the eyelid is devoid of fat and is the locus of the orbicularis oculi. This tissue is especially loose in construction and very sensitive to any increase in tissue fluid pressure which is seen as puffiness of the eyelids.

The palpebral fissure, the interval between the lids, is oval when the eyes are open. The margin of the upper lid should cover the upper limbus by about 2 mm, while the lower lid usually rests at the level of the lower limbus. As the eyes are closed by the orbicularis oculi, the upper lid descends, while the lower lid moves slightly medially, but changes little in vertical position.

The eyelids are supplied by the palpebral branches of the ophthalmic artery which pierce the orbital septum to form arcades near the margins of the lids. The subconjunctival veins drain to the ophthalmic veins; in contrast, the subcutaneous veins drain to the facial and superficial temporal drainage areas. The skin of the upper lid is innervated by branches of the ophthalmic division of the trigeminal nerve (V_1) and the lower lid by branches of the maxillary division (V_2). The passage of these structures through the various orbital fissures and canals is outlined in Table 18–1.

SIGNS AND SYMPTOMS OF ORBITAL DISEASE

Exophthalmos (Proptosis): Exophthalmos is a familiar sign of orbital disease. As the orbit is a bony pyramid with rigid sides everywhere except anteriorly, the path of least resistance to any expansive process within the orbit is forward. Thus any process that increases the volume of the orbital contents will cause forward protrusion of the globe (exophthalmos or proptosis), other orbital tissues, or both. To some extent, the direction of the proptosis is suggestive of the location of the orbital process. Because the majority of orbital masses is located superiorly, the most frequent direction of proptosis is downward. Inferior orbital masses such as lymphoma or maxillary sinus pathology cause upward displacement. Anterior masses are likely to cause more displacement then

exophthalmos, whereas posterior masses cause more exophthalmos than displacement. Primary optic nerve tumors such as optic nerve glioma and optic nerve sheath meningioma almost always cause a decrease in visual acuity before exophthalmos.

Obviously, the critical relationship is that between the volume of the orbital contents and the volume of the orbit. Any disproportion that results in an increase in the volume of the orbital contents relative to the orbital cavity will cause an apparent proptosis. Thus, it is important to rule out causes of pseudoproptosis before embarking on an extensive workup for exophthalmos. Pseudoproptosis may occur when the eyeball is enlarged, as in high myopia, posterior staphyloma, or congenital glaucoma (buphthalmos). Occasionally, the eye falsely may appear to be proptotic with lid retraction, widening of the palpebral fissure, or contralateral enophthalmos; however, measurement of the position of the cornea will reveal a lack of true protrusion of the eye. An apparent proptosis can occur when the orbits are small, as in craniofacial anomalies (such as Apert's syndrome and Cruzon's disease), or when the bony orbit encroaches upon the orbital contents (as in fibrous dysplasia or sphenoid ridge meningioma).

In contrast to exophthalmos, **enophthalmos** is a relatively rare presentation of orbital disorders (Table 18–2). It occurs most frequently when a blowout fracture enlarges the orbital space or allows the orbital contents to herniate outside the normal bony

TABLE 18–2. ETIOLOGY OF ENOPHTHALMOS

Structural abnormality	Trauma
	Asymmetry
	Destruction of the orbital floor
	Absence of sphenoid wing (von Recklinghausen neurofibromatosis–NF-1)
	Sympathetic paresis
Atrophy	Posttraumatic
	Following irradiation
	Lipodystrophy
	Varix
	Marasmus and senility
	Phthisis
Cicatrization	Posttraumatic
	Following inflammation (sclerosing pseudotumor)
	Metastatic schirrous carcinoma
	Postsurgical shortening "Nystagmus" retractorius
	Linear scleroderma
	Progressive facial hemiatrophy (Parry-Romberg syndrome)

From Rootman J. Frequency and differential diagnosis of orbital disease. In: Rootman J, ed. Diseases of the Orbit: A Multidisciplinary Approach. New York: Lippincott, 1988:131.

orbit. More rarely, atrophy of orbital fat following trauma or associated with hemifacial atrophy causes enophthalmos. Two additional etiologies are (1) scirrhous carcinoma of the breast metastatic to the orbit; and (2) sclerosing pseudotumor; both of which are associated with very firm orbits, usually significant limitation of motility, and (at times) chemosis or other signs of inflammation.

Diplopia is another important symptom of orbital disease. In fact, thyroid orbitopathy is one of the most frequent causes of acquired diplopia in adulthood, especially when the limitation of motility does not conform to the pattern of an ocular motor nerve palsy. Although cranial nerve palsies occur in orbital disease, restrictive limitations of eye movement—such as those caused by thyroid orbitopathy, orbital pseudotumor, trauma, and orbital masses—are much more common. **Forced duction** testing (see Chapter 15) is important for confirmation of the motility restriction.

Alterations in lid position. Lid position changes offer important clues to orbital disease. Lid retraction is essentially pathognomonic of thyroid orbitopathy, but can occur in sclerosing lesions and

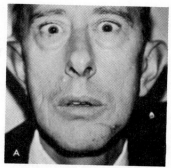
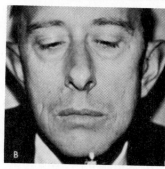
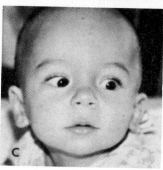

Figure 18-8. Pathologic lid retraction (Collier's sign) in rostral mesencephalic disorders. **A.** Patient with penealoma. Note position of lids in forward gaze. Pupils are mid dilated and light fixed. **B.** On downward gaze lids follow eyes smoothly without retraction. **C.** "Setting sun" sign with lid retraction, associated with infantil hydrocephalus. *From Glaser, J.S. Neuro-ophthalmic Examination. In: Duane, T, ed. Clinical Ophthalmology, Hagerstown, Md: Harper & Row, 1976; 2, with permission.*

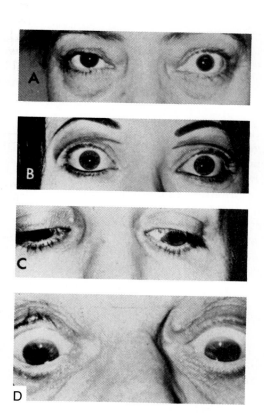

Figure 18-7. Spectrum of lid retraction in dysthyroidism. **A.** Mild unilateral retraction. **B.** Moderate bilateral "stare." **C.** Modest unilateral lid lag on downward gaze. **D.** Marked lid retraction in downward gaze. *From Glaser, J.S. Neuro-ophthalmic Examination. In: Duane, T, ed. Clinical Ophthalmology, Hagerstown, Md: Harper & Row, 1976; 2, with permission.*

(rarely) in cirrhosis. True lid retraction must be differentiated from the apparent lid retraction that occurs in attempted upgaze when there is a paresis of upward gaze (Collier's sign) or tonic downward deviation of the eyes (setting sun sign) (Figs. 18–7, 18–8). Exophthalmos may give a false impression of lid retraction as may contralateral enophthalmos. Ptosis occurs in involvement of the lid and levator by orbital masses as well as with third-nerve palsies and Horner's syndrome.

Visual loss. Visual loss from optic nerve compromise occurs either primarily (optic nerve tumors) or secondarily (compression, inflammation, or ischemia). On ophthalmoscopic examination, chronic optic nerve damage may be heralded by optic atrophy and retinal nerve fiber layer changes. Disc swelling occurs in optic nerve involvement or obstruction of venous outflow from the globe or orbit. The triad of exophthalmos, optic atrophy, and an associated optociliary shunt vessel at the disc, if associated with decreased visual acuity, is nearly pathognomonic of an optic nerve sheath meningioma. Rarely, an enlarged blind spot or visual field defect will be the presenting symptom of orbital pathology.

Another ophthalmoscopic finding in orbital disease is **choroidal fields.** (See Chapter 3).

Chemosis or edema of the conjunctiva usually indicates venous stasis or inflammation. In the latter case, pain and suffusion of the conjunctiva as well as swelling are present. In thyroid orbitopathy, a typical "finger" edema of the lids is often present.

Pulsation: Vascular lesions, carotid–cavernous or dural fistulas, and ateriovenous malformations with large flow, have orbital and ocular pulsations synchronous with the pulse. Defects in the orbital walls may be associated with similar pulsations, show protrusion with increased venous pressure or the Valsalva maneuver, or trasmit cerebrospinal fluid pulsations, as in sphenoid wing defects associated with neurofibromatosis (Table 18–3). Rarely, a defect in the lateral orbital wall permits contraction of the temporalis muscle to be transmitted to the orbit.

EVALUATION OF ORBITAL DISEASE

History: The history, in addition to detailing the onset and progression of symptoms, should also explore the tempo of the process, whether it is intermittent or otherwise episodic and whether there are any systemic disorders that might be associated with the orbital pathology. Defects of the sphenoid bone—congenital as in neurofibromatosis, surgical, or acquired as in intracavernous aneurysms—may cause pulsating exophthalmos. Venous vascular abnormalities (lymphangioma), especially in children, following upper respiratory tract infections, are infrequently associated with repeated orbital hemorrhages and proptosis. A history of sinus disease or recent nasal drainage may give an important clue as to the etiology of an orbital inflammatory process or a mass such as a mucocele. Primary tumors elsewhere in the body, of course, may metastasize to the orbit, and the orbit may be affected in systemic processes such as neurofibromatosis, Albright's disease, and Wegener's granulomatosis. Many orbital disorders are age specific in their presentations. A history of trauma should be sought.

Pain is a nonspecific symptom seen most frequently with inflammatory processes and with rap-

TABLE 18–3. DYNAMIC LESIONS OF THE ORBIT (PULSATING EXOPHTHALMOS)

Bone Defects	Congenital absence of sphenoid wing (neurofibromatosis)
	Meningoencephalocele
	Potentially destructive lesions of bone
	Massive frontal mucocele
	Aneurysmal bone cyst
	Reparative granuloma
	Xanthomatous lesion of bone
	Posttraumatic or postsurgical bone dehiscence
	Dermoid and other orbital cysts, especially with rupture or inflammation
	Metastatic lytic tumors of bone
	Histiocytosis X
AV Shunts	Capillary hemangioma
	High-flow congenital and acquired shunts (carotid–cavernous sinus fistulae, arteriovenous malformations)
	Vascular tumors
	Thyroid carcinoma
	Nephroblastoma
	Prostatic carcinoma
Venous Anomalies	Distensible varices
	Venous angiomas, "lymphangioma"

Modified from Rootman J. Anatomy of the orbit. In: Rootman J, ed. Diseases of the Orbit: A Multidisciplinary Approach. New York: Lippincott, 1988:131.

idly expansive lesions either primary in the orbit or metastatic (eg, adenocarcinomas of bowel and sometimes breast or bony invasion).

Examination: Examination of the orbital disease patient begins with observation and palpation. Note the position of the globe in the orbit and the positions of the lids. Also note any abnormalities or asymmetry of the orbital adnexae. Determine the best corrected visual acuity; evaluate color vision and the visual field. Palpation will give clues about the nature of the disease process by detecting masses, irregularities, tenderness, warmth (in acute anterior infections), and pulsation of the globe or orbital contents (directly or indirectly, eg, on tonometry). Evaluate the pupils and motility.

The ease of **retropulsion** of the globe is assessed by gentle pressure or ballotment. The character of the palpated mass (eg, hard, ropey, or fluctuant) may also be of assistance in determining the etiology and pathology. The orbit and temporal area should be auscultated for bruits.

Especially in cases of intermittent proptosis, the

patient should be asked to perform a *Valsalva maneuver* in order to attempt to fill any venous channels contributing to the proptosis.

In addition to detecting disc swelling, optic atrophy, and cilioretinal shunt vessels, *fundoscopy* may reveal primary intraocular masses, high myopia, posterior staphyloma, or buphthalmos, or involvement of the globe with orbital processes such as pseudotumor. Retinal striae, choroidal folds, or acquired hyperopia suggests a mass deforming the posterior aspect of the globe or tethering the optic nerve.

Rubor usually indicates an inflammation or infectious process. Local infiltration by lymphoproliferative disease or rapidly invasive tumors, such as rhabdomyosarcomas and metastatic carcinoma, also cause lid rubor and chemosis. Lid ecchymoses are found in orbital hematomas and leukemia, whereas metastases of neuroblastoma cause a similar but more violaceous color of the lids.

Injection of the conjunctiva or dilation of conjunctival veins may occur with or without chemosis and is typical of inflammatory processes and vascular abnormalities (Table 18–4).

Verify any apparent *exophthalmos* by examining the globes from above (looking over the brows from a position above the patient's head to see if there is actual protrusion or asymmetry of the globe position) and quantify by exophthalmometry.

Many methods have been devised to measure the position of the globe relative to some landmark, usually a portion of the skull. None of the methods is perfect because some of the disease processes that cause exophthalmos also cause or are associated with deformities of the bony skull (eg, fibrous dysplasia or absence of the orbital rim following a lateral orbitotomy).

A most common and practical means of measuring the position of the globe in the frontal plane is to measure the horizontal and vertical position of the globe by placing a clear ruler across the bridge of the patient's nose. Align the edges of the ruler with the lateral canthus (obviously, any distortion of the lateral orbital rim will decrease the reliability of this method). Any vertical displacement of the globe is evident immediately. Then, measure the distance from the center of the nose to each nasal limbus to detect any horizontal displacement (Fig. 18–9A, B).

Exophthalmometry: Many instruments have been devised to measure exophthalmos. Most of them measure displacement in an anterior posterior plane by measuring the difference between the apex of the cornea and a point on the bony margin of the orbit.

The instrument most commonly used for assessment of exophthalmos is a Hertel exophthalmometer or one of its variants. In these devices, foot plates rest on the lateral orbital rims, and by means of mirrors the reflection of the cornea is superimposed on a measuring scale, with measuring lines drawn to correct for parallax (Fig. 18–9C).

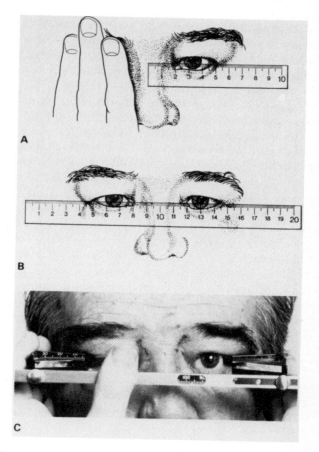

Figure 18–9. A. Measurement of horizontal displacement of eye by recording distance (in millimeters) at level of canthi from center of nose to medial edge of limbus. **B.** Measurement of vertical displacement of eye by recording position of globe above or below level of canthi. **C.** Measurement of proptosis with exophthalmometer; with other eye occluded, patient looks along central axis. *(From Rootman J. An Approach to diagnosis of orbital disease. Can J. Ophthalmol. 1983;18:103.)*

TABLE 18–4. CAUSES OF ACUTE ORBITAL INFLAMMATION

Cellulitis (bacterial or fungal)
Graves' disease
Idiopathic inflammatory pseudotumor
Retained orbital foreign body
Orbital thrombophlebitis
Ruptured dermoid
Vasculitis
Collagen disease
Orbital hemorrhage
Lymphangioma
Metastatic neuroblastoma and leukemia

From Jones IS, Jakobiec FA, Nolan BT. Patient Examination and Introduction to Orbital Disease. In: Duane T, ed. Clinical Ophthalmology. Hagerstown, MD: Harper & Row, 1976;2;29.

One of the simplest devices is the Luedde exophthalmometer, which is simply a piece of plastic ruled on both sides. It is held against the lateral orbital rim and parallel to the visual axis while the patient looks straight ahead. The distance from the orbital rim to the apex of the cornea is measured and, if the scales on both sides are properly aligned, the problem with parallax is eliminated.

The Mutch exophthalmometer has the advantage that it measures from the brow and cheek and, therefore, is of value when the lateral orbital rim is distorted by the pathologic process or surgery.

Normally, the corneal apex extends about 16 mm anterior to the lateral orbital rim. Values from 10 to 22 mm are within the normal range. There appear to be some racial differences with blacks having relatively more protuberant eyeballs, such that a reading of 24 mm may still be within the normal range. Readings outside this range are abnormal and differences of more than 2 mm between the two eyes are also abnormal.

The attitude of the head is also of importance, as the globe falls approximately 2 mm into the orbit in the supine position. The absence of this descent has been used diagnostically in cases of orbital tumors and endocrine exophthalmos.

Radiographic estimates of ocular protrusion have often been made, especially in an attempt to find a more reliable reference point than the lateral orbital rim. However, most of these are expensive and impractical for daily use. Modern neuro-imaging allows such accurate depiction of orbital topography that these elaborate methods have no practical advantage over the simpler ones.

ORBITAL DISORDERS

Differential Diagnosis of Exophthalmos

The differential diagnosis of exophthalmos begins by grouping the disorders into several large categories: inflammatory disorders (Fig. 18–10).

Infectious and Inflammatory Orbital Disorders. Infectious and inflammatory diseases of the orbit cover a wide spectrum (Fig. 18–11 and Table 18–4). They may be explosive or insidious in onset; they may involve the orbit diffusely, isolated tissues within the orbit, or multiple tissues in one geographic portion of the orbit; the etiologies range from common to obscure; the orbit may be involved in isolation or in contiguity with surrounding structures such as the sinuses or intracranial contents. One entity, idiopathic inflammatory pseudotumor, is an inflammation, acts like a tumor, and histopathologically merges almost imperceptibly with orbital lymphomas. All these processes may present with proptosis, ptosis, motility disturbance, and visual loss. The degree of lid erythema, edema, conjunctival injection, chemosis, and pain is usually related to the degree of inflammation present.

Thyroid orbitopathy: This autoimmune disorder is the most frequent cause of both unilateral and

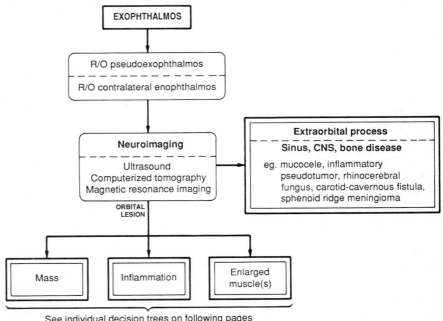

Figure 18–10. Decision tree of exophthalmos.

See individual decision trees on following pages

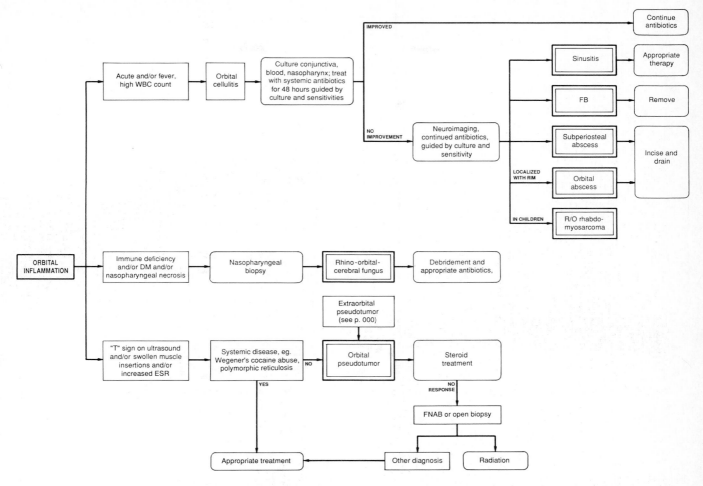

Figure 18–11. Decision Tree of orbital inflammation.

bilateral exophthalmos. In most cases, an apparent unilateral exophthalmos is really an asymmetric involvement of the two orbits, as the orbits are bilaterally involved. Thyroid orbitopathy also is probably the most frequent cause of acquired diplopia unrelated to extraocular muscle palsy. Even when there is no clear history of thyroid disease, the associated signs will almost always establish the diagnosis. Lid retraction is present in a majority of patients. Lid lag is also frequently seen, as are chemosis, injection over the insertions of the recti muscles, and a peculiar finger edema of the lids (Fig. 18–12).

If the onset of symptoms is rapid, especially if the inflammatory changes predominate and the asymmetry is marked, the clinical picture must be differentiated from idiopathic orbital inflammation (which is usually unilateral) in adults and from rhabdomyosarcoma and orbital cellulitis in children.

The associated motility disorder is a restrictive myopathy that clinically involves upgaze (the inferior rectus) most frequently. However, on neuroimaging, the medial rectus is enlarged more often than the inferior rectus. The motility disorder must be distinguished from other myopathies, primary myositis, dural fistulas, and the effects of certain pituitary tumors, especially those that produce acromegaly (Fig. 18–13). All these entities produce enlarged extraocular muscles and chemosis. Maxillary antral carcinoma invasive into the floor of the orbit and orbital trauma with entrapment of connective tissue or muscles also cause restrictive myopathies. Neurogenic causes of upgaze limitation such as double-elevator palsy and skew deviation are more easily differentiated, often by the frequently associated neurologic concomitants and, especially, by forced duction testing, which is abnormal in restrictive myopathies and normal in ocular motor nerve palsy, strabismus, myopathy, skew, and so forth.

The exact relationship of the orbitopathy to thy-

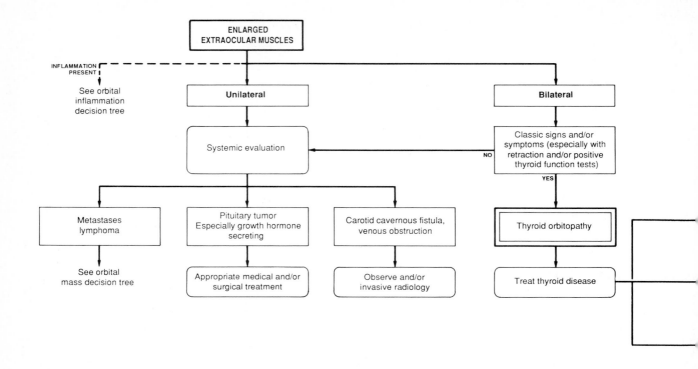

Figure 18–12. Decision Tree of enlarged extraocular muscles.

roid dysfunction is unclear; in fact, it is not even known whether the orbitopathy occurs in the absence of disease of the thyroid gland or pituitary–thyroid axis. Personal observations suggest that the orbitopathy occurs when the level of thyroid function changes, whether it be from normal to abnormal or vice-versa. Thus, patients who are euthyroid and become hyperthyroid, patients who are euthyroid and become hypothyroid, or patients who are hyperthyroid and become euthyroid, all exhibit thyroid orbitopathy. Nearly all patients with Graves' disease have some ophthalmopathy but it is clinically evident in only about 40%. It is widely recognized that the orbital changes may become apparent shortly after the treatment of classical thyrotoxicosis. Thus, patients may show no systemic symptoms of thyroid disorder; may be hyperthyroid with weakness, weight loss, nervousness, and palpitations; or may be hypothyroid with cold intolerance, lethargy, and constipation. In all, about 80% of patients develops orbital involvement during or after an episode of hyperthyroidism. Approximately 75% develops orbital involvement within a year prior to or after the appearance of the hyperthyroidism. Thereafter, significant progression of the orbitopathy is uncommon,

although exacerbations often occur following antithyroid therapy. Whether this is coincidental or a result of therapy remains controversial.

Pathogenesis. Although we continue to learn about thyroid orbitopathy and associated thyroid disorders, the precise mechanisms involved in its pathogenesis remain obscure. There is infiltration of the extraocular muscles, orbital fat, and skin by lymphocytes, plasma cells, macrophages, and mast cells with increased deposition of mucopolysaccharides, especially hyaluronic acid released by proliferating fibroblasts. Their hydrophilic nature contributes to the tissue swelling. All this occurs on an autoimmune basis. Ultimately, there is collagen deposition and muscle degeneration. Classic Graves' disease is associated with multiple antibodies to thyroid cell membranes and/or thyroid-stimulating autoantibodies to the thyrotropin receptor. Patients with thyroid orbitopathy possess serum autoantibodies to eye muscle membrane antigens and orbital fibroblasts, which also produce cytotoxic effects on extraocular muscle. In some studies, the antibody level is proportional to the severity of orbital disease. How antibodies to cell membranes produce hyperthyroidism and/or its orbital concomitants is not understood.

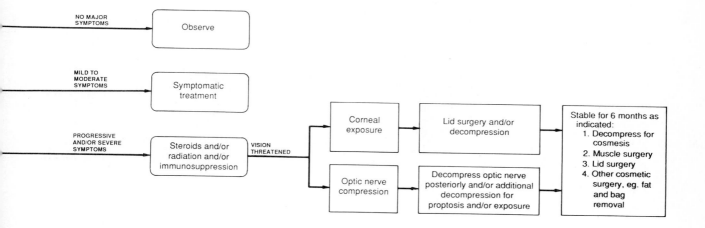

Wall has hypothesized that the antibody–antigen reaction on the cell membrane exposes orbital proteins to further antibody production and leads to tissue damage by the action of killer cells, rather than being the direct cause.

Diagnosis. Patients with a clinical presentation suggestive of thyroid orbitopathy should be evaluated for thyroid disease. The "sensitive" thyroid-stimulating hormone (TSH) assays (immunoradiomimetic IRMA) give the most accurate assessment of thyroid function, replacing not only the free thyroxin index (FTI) but also thyrotropin-releasing hormone (TRH) stimulation and T_3 suppression for evaluation of TSH levels. A normal "sensitive" TSH assay is a reliable prediction of euthyroidism; an increase in free thyroxine indicates thyrotoxicosis and a decrease indicates hypothyroidism.

Despite the sensitivity of modern assays, there is still a significant number of patients (about 15%) who appear to have Graves' orbitopathy without evidence of disturbance of the hypothalamic–thyroid axis or thyroid hormones. Almost all of these patients will show characteristic findings on ultrasound, computed tomography (CT), or magnetic resonance imaging (MRI).

Because of the high prevalence of thyroid eye disease, thyroid function testing should also be performed in patients with otherwise unexplained exophthalmos or motility disorders. In addition, this group of patients should have a baseline visual evoked potential evaluation, which may be the most sensitive indication of an associated optic neuropathy. Usually the clinical diagnosis of thyroid orbitopathy will be confirmed by ultrasound, CT scan, or MRI. Ultrasonography, because there are quantitative norms established for the maximum diameters of the extraocular muscles, is probably the most sensitive. CT and MRI have the advantage of being able to display both orbits simultaneously and in coronal sections. This gives an excellent overview of the status of the extraocular muscles. In addition, CT and MRI are superior in imaging the orbital apex for evaluation of possible optic nerve compression. Interestingly, patients with optic neuropathy have less proptosis, perhaps because of a firmer orbital septum. These patients may also be older and have diabetes. Quantitative studies have been done with CT scanning, but most facilities do not take the time for this more demanding method. Usually, when multiple muscles of both orbits are involved, the diagnosis of thyroid orbitopathy is established. Rarely, the my-

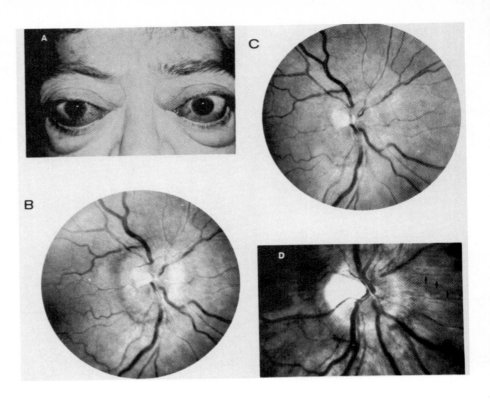

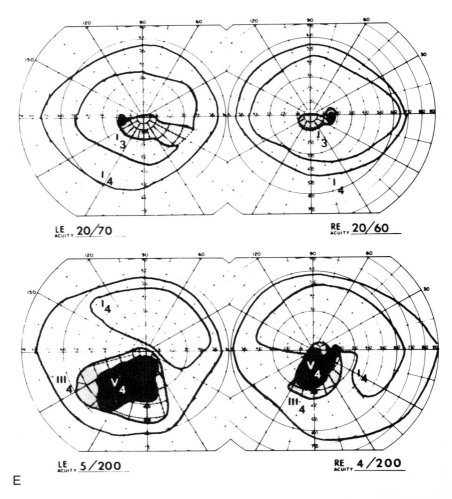

Figure 18–13. Dysthyroid optic neuropathy. **A.** Patient with four years of stable ophthalmopathy noted progressive right visual loss to 20/80 (6/24). **B.** Right disc is edematous and elevated. Lateral orbital decompression with floor fracture was performed. Within 48 hours vision was 20/25, and disc detumesced **(C) D.** Fundus of different patient demonstates hypermic edematous disc, and retinochoroidal folds (*arrows*). **E.** Dysthyroid optic neuropathy. **(Top)** Central nerve fiber bundle defects. Arcuate pattern in left field mimics glaucoma. Patient was a 53-year-old woman with moderate bilateral proptosis and lid retraction, who noted slowly progressive loss of color appreciation. Visual defects cleared rapidly and completely on large doses of systemic corticosteroids. Discs were at all times normal. **(Bottom)** a 57-year-old woman with moderate congestive ophthalmopathy experienced diminution of vision from 20/25 (6/7.5) OU to 20/100 (6/30) OU in 6 weeks and 4/200 (1.2/60) to 5/200 (1.5/60) by 10 weeks. The right disc was swollen and elevated with several hemorrhages; the left disc was normal. Massive doses of systemic steroids resulted in slow improvement to 20/200 (6/60) and 20/400 (6/120). (*From Glaser, J.S.* Topical Diagnosis: Prechiasmal Visual Pathways. *In: Duane, T, ed.* Clinical Ophthalmology, *Hagerstown, Md: Harper & Row, 1976; 2, with permission.*)

ositic form of idiopathic orbital inflammation can involve both orbits. However, inflammatory pseudotumor usually involves the muscles right up to their insertions, whereas in thyroid orbitopathy, the muscle insertions are not enlarged. Other causes of enlarged extraocular muscles (such as carotid–cavernous fistulae and pituitary tumor) and of restrictive myopathy (such as sinus disease, metastases, and trauma) will almost always be detected easily by these two scanning modalities.

Treatment: Most patients have a myriad of ocular symptoms, most of them related to corneal exposure and restrictive myopathy. Although troubling to the patient, the majority of symptoms is mild to moderate in severity and needs to be treated only symptomatically. Treatment (Table 18–5) aims to relieve pain and discomfort, protect visual acuity, minimize diplopia, and improve cosmesis. Ocular lubricants and protective shields are the first line of defense. Resistant dry eye symptoms are often helped by 0.1% sodium hyaluronate drops. Additional pillows may be used to ameliorate orbital and periorbital swelling. If this is not sufficient, the head of the patient's bed may be elevated on blocks.

Exposure problems are accentuated and compounded by the lid retraction, exophthalmos, and decreased blinking (Stellwag's sign). A poor tear film often coexists with these problems. Using moist chambers or taping the lids shut at night may be helpful, as may be the use of side shields or wraparound lenses on glasses. In dry climates, humidifiers can also be useful. Various epidermal growth factors to maintain corneal integrity are under investigation and these may prove helpful in cases of repeated corneal breakdown, although they appear to lose their effectiveness in long-term use. Topical corticosteroid drops are *absolutely* contraindicated as they often combine with the factors above to cause a dramatic deterioration of the cornea. The lid lag and retraction often respond to treatment of hyperthyroidism. The lid retraction also may be ameliorated by sympatholytic drugs such as guanethidine, bethanidine, and thymoxamine.

If diplopia is minimal and limited to one or two directions of gaze, it can sometimes be treated effectively by prisms. Otherwise, frosting or taping one lens in a pair of eyeglasses or a patch over one eye will eliminate the diplopia.

After control of hyperthyroidism, less than 20% of patients requires more than symptomatic treatment.

In acute disease posing a threat to vision, such as optic nerve compression and corneal exposure, oral steroids and irradiation are the next alternatives. Steroids seem most effective and are usually given in divided doses, totaling 60 to 120 mg of prednisone

TABLE 18–5. AVAILABLE THERAPIES FOR THYROID-ASSOCIATED OPHTHALMOPATHY

Aims	Modes	Mechanism of Effect
Protection of cornea	Lubricants Taping eyelids shut Protective eye patches Dark spectacle lenses Tarsorrhaphy Müller myotomy Scleral graft insertion in eyelids	Prevent corneal drying and exposure
Reduction of intra-orbital soft tissue volume	Diuretics	Nonspecific fluid elimination
	Radiotherapy	Kills pathogenic retro-ocular lymphocytes
	Plasmapheresis	Removes pathogenic antibodies
	Thyroid ablation	Removes source of putative antigen stimulating production of cross-reacting antibodies
	Steroids (retrobulbar and systemic), cyclosporine, azothioprine, cyclophosphamide	Exert relatively nonspecific immune suppression, anti-inflammatory effects
Expansion of orbital space	Decompression by transantral, transfrontal, lateral, medial, or anterior inferior approaches	Relief of intraorbital pressure by allowing expansion of orbital tissues into adjacent areas
Correction of diplopia	Extraocular muscle surgery	Modifies tension to allow realignment of eyes deviated and/or restricted by extraocular muscle fibrosis
Improvement of appearance	Eyelid surgery	Corrects eyelid malposition

Modified from Bahn RS, Gorman CA. Choice of therapy and criteria for assessing treatment outcome in thyroid-associated ophthalmopathy. Endocrinol Metab Clin North Am. 1987;16:391–407.

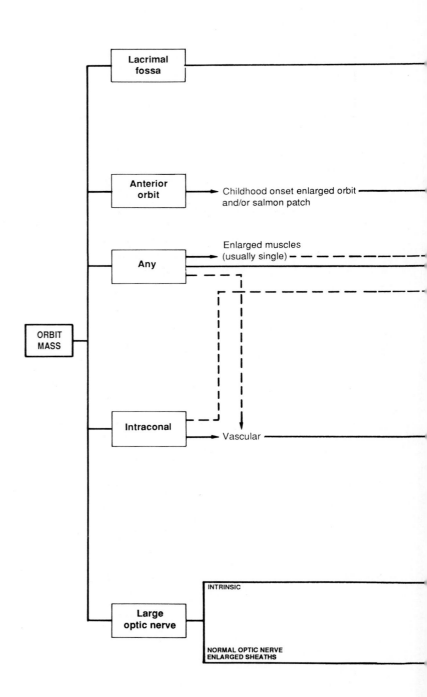

Figure 18–14. Decision tree of the location, probable diagnosis, further considerations and treatment of orbital mass.

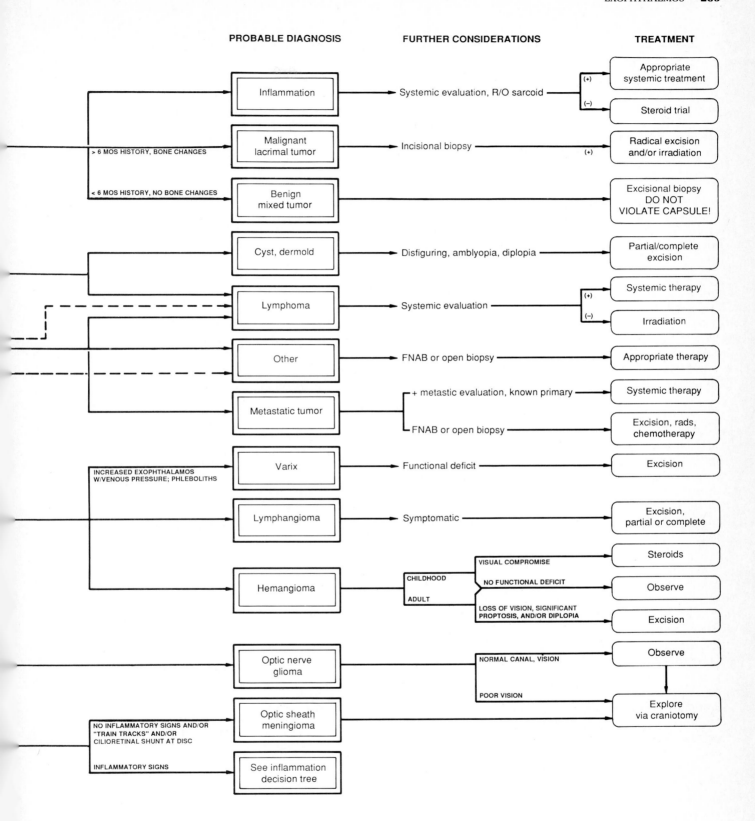

PROBABLE DIAGNOSIS | FURTHER CONSIDERATIONS | TREATMENT

> 6 MOS HISTORY, BONE CHANGES

< 6 MOS HISTORY, NO BONE CHANGES

- **Inflammation** → Systemic evaluation, R/O sarcoid → (+) Appropriate systemic treatment / (−) Steroid trial
- **Malignant lacrimal tumor** → Incisional biopsy → (+) Radical excision and/or irradiation
- **Benign mixed tumor** → Excisional biopsy DO NOT VIOLATE CAPSULE!
- **Cyst, dermold** → Disfiguring, amblyopia, diplopia → Partial/complete excision
- **Lymphoma** → Systemic evaluation → (+) Systemic therapy / (−) Irradiation
- **Other** → FNAB or open biopsy → Appropriate therapy
- **Metastatic tumor** → + metastic evaluation, known primary → Systemic therapy / FNAB or open biopsy → Excision, rads, chemotherapy

INCREASED EXOPHTHALAMOS W/VENOUS PRESSURE; PHLEBOLITHS

- **Varix** → Functional deficit → Excision
- **Lymphangioma** → Symptomatic → Excision, partial or complete
- **Hemangioma** → CHILDHOOD / ADULT
  - VISUAL COMPROMISE → Steroids
  - NO FUNCTIONAL DEFICIT → Observe
  - LOSS OF VISION, SIGNIFICANT PROPTOSIS, AND/OR DIPLOPIA → Excision

NO INFLAMMATORY SIGNS AND/OR "TRAIN TRACKS" AND/OR CILIORETINAL SHUNT AT DISC

INFLAMMATORY SIGNS

- **Optic nerve glioma** → NORMAL CANAL, VISION → Observe
- **Optic sheath meningioma** → POOR VISION → Explore via craniotomy
- **See inflammation decision tree**

daily. One expects to see an effect within 1 to 2 weeks. Pulse IV methylprednisone (1 g daily for 3 days) has recently produced good results. Somewhat lower doses (20 to 40 mg/day for 1 month with tapering doses over the next 3 months) may prevent exacerbations occurring after radioiodine therapy.

With **irradiation,** one doesn't expect the effect for 3 to 4 weeks, and maximal improvement is not reached for 3 to 4 months. Caution must be taken to avoid cataractogenic doses to the lens (which may be as low as 2 to 5 Gy); thus, well-collimated supervoltage treatment is usually suggested. The Stanford protocol uses 1000 to 2500 cGy over 2 to 3 weeks. Both steroids and irradiation are thought to work by reducing inflammation and are usually most effective in early stages of disease when the inflammatory aspects are predominant. The soft tissue changes and proptosis improve most; ophthalmoplegia responds less well. Some observers even believe that they may hasten, and/or worsen, the fibrotic stage of the disease. Low-dose cyclosporine and bromocriptine have been suggested for resistant cases. A combination of cyclosporine and prednisone proved effective in patients who did not respond to either drug alone.

When a threat to vision persists after medical therapy, or if delay cannot be tolerated (Fig. 18–14), immediate decompression is needed.

The **surgical approach** and the extent of decompression depend upon the desired results. If the major problem is optic nerve compression because of apical enlargement of the muscles, then it is critical to decompress the apex of the orbit. This is done most effectively by decompressing the posterior medial wall with removal of the apical periorbita. Depending on the degree of exophthalmos, decompression of the floor, lateral wall, or both, may be added. It is interesting that the optic neuropathy usually occurs in orbits with significantly enlarged muscles in the apex, but not in those orbits with the most dramatic proptosis.

In extravagant exophthalmos with massively increased extraocular muscle and orbital fat volume, gain maximal decompression by removing not only the floor of the orbit but also the medial and lateral walls and even, if necessary, the roof. The bifrontal approach is good for simultaneous treatment of both orbits. The effectiveness of the decompression into each wall is approximately in the order given.

When vision is not threatened, it is best to postpone surgery until the orbitopathy has stabilized and the patient has been free of steroids for 6 months. Decompression for cosmetic reasons may be considered at this point. Generally, decompression precedes extraocular muscle surgery. The final step is lid surgery.

When appropriate muscle surgery is indicated,

holding sutures are often useful in maintaining the surgical correction in the immediate postoperative period. Adjustable sutures are found to be very helpful by some, and are disliked by others.

Definitive lid surgery, including medial canthoplasty and recession of the lid retractors, may make the lid position more favorable and provide better corneal protection; eye bank scleral grafts or tarsal transplants are used if necessary. Again, the effectiveness of the surgery increases by using holding sutures to keep the lids from returning to their previous positions. In the upper lid, disinsertion of Müller's muscle will give 2 mm of lid drop. Disconnecting both the levator and Müller's muscle will give a 4-mm drop. Scleral implants or tarsal transplants may augment the result in both the upper and lower lids. In recessing the inferior rectus, be careful not to create lower lid retraction by posterior displacement of the lower lid retractors. If during muscle surgery, repeated intraoperative forced duction testing reveals that recession alone is not adequate to obtain binocular vision in primary position, marginal myotomy, free tenotomy, or massive recessions may be performed. Aim for single binocular vision in primary position and for the first 15 to 20 degrees of downgaze with as large a possible binocular field. Patients who gain motility but lose binocular field are unhappy, as are those who cannot lower their eyes to read or negotiate stairs and curbs.

Of course, all the ophthalmic remedies should be accompanied by concomitant efforts to effectively treat any underlying thyroid disorder.

Idiopathic orbital inflammatory pseudotumor: Following thyroid orbitopathy, nonspecific orbital inflammatory pseudotumor is the most frequent inflammatory process affecting the orbit, consistently producing proptosis and orbital pain (Table 18–6). It may affect any portion or group of tissues in the orbit, singly or in isolation. It also merges impercepti-

---

TABLE 18–6. CONDITIONS CAUSING ORBITAL PAIN

Orbital cellulitis
Retrobulbar neuritis
Idiopathic inflammatory pseudotumor
Adenoid cystic carcinoma of lacrimal gland
Superior orbital fissure (Tolosa-Hunt) syndrome
Cluster headache and migraine
Sinusitis and mucocele
Nasopharyngeal and sinus carcinoma
Metastatic carcinoma
Intracranial aneurysm
Other referred intracranial pain
Posterior scleritis

From Jones IS, Jakobiec FA, Nolan BT. Patient examination and introduction to orbital disease. In: Duane T, ed. Clinical Ophthalmology. Hagerstown, MD: Harper & Row, 1976;2;29.

bly with inflammatory processes of the orbital apex and the anterior cavernous sinus, including superior orbital fissure syndromes, the orbital apex syndrome, and the Tolosa-Hunt syndrome. On occasion, identical nonspecific inflammatory lesions in contiguity with the orbital process are found, in either the sinuses or the intracranial fossae.

Most often, there is generalized orbital inflammation, acute or subacute in presentation, with proptosis, pain, and limitation of ocular motility. The more acute varieties have extensive chemosis and injection. Involvement of the globe may include uveitis, usually posterior, and frequently scleritis and/or tenonitis. Involvement of the optic nerve, either primarily by an inflammatory process or by compression by swollen tissues, may decrease vision. In the anterior orbit, involvement of the lacrimal gland is frequent and may be involved in isolated presentation. In the myositic form one or more muscles are affected primarily.

Inflammatory pseudotumor usually is a unilateral process, in contrast to thyroid orbitopathy. However, it may be bilateral, especially in children in whom the disease frequently takes a more aggressive course. When it does present unilaterally in a child in the explosive inflammatory form, biopsy is necessary to differentiate it from rhabdomyosarcoma. In adults, it must be distinguished from lymphoma.

Evaluation by the imaging modalities usually etablishes the diagnosis. On **ultrasonography,** the most frequent picture is diffuse infiltration of the orbit, blending the orbital structures together in a mass that is predominantly of low reflectivity. When Tenon's capsule is involved, the characteristic "T-sign" is seen at the posterior sclera. Involvement of the sclera and intraocular structures is seen as a continuous area of low reflectivity associated with intraocular inflammation—vitreous opacities and thickening of the choroid. Optic nerve involvement is frequently detected by broadening of the cerebrospinal fluid space of the perioptic meninges. The extraocular muscles are diffusely thickened with inflammatory changes that persist right to their insertions. In contrast, in thyroid orbitopathy the swelling is usually fusiform and does not involve the tendinous insertions. The myositis may involve only one muscle; single muscle involvement is exceedingly rare in thyroid orbitopathy. When myositis involves the tendon of the superior oblique, a pseudo-Brown's syndrome may result. Similar findings are seen on CT scanning or MRI. The scanning modalities can also demonstrate contiguous involvement of the sinuses or intracranial cavities, and concomitant sinus or nasopharyngeal disease (Wegener's granulomatosis or polymorphic reticulosis—formerly lethal mid-

line granuloma), or infectious processes such as sinusitis or rhino–cerebral fungus.

A systemic workup should be done, especially in bilateral cases and in children, looking for collagen vascular diseases and sources of metastases or lymphoma. A foreign body must also be kept in mind, as should the possibilities of inflammatory reactions to other orbital processes such as dermoids, sclerosing hemangioma, or hemorrhage into a lymphangioma. Occasionally, metastatic disease has a significant inflammatory component and looks quite similar.

Treatment. In most cases, firm suspicion of idiopathic orbital pseudotumor merits a trial of steroids, to which this inflammatory process is usually very sensitive. However, it must also be kept in mind that infectious processes, lymphoma, and metastatic disease may also respond favorably to steroids. Biopsy is reserved for those cases in which there is considerable doubt about the diagnosis, as the results of a biopsy can be disastrous, especially in cases with marked inflammatory reaction. Fine-needle aspiration biopsy (FNAB) may provide a tissue diagnosis without evoking the same degree of inflammatory reaction as an open biopsy.

Occasionally these processes, especially the sclerosing subset, become steroid resistant and progress despite large doses of prednisone. In these cases, low-dose orbital irradiation with protection of the globe usually stabilizes the process. Immunosuppressive agents, including cyclosporin, are sometimes successful in resistant cases, and indomethacin has been reported to give a good result. One therapeutic approach is given in Table 18–7.

Histopathologically, the diagnosis of idiopathic inflammatory pseudotumor embraces a range of pictures comparable to the range of clinical presentations. When the infiltrate is polymorphous with plasma cells and a significant reactive fibrovascular component, the diagnosis of pseudotumor is certain. However, varieties that appear granulomatous must be differentiated from sarcoid and tuberculosis, whereas those that present with a monomorphous lymphocytic infiltrate make it almost impossible to differentiate between the histology of benign lymphoid hyperplasia and lymphoma.

Specific arteritides, such as Wegener's granulomatosis and systemic involvements such as polymorphic reticulosis and Lyme disease, can present an identical clinical picture.

Orbital infections are proportionately more frequent in children. The most common infection is a preseptal cellulitis, localized in the eyelid anterior to the orbital septum with involvement of the orbital tissues per se; it is usually associated with an adjacent sinusitis, especially an ethmoid sinusitis. Any

TABLE 18–7. TREATMENT PROTOCOL FOR ORBITAL INFLAMMATORY DISEASE

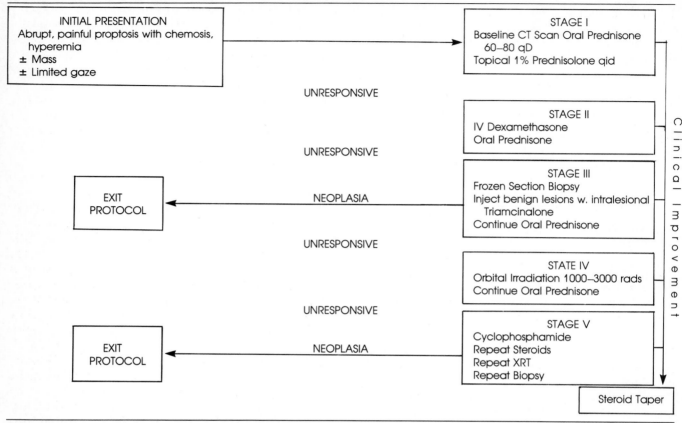

From Leone C. Treatment protocol for orbital inflammatory disease. Opthalmol. 1985; 92:1325–1331.

systemic signs or symptoms, if present, usually consist only of slight fever and a minimal leukocytosis. Appropriate antibiotic treatment is usually curative (Table 18–8). Any persistent underlying sinusitis should be appropriately treated.

Infections that involve the orbit itself are much more serious. Like other significant infections of the face and anterior cranial cavity they pose a threat of life-threatening cavernous sinus thrombosis. The patient with an infected orbit is usually ill with fever, leukocytosis, erythema and edema of the lids, and proptosis. Chemosis, limitation of ocular motility, and visual loss are variable. The deeper orbital infections—especially those that are bacterial, like preseptal cellulitis—most frequently are associated with sinus infection. Evaluation by CT or MRI will usually establish the diagnosis. Appropriate IV antibiotic therapy should be started immediately, including coverage for *Haemophilus influenzae* in children under the age of 5 years. If the response is not prompt (significant within 24 to 48 hours) or if there is progression, any localized fluctuant area, localized ring abscess on CT or MRI, or any subperiosteal collection, the patient should be treated surgically with incision and drainage. The appear-

ance of ophthalmoplegia or optic nerve involvement, if not previously present, may herald the backward extension of infection from the face or neck. Development of contralateral involvement, especially a sixth-nerve palsy in a quiet orbit, is especially worrisome for the onset of cavernous sinus involvement.

Rarer infections include a host of infestations. One must always be on the lookout for tuberculosis, sarcoidosis, and syphilis; be suspicious of foreign bodies, especially with a history of trauma; and consider the possibility of a ruptured vascular malformation or dermoid. Most of these diagnoses should be obvious on appropriate systemic workup and imaging studies.

Fungal involvement of the orbit is uncommon and has been thought to occur predominantly in diabetic, debilitated, and immunosuppressed patients. Prompt recognition of fungal invasion of the orbit is critical as aggressive amphotericin therapy and surgery now achieves significantly better results than expected previously. Because fungi invade tissues through the arterioles, necrosis is usually a predominant finding; but clinical manifestations of necrosis may not be obvious if the infection is deep seated. Nearly always, infection gains access to the orbit

TABLE 18–8. EMPIRIC ANTIMICROBIAL REGIMENS FOR ORBITAL CELLULITIS

Clinical Type	Predominant Organism	Recommended Regimens
Preeptal (periorbital)	*H. influenzae,* group A streptococci, *S. aureus*	Pen G + cloxacillin Chloramphenicol + cloxacillin Cefamandole or cefaclor
Orbital (sinusitis related)	Streptococci Pneumococci *H. influenzae* Bacteroides Fusobacterium Anaerobic cocci (coliforms are uncommon)	Penicillin or clindamycin Cefotaxime (Surgical drainage essential if abscess)
Trauma or foreign-body related	*S. aureus* *S. epidermidis* Streptococci	Cloxacillin, cefazolin, or vancomycin

From Rootman J, et al. Inflammatory diseases. In: Rootman J, (ed) Diseases of the Orbit: A Multidisciplinary Approach. New York: Lippincott, 1988:152.

from the sinus, or more rarely from the cranial cavity; imaging studies will reveal contiguous involvement. Perineural involvement is also frequent and pain is usually a prominent sign. Usually, careful examination of the nose and sinuses will reveal black necrotic patches from which a diagnostic biopsy may be taken. Prompt therapy with IV amphotericin-B should be instituted and any and all necrotic tissue debrided. Systemic disease should be treated aggressively (eg, control of blood sugar, hydration, and hyperalimentation as indicated).

With the advent of more aggressive therapy and earlier diagnosis, this previously fatal entity now often is treated successfully. In fact, with prompt treatment, limited extirpation of the affected orbital contents can sometimes avoid exenteration. Whether the success of less radical treatment implies a less aggressive entity is not clear, but cases following a much more benign course have been identified in generally healthy individuals.

Aspergillosis may present a similar picture, but is less aggressive.

Orbital Tumors

Orbital tumors arise from any of the orbital contents, bones, surrounding sinusus and also pharynx, cranial cavities, facial structures, and metastases.

Orbital lymphoma. This tumor of hematogenous origin is included in proximity to the infiltrative and inflammatory orbital disorders because of the frequent difficulty in differentiating it histopathologically from orbital pseudotumor. Orbital lymphomas

usually involve the anterior orbit, and when a typical salmon patch lesion of the conjunctiva is seen, the diagnosis is easy. Other anterior orbital masses that are more infiltrative and that on ultrasound, CT, and MRI studies appear similar to the mildly inflammatory forms of idiopathic inflammation, are difficult to diagnose. These patients should have a workup for systemic disease, but it may be necessary to proceed to biopsy for definitive diagnosis. The proliferation of increasingly refined cytochemical and immunohistopathologic methods of tissue analysis allows more accurate definition of the tumorous cell types. However, this explosion of information has yet to be translated into a practical clinical tool for diagnosis, treatment, and prognosis (Table 18–9).

The occurrence of orbital lymphomas has always been a bit of a puzzle, as the orbit is said to be free of lymphoid tissue. There are lymphatics in the lids and there appears to be some lymphoid tissue in contiguity with the lacrimal gland. This is probably why the lacrimal gland is frequently a site of involvement with lymphoma. A thorough systemic workup is indicated to rule out generalized lymphoma.

Once the diagnosis has been established, these tumors are usually exquisitely sensitive to low doses of radiation (15 to 25 cGy).

Vascular disorders of the orbit. Vascular tumors of the orbit are the most common true orbital neoplasms, and hemangiomas are the most common vascular tumors.

TABLE 18–9. CELL IDENTIFICATION BY IMMUNOLOGIC METHODS

Immunologic Markers	Cell Types
Surface immunoglobulins	B lymphocytes
Polyclonal	Benign proliferations
Monoclonal	Malignant proliferations
Cytoplasmic immunoglobulins	Plasma cells, immunoblasts
Polyclonal	Benign proliferations
Monoclonal	Malignant proliferations
Receptor for sheep erythrocyte	T lymphocytes
E rosettes	
Receptor for complement (C_3)	B lymphocytes
EAC rosettes (erythrocytes-IgM-complement)	
Receptor for Fc-fragment	Monocytes, histiocytes
EA rosettes (erythrocytes-IgG)	
T lymphocyte antigen	T lymphocytes
Anti T lymphocyte heterologous antisera	

From Rootman J, et al. Lymphoproliferative and leukemic lesions. In: Rootman J, ed. Diseases of the Orbit: A Multidisciplinary Approach. New York: Lippincott, 1988:208.

Capillary hemangiomas are tumors of early childhood that frequently present within the first year of life, hypertrophy for several months, and then involute. When they appear on the skin, they form the so-called "strawberry nevus." Their natural history is to involute within the first few years of life. Usually they are only of cosmetic significance. However, when the lid is massively involved and threatens amblyopia because of irregular astigmatism or occlusion of the visual axis, or when the orbit is significantly involved, treatment is indicated. The congenitally involved orbit may be enlarged and there may be other associated cutaneous and occasionally central nervous system hemangiomas. Both systemic steroid treatment and intralesional injections of steroids have been advocated as has been superficial radiotherapy.

In adults, **cavernous hemangioma** is the most common benign orbital tumor. This tumor is slowly progressive and usually presents with proptosis in the second or third decade. It is usually a round, homogeneous intraconal mass on all imaging modalities. By A-scan echography, spontaneous movements within the mass and compressibility may be documented. Excision, although easily accomplished, is not indicated unless the proptosis is disfiguring or other problems such as optic nerve compression or diplopia occur.

Lymphangiomas are much rarer and usually occur in young patients. Involvement of the conjunctiva may lead to an early diagnosis. Surgical excision may be done for reasons of cosmesis. These superficial tumors are often limited in extent and can be relatively easily resected. On the other hand, in slightly older children, hemorrhage following upper respiratory tract infection frequently causes sudden proptosis, which at surgical exploration is seen to be caused by a so-called "chocolate cyst." MRI should clearly demonstrate the hemorrhagic nature of these "cysts," and identification of an enhancing vascular component by CT or contrast MRI enables optimum surgical planning to prevent postoperative hemorrhage. Diagnostic imaging usually shows a more diffuse involvement of the orbit than with hemangiomas.

Venous vascular malformations may present very similarly to lymphangiomas, in fact there is discussion among ophthalmic pathologists as to whether these are truly two distinct entities. Those venous malformations that cause a truly intermittent proptosis associated with increased vascular pressure caused by straining, the Valsalva maneuver, or standing on one's head, certainly are at one end of the spectrum. Sometimes over time these orbital varices compress the orbital tissues sufficiently that an enophthalmos ensues, alternating with the exophthalmos caused by increased venous pressure. These masses may be difficult to demonstrate by imaging modalities, even during the Valsalva maneuver. The finding of phleboliths is characteristic.

Both of these tumors may cause enlargement of the orbit and insinuate themselves throughout the orbital tissues and prove a real challenge to the orbital surgeon. When surgery is necessary, serious consideration should be given to removing only those portions of the tumor that are most troublesome, not trying to achieve complete removal, which sometimes is impossible. The CO_2 laser has proven useful in the subtotal removal of lymphangioma (personal communication, J. Kennerdell). Rarer vascular tumors include hemangiopericytoma, hemangioendothelioma, Kaposi's sarcoma, and Kimura's angiomyomata (usually the lid and conjunctiva are the only tissues involved).

Developmental orbital tumors. Dermoid and epidermoid cysts are common developmental tumors of the orbit that generally present during childhood, if not at birth. Epidermoid cysts are more frequently found in the skin of the periorbital area, and dermoids are more characteristically found within the orbit itself. The epidermoids arise in the lateral portion of the brow as firm, painless subcutaneous masses. Rarely, they may present acutely with swelling and inflammation following spontaneous rupture. Characteristic cystic defects in the orbital bones are frequently seen on imaging studies.

Dermoid cysts also predominate temporally and in the superior orbit. It is not unusual for these tumors to extend posteriorly and even into the intracranial cavity. These tumors rarely cause significant symptoms except for mild proptosis; surgery is most often performed for cosmetic reasons. Where possible, total extirpation should be undertaken, with care not to rupture the cyst contents which can excite an inflammatory reaction. When the tumor does dive into the posterior reaches of the orbit, it is usually best not to attempt total removal.

Neural tumors of the orbit. The primary neural tumors are optic nerve glioma and optic nerve sheath meningioma.

The optic nerve gliomas may be classified into the **optochiasmatic gliomas of childhood** and the **malignant glioma of adulthood.** The former tumors are low-grade astrocytomas, which present primarily with visual loss and disc swelling or optic atrophy; proptosis is a later development. Often there is an enlargement of the optic canal. This tumor is considered more extensively in Chapter 5. The **malignant glioma of adulthood** initially presents as an optic neuritis, except that over weeks to months it inexorably decreases visual acuity to no light perception. By this time, the other orbit is involved;

intracranial extension and death follow. This is an ocular form of glioblastoma multiforma.

Meningiomas of the orbit originate predominantly from the optic nerve sheaths. Primary ("ectopic") meningiomas of the orbit originating from other neural structures are very rare. In addition, the orbit may be involved in sphenoid ridge meningiomas (discussed later in the chapter).

Similar to optic nerve gliomas, optic nerve sheath meningiomas generally present with visual loss prior to proptosis. These tumors tend to occur in middle-aged women, may have optociliary shunt vessels at the optic disc, and have characteristic ultrasonographic, CT, and MRI findings (see Chapter 5 for more details).

The other common neural mass of the orbit is the plexiform neuroma associated with neurofibromatosis. Although the incidence of optic gliomas and meningiomas may be increased in this disease, the plexiform neurofibroma of the orbit is pathognomonic. It may present with a spectrum of changes ranging from mild localized involvement to massive and extensive infiltration of the orbital soft tissues. Most frequently, the lid shows a typical wormy enlargement. Massive enlargement of the intraorbital nerves can carry backwards through an enlarged superior orbital fissure to similar massive enlargement of the cavernous sinus.

Thin-section CT scanning can demonstrate involvement of nearly every orbital structure.

Less common neural tumors include schwannomas (neurilemomas), neurofibromas, and postamputation neuromas, which on rare occasions may be associated with significant orbital pain.

Solitary neural tumors of the orbit present with painless and slowly progressive proptosis. They can rarely be diagnosed definitively without orbital biopsy.

Meningoceles and encephaloceles may occasionally present as orbital, ethmoidal, or frontal masses in early childhood. Adequate CT or MRI study should be done to define the extent of any cystic orbital mass, to be sure that one is not surprised by finding cerebrospinal fluid or brain tissue in an attempt to biopsy or extirpate the lesion.

Mesenchymal orbital tumors. The most dramatic of these tumors and the most common primary malignant orbital tumor in childhood is the **rhabdomyosarcoma.** Most occur before 10 years of age. This tumor usually presents acutely as a rapidly progressive exophthalmos associated with inflammatory signs. Ptosis is frequently an early manifestation. Rhabdomyosarcomas are virtually always unilateral.

In a child, any rapidly expansile orbital mass not conclusively identified as infectious or inflammatory should be biopsied immediately. These tu-

mors are now managed with combined radiotherapy and chemotherapy with quite good results (95% 5-year survival). However, the prognosis is poor for maintaining significant vision in the involved orbit. In 75 to 80% of patients, severe corneal, lens, or retinal changes impair vision. Facial asymmetry usually results from irradiation of the immature skull.

Lacrimal gland tumors: Patients with lacrimal gland masses present with swelling in the region of the lacrimal gland and often a characteristic S-shaped deformity of the upper lid. Statistically, 50% of these lesions is inflammatory or lymphoid in origin and 50% are epithelial tumors. Of the latter, 50% are benign mixed tumors and 25% adenoidcystic carcinomas.

Benign mixed tumors are relatively slow-growing tumors. Benign mixed tumors are usually present with a 3- to 5-year history of a painless mass, in the later stages associated with inferonasal displacement of the globe. Pain and diplopia are relatively rare. Because of the slow growth of the tumor, there is usually bony fossa formation demonstrated on CT or MRI studies of the orbit. The clinical and radiographic findings usually give a picture highly suggestive of this tumor. When a benign mixed lacrimal gland tumor is the primary consideration, it should be removed carefully and en toto through a lateral orbitotomy with its capsule intact because of the potential to reemerge as a malignant mixed-cell tumor. *Incomplete excision or incisional biopsy is absolutely contraindicated.*

Adenoidystic carcinoma is the most common of the lacrimal gland malignancies. This tumor has a much more acute course, (rarely more than a few months), significant pain (related to perineural and bony invasion), and irregular destruction of the bone of the lacrimal fossa. Even if not clinically involved, when examined histopathologically the bone is almost universally invaded. If this tumor is suspected, it should be biopsied through the lid in order to substantiate the diagnosis. Once the diagnosis is established, most orbital surgeons currently perform extended exenterations to control this relentlessly recurrent and nearly uniformly fatal tumor. However, because of the lengthy natural history to eventual demise (10 to 15 years), there has not been sufficient time to assess the efficacy of radical orbitectomies.

Lymphomatous invasion of the gland is also common and best diagnosed by biopsy.

Inflammatory lesions of the lacrimal gland include infection, sarcoid, pseudotumor, and involvement in Sjögren's syndrome. **Infectious involvement of the lacrimal gland** can usually be identified by the mucopurulent discharge. The other inflammatory disorders, in analogy to orbital pseudotumor, can be treated with steroids and biopsied if they recur or do not respond. In the latter cases, systemic workup is also indicated.

For discussion of rarer orbital tumors, most of which can be diagnosed only by biopsy, see the general references included in the bibliography.

Metastases. Metastatic disease of the orbit is not uncommon, but usually does not pose a diagnostic dilemma, especially when a primary tumor has been identified; however, in about 25% of patients the orbital tumor is the initial presentation. In children, neuroblastoma and Ewing's sarcoma are the most common tumors to metastasize to the orbit. They both present with exophthalmos and lid ecchymosis. The metastases of neuroblastoma are more frequently bilateral and cause a violaceous hue to the lids as well as ecchymosis.

In adults, the most comon metastatic orbital tumors are breast carcinoma in women and lung carcinoma in men. Prostatic carcinoma also metastasizes to the orbit relatively frequently, often involving the frontal bone.

These tumors may present acutely with rapid proptosis and inflammatory signs, but more often with infiltration, slowly progressive proptosis, or disorders of ocular motility or optic nerve function. Diagnosis by fine-needle aspiration biopsy can be especially useful when visual acuity has been significantly affected. Histologic confirmation of tumor type should be obtained in all patients with a reasonable life expectancy. **Schirrous carcinoma** of the breast can actually cause enophthalmos and a frozen orbit.

Orbital involvement with diseases of the paranasal sinusus. Inflammatory and infectious processes involving both the sinuses and the orbit have already been discussed (see above). In addition, the orbit is not infrequently involved in other sinus pathology; it is eventually involved in the large majority of malignant tumors of the sinuses. The most common site of origin is the maxillary sinus. Typical destruction of bone is well demonstrated on CT and parenchymal extension on MRI imaging. Tumors arising from the maxillary sinus invade the floor of the orbit, pushing the globe upward; they may also cause numbness of the cheek if the infraorbital nerve is involved, or present with tearing if the lacrimal ducts or sac is invaded. **Malignant tumors of the nasopharynx** may act similarly but more often invade the posterior orbit and base of the skull.

Recurrent inflammation of the sinuses obstructing their ostia may cause the formation of a **mucocoele** or **mucopyocoele.** When these enlarge toward the orbital space, they produce the familiar symptoms of an orbital mass. Ultrasonograms, able to penetrate through the low reflectivity of these masses,

show pathognomonic findings and demonstrate extension beyond the orbital cavity. The surgical approach to these masses necessitates complete removal of the lining of the cyst and restoration of drainage from the affected sinus.

Osteomas are the most common tumors of bone to involve the orbit and most often arise from the frontal and ethmoidal sinuses. These rock-hard calcified masses are easily identified on CT scans. Removal of a tumor is curative, although it can recur, especially in young patients.

Other bony tumors. Primary tumors of the bone are uncommon. However, in children, unilocular or multilocular manifestations of histiocytosis X must be considered. The orbit is also a site of fibrous dysplasia, Albright's disease, Paget's disease, Engleman's syndrome, osteopetrosis, orbitofrontal cholesterol granuloma, and other similar processes. They may present with optic nerve compression as well as proptosis. Special mention should be made of osteosarcoma arising in orbits that have been irradiated for retinoblastoma. This is probably the result of the clastogenic nature of the retinoblastoma gene, rather than merely a complication of radiotherapy.

Involvement of the orbit by intracranial processes. Possibly the most common orbital involvement of intracranial disease is the proptosis that occurs in **sphenoid ridge meningiomas.** In contrast to the early visual loss in optic nerve sheath meningiomas, sphenoid ridge meningiomas frequently present with exophthalmos before visual acuity is affected. CT scanning with obvious hyperostosis and MRI imaging are usually diagnostic. Although these tumors are relatively benign in adults, their extent can be surprising and complete removal may be impossible. The benefits of total extirpation must be carefully weighed against the risk to surrounding structures such as the optic nerve and cavernous sinus. Recent advances in basofrontal multidisciplinary surgical approaches to these and similarly located masses are often extremely effective.

Other common intracranial problems causing orbital manifestations originate in the cavernous sinus. **Carotid–cavernous fistulas** and **dural fistulas** may cause proptosis, enlargement of the orbital muscles, and suffusion of the orbital tissues (Table 18–10). Frequently a bruit can be heard by the examiner or the patient and characteristic corkscrew-like arterialized veins are obvious on the conjunctiva. Ultrasound, CT, and MRI will usually all show an enlarged supraorbital vein; CT and MRI will show involvement of the cavernous sinus. The smaller-flow dural shunts frequently occur spontaneously and approximately one third of them will disappear spontaneously as well. They are more likely to occur

TABLE 18–10. MANIFESTATIONS OF CAROTID–CAVERNOUS FISTULA

Engorged and arterialized retinal veins
Dilated retinal veins +/– ischemic retinopathy
Glaucoma
Bruit
Cataract
Motility disturbances
Keratopathy
Uveitis
Cranial nerve palsies
Enlarged extraocular muscles

in elderly women. Conjunctival engorgement, arterialized venous loops, orbital pain, and intraocular pressure are also typical. Higher-flow shunts are less likely to disappear and more likely to be traumatic; they more frequently necessitate surgical intervention. The definitive study in these cases is four-vessel angiography, as the shunt often involves an extensive network of feeding and draining vessels. This study should not be undertaken until a definitive procedure is seriously considered, as the hemodynamics frequently change over time. Currently, invasive neuro-radiologic techniques using assorted types of obstructive elements, balloons, and emboli are often effective in obliterating the shunt.

Giant aneurysms arising within the cavernous sinus usually do not cause damage by rupturing (perhaps because they are invested with the several layers of sinus tissue), but rather by causing a large mass effect. They may erode into the pituitary fossa as well as the orbit. When they erode anteriorly into the orbit, they usually enlarge the superior orbital fissure and occasionally the optic canal. If they enlarge acutely, they present with pain, proptosis, and ophthalmoplegia, sometimes accompanied by visual loss, and must be differentiated from pituitary apoplexy and other causes of painful ophthalmoplegia. Again, CT scan and especially MRI imaging are diagnostic. Usually, after an abrupt period of acute enlargement, intracavernous aneurysms tend to stabilize. Because there is no definitive treatment, attempts to restrict the blood supply should be limited to those aneurysms that are continuing to cause excessive pain or that are growing relentlessly.

Less commonly, the orbit is invaded by **tumors arising around the face,** especially squamous cell carcinoma. This tumor has a predilection for infiltrating along nerves and may involve the orbit, generally causing unrelenting pain, sometimes loss of sensation, and sometimes ophthalmoplegia without much proptosis. A history of removal of a squamous cell carcinoma from the face should be sought, because the invasion may be only a few cell layers thick and difficult to demonstrate by imaging techniques. Usually by the time the orbit is invaded, the nasopharynx, pterygoid fossa, or intracranial cavity, or a combination of these locations, is involved as well. Definitive treatment is rarely possible and chemotherapy is used for palliation.

BIBLIOGRAPHY

General

Rootman J. *Diseases of the Orbit: A Multidisciplinary Approach.* New York: Lippincott, 1988.

Anatomy

Burde RM. Direct parasympathetic pathway to the eye: revisited. *Brain Res.* 1988;463:158–162.
Doxanas MT, Anderson RL. *Clinical Orbital Anatomy.* Baltimore: Williams & Wilkins, 1984.
Jakobiec FA, ed. *Ocular and Adnexal Tumors.* Birmingham, AL: Aesculapius, 1978.
Jones IS, Jakobiec FA, Nolan BT. Patient Examination and Introduction to Orbital Disease. In: Duane T, ed. *Clinical Ophthalmology.* Hagerstown, MD: Harper & Row, 1976;2.
Koorneef L. *Spatial Aspects of Orbital Musculo-fibrous Tissue in Man.* Amsterdam: Swets & Zeitlinger, 1977.
Woolf S. *Anatomy of the Eye and Orbit.* 6th ed. Revised by EJ Last. London: Lewis, 1968.

Exophthalmos and Exophthalmometry

Bullock JD, Bartley GB. Dynamic Proptosis. *Am J Ophthalmol.* 1986;102:104–110.
Drews LC. Exophthalmometry and a new exophthalmometer. *Trans Am Ophthalmol Soc.* 1956;54:215–252.
Migliori ME, Gladstone GJ. Determination of the normal range of exophthalmometric values for black and white adults. *Am J Ophthalmol.* 1984;98:438–442.

Thyroid

Autoimmune thyroid disease. *Endocrinol Metab Clin North Am.* 1987;16:229–473.
Bartalena L, Marcocci C, Bogazzi F et al. Use of corticosteroids to prevent progression of Graves' ophthalmopathy after radioiodine therapy for hyperthyroidism. *N Engl J Med.* 1989;321:1350–1352.
Guy JR, Fagien S, et al. Methylprednisone pulse therapy in severe dysthyroid optic neuropathy. *Ophthalmology.* 1989;96:1048–1053.
Hartel WC, Kennerdell JC. Dysthyroid orbitopathy. In: Spoor TC, ed. *Modern Management of Ocular Disease.* Thorofare, NJ: Slack, 1985.

Lopatynsky JO, Krohel GB. Bromocriptine therapy for thyroid ophthalmopathy. *Am J Ophthalmol.* 1989;107:680–683. Letter.

Neigel JM, Rootman J, et al. Dysthyroid optic neuropathy: The crowded orbital apex syndrome. *Ophthalmology.* 1988;95:1515–1521.

Newman NM, et al. CT evaluation of "thyroid" orbitopathy (St. Yves syndrome): A quantitative approach. Unpublished data from 4700 CT scans, Centre Nationale D'Ophthalmologie, Hôpital Quinze Vingts, Paris.

Prummel MF, Mourits MP, Berghout A, et al: Prednisone and cyclosporine in the treatment of severe Graves' ophthalmopathy. *N Engl J Med.* 1989;321:1353–1359.

Wall JR. Humoral mechanisms in relationship to Graves' ophthalmopathy. In: Walfish PG, Wall JR, Volpe R, eds. *Autoimmunity and the Thyroid.* Orlando: Academic Press, 1985.

Tumors

Henderson JW. *Orbital Tumors.* New York: Decker, 1980.

Lacrimal

Stewart W, Krohel GB, Wright JE. Lacrimal gland and fossa lesions: An approach to diagnosis and management. *Ophthalmology.* 1979;86:886–895.

Neurofibromatosis

Reed D, Robertson WD, Rootman J, Douglas G. Plexiform neurofibromatosis of the orbit: CT evaluation. *Am J Neuroradiol.* 1986;7:259–263.

Idiopathic Orbital Inflammatory Disease (Orbital Pseudotumor)

Diaz-Llopis M, Menezo JL. Idiopathic inflammatory orbital pseudotumor and low-dose cyclosporin. *Am J Ophthalmol.* 1989;108:547–548. Letter.

Noble AG, Tripathi RC, Levine RA. Indomethacin for the treatment of idiopathic orbital myositis. *Am J Ophthalmol.* 1989;108:334–338. Letter.

Section IV
Headaches and Functional Disorders

CHAPTER 19

HEADACHES, PAIN, AND THE EYE

The "headache" patient consults ophthalmologists and neuro-ophthalmologists on the mistaken assumption that refractive errors cause headaches.

Eyestrain, fatigue, and aching do occur with refractive errors and muscle imbalance, but they usually are mild discomforts (see "Eye Pain" later in the chapter). Despite this, headache is a frequent and important symptom of neuro-ophthalmic problems, and may herald life-threatening and vision-threatening disorders (Table 19–1).

Headaches are ubiquitous; they affect most of us at some time and for about half of us they are occasionally severe. Because they are universal, because it is easy to be cavalier about them, because the mechanism of headache is poorly understood, and because mental set plays a large role in the precipitation of headaches, it is critical to differentiate accurately the threatening from the trivial. Although most headaches are benign (Table 19–2), headache is frequently a presenting symptom of brain tumor, subarachnoid hemorrhage, and giant-cell arteritis. Even if the headache is not a manifestation of a life-threatening illness, the headache patient is a significant part of neuro-ophthalmic practice. Correct diagnosis leads to effective therapy, avoiding substantial discomfort and disability.

As with all of neuro-ophthalmology, obtaining a complete and accurate history is critical to correct diagnosis and appropriate treatment (Table 19–3).

THE TRIGEMINAL NERVE

Ophthalmic Division (V_1). Most pain-sensitive areas of the eye, face, and head are innervated by the three divisions of the trigeminal nerve (V)—the ophthalmic, maxillary, and mandibular divisions. The trigeminal nerve is the largest of the cranial nerves (Figs. 19–1, 19–2).

The major nerves from the eye and orbit are branches of its **ophthalmic division** (V_1). The ophthalmic division has three branches: the frontal, nasociliary, and lacrimal nerves. **The frontal nerve**, the largest, runs under the orbital roof, over the levator, and gives rise to two major branches in the orbit, the supratrochlear and supraorbital branches (Fig. 19–1). The mesial upper lid and conjunctiva are innervated by the supratrochlear branch; and the forehead, scalp, and frontal areas by the supraorbital branch (Fig. 19–3).

The **lacrimal nerve** supplies the skin and conjunctiva contiguous to the lacrimal gland, and via an anastomosis with the zygomatic nerve (V_2) also carries postganglionic parasympathetic fibers to the lacrimal gland for reflex lacrimation. It runs laterally in the orbit.

The sensory supply to all of the eyeball, the sphenoid and ethmoid sinuses, nasal mucosa, skin of the tip of the nose, and medial and inferior orbital structures and lid is carried in the **nasociliary nerve**, the medial branch of the ophthalmic division.

The frontal, lacrimal, and nasociliary nerves pass through the superior orbital fissure (SOF) and join in the anterior cavernous sinus to form the ophthalmic division (V_1) of the trigeminal nerve, which runs in the lateral wall of the cavernous sinus (below the oculomotor and trochlear nerves and lateral to the sixth nerve) to the Gasserian ganglion (see Fig. 13–5). Recurrent branches to the pain-sensitive structures of the supratentorial cranial cavity (dura, venous sinuses, and blood vessels) are the basis for pain referred to the eye and orbit. For example, recurrent branches supply the tentorium and dura over the posterior pole of the cerebral hemisphere; they are thought to mediate referred pain to the inner can-

TABLE 19–1. DIFFERENTIAL DIAGNOSIS OF HEADACHE

	Headache			Character of Pain	
	Intensity	*Quality*	*Location*	*Frequency*	*Duration*
Vascular					
Migraine	+ +–+ + +	Throbbing	Often unilateral	Episodic 1–2/month	18–36 hr
Cluster	+ + + +	Boring, excruciating	Orbit, temple	Nearly daily for periods of weeks	1–2 hr
Raeder's syndrome	+ + +	Dull	Unilateral retro-orbital	Persistent	Persistent
Temporal arteritis	+ + +	Boring	Temple, often unilateral	Persistent until treated	Persistent until treated
Carotid dissection	+ +	Dull	Neck, throat, face	Persistent until thrombosis or dissection stops	Persistent
Tension/Muscular					
	+–+ +	Band-like, heavy	Generalized frontal, nuchal	Daily	Chronic
Neuralgic					
Trigeminal neuralgia (tic doloreaux)	+ + + +	Lancinating, sharp, jabbing	Unilateral; V_2, $V_3 > V_1$	Multiple/day	Waves lasting secs to minutes
Postherpetic neuralgia	+ + + +	Burning	V_1	Daily	Continuous
Atypical facial pain	+ +–+ + +	Boring	"Deep" dermatomal	not always	Constant, lasting days to months
Orbital Pain					
	+ +	Aching	Orbit	—	Until treated
Ocular Pain					
	+–+ + +	Aching	Eye	—	Until treated
CNS Disease					
Subarachnoid hemorrhage	+ + + +	Crushing	Variable	—	Until blood gone
Mass	+ +	Aching	Supratentorial: anterior, face	Intermittent to constant	Until treated
Meningitis	+ + +	Aching	Infratentorial: occipital, cervical	Constant	Until treated
Pseudotumor cerebri	+ +	Aching	Variable	Relatively constant	Until treated
Posttraumatic headache	+ +	Dull	Diffuse	Daily	Often 1–2 yr
Systemic Disease					
Infection	+ +	Throbbing	Frontal, nuchal	Constant	Until treated
Sinus	+ +	Aching	Frontal	Starts PM	Until treated
Pheochromocytoma	+ + +	Throbbing, severe	Bilateral, often occipital	1–3/day	< 1 hr, often on awakening

+, present; + +, marked; + + +, severe; + + + +, very severe or characteristic of diagnosis; ±, variable; AD, autosomal dominant; CSF, cerebrospinal fluid; ESR, erythrocyte sedimentation rate; ETOH, alcohol; FH, family history; ICP, intracranial pressure; PMR, polymyalgia rheumatica; SAH, subarachnoid hemorrhage.

Age at Onset	FH	Associated Symptoms	Initiating Factors	Other
Child to teens	+ + + AD	Nausea, vomiting, photophobia, autonomic symptoms	Stress, foods, hormones, nitrates, etc	Aura
Middle age	0	Nasal congest., Horner's syndrome, lacrimation	ETOH, vasodilators in cluster period	Nocturnal, months of pain-free intervals
Older	0	Horner's syndrome; if V_1, V_2, or other cranial nerves affected, rule out brain tumor	—	Cluster variant but beware of tumor
Elderly	0	Polymyalgia, tender scalp, jaw claudication, PMR		High ESR, anemia
Varies	0	Horner's syndrome	Trauma	Anticoagulation
Any	+/−	May overlap vascular headache	Stress	Tenderness of occipital ridge
50–60 Mostly elderly	0	If hypaesthesia, rule out brain tumor rule out multiple sclerosis	Cold air, touch	Trigger point
Usually elderly	0	—	—	History of herpes zoster ophthalmicus
Young adult	0	—	—	Frequent drug problems, psychopathic personality
—	0	—	—	Proptosis, ophthalmoplegia
—	0	—	—	Ocular inflammation, photophobia
Middle age	+/−	Stiff neck	Hypertension	Blood in CSF
Any	0	Neurologic	—	
Any	0	Nuchal Rigidity	—	Cells in CSF
3–4 decades	0	Papilledema	Drugs, vitamin A, venous thrombosis	Increased ICP
Any	0	Residua of trauma, spasm of near reflex	Trauma	—
Any	0	—	—	Fever, malaise, photophobia
Any	0	—	—	Sinus tenderness
Any	+/−	Sweating, pallor, tachycardia, hypertension	Change is positive	No symptoms when supine

TABLE 19–2. THE FINAL DIAGNOSES IN PATIENTS ATTENDING TWO HEADACHE CLINICS

1152 Patients		200 Patients	
Diagnosis	*Percentage*	*Diagnosis*	*Percentage*
Migraine	53	Migraine	44.5
Tension headache	41	Depression	14.5
Cluster headache	1	Tension headache	11.5
Brain tumor	< 1	Cluster headache	8
Disorders of cervical spine, sinuses, systemic and psychiatric disorders	5	Posttraumatic syndrome	8
		Eye disorders	5
		Brain tumors	3
		Cervical spondylosis	2.5
		Temporal arteritis	2
		Sinusitis	1

Data on 1152 patients from Lance JW, Curran DA, Anthony M. Investigations into the mechanism and treatment of chronic headache. Med J Aust. 1965;2: 909–914. Data on 200 patients from Carroll JD. Diagnostic problems in a migraine clinic. In: Cummings JN, ed. Background to Migraine, Fourth Migraine Symposium. New York: Springer-Verlag, 1971:14–24.

thus associated with occipital lobe infarcts (posterior cerebral artery occlusion). Other recurrent branches refer pain to the forehead and temple. In contrast, pain from infratentorial structures is referred to the occiput, ear, and retroauricular area.

Maxillary division (V_2). The infraorbital nerve that supplies the skin of the lower eyelid, midface, and upper lip traverses the inferior orbital fissure to the pterygopalatine fossa, joining with other fibers (eg, from the sphenopalatine ganglion) to form the *maxillary division* (V_2) of the trigeminal nerve (Fig. 19–2A). It passes into the skull via the foramen rotundum, also entering the lower portion of the wall of the cavernous sinus, and runs with the fibers from V_1 to the Gasserian ganglion. Its intracranial branches supply the dura and vessels of the middle cranial fossa.

Mandibular division (V_3). The *mandibular division* (V_3) of the fifth nerve (Fig. 19–3) supplies both sensory function to the lower face and motor

TABLE 19–3. THE HEADACHE HISTORY

History of headache	Age at onset, duration of symptoms, frequency of headache, more than one type of headache, headache-free intervals
Characteristics of pain	Location, intensity, frequency, quality, time of day, duration, rapidity of onset/offset
Patient history	Family history, medical history, allergic history
Associated symptoms	Aura, autonomic, photophobia, neurologic
Precipitating factors	Food, hormones, activity, stress and relief from stress, sexual intercourse
Relief of headache	Medications and maneuvers taken and response to avoid/control headache
Relation to	Menstruation, Sleep
Effect of Valsalva Maneuver	Cough, sneeze, bearing down at bowel movement, sexual intercourse
Presentation	Rapidity of onset/offset

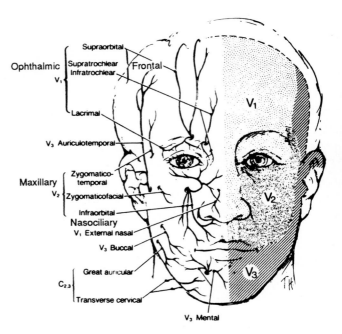

Figure 19–1. Sensory nerves of the face and scalp. Note the distribution of the three divisions of the trigeminal nerve and their areas of overlap. (*From Miller NR, ed.* Walsh and Hoyt's Clinical Neuro-ophthalmology. *Baltimore: Williams & Wilkins, 1985; 2; with permission.*) N.B. external nasal branch of nasociliary artery is a branch of V_1 This is the anatomical reason that involvement of the tip of the nose with Herpes Zoster often heralds involvement of the eye.

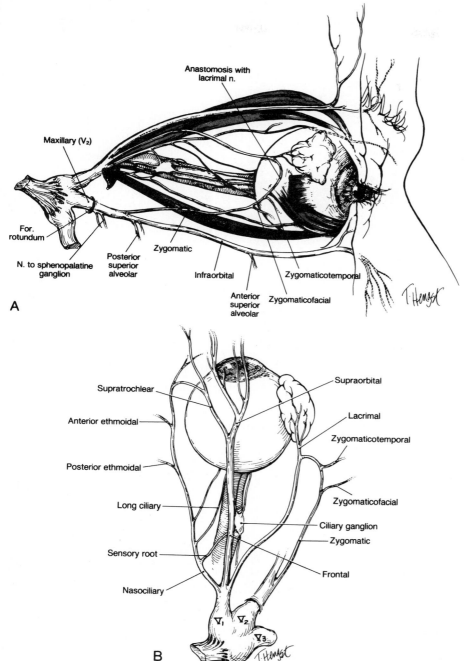

Anastomosis with
lacrimal n.

Maxillary (V₂)

For.
rotundum

N. to sphenopalatine
ganglion

Posterior
superior
alveolar

Zygomatic

Infraorbital

Anterior
superior
alveolar

Zygomaticofacial

Zygomaticotemporal

A

Supratrochlear

Anterior ethmoidal

Posterior ethmoidal

Long ciliary

Sensory root

Nasociliary

Supraorbital

Lacrimal

Zygomaticotemporal

Zygomaticofacial

Ciliary ganglion

Zygomatic

Frontal

V₁ V₂ V₃

B

Figure 19–2. Trigeminal nerve branches. **A.** Lateral view. **B.** View from above. (*From Doxanas MT, Anderson RL. Lacrimal system. In: XY, ed.* Clinical Orbital Anatomy. *Baltimore: Williams & Wilkins, 1984, with permission.*)

function to the muscles of mastication; it enters the skull through the foramen ovale and does *not* enter the cavernous sinus. The sensory fibers join the Gasserian ganglion; the **motor root** enters the brain stem directly.

The **Gasserian (trigeminal, semilunar) ganglion** lies on the anterior superior surface of the petrous bone surrounded by a pouch of arachnoid and dura. It is analogous to a spinal root ganglion and contains

the bodies of the sensory axons of all three divisions of the trigeminal nerves. The major root of the fifth nerve carries the sensory fibers and the minor root carries the motor fibers from V₃ into the brain stem.

The fibers of the sensory root leave the Gasserian ganglion posteriorly, traverse the pontine cistern to enter the anterolateral pons, and then cross the basal pons to the sensory trigeminal nuclear complex. The fibers of the motor root form a bundle in the mesen-

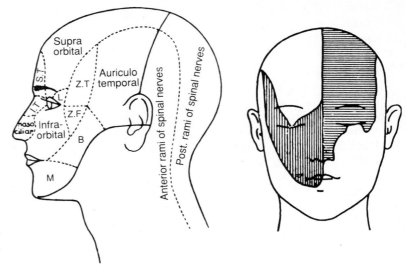

Figure 19–3. A. The sensory nerves of the skin of the head. **B.** Cutaneous distribution of the maxillary (right) and ophthalmic (left) divisions of the trigeminal nerve. (*From Duke-Elder S.* System of Ophthalmology. *Vol 12 in* Neuro-ophthalmology. *St. Louis: Mosby, 1971, with permission.*)

cephalic root of the fifth nerve but apparently do **not** end in the **motor nucleus,** which lies medial to the main sensory nucleus at the level of the midpons (Figs. 19–4B, C).

The **sensory nucleus of the trigeminal nerve** extends from the midbrain to the cervical spinal cord (Figs. 19–4A–C). It has three divisions:

1. The spinal tract and nucleus subserve pain and temperature; their separation from the

nuclei for other sensations and accessibility to surgical intervention are the basis for medullary spinal tractotomy.
2. The main (principal) nucleus subserves touch.
3. The mesencephalic nucleus subserves proprioception from the muscles served by V_3.

Short interneurones form connections with the other brain-stem nuclei, which are the bases of the reflexes

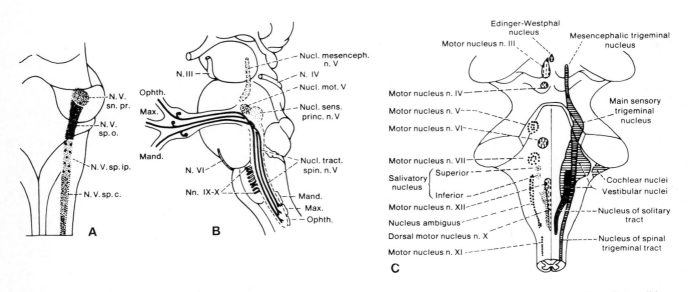

Figure 19–4. A. Subdivision of the **trigeminal sensory nuclei.** The upper region (NV snpr) is the main sensory nucleus. Below this follow the three subdivisions of the spinal nucleus: the oralis (NV spo), the interpolaris (NV spip), and the caudalis (NV spc). The latter continues caudally into the dorsal horn. **B.** Topical arrangement within the **spinal trigeminal tract** of the fibers belonging to the main divisions of the trigeminal nerve. The fibers terminate in the nuclei according to the same pattern. The successive rostrocaudal termination of the three groups shown in the diagram is disputed. **C.** Columnar arrangement of the cranial nerve nuclei. The nuclei belonging to the same categories are indicated by identical symbols. (*From Brodal A.* Neurological Anatomy in Relation to Clinical Medicine. *2nd ed. New York: Oxford, 1969, with permission.*)

mediated by the fifth nerve. In addition, convergence of stimuli from both trigeminal and cervical regions on the same cell bodies in the fifth nerve nucleus explains eye and orbital pain with cervical irritation or vice-versa.

The pathways ascending from the trigeminal nuclei decussate, traveling with the medial lemnisci and spinothalamic tracts to the medial ventral posterior thalamic nuclei (NVPM). A secondary ascending tract passes more dorsally and decussates only partially. As a result, pontine and tegmental lesions *cannot* cause total loss of sensation on only one side of the face. Thus, *unilateral trigeminal sensory loss occurs only when nuclear or peripheral V nerve fibers are damaged.* After a synapse in the posterior ventral thalamus, the sensory fibers project to the primary sensory cortex of the paracentral and postcentral gyri of the parietal lobe via the posterior limb of the internal capsule.

Trigeminal Reflexes

The connections of the trigeminal complex nuclei with other cranial centers and brain-stem nuclei form the basis of numerous trigeminal reflexes (Table 19–4).

The **blink reflex** is an important protective reflex; its afferent arc is the ophthalmic division of the trigeminal nerve and its efferent arc the facial nerve fibers to the orbicularis oculi. In everyday life it is elicited by potential threats to the eye: physical movement, bright light, touching the cornea or the skin of the eyelids, and so forth. It is an important part of the neuro-ophthalmic examination that may be used to test both fifth and seventh nerve function. Compressive lesions affect the **corneal reflex** (the blink reflex in response to touching the cornea) before other functions of the fifth nerve. Therefore, a diminished corneal reflex may be the first objective sign of tumor compressing the fifth nerve.

Another important, potentially dangerous trigeminal reflex is the **oculocardiac reflex.** The afferent arc is again V_1; the outflow causes slowing of the heart via the vagus nerve. The oculocardiac reflex should be remembered during ophthalmic surgery where traction on the extraocular muscles, pressure on the globe, or increased intraocular pressure may cause cardiac slowing, heart block, or even cardiac arrest. Attacks of narrow-angle glaucoma with extremely high intraocular pressure can do the same.

The oculocardiac reflex is also used beneficially. It is well known that pressure on the eyeball can cause reflex slowing of the heart and may be used to halt attacks of paroxysmal atrial tachycardia (PAT).

A number of trigeminal reflexes is tested in the neurlogical examination. Many are release phenomena, the result of bilateral interruption of the corticobulbar projections to the trigeminal motor nucleus. They include the corneo-mandibular reflex, jaw jerk, and snout reflex.

In the **photic sneeze reflex,** shining light into the

TABLE 19–4. TRIGEMINAL REFLEXES

Name	Stimulus	Afferent Arc	Efferent Arc	Response	Clinical Significance
Blink	Threat to eye, touch to lids, cornea; bright lights, wind	V_1	VII (to orbicularis)	Blink	Tests both V_1 and seventh-nerve corneal reflex lost early in fifth-nerve compression (eg, CPA tumor)
Oculocardiac	Increased IOP, traction on eye muscles, pressure on globe	V_1	Vagus	Cardiac slowing, heart block, cardiac arrest	Important to be wary during eye surgery, esp. muscle surgery Occurs in NAG attacks, can halt PAT
Corneo-mandibular	Touching cornea (V_1)	V_1	V_3	Jaw jerk to opposite side	
Jaw Jerk	Tap on chin	V_3 sensory	V_3 motor	Jaw Jerk	Bilateral corticobulbar lesions Release phenomena
Snout	Tap on upper lip	V_3 sensory	VII	Lips purse	

CPA, cerebellar pontine angle; IOP, intraocular pressure; NAG, narrow-angle glaucoma; PAT, paroxysmal atrial tachycardia.

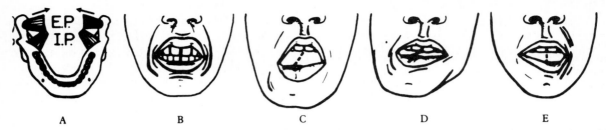

A   B   C   D   E

Figure 19–5. A. Anatomy of the pterygoid muscles; the direction of pull by the muscles is indicated by the arrows. (EP, external pterygoid; IP, internal pterygoid.) **B–E.** Paralysis of the right pterygoid muscles. **B.** At rest the jaw does not deviate. **C.** When the patient attempts to open the mouth, the jaw deviates to the right as a result of the unbalanced action of the left pterygoid muscles. **D.** When asked to move the jaw toward the right, the patient is able to do so. **E.** When asked to move the jaw to the left, the patient is unable to do so. (*From Rengarchy SS. Cranial nerve examination. In: Wilkins RH, Rengachary SS, eds.* Neurosurgery. *New York: McGraw-Hill, 1985; 1; with permission.*)

eyes causes reflex sneezing. The mechanism for this is not clear.

The **Marcus Gunn jaw-winking synkinesis** consists of ptosis, nearly always congenital, associated with elevation of the lid when the jaw moves. This synkinesis between the pterygoid nerve (V_3) and the levator muscle (III) probably results from a congenital misdirection of a branch of V_3 into the superior division of the third nerve. It is usually noted soon after birth when the lid elevates rhythmically as the baby feeds. The Marcus Gunn phenomenon is often associated with other oculomotor abnormalities, most commonly double-elevator palsy and superior rectus palsy.

Clinical Evaluation of the Trigeminal Nerve

Corneal and facial sensation is tested by a light touch with a small piece of cotton or Q-tip drawn to a fine point. Both the patient's subjective report and, in the case of the cornea, observation of the blink reflex are recorded. Cutaneous sensation should be tested for all three divisions of the trigeminal distribution. Discrepancies should be sought between the right

and left sides, between the objective and subjective responses, and between the three divisions of the trigeminal nerve. A corollary objective sign of trigeminal integrity, analogous to the blink reflex, is using a cotton or facial tissue "wick" as an intranasal stimulus. The reflex raising of the head and movement of the nose away from the vibrissae stimulus is called **nudation.** Asymmetry of this response is another **objective** sign of loss of trigeminal sensation. The motor functions of V_3 are tested by having the patient clench the jaw shut while palpating the temporal and masseter muscles, by sensing any asymmetry in pushing the jaw from side to side against resistance, and by looking for asymmetry as the lower jaw is pushed forward by the patient. Remember, pterygoid contraction causes deviation of the jaw to the opposite side; for example, a lesion of V_3 on the right will cause the jaw to deviate to the right and exhibit weakness against pressure from the left (Fig. 19–5).

If a brain-stem lesion is suspected, testing pain (with pin prick), temperature, vibration, two point, and so forth, may be helpful in localizing trigeminal

Figure 19–6. TOP Lateral view of the area of the cavernous sinus and its relation to the sphenoid sinus. The oculomotor (III) and trochlear (IV) nerves are seen above. The intracavernous portion of the carotid artery is seen medial to the trigeminal root (I) and the ophthalmic (V_1), maxillary (V_2), and mandibular (V_3) divisions of the trigeminal nerve. The opening into the sphenoid sinus is located between the first and second trigeminal divisions. (*From Rhoton AL Jr. Microsurgical anatomy of the sellar region. In: Wilkins RH, Rengachary SS, eds.* Neurosurgery. *New York: McGraw-Hill, 1985;1; with permission.*)

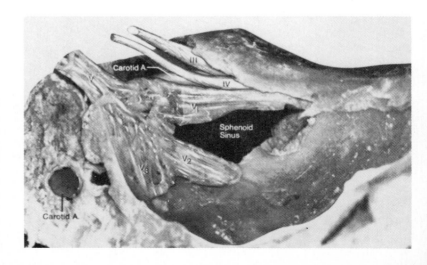

TABLE 19–5. CAUSES OF CORNEAL HYPESTHESIA

Trigeminal Nerve

Compression or invasion by tumor

Systemic disease (sensory neuropathies): diabetes mellitus, leprosy, hypovitaminosis A, connective tissue disease

Toxic exposure: Carbon disulfide, hydrogen sulfide, trichloracetic acid

Pharmacologic: Stilbamidine

Congenital (rare)
  Idiopathic
  Familial: Riley-Day syndrome (associated with painless corneal erosion and scarring)

Ocular

Corneal herpes simplex and zoster

Contact lens wear (especially hard lenses)

Refractive surgery, corneal transplantation, cataract surgery

Corneal dystrophy

Some glaucoma medications

nuclear lesions. Trigeminal sensory functions are separately represented in the brain-stem nuclei: The spinal nucleus subserves pain and temperature; the main nucleus, touch; and the mesencephalic nucleus, proprioception.

In disorders of the fifth nerve causing hypesthesia, sensation rarely changes abruptly at the midline. Thus, any patient reporting a clear-cut, instantaneous change in sensation exactly at the midline is suspect for malingering, as are patients who include the ear lobe or angle of the jaw in the area affected, or whose loss of sensation ends at the hairline rather than at the vertex of the scalp (see Fig. 19–2). Lesions of the cavernous sinus and orbit spare V_3 sensation and motor function because the mandibular branch exits through the foramen ovale without entering the cavernous sinus. About 10% of the time V_2 lies unprotected in the wall of the sphenoid sinuses (Fig. 19–6).

TABLE 19–6. FIFTH-NERVE LESIONS[a]

Location	Etiology	Associated Findings	Special Characteristic
Intrinsic Brain-stem Lesions			
Medulla	Syringobulbia, Wallenberg's syndrome, PICA or vertebral artery occlusion	Hiccups, hoarseness, Horner's syndrome, lateropulsion of eye movements, crossed, sensory loss	Occasionally characterized as stinging or "salt and pepper" pain Early pain in face, masseter spasm
Thalamus—Dejerine-Roussy syndrome	Thalamogeniculate artery occlusion (branch of PCA)	Transient homonymous hemianopia, contralateral pain	Esp. disagreeable quality to pain; rx: Tegretol
Basal Lesions			
Gradenigo's syndrome	Chronic otitis with petrous apex inflam.	VI	Pain in distribution of V
	CPA tumor, aneurysm, trauma	VII, VIII	
	Meningeal lesions, carcinomatosis, or sarcoidosis		Multiple cranial nerve palsies; may vary in involvement, intensity
Orbit			
Isolated neuropathy	Trauma, sinus infection (rare), invasion by tumor	V_2 hypesthesia, proptosis	Tingling or prickly numbness of the cheek
	Idiopathic	Cornea spared	Remitting
	Congenital	Painless corneal erosion, opacity	Bilateral
	Toxic	Nasal erosion, dysesthesias	Hydrogen sulfide, carbon disulfide, stilbamidine, trichlorocetic acid
	Systemic diseases	Paresthesias	Leprosy, diabetes mellitus, vitamin A deficiency, connective tissue disease, multiple sclerosis
V₃, mental nerve only	Intrinsic tumor Mets, lymphoproliferative disease		Numb chin

CPA, cerebellar pontine angle; PCA, posterior cerebral artery; PICA, posterior inferior cerebellar artery.
[a] Cause loss of sensation unless otherwise noted.

TABLE 19–7. TYPE AND DISTRIBUTION OF LESIONS CAUSING FIFTH CRANIAL NERVE SYMPTOMS

Location/Type	No. (%)
Brain Stem	
Multiple sclerosis	4
Glioma	4
Stroke	3
Metastasis	1
Cavernous angioma with hemorrhage	1
Syringohydrobulbia	1
Total	14 (18)
Preganglionic Segment	
Vascular compression	4
Arteriovenous malformation	3
Meningioma	2
Epidermoid	2
Acoustic neuroma	1
Metastasis	1
Surgical sectioning	1
Total	14 (18)
Gasserian Ganglion	
Metastasis	3
Trigeminal schwannoma	3
Total	6 (8)
Cavernous Sinus	
Cavernous carotid aneurysm	3
Metastasis	2
Total	5 (7)
Peripheral Divisions[a]	
V₁–V₃	
Neurofibroma	1
Spindle cell skin carcinoma	1
Tongue squamous cell carcinoma	1
V₁ and V₂	
Nasopharyngeal squamous cell carcinoma	1
Sphenoid wing meningioma	1
Neurofibroma	1
V₂ and V₃	
Malignant salivary gland tumors	4
Lymphoma	2
Lip squamous cell carcinoma	1
Poorly differentiated skin carcinoma	1
Rhabdomyosarcoma	1
V₁ and V₂	
Metastasis	1
V₂	
Nasopharyngeal squamous cell carcinoma	2
Skin squamous cell carcinoma	1
Maxillary sinus squamous cell carcinoma	1
Chondrosarcoma	1
Sphenoid mucocele	1
Maxillary sinusitis	1
Malignant salivary gland tumor	3
Malignant schwannoma	2
Lymphoma	2
Osteomyelitis	1
Abscess	1
Nasopharyngeal squamous cell carcinoma	1
Oropharyngeal squamous cell carcinoma	1
Ewing sarcoma	1
Chondrosarcoma	1
Metastasis	1
Total	37 (49)

[a] Lesions in the V₁ peripheral division are classified under cavernous sinus.
From Hutchins LG, et al. The radiologic assessment of trigeminal neuropathy. Am J N R. 1989;10:1031–1038.

Loss of Sensation in the Trigeminal Nerve Distribution

Most afflictions of the trigeminal nerve, central and peripheral, produce hypesthesia (Table 19–5) rather than (or in addition to) pain or headache. Compression, demyelination, and infection or inflammation cause essentially indistinguishable sensory loss. Thus, the differential diagnosis of fifth nerve lesions largely depends on accompanying signs and symptoms (Table 19–6). Thorough evaluation of adjacent cranial nerves is paramount, because most intracranial space-occupying lesions cause more than an isolated trigeminal neuropathy. For example, because the ophthalmic fibers are ventral as the root enters the pons, loss of the corneal reflex is frequently the first sign of fifth-nerve compression by acoustic neuromas and other cerebellopontine angle (CPA) tumors. The seventh and eighth nerves are usually affected as well. The exception is an isolated tumor of the nerve itself, which may be intra- or extracranial.

In general, the type and distribution of symptoms are disappointingly inaccurate for localization of trigeminal lesions, although pain and numbness tend to be associated with peripheral fifth nerve lesions (Tables 19–7 to 19–9). Magnetic resonance imaging (MRI) is the diagnostic test of choice for trigeminal neuropathy.

Isolated fifth nerve palsies are usually caused by an otherwise unexplained trigeminal neuropathy (which may be evanescent or remitting) and multiple sclerosis. Isolated neuropathies often are purely sensory and tend to preserve the corneal reflex. In contrast, most compressive or invasive lesions involve the corneal reflex early and worsen with time. Rarely, trigeminal neuropathies are associated with systemic diseases such as diabetes and leprosy, vitamin A deficiency, and connective tissue disease; or are toxic (carbon disulfide, hydrogen sulfide). Congenital neuropathies are rare, bilateral, and associated with painless corneal erosion and opacity. Lesions of the peripheral branches of the fifth nerve are relatively uncommon and usually are caused by trauma or tumors

Lesions of the infraorbital nerve (V₂) are especially prone to cause loss of sensation around the orbit, and include facial and lower face etiologies and orbital trauma (eg, blowout fractures) and nasopharyngeal, maxillary sinus, or cutaneous carcinoma invading along the infraorbital nerve. Ask for history of removal of a skin lesion from the face. Infiltrating tumors may also involve the branches of the seventh nerve. Frequently, these tumors—especially squamous cell carcinoma of the skin, sinus, and nasopharynx—infiltrate so subtly along the nerve that imaging studies may be unrewarding;

TABLE 19–8. DISTRIBUTION OF CLINICAL SIGNS ACCORDING TO LESION LOCATION[a]

Distribution of Symptoms	Lesion Location				
	Brain Stem	Preganglionic Segment	Gasserian Ganglion	Cavernous Sinus	Peripheral
V_1–V_3	7	4	2	1	1
V_1 and V_2	2	2	1	0	3
V_1 and V_3	2	4	2	1	9
V_1 and V_3	0	0	0	0	0
V_1	0	0	0	2	—[a]
V_2	1	1	0	1	7
V_3	1	1	0	0	16
Not known	1	2	1	0	1
Total	14	14	6	5	37

Note—The distribution of clinical signs was determined by history and physical examination.
[a] See cavernous sinus.
From Hutchins LG, Harnsberger XY, et al. The radiologic assessment of trigeminal neuropathy. Am J N R. 1989;10:1031–1038.

nevertheless, the pterygopalatine fossa and foramen rotundum especially should be studied for evidence of neural thickening. Tumors of the maxillary sinus may cause nasal stuffiness, tearing, or both, long before significant hypesthesia occurs. Boring, difficult-to-control pain is common in infiltrative squamous cell carcinomas.

Dissociated sensory loss characterizes trigeminal tract and nuclear lesions within the brain stem. The extension of the three trigeminal nerve sensory nuclei through the length of the brain stem and into the cervical cord as well as the separation of sensory function in the three nuclei (mesencephalic nucleus for proprioception, main nucleus for touch, and spinal tract and nucleus for pain and temperature) leads to this dissociation, as lesions rarely involve all three nuclei. In addition, the varied levels at which the different sensory fibers cross the midline not infrequently give rise to crossed as well as dissociated sensory loss. For example, **the lateral medullary syndrome of Wallenberg** is due to infarction of the posterior inferior cerebellar artery (PICA) or other vertebrobasilar branches. It is associated with loss of pain and temperature but touch (the corneal reflex) is preserved. Pain in the face may be the primary complaint. Lesions in the pons are usually associated with disorders of ocular motility in addition to loss of sensation.

The supratrochlear branch of V_1 is especially prone to damage in frontal and ethmoid sinus surgery. Metastases or lymphoproliferative disease often involve the mental branch of V_3, causing a numb chin.

Isolated loss of corneal sensation usually indicates local (ocular) disease and warrants a careful search for a history of previous ocular surgery, such as cataract extraction, and a meticulous slit-lamp exam for evidence of herpes simplex or, less com-

TABLE 19–9. PRESENTING SYMPTOMS OR SIGNS BY LESION LOCATION

Symptom or Sign	Lesion Location				
	Brain Stem	Preganglionic Segment	Gasserian Ganglion	Cavernous Sinus	Peripheral[a]
Pain	2	6	1	1	8
Numbness	11	5	3	3	13
Pain and numbness	0	0	0	1	11
Other	0	1[b]	0	0	1[c]
Not known	1	2	2	0	4

[a] In five patients with malignant lesions, trismus was part of the symptom complex.
[b] Hyperactive jaw reflex was the only fifth cranial nerve manifestation in a patient with a large cerebellopontine angle meningioma.
[c] Jaw weakness and trismus were the only fifth cranial nerve manifestations in a patient with a deeply invasive, mixed malignant minor salivary gland tumor extending from the base of the skull to the angle of the mandible.
From Hutchins LG, et al. The radiologic assessment of trigeminal neuropathy. Am J N R. 1989; 10:1031–1038.

monly, corneal dystrophy. Some contact lens wearers may exhibit a noticeable decrease of corneal sensitivity, which is symmetrical if lenses are worn in both eyes. Timolol or propranolol drops used to treat glaucoma may also cause diminished corneal sensation.

Neuroparalytic keratitis may occur following loss of corneal sensation, especially following intracranial trigeminal nerve or (rarely) nucleus lesions (eg, destructive treatments for trigeminal neuralgia, cerebellopontine angle tumors, and so forth). Corneal haze, conjunctival hyperemia, and iritis are often associated. The loss of protective reflexes (eg, blink reflex, reflex tearing) certainly contributes to the disorder; the cornea not only becomes vulnerable to breakdown and infection, but seems unable to repair itself normally. Therapy is by lubricants, moist chambers, bandage contact lenses, patching, and tarsorrhaphy or medial canthoplasty if necessary. This problem can be especially vexing when fifth nerve palsies are associated with seventh nerve palsies causing exposure.

Facial Dysesthesia

In lesions of the fifth nerve, dysesthesias are rarer than pain or diminished sensation. Usually associated with a degree of hypesthesia, they frequently follow trauma and may be associated with amputation neuromas. Facial dysesthesia can occur following orbital surgery. An especially vexing discomfort (anesthesia dolorosa) may follow surgical attempts to cure trigeminal neuralgia. Sometimes in an attempt to get rid of the pain, the patient picks away at the nose and may destroy the ala nasae on the affected side. A similar pain is associated with infiltrative carcinomatous neuropathy such as that caused by squamous cell carcinoma. Multiple sclerosis (MS), toxic exposures to trichloracetic acid, and stimbamidine treatment for tic douloureux also cause dysesthesia. Occlusion of the thalamogeniculate artery (a branch of the posterior cerebral artery) can lead to the Dejerine-Roussy syndrome, in which an especially disagreeable pain sensation and hypesthesia are associated with a homonymous hemianopsia, all contralateral to the lesion. These patients frequently withdraw from all usual contact and may become hermit-like, carefully shielding the painful extremity or soaking a limb in water.

Trigeminal Neuralgia (Tic Douloureux)

Paroxysms of excruciating pain ("lancinating pain") localized to one or more divisions of the trigeminal nerve and lasting seconds characterize **trigeminal neuralgia.** Frequently, "trigger" zones exist near the eye, nose, or mouth, where the slightest stimulus

TABLE 19–10. SYNDROMES CAUSED BY VASCULAR CROSS-COMPRESSION OF CRANIAL NERVES

Tic douloureux
Hemifacial spasm
Glossopharyngeal neuralgia
Sphenopalatine neuralgia

induces a paroxysm of pain so severe it is impossible for the patient to talk, eat, or drink. Yet paradoxically, people with tic frequently "play" with their trigger zones. Not uncommonly, signs of autonomic irritation, (lacrimation, conjunctival injection, salivation, flushing) are seen as well. Sensation is normal and the disorder is almost exclusively unilateral. This disease affects predominantly the middle aged and it involves V_2 and V_3 much more often than V_1. At their onset, the attacks are usually spaced well apart; as time passes, they increase in frequency, although remissions do occur.

Etiology. Current theory classifies trigeminal neuralgia as one of the neuropathies associated with cross-compression of nerve roots by aberrant, ectatic, or otherwise abnormal blood vessels (listed in Table 19–10). Other causes of the axonal and myelin disruption seen histologically are rarer (Table 19–11). Those not visible at the time of surgery are less well defined.

Differential Diagnosis. Although classical tic-like symptoms are rarely caused by tumor, cases of atypical tic—especially if associated with hypaesthesia—may be caused by posterior fossa tumor. Look for atrophy of the muscles of mastication (V_3) which

TABLE 19–11. OPERATIVE FINDINGS IN 125 PATIENTS WITH TRIGEMINAL NEURALGIA

Abnormality	Number of Patients
Compressing vessel	90[a]
Superior cerebellar artery	75
Anterior inferior cerebellar artery	14
Posterior inferior cerebellar artery	1
Basilar artery	1
Vein	15
Aneurysm	2
Tumor	5
Abnormal nerve root	2
None	26

[a] In 16 patients, two vessels appeared to distort the trigeminal nerve root. *From Zorman G, Wilson CB. Outcome following microsurgical vascular decompression of partial sensory rhizotomy in 125 cases of trigeminal neuralgia. Neurology. 1984; 34:1362–1365.*

never occurs in true tic. Symptoms of tic in patients less than 50 years old suggest multiple sclerosis.

Tic douloureux occurs in 2 to 5% of patients with MS (conversely, MS occurs in 2 to 5% of tic patients). Tic is usually an early symptom in the MS patient but rarely is the very first symptom. In contrast to "idiopathic" or compressive tic, in MS the pain may be bilateral.

Evaluation. Every patient with tic neuralgia should undergo thorough neurologic and neuro-imaging evaluation to rule out MS, tumor, and other possible causes of facial pain. MRI is most sensitive.

Treatment. Control of pain by medications such as Tegretol (carbamazepine), Baclofen, and Dilantin is moderately successful; about 25% becomes pain free and about 95% obtains some relief (Table 19–12). However, the 25 to 50% of patients that develops resistance to medical therapy will need surgical therapy (Table 19–13). Tegretol is so effective initially that if 600 to 800 mg/day do not produce some relief you should doubt your diagnosis. On the whole, it has fewer side effects than Dilantin, but occasionally

TABLE 19–13. SUMMARY OF THE MANAGEMENT OF TRIGEMINAL NEURALGIA

Use of Carbamazepine	1. Establish diagnosis. 2. Carbamazepine, 100–200 mg tid, increase to 1000 mg/day if indicated. 3. Obtain serum levels in 1 week. 4. Follow complete blood count monthly. 5. If pain control is insufficient, add baclofen, 10 mg tid; increase if indicated.
Ancillary Drugs	1. Phenytoin, 100 mg qid; stop other medications first. 2. Chlorphenesin, 400 mg tid; can use in combination with other drugs.
Surgery Considered[a]	1. If pain is unresponsive to drugs or recurs. 2. If there are toxic reactions to drugs. 3. As an alternative to medical therapy.

[a] Glycerol rhizolysis, microcompression, vascular decompression.
Modified from D'Allessio DJ, ed. Wolff's Headache and Other Head Pain. *5th ed. New York: Oxford, 1987:274.*

TABLE 19–12. DRUGS USED FOR TREATMENT OF TRIGEMINAL NEURALGIA

Generic Name	Brand Name	Dose Range (mg)	Usual Therapeutic Plasma Conc. (μg/mL)	Approximate Half-life (hr)	Common Side Effects	Effectiveness Short Term (1–2 yr)	Long Term (> 2 yr)
Initial Therapy							
Carba-mazepine	Tegretol	400–1600	4–12	12	Drowsiness, light-headed-ness, ataxia	70–80%	50–60%
Phenytoin	Dilantin	300–600	10–12	24	Ataxia, skin rash, diplopia		10–30%
For Resistant Patients							
Baclofen	Lioresal	40–80	?	4	Drowsiness, ataxia, confusion, insomnia		50% (sometimes in combina-tion with initial therapy)
Valproic acid	Depakote	500–2000	50–100	15	Nausea, tremor, weight gain, alopecia		60% resistant
Clonazepam	Klonopin	2–8	0.02–0.08	28	Drowsiness	60%	
Chlorphenesin	Myolate	800–2400	?	?	Drowsiness, weakness, nausea	?	

From Raskin NH. Headache. *2nd ed. New York: Churchill Livingstone, 1988:340.*

these can be serious (bone marrow, liver, kidney toxicity) in addition to nausea and dizziness.

Surgical therapy for trigeminal neuralgia includes efforts to interrupt the fibers of the appropriate division of the nerve at the Gasserian ganglion, to sever or decompress the nerve root, and procedures on the intrinsic central nervous system pathways—the fifth nerve nuclei and mesencephalic tract (Table 19–14). A properly chosen neurosurgical procedure can nearly always relieve the pain of tic and should be performed promptly when pharmacotherapy is exhausted. The goal of surgical therapy is relief of pain with minimal sensory loss. The major complication of surgery is denervation of the face and eye. Figure 19–7 summarizes the management of trigeminal neuralgia.

Percutaneous radiofrequency trigeminal rhizotomy (PRTR) is relatively safe, simple, and inexpensive when compared to procedures necessitating cord section or craniotomy. An insulated needle is threaded from the cheek (through the foramen ovale) to the ganglion and its roots. A radiofrequency current is passed through the needle to cause thermal damage to the ganglionic roots. Pain recurs in 10 to 25% of patients. Muscle weakness occurs in a quarter of patients but usually resolves in months. Ten percent of patients suffer profound numbness including loss of corneal sensation; anesthesia dolorosa is rare. Other cranial nerve palsies can follow the procedure, but in experienced hands, complications are infrequent. It is currently the procedure of choice in patients too ill or elderly to safely undergo a major neurosurgical procedure.

Procedures on the nerves and sensory root other than PRTR are now rarely performed because of relatively high failure rates and significant incidence of corneal anesthesia and anesthesia dolorosa. However, they have the advantage of being relatively minor surgical procedures.

Attacks on the trigeminal ganglion by injection of glycerol and percutaneous microcompression by balloon catheter are newer procedures that combine a high degree of effectiveness and low complication rate. Currently they are performed in relatively few centers. Variations in the results obtained by glycerol injection are attributed to differing osmolalrity among glycerol preparations. More information is needed to properly deploy these procedures in the attack on trigeminal neuralgia. Percutaneous balloon compression also appears effective in pain related to temporal mandibular joint disorders associated with tenesmus.

Microsurgical decompression of the vessel causing cross-compression is best done early. If done when tic douloureux has been present less than 9 years there is an 88% cure rate. If done following a greater than 9-year history, there is a 42% incidence of cure. If done as the first procedure, there is a 92% success rate; but if done after PRTR, only 43% improves. If there is a history of herpes zoster, there is a high incidence of recurrence possibly prevented by pretreating with interferon. Direct exploration, usually done by the suboccipital route, also has the advantage that it may disclose a previously undiagnosed tumor (but tumor **rarely** gives the clinical picture of true tic douloureux). Anesthesia dolorosa, corneal anesthesia, and neuroparalytic keratitis are very rare. If the procedure fails, PRTR will still be effective in a majority of patients.

Medullary tractotomy preserves corneal sensitivity, because the medullary spinal nucleus serves pain and temperature. The primary nucleus separately located in the brain stem serves touch.

OTHER NEURALGIAS

Other cranial neuralgias include sphenopalatine, geniculate, glossopharyngeal, and greater occipital neuralgias—a mixed bag of pain syndromes.

TABLE 19–14. COMPARISON OF OPERATIVE TECHNIQUES FOR TRIGEMINAL NEURALGIA[a]

Technique	Description	Complications
Radio-frequency rhizotomy (PRTR)	90% effective, minor percutaneous needle procedure, brief hospital stay	Facial sensory loss is frequently quite severe, corneal hypesthesia (10–15%), occasional masseter weakness
Glycerol injection	85% effective, minor percutaneous needle procedure, brief hospital stay	Facial sensitivity loss is slight; persistent corneal hypesthesia 5–15%, up to 50% has persistent or recurrent pain, masseter weakness is rare
Percutaneous microcompression (balloon)	90% effective, minor procedure, brief hospital stay, anesthesia w/o intubation	Facial sensory loss, loss of corneal sensation, anesthesia dolorosa rare
Microvascular decompression	90% effective, major craniotomy, 4–10 day hospital stay	Approximately 4% serious postoperative complications, 1% mortality

[a] Each of the procedures is associated with a modest recurrence rate. The recurrence rate is least with microvascular decompression and modestly greater with radiofrequency rhizotomy, balloon compression, and glycerol injection.
Modified from D'Allessio DJ, ed. Wolff's Headache and Other Head Pain. *5th ed. New York: Oxford, 1987;274.*

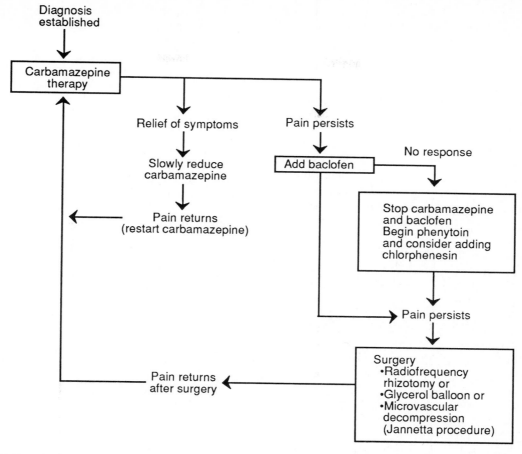

Figure 19–7. Management of trigeminal neuralgia. (*From D'Allessio DJ, ed. Wolff's Headache and Other Head Pain. 5th ed. New York: Oxford, 1987, with permission.*)

Sphenopalatine and glossopharyngeal neuralgias are analogous to trigeminal neuralgia, occurring in the middle aged and consisting of paroxysms of pain frequently set off by touching a trigger point. These neuralgias consist of one or a combination of tongue, palate, tonsil, or ear pains, similar to the pain of tic but sometimes longer lasting. Vagal symptoms such as slowing of the pulse (which may lead to heart block and cardiac arrest) often are associated. The sensitivity of the trigger points can be so pervasive as to provide the basis of a diagnostic test: 10% cocaine is applied to the tonsil and pharynx. This should provide 1 to 2 hours of relief from the painful paroxysms. Especially if the cocaine test is negative, an evaluation by an ears, nose, and throat specialist is in order, to be sure that a small carcinoma of the tonsil or posterior third of the tongue is not overlooked.

Tegretol is the best medical therapy for these neuralgias, but appears to be somewhat less effective than in trigeminal neuralgia, necessitating more frequent surgical therapy. Also, as with trigeminal neu-

ralgia, microvascular cross-compression of the nerve roots is thought to be a cause of the symptoms. Microsurgical decompression is probably the procedure of choice when medical therapy does not succeed, even though it is less successful than in trigeminal neuralgia. Tumors are more often associated with glossopharyngeal neuralgia than with tic douloureux.

Geniculate neuralgia (the Ramsay-Hunt syndrome) has an entirely different cause; it is a manifestation of Herpes zoster, which presents with pain in the ear and seventh-nerve paresis. The herpetic lesions may occur in the external auditory canal, behind the ear, on the tympanic membrane, and in the C_2C_3 distribution.

Occipital neuralgia is frequently accompanied by referral of pain to the eye, orbit, and temple. There usually is associated tenderness in the region of the cervical spine (sometimes associated with arthritis or malformations) or the tendinous insertion of the splenius capitus on the occipital ridge. Inflammation or entrapment of the greater occipital nerve ensue.

The pain is often controlled with injections of local anesthesic (eg, Bupivicaine 5%, 0.5 cc).

ATYPICAL FACIAL PAIN

Atypical facial pain does not follow a nerve distribution. It is bilateral, occurs in a specific location, is nearly constant, and has no trigger point. Usually given a "deep localization," it frequently seems to be of psychogenic origin, as drug addiction and psychopathic personalities are frequent concomitants. Rarely an etiology is discovered, such as sinus infection, dental infection, malocclusion, temporal mandibular joint disorder, deep-seated tumor, or infection.

Work up these patients by neuro-imaging, as organic disease must be ruled out. The differential diagnosis includes temporal arteritis, carotid occlusion, carotid dissection, and temporal mandibular joint problems. Treatment is not very successful, although recent reports suggest some success with transcutaneous electric stimulation. Some patients respond well to medications for migraine and cluster headache, phenelzine and tricyclic antidepressants. After appropriate psychologic evaluation, tractotomy may help severe unremitting pain.

HERPES ZOSTER

The ophthalmic division of the trigeminal nerve is the most common site of dermatomal zoster (16% of all cases) and sustains a higher frequency of complications than elsewhere (about 55%, or 75% if the nasociliary nerve is involved). There also is a higher incidence of postherpetic neuralgia.

The Herpes zoster virus has been demonstrated to reside in the Gasserian ganglion. Intermittently it becomes activated with consequent inflammation of the ganglion, necrosis of ganglion cells, leptomeningitis, and associated alterations of the sensory root and pons adjacent to its entry zone.

Trigeminal herpes zoster affects the cornea most often of the ocular structures. The facial pain may precede the vesicles by 2 to 3 days. Their appearance at the tip of the nose signals involvement of the nasociliary branch of the fifth nerve usually associated with corneal involvement. The entire eye may be involved with herpes zoster: iritis, panuveitis, and optic neuritis are not infrequent. More rarely, intracranial (presumably) spread of the virus may affect one or more of the oculomotor nerves, causing an associated ophthalmoparesis. An associated arteritis may cause stroke and hemiparesis. Men are affected more often than women. The initial pain is steady and typically lasts 2 to 3 weeks. The patient is frequently left with significant dermatomal scarring, depigmentation, and hyperpigmentation.

The numbness that follows the resolution of the infection is due to the ganglion cell damage; the resultant scarring in the ganglion is thought to provide a nidus of irritation to surrounding ganglion cells to account for the vexing **postherpetic neuralgia,** which may be severe and last for years. It occurs in about one fourth of patients and may occur immediately following the primary neuralgia or follow a pain-free interval of weeks to months. Treatment of both the acute and chronic problems is disappointing. The efficacy of steroid treatment remains in dispute; oral Acyclovir is effective in the acute outbreak, especially if started promptly, and recent reports suggest a role for interferon (especially prior to surgical therapy) and levodopa. No entirely successful medical treatment of the neuralgia exists, although recently small numbers of patients are reported to respond well to topical Lidocaine spray or gel, Capsicum, and amitryptyline. Usually, symptomatic therapy with analgesics and amitryptyline is all we can offer. The same surgical procedures that are used in trigeminal neuralgia have been used in severe cases of postherpetic pain but with much less success; transcutaneous nerve stimulation also appears to have some success.

VASCULAR HEADACHES

Migraine and Migraine Equivalents

Migraine is very common, affecting at least 20% of the population. It is hereditary (20 to 90%), paroxysmal, periodic, and affects women more than men by a factor of at least two to one. Migraine consists of a phase of intracerebral arterial constriction followed by a phase of extracerebral arterial dilatation. Its exact etiology is not understood, but is thought to relate to abnormal cerebrovascular reactivity (Fig. 19–8). It usually has its onset in childhood (often with car sickness, night terrors, ice cream headaches, autonomic and basilar symptoms) or the mid-third decade (Table 19–15). Any migraine-like syndrome starting after 50 years old should arouse suspicion of another cause. Susceptibility to precipitating factors is the rule; these include stress, hormonal changes, alcohol, contraceptive pills, caffeine, certain foods, and coexistence with tension and muscular headaches.

Classification of Migraine

The International Headache Society has recently reclassified headache and migraine, eliminating many familiar designations. The new terms are enclosed in parentheses in the following paragraphs.

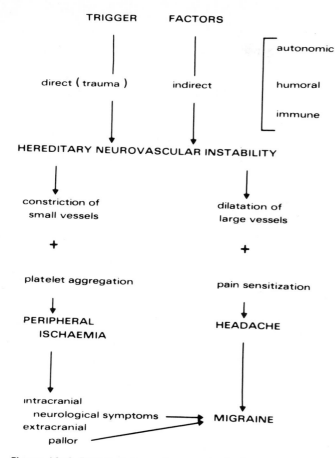

Figure 19–8. Factors in the pathogenesis of migraine. Outline of humoral–vascular theory of migraine. (*From Lance JW. The Mechanism and Management of Headache. 3rd ed. London: Butterworths, 1978, with permission.*)

TABLE 19–16. SYMPTOMS ACCOMPANYING MIGRAINE ATTACKS IN 500 PATIENTS

Symptom	Percentage Affected
Nausea	87
Vomiting	56
Diarrhea	16
Photophobia	82
Visual disturbances	36
Fortification spectra	10
Photopsia	26
Paresthesias	33
Scalp tenderness	65
Lightheadedness	72
Vertigo	33
Alteration of consciousness	18
Seizure	4
Syncope	10
Confusional state	4

Modified from Selby G, Lance JW. Observations on 500 cases of migraine and allied vascular headache. J Neurol Neurosurg Psychiatry. 1960; 23:23–32; Lance JW, Anthony M. Some clinical aspects of migraine. A prospective survey of 500 patients. Arch Neurol. 1966; 15:356–361.

premonitory or concomitant focal neurologic disturbances. Successive attacks frequently alternate from one side of the head to the other. Often, the migraineur seeks relief by holding the head or retreating to a dark, quiet room. Autonomic symptoms are frequent.

Classic migraine occurs in only about 10% of migraine patients have classic migraine, the type associated with the "scintillating scotoma" (Fig. 19–9) usually as a premonitory sign. The scotoma is present in homonymous fields of both eyes (in contrast to amaurosis fugax associated with carotid transient ischemic attacks [TIAs], which is monocular). The scintillating scotoma usually begins as a small paracentral scotoma that spreads peripherally, sometimes producing typical "fortifications," with or without colored aspects. It may also be described as shimmering or heat waves. The visual symptoms of migraine nearly always persist with the eyes closed. Many of these descriptions are accompanied by a typical bilateral gesture with the hand—the migraine "hello" (Fig. 19–10). The speed of enlargement of the classic scotoma corresponds to the speed with which "spreading depression" travels over the visual cortex; it usually lasts a total of about 20 minutes and is followed by a migraine headache. Especially in older patients, the visual symptoms may occur without the associated headache, so-called "acephalgic migraine."

Complicated migraine. Patients with other focal neurologic symptoms accompanying migrainous episodes are said to have complicated migraine. Usu-

Common migraine (migraine without aura) is the headache syndrome experienced by most migraineurs. They suffer the "typical" headache—a pulsating, frequently lateralized, often severe headache associated with nausea, vomiting, phonophobia, and photophobia that lasts from hours to days (Table 19–16). They do *not* experience distinctive

TABLE 19–15. AGE AT ONSET OF MIGRAINE IN 496 PATIENTS

Age at First Attack (Years)	Percentage of Patients
0–10	21
10–20	25
20–30	27
30–40	19
40–50	6
50–60	2

From Selby G, Lance JW. Observations on 500 cases of migraine and allied vascular headache. J Neurol Neurosurg Psychiatry. 1960; 23:23–32.

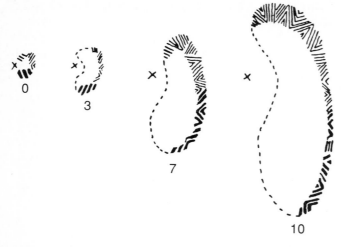

Figure 19–9. Lashley's progression of fortification spectra in migraine. Lashley's (1941) maps of the progression of his own fortification spectra at varying time intervals after the onset of a migrainous attack. The "X" in each instance indicates the visual fixation point. The numbers represent minutes. (*From Raskin N, Appenzeller O. Migraine: Clinical aspects. In: Smith LH Jr, ed. Headache. Vol 19 in Major Problems in Internal Medicine: Philadelphia: Saunders, 1980, with permission.*)

ally, as with classic migraine, these symptoms are transient but can be persistent, as in hemiplegic migraine. On T_2-weighted MRI studies, 41% of classic and 67% of complicated migraine patients have well-defined lesions. Two special types of complicated migraine of neuro-ophthalmic importance are:

1. **Retinal migraine.** Vasospasm presumably affects the ocular or orbital vasculature, resulting in a uniocular transient visual field defect or visual loss followed or accompanied by the migraine headache; the visual loss sometimes is described as a "whiteout," which is unusual during ocular TIAs or other causes of transient visual loss.

2. **Ophthalmoplegic migraine.** Usually manifested even more rarely as a third nerve palsy; it often *follows* the migraine headache. This entity frequently affects children; the ophthalmoplegia may last for weeks; rarely, the deficit becomes permanent or may be associated with aberrant regeneration of the third nerve. It must be differentiated from other causes of ophthalmoplegia (which are rarely recurrent) and painful ophthalmoplegia (like the Tolosa-Hunt and orbital apex syndromes, aneurysm, and vascular third nerve palsy); (see Chapter 13 on "Orbital Pain" and Table 19–27 later in the chapter).

In both retinal and ophthalmoplegic migraine, a previous history or family history of migraine is very helpful in making the diagnosis. Without such a history, opinion is divided as to the need for neuroimaging workup. It probably is indicated, especially in the face of an acute third nerve palsy with involvement of the pupil and associated headache.

Hemiplegic migraine frequently is familial. As in other complicated migraines, the neurologic symptoms accompany or follow rather than precede the headache. A less common, neuro-ophthalmic form of hemiplegic migraine is a persistent homonymous hemianopia.

Basilar migraine. In these patients the ischemic symptoms are in the distribution of the vertebral

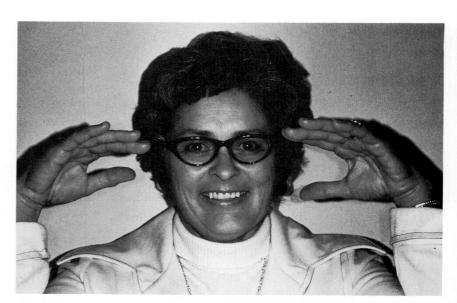

Figure 19–10. Migraine "hello."

basilar system. Visual symptoms sometimes involve both hemispheres and therefore cause defects in both visual fields including total blindness. More frequent symptoms include tinnitus, vertigo, ataxia, and diplopia. Headache may or may not occur; it is usually bioccipital and severe if somewhat short-lived (45 to 75 minutes).

Migraine equivalents (migraine aura without headache): Focal neurologic deficits unassociated with headache are usually classified as migraine equivalents when they occur in patients with a migraine history, especially when similar symptoms accompanied typical migraine headaches in the past. These tend to occur in older patients (perhaps those whose extracranial blood vessels are arteriosclerotic and less distensible because of atheroma than at an earlier age). Again, if the patient has a previous history of such symptoms accompanied by headache, the diagnosis is relatively easy. Lacking such a history only the repetitive and benign nature of the symptoms may suggest the diagnosis. Basilar equivalents are most common. "Abdominal" and pelvic migraine are seen in children and young women. Some people think that Prinzmetal's vasospastic angina is a cardiac equivalent of migraine.

Childhood migraine: Migraine is probably the most frequent cause of recurrent headache in children; many migraineurs experience their first symptoms as children. In childhood 60% of the patients is male, attacks are brief, and basilar symptoms are more frequent. In fact, the male predominance in childhood, in contrast to the female predominance after puberty, lends credence to the imputed role of estrogens in migraine. Common precipitants of the headache in children are school stress and light sensitivity. Cyclic vomiting and periodic abdominal pain are migraine equivalents of childhood.

Migraine is associated with epilepsy (but many migraineurs have abnormal electroencephalograms without a history of seizures) and episodic pupillary dilation (unilateral dilation sometimes alternating sides and usually occurring in otherwise asymptomatic young women with a migraine history). Other ocular pathologies statistically associated with migraine include optic nerve head drusen and low-tension glaucoma. Migraine also is associated with mitral valve prolapse and prosthetic cardiac valves.

Although the periodic neurologic deficits associated with migraine nearly always resolve, sometimes they do not. Many strokes in patients younger than 50 are migraine associated. Abnormal clotting factors and unsuspected embolic sources may act in conjunction with the migrainous vascular instability (see Chapter 8).

Differential Diagnosis. Usually the stereotyped headache and autonomic symptoms combined with a family history make the diagnosis of migraine fairly obvious. Most patients have made the diagnosis themselves, and if they have classical or complicated migraine, appear relatively calm about their symptoms. Migraine headaches often affect one side predominantly but do shift sides, generalize, or both. Alternation of sides is something headaches rarely do that are associated with arteriovenous malformations or leaking aneurysms. Only rarely do leaking occipital arteriovenous malformations or TIAs duplicate the scintillating scotomata of classic migraine, but on rare occasions carotid occlusion, vascular occlusion secondary to systemic lupus erythematosus, and metastatic tumors may do so. Occipital arteriovenous malformations (AVMs), on the other hand, are usually associated with monotonously unilateral headaches, occipital epilepsy, or occipital apoplexy.

In occipital epilepsy, the focal seizures associated with AVMs are elementary, unformed visual sensations, lasting only seconds to a minute or two. Occipital apoplexy presents as severe headache and homonymous visual loss. It is important to recognize occipital epilepsy and to treat it appropriately. Even more important is the identification of occipital apoplexy, because prompt surgical intervention can often reverse the effects of compression by hematoma.

Evaluation. The typical migraine history and symptoms are usually sufficient for diagnosis. Where history or symptoms are atypical, computed tomography (CT), magnetic resonance imaging (MRI), or both, and occasionally angiography, may be indicated to rule out carotid artery disease, aneurysm, or AVM; however, it should be kept in mind that migraineurs may be especially susceptible to vasospasm and subsequent stroke with dye injection. Unfortunately, no objective study exists that can establish the diagnosis of migraine.

Patients with mitral valve prolapse (MVP) may experience migraine-like episodes. The basis for the association is not understood. Perhaps the abnormal mitral valve affects platelet integrity and facilitates serotonin release. Additionally, young patients who suffer a stroke have an increased incidence of MVP, possibly related to thrombi forming on the abnormal valve. The young stroke patient and the atypical migraine patient deserve careful cardiologic evaluation and echocardiography.

Treatment. Primary therapy for the migraine patient is establishment of a trustful and supportive relationship, reassuring the patient that an appropriate

TABLE 19–17. PRINCIPLES OF MIGRAINE THERAPY

Avoid exciting factors

Simple analgesia

Anticonvulsives especially effective in children

Frequent attacks—prophylaxis with vasoactive drugs: extracranial vasoconstrictors, serotonin antagonists, propanolol, amitryptyline, phenelzine, papaverine

Acute attack—ergotamines IV (89% headache free, 5% improved)

Ergotamines contraindicated in anterior ischemic optic neuropathy

and successful therapy is available (Table 19–17). Ninety percent of patients obtains relief with medical treatment. However, all therapy must be individualized. The more quickly each acute migraine attack is treated, the greater the chance of aborting or significantly diminishing it.

Simple analgesics should be tried first. If they are not effective, the next line of therapy is dependent upon the frequency and type of attack. Relatively spread-out attacks, especially those preceded by an aura, may be effectively treated with ergot preparations taken at the onset of the aura to abort the attack (Table 19–18). Frequent, severe, or long-lasting attacks may be treated with prophylactic measures: methysergide, beta blockers, antidepressants, anticonvulsants (especially in children), monoamine oxidase inhibitors, antiinflammatory drugs, serotonin antagonists, lithium, and calcium channel blockers (Tables 19–19 and 19–20). Methysergide may cause retroperitoneal and other fibrotic syndromes unless the drug is discontinued periodically (eg, one month in four), but is considered a very effective prophylactic drug, especially in young patients. In any patient with ischemic symptoms (eg, angina or completed ischemic events such as ischemic optic neuropathy or stroke), ergot preparations should be used *very* cautiously. Calcium channel blockers seem to be effective in many patients unresponsive to other treatments, especially young patients; they may be the therapy of choice in complicated and hemiplegic migraine because they vasodilate and increase cerebral blood flow. Concomitant use of sedatives seems to increase the effectiveness of analgesics.

Precipitating agents (Tables 19–21 and 19–22) (eg, foods [red wine and other alcohols, chocolate, dairy products, MSG, citrus fruits], stress, certain medications) should be avoided. For young women patients who develop new or more severe headaches after beginning oral contraception (with a migraine or headache history or family history), estrogen-containing medications are absolutely contraindicated. Occasionally a migrainous woman will be placed on "the pill" and will have relief or improvement of headaches. Similar symptoms or history in a menopausal woman are likewise a relative contraindication to estrogen use, although in the older age

TABLE 19–18. COMMON PHARMACEUTICAL PRODUCTS USEFUL IN MIGRAINE, ABORTIVE THERAPY

Route	Drug	Dosage
Oral	Ergotamine tartrate (Gynergen)	1 tablet immediately, repeat every ½ hr if necessary; minimum of 6 tablets per attack.
	Ergotamine, caffeine, phenacetin, and belladonna (Wigraine)	
	Ergotomine and caffeine (Cafergot)	2 tablets immediately, repeat 1 every ½ hr to a maximum of 10 per week.
	Ergotomine tartrate, cyclizine, and caffeine (Migral)	2 tablets at onset. May repeat every ½ hr up to 6/day, 10 per week.
	Isometheptene mucate, dichloralphenazone, and acetaminophen (Midrin)	2 capsules at once, followed by 1 capsule every hour until relieved, up to 5 capsules in a 12-hr period.
Sublingual	Ergotamine (Ergomar, Ergostat)	1 tablet immediately, under the tongue; repeat at ½-hr intervals if necessary, but not more than 3 tablets in any 24-hr period.
Inhalation	Ergotamine (Medihaler Ergotamine)	One dose immediately; repeat every 5 min to a maximum of 6 per day, if necessary.
Intramuscular	Ergotamine tartrate (Gynergen)	½ to 1 cc immediately; no more than 3 cc per week.
	Dihydroergotamine (DHE-45)	1 cc at hourly intervals, up to 3 cc per day, if necessary.
Rectal	Ergotamine and caffeine (Cafergot, Cafergot-PB)	Insert 1 suppository in rectum immediately; repeat in 1 hr if necessary.
	Ergotamine, caffeine, phenacetin, and belladonna (Wigraine)	

From D'Allessio DJ, ed. Wolff's Headache and Other Head Pain. 5th ed. New York: Oxford, 1987:134.

TABLE 19–19. MIGRAINE PROPHYLAXIS

Drug	Dose (mg/day)	Side Effects
Beta blockers		
Propranolol (Inderal)	80–320	Exacerbation of asthma Synergism with ergot medication Lethargy, insomnia, constipation, light-headedness, nightmares, depression, migraine-like scintillations
Atenolol (Tenormin)	50–100	
Nadolol (Corgard)	40–160	
Metoprolol (Lopressor)	100–200	
Timolol	20–30	
Calcium-channel blockers		
Verapamil (Isoptin, Calan)	320–480	Hypotension, constipation, light-headedness, nausea, fluid retention
Nifedipine (Procardia)	40	Constipation
Nimodipine	Not released	
Diltiazem	30–90	
MAO inhibitors		
Phenelzine sulfate	15	
Ergonovine	0.2	Nausea, abdominal pain, leg "tiredness"
Ergot-belladonna	1–4 tablets	Nausea, sedation
Flunarizine	5–15	Sedation, weight gain
Phenelzine	15–75	Insomnia, light-headedness, constipation, orthostatic hypotension
Papaverine	150, 300	Nausea
Antidepressants		
Amitriptyline (Elavil, Endep)	75–150	Anticholinergic effects; increased appetite Start slowly to avoid soporific side effects Sedation, dry mouth, weight gain
Doxepin (Adapin, Sinequan)	25–100	
Antiinflammatory Drugs		
Indomethacin (Indocin)	75–150	
Ibuprofen (Motrin, Rufen, Advil)	1200–1800	
Naproxen sodium (anaprox)	1100	Epigastric burning, nausea, abdominal pain, fluid retention
Aspirin		
Serotonin Antagonists		
Methysergide (Sansert)	4–8	Ergotism, abdominal pain, muscle cramps, weight gain, edema, peripheral vasoconstriction
Cyproheptadine (Periactin)	6–8	Sedation, weight gain, fibrosis
Lithium		
Lithium Carbonate (Eskalith, Lithobid)	600–900	

Modified from D'Allessio DJ, ed. Wolff's Headache and Other Head Pain. *5th ed. New York: Oxford, 1987:115.*

groups there seem to be many fewer thromboembolic episodes. Changes in sleep pattern also may precipitate migraine attacks.

Cluster Headache

Cluster headache (Table 19–23) is a stereotypical headache that occurs in the periorbital region and predominantly affects middle-aged men. It is rarer than migraine and *always unilateral.* The pain is cyclic—present for weeks to months, and then disappearing for months. This headache is excruciating and explosive in onset, reaching a crescendo in about 1 to 5 minutes; it lasts an average of ½ to 2 hours. Its severity is such that suicide is frequently contemplated. Fifty percent of attacks occurs at night. Cluster headaches are attended by homolateral lacrimation, nasal stuffiness, and vascular congestion of the conjunctiva. An ipsilateral Horner's syndrome occurs in about fifty percent of patients and may persist between attacks (Table 19–24). Patients with cluster headaches do not have the positive family

TABLE 19–20. PROPHYLACTIC TREATMENT OF MIGRAINE: COMPARATIVE RESPONSIVENESS TO DRUGS

Drug	Percentage of Patients Improved
Phenelzine	80
Amitriptyline	72
Methysergide	57
Cyproheptadine	46
Ergotamine, phenobarbital, and belladona	34
Propranolol	34
Placebo	20
Calcium channel blockers	?
Naproxen Na	?
ASA	?
Flunarizine	?

history or other associated focal neurologic symptoms that may occur in migraine.

Few headache syndromes mimic classic cluster headache, but carotid dissection can present with severe unilateral pain in the neck or lower face and a Horner's syndrome. The pain, however, is continuous and lasts several hours to days.

Therapy includes vigorous exercise or inhalation of 100% oxygen at very first sign of attack. Ergotamine aerosol can be very effective in individual bouts. Methysergide, lithium, propanolol and prednisone are variably effective for prevention. However, prednisone must be used in relatively high doses and it should not be used for longterm therapy; lithium is most effective but may be associated with

TABLE 19–21. FACTORS PRECIPITATING MIGRAINE ATTACKS

Common Factors	Less Common Factors
Stress, worry	High humidity
Menstruation	Excessive sleep
Oral contraceptives	High-altitude exposure
Glare, dazzle	Excessive vitamin A
Physical exertion, fatigue	Drugs: nitroglycerine, histamine, reserpine, hydralazine, estrogen, corticosteroid withdrawal
Lack of sleep	
Hunger	
Head trauma	
Foods or beverages containing nitrite, glutamate, salt, aspartame, tyramine, and other, as yet unidentified chemicals	Cold foods
	Reading, refractive errors
	Pungent odors: perfumes, organic solvents, smoke
	Fluorescent lighting
Weather or ambient temperature change	Allergic reactions

Data from Selby G, Lance JW. Observations on 500 cases of migraine and allied vascular headache. J Neurol Neurosurg Psychiatry. 1960;23:23–32; and Pearce J. Some aetiological factors in migraine. In: Cumings JN, ed. Background to Migraine. Fourth Migraine Symposium. New York: Springer-Verlag, 1971.

TABLE 19–22. DRUGS THAT EXACERBATE MIGRAINE

"The pill," estrogen
Trinitroglycerine and other nitrates, hydralyzine, reserpine, vitamin A, clomiphene, indomethacin
Exogenous thyroid
Dipyramidole
Beta blockers (rare)
Calcium channel blockers (also used for treatment!)
Lithium (also used for treatment!)
Fenfluramine

tremor (sometimes halted by simultaneous propranolol therapy), weakness, lethargy, nausea and hypothyroidism (Table 19–25).

Lithium increases erythrocyte choline levels which are depressed in patients with the cluster syndrome both during and between attacks. Intranasal lidocaine by drop or spray gets good results in many patients.

When the patient is bothered by the miosis and/or ptosis of a persistent Horner's syndrome, treatment with 2.5% phenlyephrine or ⅛% vasocon can enlarge the pupil and improve the ptosis.

Chronic paroxysmal hemicrania (CPH), thought to be a cluster variant, is characterized by hemicranial pain that is chronically present with 15 to 20 recurrent severe superimposed unilateral focal head pain daily. CPH is a rare headache, only recognized in the last decade as distinct from cluster headache; however, it has many features in common with cluster headache. These include the severity and the unilaterality of the headache, nasal stuffiness, rhinorrhea, tearing and conjunctival injection. Like cluster headache, migrainous prodromes and phenomena are not associated. However, in contrast to cluster headache, CPH affects women predominantly and the number of daily headaches is much higher. CPH attacks tend to be shorter and are not predominantly nocturnal. Additionally, mechanical

TABLE 19–23. CLUSTER HEADACHE

Pain	Unilateral, periorbital, paroxysmal, explosive, crescendo
Sex	Almost exclusively male (6:1)
Age	20–50
Associated Symptoms	Ipsilateral nasal stuffiness and lacrimation, rhinorrhea, red eye, ipsilateral Horner's syndrome
Clusters	1–3/night, 20 min–2 hr, in 6- to 12-week episodes, occuring 1–2 times/yr
Precipitants	Alcohol intake, ETOH, vasodilators, sleep
Family History	Negative (no migraine history)

TABLE 19–24. ASSOCIATED SYMPTOMS IN CLUSTER HEADACHE IN 180 PATIENTS

Symptom	Incidence (%)
Lacrimation	84
Conjunctival injection	58
Ptosis	57
Blocked nostril	48
Rhinorrhea	43
Bradycardia	43
Nausea	40
General perspiration	26

Data from Manzoni GC, Terzano MG, Bono G, et al. Cluster headache: Clinical findings in 180 patients. Cephalalgia. 1983;3:21–30.

elements appear to precipitate attacks; about half of the attacks are set off by flexion or rotational movements of the neck. The curative effect of Indomethacin is so dramatic that it may be used as a diagnostic test; in cluster headache, the effect of Indomethacin is minimal.

Treatment is by Indomethacin, but the dose necessary for each individual varies greatly, eg, from 25 to 250 mg per day.

Another headache responding to Indomethacin which should be mentioned is *hemicrania continua*. However, this headache is not likely to be confused with cluster headaches or CPH as it is a moderate headache, although steady and continuous.

Raeder's Paratrigeminal Syndrome

Raeder's syndrome consists of a severe unilateral persistent headache, usually involving the ophthalmic division of the trigeminal distribution, and, as in cluster headaches, an ipsilateral Horner's syndrome, nasal stuffiness and conjunctival congestion. If no other cranial nerves are involved, it may be considered a variant of cluster headache and treated accordingly—eg, ergotamine, methsergyide, lithium, corticosteroids. A similar headache, usually lower in the face or the neck associated with a Horner's syndrome but without nasal and conjunctival signs may herald carotid dissection. If there is associated numbness in the trigeminal distribution (especially if V_2 and V_3 are involved) or involvement of the oculomotor nerves, the etiology is more likely to be a space occupying lesion. In this case, neuro-imaging and ENT work-up is mandatory.

Ice Pick-like Pains (Ophthalmodynia)

These lancinating momentary jabs are frequently suffered by patients with other types of headache as well as those with no previous headache history. The "headachey" patients may be migraineurs, cluster sufferers, or patients with temporal arteritis. Those without a headache history are frequently middle-aged to elderly women. The pains are attention catching but do not have the excruciating quality of tic; they are almost never associated with any identifiable condition and do not seem to be harbingers of any vascular or neurological disaster.

Carotidynia (Lower-half Headache, Facial Migraine)

This term has been used for a symptom complex which consists of facial pain located in the jaw or neck, sometimes associated with ice pick-like jabbing pain which affects middle-aged women. Attacks occur several times a week, last minutes to hours, and are sometimes combined with a throbbing ipsilateral headache. The carotid artery may be tender and prominent and the overlying soft tissue may swell. A history of dental trauma is sometimes obtained. Carotidynia appears to respond to the same vasoactive drugs as migraine; it probably represents a migraine variant. A large proportion of migraine patients has tenderness along the carotid ipsilateral to the hemicrania. Differential diagnosis includes carotid dissection and thrombosis and temporal arteritis.

Vascular Occlusion, Ischemic Pain, Carotid Artery Dissection

Pain in the neck, throat, and face associated with headache and Horner's syndrome also may herald *carotid artery dissection*, which should be treated by immediate anticoagulation to prevent total thrombosis of the carotid or its branches. Immediate angiography with oblique views to delineate the involved artery is indicated. The rare subadventitial (as opposed to the more common subinitial) dissection is best imaged by MR angiography. Emboli from trailing thrombi may cause ophthalmic artery or retinal arterial occlusion or emboli. Occasionally, the dissection follows neck trauma; usually no proximate cause is found.

Vascular occlusion, especially internal carotid occlusion, can cause pain in and above the eye. The pain is often steady and can present for days or even weeks until it becomes stable, easing after occlusion! The pain may be due to vascular compromise of the vessels of the dura. The onset of new vascular headaches in older patients mandates evaluation of the cerebral vascular tree for aneurysm or occlusive or collagen vascular disease. If digital subtraction angiography and CT are negative, standard angiography should be performed.

Temporal Arteritis

Temporal arteritis is a disease clinically affecting nearly 1 in 1000 of those aged 60 years and above. It

TABLE 19–25. PROPHYLACTIC AGENTS IN EPISODIC CLUSTER HEADACHE

Conditions	Drug of Choice	Common Contraindications and Side Effects
Age		
Under 30	Methysergide (2 mg 3 or 4 times a day)	Cardiac and peripheral vascular disorders, extremity or chest pain, GI effects, paresthesias
30–45	Prednisone (tapering off from 40 mg/day for 3 weeks)	Ulcers, diverticulosis, high blood pressure, diabetes, infection
Over 45	Lithium carbonate (300 mg 2 to 4 times a day)	Diuretic or low-salt therapy, tremor, GI effects
Other		
Attacks in sleep	Ergotamine tartrate (2 mg on retiring)	See methysergide, above

From Kudrow L. Cluster headache: New concepts. Neurol Clin. 1983;1:379.

is one of the few true neuro-ophthalmic emergencies. The pain may be severe and usually involves the temporal artery territory with associated scalp tenderness; it may radiate into the neck, jaw, or ear; be associated with jaw claudication; and, rarely, cause necrosis of the tongue or scalp. The temporal arteries are often enlarged, tortuous, tender, and nonpulsatile; however, they may seem normal on physical exam. Caucasian women seem to be affected disproportionately but temporal arteritis should *always* be considered in any patient more than 60 years old with headache, and visual acuity is decreased.

Usually, there are associated complaints of a chronic nature, including arthralgias in the shoulder and hip girdles, anorexia, weight loss, fever, anemia, leukocytosis, and occasionally diplopia or cranial nerve dysfunction (Table 19–26). The hallmark of the disease is a high erythrocyte sedimentation rate, commonly above 80 mm/hr Westergen (Table 19–27).

If untreated, severe visual loss will occur in more than half those afflicted; in 80% of these, bilateral blindness follows. Visual loss tends to occur within 1 month following the onset of headache and frequently occurs soon after the onset of diplopia, especially diplopia without obvious cranial nerve paresis (an ominous painful ophthalmoplegia). Amaurosis fugax occasionally precedes the visual loss. Temporal arteritis may also present as an ischemic optic neuropathy preceding other symptoms (see Chapter 4 for fundus findings).

Temporal arteritis may be differentiated from small subarachnoid hemorrhages, aneurysms, and arteriovenous malformations by the frequent systemic manifestations, elderly age of the patient, and high ESR. Patients with brain tumors usually have intermittent headaches that progressively worsen, associated central nervous system symptoms and only rarely have other systemic manifestations. Carotid dissections tend to be associated with ipsilat-

TABLE 19–26. CLINICAL FEATURES OF GIANT-CELL ARTERITIS

Percentage Incidence of Common Features at Initial Evaluation		Less Common, But Characteristic Features
Headache	85	Raynaud's phenomenon of limbs or tongue
Temporal artery tenderness	70	Tender scalp nodules
Jaw claudication	65	Thick, tender occipital arteries
Lingual, limb, or swallowing claudication	20	Necrotic lesions of scalp, tongue
Brachiocephalic bruits	50	Carotid artery tenderness
Thickened or nodular temporal artery	45	Swelling of the hands
Pulseless temporal artery	40	Taste, smell disturbances
Visual symptoms	40	Distended, beaded retinal veins
Fixed blindness, partial or complete	15	Diminished or absent radial artery pulses
Polymyalgia rheumatica	40	Mononeuropathy: median, peroneal, cervical root
Weight loss > 6 kg	35	
ESR > 50 mm/hr	95	
> 100 mm/hr	60	
Fever (>37.7°C)	20	
Abnormal liver function	50	
Anemia (hematocrit <35%)	50	

From Raskin NH. Headache. 2nd ed. New York: Churchill Livingstone, 1978:319.

TABLE 19–27. ERYTHROCYTE SEDIMENTATION RATES (WINTROBE METHOD) RELATED TO AGE OF PATIENTS

Age (yr)	No. Patients	Mean (mm/hr)	Standard Deviation	Percentage > 20 mm/hr
< 30	23	9	6	0
30–39	26	12	8	12
40–49	24	15	8	21
50–59	25	15	12	24
60–69	32	19	9	47
70–79	22	23	13	46
80–89	12	27	14	47

Data from Hayes GS, Stinson IN. Erythrocyte sedimentation rate and age. Arch Ophthalmol. 1976;94:939–940.

eral Horner's syndrome and occur in a younger age group. The pain of dissection is usually in the lower half of the face and neck. Temporal mandibular joint (TMJ) problems can nearly always be distinguished by limitation of jaw opening, audible TMJ clicks, or both.

Diagnosis. Usually is confirmed by measuring the erythrocyte sedimentation rate (ESR). If visual symptoms (ischemic optic neuropathy, transient visual loss, and so forth) even suggest temporal arteritis (ischemic optic neuropathy or retinal arterial occlusion, especially in a patient over 60 years old) once blood is drawn, *immediate* treatment should be started with high-dose corticosteroids (100 mg PO qAM) (Fig. 19–11). Some advocate hospitalization with immediate treatment by pulsed IV methylprednisolone (1000 mg every 12 hours for 5 days). There is a suggestion that this aggressive therapy may occasionally restore vision. Temporal artery biopsy should be done to confirm the diagnosis. Biopsy evidence of inflammation will not be affected by steroid therapy in the first 8 to 10 days or longer. Therefore, *therapy absolutely should not be deferred pending biopsy.* Sometimes, following the biopsy, the headache disappears.

The characteristic histopathologic features include inflammation (lymphocytic and plasma cell infiltration), granulomatous reaction, and giant cells (*not* necessary for diagnosis); and hypertrophy of the intima and fragmentation and necrosis of the internal elastic lamina leading to obliteration.

Among the arteries involved are the posterior ciliary arteries, which are responsible for the visual loss. Occlusion of other orbital arteries to the extraocular muscles and the vasovasorum of the cranial nerves cause the diplopia.

Biopsy should be done even when the symptom complex is pathognomonic. Because of the occurrence of skip lesions, the contralateral artery should be biopsied if the first biopsy is negative. It is much easier on the physician to continue giving steroid therapy when the diagnosis is confirmed by a positive biopsy. However, if symptoms are typical and if you can commit to carrying out appropriate therapy for temporal arteritis without equivocation, then the biopsy may be omitted—in other words, if it will *not* affect treatment, don't do it!

Treatment. Currently, a 2- to 3-year course of treatment is considered optimal. Ideally, the symptoms and the ESR will respond to corticosteroids within a few days to weeks. The steroids are tapered (over another 1 to 2 weeks) to maintain the ESR less than 20 with a steroid dose no greater than 20 mg prednisone and, hopefully, around 5 mg PO qAM (Fig. 19–12). If this is difficult and large (>50 mg prednisone) doses of steroids are required, I will allow the sedimentation rate to be in the 30 to 50 mm range (considered normal by some for elderly adults), especially if the patient is asymptomatic. Occasional patients maintain exceedingly high (>80 mg) sedimentation rates in the face of daily steroid doses above 50 mg. In these cases, continue high-dose steroids for 3 months if there are no medical contraindications, especially if symptoms persist. At this point, there is only a small chance of further visual loss, an acceptable risk when compared to almost certain intervertebral compression fractures, hip necrosis, and other serious disabilities associated with continued high-dose steroid use in this age group (vertebral compression in 25%, steroid myopathy in 15%, and subcapsular cataracts in 5%, according to a study by Huston). Nonsteroidal anti-inflammatory agents seem to help some in suppressing the ESR, but it is not known whether they also decrease the risk of visual loss. The goal of therapy is to prevent visual loss and life-threatening complications such as aortic rupture.

The relationship of temporal arteritis to polymyalgia rheumatica (PMR) and its implications for treatment remains somewhat obscure. Certainly, many more elderly adults have PMR than temporal arteritis; probably those patients without the typical

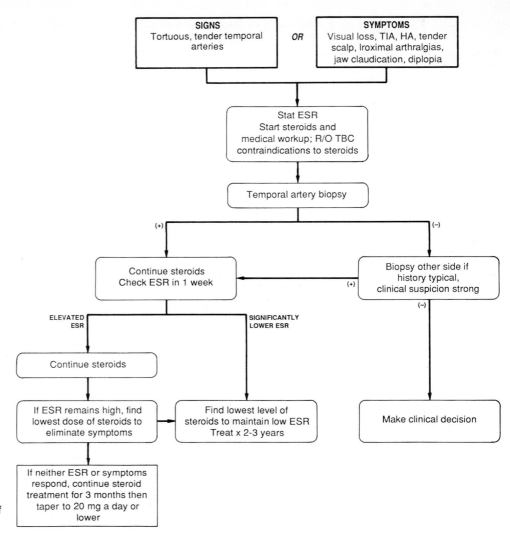

Figure 19–11. Management of temporal arteritis.

symptoms of temporal arteritis should be treated with low-dose (<20 mg) rather than high-dose steroids. However, temporal arteritis should be recognized as only one manifestation of a systemic process, a giant-cell arteritis affecting medium to large arteries with granulomatous inflammation, necrosis of the elastica, and obliteration. Other life-threatening complications include mesenteric arteritis leading to bowel necrosis and aortic arteritis.

TENSION (MUSCULAR) HEADACHES

The typical "tension headache" is a bilateral dull bandlike sensation that may affect any part of the head and waxes and wanes in intensity. It is often frontal or occipital, "band-like," and "vise-like." It may occur on nearly a daily basis and is not associated with focal neurologic symptoms.

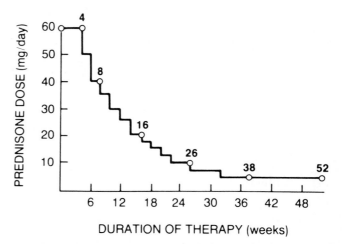

Figure 19–12. Prednisone therapy—giant-cell arteritis. An example of a prednisone treatment schedule for a patient with giant-cell arteritis. *(From Raskin NH: Headache. 2nd ed. New York: Churchill Livingstone, 1988, with permission.)*

As in migraineurs, there appears to be an increased incidence of epilepsy, and many patients experience both types of headaches. Many neurologists feel there are more similarities than differences in the two headache syndromes (Fig. 19–13, Table 19–28).

Frequently, these headaches are associated with tenderness of the trapezius and at the occipital ridge. The patient may freely admit to stress, anxiety, or depression. However, a direct link to stress is not always clear.

Therapy. For situational stress, where the problem warrants it, psychotherapy helps in tension headache, in contrast to its striking ineffectiveness in migraine. Relaxation methods are often helpful, and if simple analgesics do not provide relief, daily amitriptyline is often successful (Table 19–29).

EYE PAIN

Headache patients are a frequent part of neuro-ophthalmic practice because it is commonly believed both by referring physicians and self-referred patients that refractive errors cause headaches. Among the unusual cases where refractive errors and/or muscle imbalance do cause symptoms, myopia is almost unheard of, but hyperopia or astigmatism may cause discomfort. Headaches associated with refractive error or muscle imbalance should occur regularly after the use of the eyes. Even when this history and a refractive error are both present, correction of the refractive error causes relief of symptoms only in a small minority of cases. Thus, as in many other headache complexes, it may well be that the discomfort associated with the ocular problem becomes a precipitating factor in patients otherwise prone to muscular tension, or migraine headaches. Most ocular and orbital disorders cause pain that is sharper and more localized than the usual headache.

Pain localized to the eye itself almost always

TABLE 19–28. FACTORS SUPPORTING THE MECHANISTIC SIMILARITY OF TENSION HEADACHE AND MIGRAINE

Neck muscle contraction is found in both disorders
Nuchal muscle contraction and pain is common prodromal feature of both disorders
Cephalic hyperemia attends headache in both disorders
Increased prevalence of epilepsy occurs in both disorders
Low platelet serotonin occurs in both disorders
Psychological data for both disorders are indistinguishable
Responsiveness of both disorders to amitriptyline, ergonovine, and propranolol are similar

From D'Allessio DJ, ed. Wolff's Headache and Other Head Pain. 5th ed. New York: Oxford, 1987:224.

arises locallly. Within the eye, the cornea and iris are very pain sensitive; the uvea, sclera, and optic nerve sheath are sensitive. The retina shows minimal sensibility and the lens is insensitive.

Ocular pain is most often related to disruption of the corneal epithelium or inflammation of the eye. Narrow-angle glaucoma (NAG) usually causes eye pain, headache, or both. Ocular tumors rarely are associated with pain unless the tumor process or necrosis has led to inflammation.

In narrow angle glaucoma (NAG), there may be ocular pain, headache, or pain referred to the V_1 distribution. Very severe pain associated with NAG attacks may even be referred to the vagal distribution, and there are stories of patients in a NAG attack who have been treated for myocardial infarction or even appendicitis, or, if the pupil is dilated, with an angiogram looking for a posterior communicating artery aneurysm.

The most common causes of corneal pain are foreign bodies and other causes of corneal erosion that may be detected by fluorescein staining and that will abate instantaneously with the instillation of topical anesthesia. In the patient without an obvious cause for eye pain, *always* look for dry eyes and corneal erosion. The failure of the pain to be relieved by topical anesthesia indicates that one must look elsewhere for its etiology.

Nearly all inflammatory diseases affecting the iris produce pain, which may be very severe at times and which also may be referred to other parts of the V_1 distribution. Iritis is also frequently accompanied by photophobia. Ocular inflammation is usually accompanied by a red eye.

Photophobia is discomfort or pain occurring when the eye is stimulated with light. Its physiology is not understood, but it does not seem related to dazzle from the light stimulus alone. In general, the causes of photophobia are difficult to pinpoint. It is frequently associated with conjunctival and corneal irritation as well as uveitis, and also occurs with

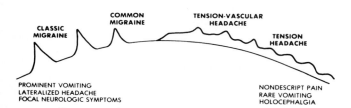

Figure 19–13. The continuum of benign recurring headaches. (*From Raskin N, Appenzeller O. Migraine: Clinical aspects. In: Smith LH Jr, ed. Headache. Vol 19 in Major Problems in Internal Medicine. Philadelphia: Saunders, 1980, with permission.*)

TABLE 19–29. TREATMENT OF TENSION HEADACHE: RESULTS WITH FIRST DRUGS ADMINISTERED

Drug	Number of Patients			
	Headache-free	*50% Improved*	*Unchanged*	*Percentage Improved*
Amitriptyline	22	38	21	73
Imipramine	6	8	15	47
Diazepam	1	5	4	60
Chlordiazepoxide	11	21	31	50
Ergotamine, phenobarbital, and belladonna	9	13	22	49
Amobarbital	2	14	27	37
Placebo	1	5	12	30

Modified from Lance JW, Curran DA, Anthony M. Investigations into the mechanism and treatment of chronic headache. Med J Aust. 1965;2:909–914.

meningeal irritation, fever, trigeminal neuralgia, and migraine. Photophobia associated with recognized organic eye disease is often associated with pupillary constriction and is relieved with mydriasis. Paradoxically, it also occurs in some patients with visual loss: in retinitis pigmentosa (RP), cone dystrophies, and following optic neuritis. Unfortunately, in most patients complaining of photophobia no organic cause is found. In these cases the symptoms may be an exaggeration of normal light sensitivity. Sometimes lightly tinted or polaroid lenses are helpful.

In 80% of retrobulbar neuritis cases eye movement elicits pain usually described as orbital or a headache rather than as eye pain.

Orbital Pain

Orbital pain is usually associated with processes that are inflammatory in nature (orbital pseudotumor or cellulitis), invade into the bone and/or the sinuses (malignant lacrimal gland and sinus tumors), or are rapidly expansile (hemorrhage). Most orbital tumors make their presence known by exophthalmos long before they become painful. Some ocular inflammatory processes, such as posterior scleritis, cause pain in the orbit. Rarely following orbital surgery an amputation neuroma may be associated with pain and paraesthesias. The orbit also may be affected by ophthalmodynia (see "Ice pick-like Pains" earlier in the chapter). Retrobulbar neuritis is frequently (80%) preceded by pain on eye movement (especially medial eye movement), which usually abates soon after visual loss commences. The orbit may also be affected by referred pain, especially by involvement of structures sharing innervation by the ophthalmic division (V_1) of the trigeminal nerve (eg, anterior cranial fossa and tentorium) and from the neck (greater occipital neuralgia). Ocular and orbital pain may precede ischemic neuropathies—anterior

ischemic optic neuropathy as well as third, fourth, and sixth nerve palsies (Table 19–30).

A large number of painful orbit processes involves the orbital apex, where they may be variously termed. One term is the **superior orbital fissure syndrome** (involving V_1, III, IV, VI and Horner's syndrome); in fact, the superior orbital fissure syndrome cannot be distinguished from similar processes involving the anterior cavernous sinus on the basis of the nerves involved. As a rule, the syndrome is incomplete. If the optic nerve is involved, the usual appellation is the **orbital apex syndrome.** Granulomatous involvement of the cavernous sinus (the **Tolosa-Hunt syndrome**) produces a similar symptom complex associated with a gnawing, boring pain. Untreated it may repeat or be recurrent; however, it is exquisitely sensitive to corticosteroid therapy, so much so that several authors have suggested the use of steroids as a diagnostic test. V_2 involvement localizes the lesion to the posterior cavernous sinus. Such lesions must be differentiated from other lesions and invasions of the cavernous sinus (eg, sellar and parasellar masses, pituitary tumor, and aneurysm). Pituitary tumors can cause similar symptoms if they push through the diaphragma sella and expand laterally at the same time; otherwise, cavernous sinus involvement is usually painless. A mild pituitary apoplexy can have an identical presentation. In ischemic lesions (ischemic optic neuropathy, pupil-sparing third nerve lesions) the pain usually precedes the visual loss or ophthalmoplegia by 1 to 2 days.

The accurate localization of these lesions necessitates a careful neuro-imaging workup with attention to the orbits, sinuses, sella, and parasellar areas and a vascular workup with serological tests for syphilis (HATTS, FTA-Abs) erythrocyte sedimentation rate (ESR), fasting blood sugar (FBS), and antinuclear antibodies (ANA). Third nerve involvement

TABLE 19–30. PAINFUL OPHTHALMOPLEGIAS

	Ophthalmoplegia	Age	Other
Orbit infection	Any	Child	Sinus disease
Orbit inflammation	Any	Any	Inflammation
Orbital apex syndrome	Any	Any	II nerve
Superior orbital fissure syndrome	Any	Middle	Decreased V_1 sensation
Tolosa-Hunt syndrome	Any	Middle	Steriod sensitive
Vascular III, IV, VI nerve lesions			
Microvascular	Pupil-sparing, III most often	Older	Headache, diabetes
Aneurysm	III with pupil	Young, middle	Severe headache
Ophthalmoplegic migraine	Recurrent	Child III	History: family history of migraine, aberrant regeneration
Raeder's syndrome	Uncommon	Older	Horner's syndrome, V
Pituitary tumor	VI first, then III, IV	Middle	Headache
Pituitary apoplexy	Any III, IV, VI	Middle	Decreased visual acuity, headache
Parasellar mass			
Aneurysm	Any	Middle	Aberrant regeneration or (rarely) neuromyotonia
Invasive pituitary adenoma	VI first		
Nasopharyngeal carcinoma, basal tumors (chordoma)	VI first	Older	Multiple cranial nerves
Sphenoid sinus mucocoele	VI		
Gradenigo's syndrome	VI	Child	Middle ear infection, otitis media
Temporal arteritis	Due to orb. vasc. occlusion, cranial nerves less commonly involved	Elderly	Tender scalp, jaw claudication, polymyalgia rheumatica, increased erythrocyte sedimentation rate, steroid response

and pain necessitates ruling out a posterior communicating artery (PCA) aneurysm (especially if the pupil is affected) and vascular third nerve palsies (often pupil sparing—see Chapter 13).

HEADACHES IN PRIMARY CNS DISEASE

Very little of the brain itself is pain sensitive, but intracranial processes that impinge on pain-sensitive structures (vessels, sinuses, meninges—Fig. 19–14) often cause headache, usually by traction on or displacement of the pain-sensitive structure. Consequently, headache is an important symptom of intracerebral tumors, even if they begin within pain-insensitive brain tissue (Fig. 19–15).

About three fourths of brain tumor patients have headache (which is even more frequent in infratentorial tumors); in half the brain tumor patients, headache is the first complaint. Additionally, 20% of pituitary adenomas presents with headache.

Headache symptoms characteristic of an intracerebral mass (Table 19–31) include:

1. The rare paroxysmal headache, maximum in 1 to 2 seconds, lasting 1 to 2 hours, highly intense and associated with loss of consciousness, drop attacks, sudden vomiting without nausea (projectile), or transient loss of vision. This type of presentation is most typical of a colloid cyst of the third ventricle, perhaps secondary to abruptly increased intracranial pressure. Colloid cysts have mental status change as the most constant feature. The tumor is rare but the headache is typical and may occur with other intracranial tumors.
2. The more common brain tumor headache may be described as "bursting" or "boring," awakens patients from sleep, and when associated with projectile vomiting (most often from posterior fossa tumors) is an ominous sign.

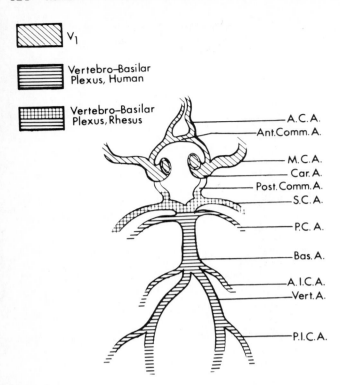

Figure 19–14. Major arterial trunks at the base of the brain according to the source of their sensory nerve supply. The ophthalmic division of the trigeminal nerve (V_1) provides the general somatic sensory nerve supply to the intracranial carotid (Car A), middle cerebral (MCA), anterior cerebral (ACA), anterior communicating (Ant Comm A), and possibly the proximal posterior communicating arteries (Post Comm A). The vertebrobasilar plexus provides a mixed sensory–autonomic nerve supply to the vertebral (Vert A), basilar (Bas A), posterior inferior cerebellar (PICA), anterior inferior cerebellar (AICA), and superior cerebellar arteries (SCA) in the human. This plexus extends more rostrally in the rhesus monkey to supply the posterior cerebral arteries (PCA) as well. The precise origin of the vertebrobasilar plexus remains unsettled. (*From D'Allessio DJ, ed. Wolff's Headache and Other Head Pain. 5th ed. New York: Oxford, 1987, with permission.*)

The headache itself has little localizing value, although there is a tendency for supratentorial masses to cause pain in the anterior head and face and for infratentorial masses to cause pain in the posterior head and neck. The more common headache associated with brain tumor is of moderate intensity, dull, and intermittent; exacerbated by exertion, change in posture, or cough; and may be associated with nausea and vomiting. Exertional headache also occurs with straining or the Valsalva maneuver, especially with posterior fossa lesions. Gliomas and other intrinsic tumors usually cause neural symptoms before headache. In contrast, extrinsic tumors such as meningiomas cause headache before other symptoms. Obviously, any patient with a headache that suggests a brain tumor needs immediate neuro-imaging workup.

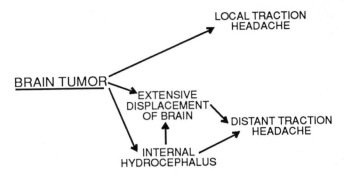

HEADACHE MECHANISMS IN BRAIN TUMOR

Figure 19–15. Schematic outline summarizing common mechanisms of brain tumor headache. (*From D'Allessio DJ, ed. Wolff's Headache and Other Head Pain. 5th ed. New York: Oxford, 1987, with permission.*)

Idiopathic Intracranial Hypertension (Pseudotumor Cerebri)

Idiopathic intracranial hypertension (IIH) (pseudotumor cerebri) (PTC) is a symptom complex that frequently presents to the ophthalmologist or neuro-ophthalmologist because of the nearly universal occurrence of papilledema in association with the other cardinal features, headache and increased intracranial pressure with normal spinal fluid contents. Other frequent visual complaints include visual obscurations secondary to the papilledema; diplopia from unilateral or bilateral sixth nerve palsy; or more rarely, divergence insufficiency. Many patients complain of intracranial noises. Symptoms often are reported on a daily basis. The large majority of IIH cases are idiopathic but occasionally a precipitating cause exists, such as sinus thrombo-

TABLE 19–31. CHARACTERISTICS OF BRAIN TUMOR HEADACHES IN 132 PATIENTS

Intensity	40% Severe, 40% moderate, 20% mild
Rhythmicity	85% Intermittent, 15% constant
Quality	25% Throbbing, 75% dull and steady
Aggravating factors	20% Stooping or lying down 25% Exertion, coughing
Timing	5% Nocturnal, 5% awakened earlier than usual 15% Upon arising
Associated features	40% Increased intracranial pressure 50% Nausea and vomiting

Data from Rushton JG, Rooke ED. Brain tumor headache. Headache. 1962; 2:147–152.

sis (Table 19–32). The cerebral spinal fluid is normal except for the increased pressure.

The typical patient is an obese woman of childbearing years, often with a recent weight gain. In addition, there appears to be a co-occurrence of pseudotumor cerebri and the empty sella syndrome. Headaches, obesity, and a female preponderance occur with equal frequency in both disorders. Because the empty sella syndrome is thought to result from the "water-hammer" pulsations of the cerebrospinal fluid transmitted to the pituitary fossa through a congenitally deficient diaphragma sella, it would not be surprising if it occurred more often in the face of the increased intracranial pressure of idiopathic intracranial hypertension. Early onset (before the age of 25) of hypertension is frequently seen in patients with IIH, but may be related to the high incidence of obesity in this population.

Differential Diagnosis. The diagnosis of IIH is one of exclusion. The obvious other causes of similar symptoms, such as real tumors and the conditions in Table 19–32, must be ruled out by appropriate neurologic and neuroradiologic evaluation. Then, a lumbar puncture must be done to document the increased intracranial pressure and check for cells or other abnormalities. Sometimes the lumbar puncture is curative.

The combination of optic nerve head drusen and headaches very frequently leads to a misdiagnosis of IIH. In an obese young woman the results of lumbar puncture are frequently borderline or elevated due to technical problems. If the patient also has visual obscurations, visual field defects, or visual evoked potential (VEP) abnormalities, all too often the patient is treated for nonexistent disease.

Idiopathic intracranial hypertension was thought to be benign and self-limiting, remitting in a period of months; commonly it is. However, nearly 50% of patients followed over a long period will suffer the only serious complication of the syndrome, visual loss; in 25%, serious detriment of vision will occur. Preventing this loss of vision is the paramount goal (Fig. 19–16, Table 19–33).

Treatment. In the early stages of the disease, relief of headache by Diamox and furosemide, prednisone, or lumbar puncture therapy is attempted. Patients treated with prednisone should be followed monthly for increased intraocular pressure. Hypertension must be carefully controlled, as high blood pressure may be a significant risk factor for visual loss in this setting, as are elevated intraocular pressure and uremia. Following the initial evaluation, the patient should be followed monthly for 3 to 6 months with

TABLE 19–32. CLINICAL CONDITIONS AND FACTORS[a] REPORTED TO BE ASSOCIATED WITH IDIOPATHIC INTRACRANIAL HYPERTENSION

Hematological disorders
  Iron deficiency anemia
  Pernicious anemia
  Polycythemia vera
  Thrombocytopenia
  Wiskott-Aldrich syndrome
Medical disorders
  Obesity[b]
  Recent weight gain[b]
  Systemic lupus erythematosus
  Histiocytosis X
  Galactosemia
  Ulcerative colitis
  Sydenham's chorea
  Lues
  Guillain-Barré syndrome
  Infectious mononucleosis
  Polycythemia vera
  Wiskott-Aldrich syndrome
  Behcet's syndrome
  Empty sella syndrome
Endocrine conditions and disorders
  Addison's disease
  Menstrual irregularities
  Pregnancy
  Hypocalcemia
  Hypoparathyroidism
  Birth control pills
  Obesity
Viral disease
  Measles
  Mumps
  Influenza
  Roseola
  Poliomyelitis
Medical/surgical conditions with impaired cerebral venous drainage
  Otitis media, mastoiditis
  Idiopathic dural sinus thrombosis
  Radical neck surgery
  Chronic pulmonary disease with venous hypertension
  Heart failure with venous hypertension
  Congenital heart disease
  Sleep apnea
Trauma (with venous sinus occlusion)
Mass lesions
  Spinal cord tumor
Dietary considerations
  Hypervitaminosis A[b]
  Hypovitaminosis A and D (?)
Common drugs
  Systemic steroids
  Systemic steroid withdrawal
  Topical steroid withdrawal (infants)
  Oral contraceptives
  Tetracycline
  Nitrofurantoin
  Sulfamethoxazole
  Nalidixic acid
  Indomethacin in Bartter's syndrome
  Dilantin (?)
  Amiodarone (?)
Heavy metals
  Lead
  Arsenic
Other toxins
  Chlordane

[a] Many of the symptoms and conditions reportedly associated with idiopathic intracranial hypertension are common in women of childbearing years and may be chance associations.
[b] Probably a true association.

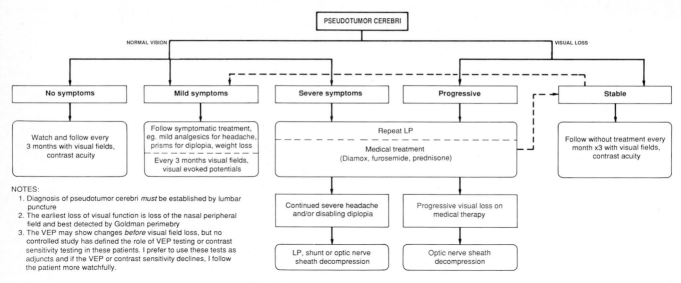

Figure 19–16. Management of idiopathic intracranial hypertension.

NOTES:
1. Diagnosis of pseudotumor cerebri *must* be established by lumbar puncture
2. The earliest loss of visual function is loss of the nasal peripheral field and best detected by Goldman perimetry
3. The VEP may show changes *before* visual field loss, but no controlled study has defined the role of VEP testing or contrast sensitivity testing in these patients. I prefer to use these tests as adjuncts and if the VEP or contrast sensitivity declines, I follow the patient more watchfully.

careful visual field and contrast sensitivity tests. In the chronic stage, if papilledema persists, it should be followed quarterly with visual field tests and yearly with VEP tests. Goldmann fields appear to be more sensitive than automated perimetry, and contrast sensitivity may be the most sensitive parameter to measure. Any complaint of dimming vision should be evaluated with utmost seriousness, because once started, visual loss can be precipitous. Progressive visual field loss or decrease in visual acuity should be aggressively treated by optic nerve decompression. Although lumbo-peritoneal shunting may seem less traumatic and risky, the long-term results are much poorer than with optic nerve decompression.

Subarachnoid Hemorrhage

Intracranial aneurysms are the most common nontraumatic cause of subarachnoid hemorrhage (SAH);

conversely, SAH is the most frequent presentation of intracranial aneurysm.

The headache of subarachnoid hemorrhage from a ruptured aneurysm is dramatic, abrupt, and excruciating. It is associated with a stiff neck and vomiting. Half of SAH victims becomes unconscious at the onset; another 25% within 15 minutes; 45% dies. Little leaks causing recurrent headache prior to the subarachnoid bleed are not rare. Thus, the onset of a new type of headache should always alert the physician to the possibility of an intracranial aneurysm. The large majority occurs in the anterior circulation in relation to the circle of Willis; in about one third of patients, aneurysms are multiple.

Giant aneurysms, in contrast, rarely bleed and usually act as space-occupying lesions, causing distortions of structures at the base of the skull; they occur most often at the bifurcations of the internal carotid and basilar arteries.

A **bleeding arteriovenous malformation** (AVM) may present a similar picture. There may also be a bruit and a history of recurrent and focal seizures (occipital epilepsy), stereotyped and unilateral. Occipital apoplexy occurring without the aura or symptoms of migraine and in patients with no family history of migraine should suggest hemorrhage into an occipital AVM. Most AVMs become symptomatic prior to middle age.

Meningitis

Meningitis causes retro-orbital pain, markedly exacerbated by eye movement and head movement. It is associated with cervical rigidity. Lumbar puncture is diagnostic.

TABLE 19–33. SERIAL NEURO-OPHTHALMOLOGIC EVALUATION OF PATIENTS WITH IDIOPATHIC INTRACRANIAL HYPERTENSION

Obtain best corrected visual acuity.
Examine visual fields by formal perimetry.
Note presence or absence of spontaneous venous pulsations.
Obtain stereo optic disc and red-free nerve fiber layer photographs.
Examine for evidence of sixth-nerve paresis.
Monitor intraocular pressure if patient is on corticosteroids.
Perform slit-lamp examination of the lens for evidence of cataracts if the patient is treated with corticosteroids.
Check serum electrolytes if patient is taking acetazolamide.
Check visual evoked response on initial evaluation; repeat later if the patient's visual field testing is unreliable.

Adapted from Wall M. Pseudotumor cerebri. In: Johnson RT, ed. Current Therapy in Neurologic Disease 1985–1986. Philadelphia: Decker, 1985:229.

Meningeal Traction

Lumbar puncture (LP) headache may occur following LP due to movement of intracranial contents and pulling on the meninges. The patient should be put flat in bed and given a high fluid intake. Persistent headache may necessitate patching the dural leak with a blood patch.

Posttraumatic Headaches

Patients with posttraumatic symptoms frequently find their way to neuro-ophthalmologic evaluation because of complaints of headache, vertigo, unsteadiness, and blurred vision.

Forty to sixty percent of patients hospitalized for closed head injury experiences headaches lasting longer than 2 months (Table 19–34). These headaches are dull, aching, generalized, and occur daily. The patient shows some features of vascular headache, including occasional scintillating scotomata and exacerbation with straining. The severity of the headache does not necessarily correlate with the severity of the trauma.

Posttraumatic headaches are usually associated with decreased concentration, memory difficulties, and irritability in adults. In children, headache is rarer, as is vertigo. Children become hyperkinetic and show poor control of anger, a decreased attention span, and eneuresis.

Therapy consists of reassurance and relaxation therapy. Ergot preparations may be helpful.

Objective evidence for the syndrome can be obtained from prolongation of the VEP with rapid stimulus rates, abnormal electroencephalograms (50%), and ENG testing (rarely normal). The blurred vision is often due to spasm of the near reflex (see Chapter 10).

HEADACHES IN SYSTEMIC ILLNESS

Headache as a symptom of systemic illnesses is much less common than is generally believed even by physicians—for example, it is rarely associated with hypertension, thyroid disease, or hypoglyce-mia. It is probably not typical of uncomplicated hypertension (unless >140 diastolic). Nevertheless, with sustained diastolic pressure above 140, headache is often present, but in these cases it is usually associated with hypertensive encephalopathy, fundus changes, and increased blood urea nitrogen. It is less common with sustained hypertension even at these levels than with paroxysmal increases in blood pressure such as occur in pheochromocytoma. Eighty percent of these patients has headaches, which typically crescendo in minutes. The association with perspiration, pallor and palpitations, nausea, tremor, or paroxysms of hypertension is pathognomonic (Table 19–35).

The most frequent association of headache with systemic disease is in various acute infections, febrile and other disease usually accompanied by vasodilation: fever (especially in infectious disease such as mononucleosis, toxoplasmosis, and other subacute systemic infections; meningitis and subacute systemic infections; meningitis and subacute bacterial endocarditis); alcohol intoxication and CO_2 retention. Other illnesses associated with alterations in blood gases, such as chronic obstructive pulmonary disease, may also be associated with headache, but usually the systemic disease is obvious. Hematologic causes include polycythemia and anemia. And of course the vasodilation headache associated with nitrite therapy is well known (Table 19–36).

"SITUATIONAL HEADACHES"

Altitude headache is one of the most prominent signs of mountain sickness, which in its severe form may also include pulmonary or cerebral edema. All are probably responses to hypoxia or decreased barometric pressure. To a degree, high altitudes over 10,000 feet are associated with an increasing frequency of symptoms; at 15,000 feet about 90% of people will develop headache. Prior acclimatization does not seem to have a protective effect, nor do

TABLE 19–34. DURATION OF THE POSTCONCUSSION SYNDROME IN 100 PATIENTS

Duration	%
Less than 30 days	10
Less than 1 year	70
Less than 2 years	80
Less than 3 years	85

Data from Denker PA. The post-concussion syndrome: Prognosis and evaluation of the organic factors. NY State J Med. 1964;44:379–384.

TABLE 19–35. CLINICAL HINTS OF PHEOCHROMOCYTOMA

Unusual lability of blood pressure
Paroxysms of hypertension and tachycardia
Spells of headache, palpitations, pallor, perspiration
Accelerated hypertension
Hypermetabolism and weight loss
Abnormal carbohydrate metabolism
Pressor response to induction of anesthesia or to antihypertensive or sympathomimetic drugs
Suprarenal or midline abdominal mass

From Bonowitz NL. Pheochromocytoma: Recent advances in diagnosis and therapy. West J Med. 1988;148:561–567.

TABLE 19–36. CAUSES OF "TOXIC" VASCULAR HEADACHES

Pathologic Conditions		Toxic Substances		Withdrawal from Drugs
Febrile	*Other*	*Nonpharmacologic*	*Pharmacologic*	
Pneumonia	Alcohol	Carbon monoxide	Nitrates	Ergot
Tonsillitis	Hypoglycemia	Lead	Indomethacin	Caffeine
Septicemia	Hypoxia	Benzene	Oral progestational	Amphetamines
Thyphoid fever	Altitude	Carbon tetrachloride	Oral vasodilators	Many phenothiazines
Tularemia	Hypercarbia	Insecticides		
Influenza	Effort	Nitrates		
Measles				
Mumps				
Poliomyelitis				
Infectious mononucleosis				
Malaria				
Trichinosis				

From D'Allessio DJ, ed. Wolff's Headache and Other Head Pain. 5th ed. New York: Oxford, 1987:8.

headaches always recur in the same individuals at the same altitude. When the eyes have been examined, retinal hemorrhages frequently accompany the headaches. In the few cases examined at autopsy petechial hemorrhages and cerebral edema have been found. Immediate descent usually alleviates the symptoms; sometimes even a loss of a few hundred feet is sufficient. Opinion is divided as to whether acetazolamide started a few days before ascent can prevent altitude sickness.

Hangover is an all too well known syndrome of headache, malaise, nausea, and light-headedness, often associated with other autonomic symptoms. It occurs several hours after the height of blood alcohol levels and lasts 5 to 10 hours, long after all alcohol has disappeared from the body.

Ice cream headache occurs when ice cream (or other very cold food or liquid) coats the roof of the mouth. The pain can be very intense, is usually frontal, and lasts only a few seconds if the cold stimulus is removed. It, like many other headaches, is significantly more frequent in migraine patients.

A number of other food elements is recognized as headache inducers, again especially in patients with a history of vascular headaches. Tyramine (cheese), phenylalanine (chocolate), mace, nitrite ("hotdog headache"), monosodium glutamate ("Chinese restaurant syndrome"), and alcohol are all frequent offenders.

SUMMARY

Relatively few of the numerous individuals suffering from headache seek help from a physician. Those who do expect an answer. It is incumbent on us to

(1) understand the mechanism of headache, (2) rule out or diagnose significant systemic or neurologic disease, (3) reassure the patient that the headache can and will be successfully treated, and (4) dispel fears of brain tumor or other serious illness.

The large majority of headaches will fall into the muscle contraction and tension group; the next largest group is the vascular headaches. Nearly all of these headaches can be accurately classified and treated without specialized testing or a multimillion-dollar neuro-imaging workup. However, their recognition is dependent on a detailed history and careful neuro-ophthalmic examination; it is dependent on familiarity with the important differences between those headaches that pose severe threats to life, vision, or neurologic function and those that are more benign. Additionally, appropriate treatment of relatively nonthreatening headaches is dependent on recognizing the type of headache to be treated.

BIBLIOGRAPHY

General

Behrens MM. Headache and head pain associated with diseases of the eye. *Res Clin Stud Headache.* 1976;4:18–36.

D'Allessio DJ, ed. *Wolff's Headache and Other Head Pain.* 5th ed. New York: Oxford, 1987.

Florence Headache 1987. Proceedings of the third congress of the International Headache Society. Florence, Italy, September 22–25, 1987. *Cephalgia:* (supplement 7) 6:1–551, 1987.

Knox DL, Cogan DG. Eye pain and homonymous hemianopia. *Am J Ophthalmol.* 1962;54:1091.

Lance JW. *The Mechanics and Management of Headache.* 4th ed. London: Butterworth, 1982.

Miller NH, ed. *Walsh and Hoyt's Clinical Neuro-ophthalmology.* 4th ed. Sensory innervation of eye and orbit. Baltimore: Williams & Wilkins, 1985;2.

Raskin NH. *Headache.* 2nd ed. New York: Churchill Livingstone, 1988.

Ziegler DK, Hasainen RS, Couch JR. Characteristics of life headache histories in a non-clinic population. *Neurology.* 1977;27:265–269.

Herpes Zoster

Bucci FA, Gabriels CF, Krohel GB. Successful treatment of postherpetic neuralgia with capsaicin. *Am J Ophthalmol.* 1988;106:758–759.

Cobo LM et al. Oral Acyclovir in the treatment of acute herpes zoster ophthalmicus. *Ophthalmology.* 1986;93:763–770.

Kernbaum S, Hauchecorne J. Administration of levodopa for relief of herpes zoster pain. *JAMA.* 1981;246:132–134.

Kissin I, McDanal J, Xavier A. Topical lidocaine for relief of superficial pain in postherpetic neuralgia. *Neurology.* 1989;39:1132–1133.

Max MB, Schafer SC et al. Amitriptyline, but not lorazepam, relieves postherpetic neuralgia. *Neurology.* 1988;38:1427–1432.

Temporal Arteritis

Behn AR, et al. Polypyalgia rheumatica and corticosteroids: How much for how long? *Ann Rheumat Dis.* 1983;42:324–328.

Hollenhorst RW. Effects of posture on retinal ischemia from temporal arteritis. *Arch Ophthalmol.* 1967;78:569–577.

Hollenhorst RW, et al. Neurological aspects of temporal arteritis. *Neurology.* 1960;10:490–498.

Huston KA. Temporal arteritis: A 25-year epidemiological, clinical and pathologic study. *Ann Int Med.* 1978;88:162–167.

Rosenfeld SI, et al. Treatment of temporal arteritis with ocular involvement. *Am J Med.* 1986;80:143–145.

Pseudotumor Cerebri

Corbett JJ. Problems in the diagnosis and treatment of pseudotumor cerebri. *Can J Neurol Sci.* 1983;10:221–229.

Corbett JJ, Thompson HS. The rational management of idiopathic intracranial hypertension. *Arch Neurol.* 1989;46:1049–1051.

Guiseffi V, Wall M, Siegel PZ, Rojus PB. Symptoms and disease associations in Idiopathic Intracranial Hypertension (pseudotumor cerebri): A case control study. *Neurology.* 1991;41:239–244.

Guy J, Johnston PK, Corbett J, Day A, Glaser J. Treatment of visual loss in pseudotumor cerebri associated with uremia. *Neurology.* 1990;40:28–32.

Ireland B, Corbett J, Wallace R. The search for causes of idiopathic intracranial hypertension: A preliminary case-control study. *Arch Neurol.* 1990;47:315–320.

Wall M. Pseudotumor Cerebri. In: Johnson RT, ed. *Current Therapy in Neurologic Disease, 1985–1986.* Philadelphia: Decker, 1985.

Parasellar

Thomas JE, Yoss RE. The parasellar syndrome: Problems in determining etiology. *Mayo Clin Proc.* 1970;45:617–623.

Raeder's Syndrome

Grimson BS, Thompson HS. Raeder's syndrome: A clinical review. *Surv Ophthalmol.* 1980;24:199–210.

Internal Carotid Artery Dissection

Fisher CM, Ojemann RG, Rohn LH. Spontaneous dissection of cervical cerebral arteries. *Can J Med Sci.* 1978;5:9–19.

Carotidynia

Raskin NH, Prusiner P. Carotidynia. *Neurology.* 1977;27:436.

Ocular Pain

Cameron ME. Headaches in relation to the eyes. *Med J Aust.* 1976;1:292–294.

Subarachnoid Hemorrhage

LeBlanc R. The minor leak preceding subarachnoid hemorrhage. *J Neurosurgery.* 1987;66:35–39.

Mohr JP et al. Intracranial aneurysms in stroke. In: Barnett HJM et al., eds. *Pathophysiology: Symptoms, Diagnosis, and Management.* New York: Churchill Livingstone, 1987.

Altitude Headache

Hamilton AJ et al. High altitude cerebral edema. *Neurosurgery.* 1986;19:841–849.

Migraine

Anderson AR et al. Delayed hyperemia following hyperperfusion in classic migraine. *Arch Neurol.* 1988;45:154–159.

Corbett JJ. Neuro-ophthalmic complications of migraine and cluster headaches. *Neurol Clin.* 1983;1:973–995.

Soges L, Cacayorin E, Petro G, Ramachandran T. Migraine: evaluation by MR. *Am J Neuroradiol.* 1988;9:425–429.

Pheochromocytoma

Duncan MW et al. Measurement of norepinephrine and 34-dihydroxy phenylglycol in urine and plasma for the diagnosis of Pheochromocytoma. *N Engl J Med.* 1988;39:136–142.

Corneal Hypaesthesia

Martin XY, Safran AB. Corneal hypaesthesia. *Surv Ophthalmol.* 1988;33:28–40.

Trigeminal Neuralgia

Burchiel KJ. Percutaneous retrogasserian glycerol rhizolysis in the management of trigeminal neuralgia. *J Neurosurg.* 1988;69:361–366.

Lichtor T, Mullan J. A 10-year follow-up review of percutaneous microcompression of the trigeminal ganglion. *J Neurosurg.* 1990;72:49–54.

Sahni KS, Pieper DR, Anderson R, Baldwin N. Relation of hypesthesia to the outcome of glycerol rhizolysis for trigeminal neuralgia. *J Neurosurg.* 1990;72:55–58.

Trigeminal Neuropathy

Hutchins LG, Harnsberger, et al. The radiologic assessment of trigeminal neuropathy. *Am J Neuroradiol.* 1989;10:1031–1038.

CHAPTER 20

FUNCTIONAL DISORDERS, HYSTERIA, AND MALINGERING

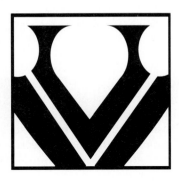

More and more frequently we encounter patients with complaints that seem not to be explained by any conceivable pathophysiologic process. More than ever, forewarned is forearmed with these patients. The patient referred by a lawyer, insurance company, or from workmen's compensation, or the patient self-referred following a motor vehicle or industrial accident, always *raises the question* of a functional complaint. The patient whose history reveals obvious secondary gain or emotional problems sufficient to account for hysteria should cause you to plan your examination even more carefully than usual. Other situations that alert you to a possible functional disorder are an aura of hostility or strange indifference, or the rare case that seems predestined for publication. Other *clues* are symptoms of a severity that clearly exceeds the obvious pathology or trauma, symptoms (especially loss of visual acuity or field) that have their onset or progress at an inappropriate temporal distance from the pathology or trauma, and symptoms that suddenly appear weeks after the injury without physical findings to explain the visual loss.

Of course, not all patients in these categories will be malingering or hysteric; functional problems do exist in patients with no obvious background for a functional complaint. Nevertheless, a high index of suspicion is very helpful in planning an examination to detect *positive* evidence of nonphysiologic or inconsistent responses. If your suspicions are not confirmed, then you must work even harder to document positive evidence of pathology.

Functional disease runs the gamut of ophthalmologic and neuro-ophthalmologic disorders and presents one of neuro-ophthalmology's greatest challenges.

Malingerers, especially, want to cooperate and please. Encourage them down the garden path of nonphysiologic anomalies.

FUNCTIONAL DISORDERS OF THE VISUAL AFFERENT PATHWAYS

Functional monocular visual loss. Functional monocular visual loss is relatively easy to evaluate. Monocular visual loss must be caused by a lesion anterior to the optic chiasm. Alterations in the media or retina should be visible to the examiner, especially when visual acuity is reduced significantly (< 20/40). Where media changes exist, in general, the examiner's view of the retina should be equivalent to the patient's visual acuity (patient's view out). Early and subtle lesions may need to be evaluated by contrast sensitivity and color-vision testing, red-free photography, visual field testing, fluorescein angiography, and electrophysiologic testing. Among lesions that can be difficult to detect are solar retinopathy, central serous retinopathy (CSR), cystoid macular edema (CME), and early cone dystrophy, and early Stargardt's retinopathy (fundus flavimaculatus) especially if they are asymmetric in their earliest manifestations.

Solar retinopathy usually shows a characteristic edema and reddish parafoveal discoloration early and pigment clumping as the lesion evolves. The mature lesion shows only the pigment alterations.

Central serous chorioretinopathy can usually be identified (1) from the patient's history; (2) by the characteristic positive scotoma, often pink or purple tinged; (3) by distortion on Amsler grid testing; and (4) by a very positive photostress test. In the area of the lesion, the retina usually has lost the normal reflexes and there is one or more slightly elevated gray disciform areas (areas of retinal pigment epithelium detachment). Fluorescein angiography shows a highly characteristic pooling of fluorescein and usually shows a leak from the choriocapillaris.

Cystoid macular edema may be difficult to detect on clinical examination alone. Again, posterior pole contact lens examination and fluorescein angiography can be very helpful, revealing the pathognomonic petalloid pooling of fluorescein in Henle's layer around the fovea.

Cone dystrophies may be asymmetrical at onset. Central acuity and color vision are decreased; there are subtle alterations in macular appearance and the foveal reflex; later, pigment mottling is seen. Photophobia frequently accompanies these complaints and seems disproportionate to the degree of visual difficulty. Onset is usually in the second or third decade. The diagnosis may be confirmed by the presence of a diminished flicker (scotopic) electroretinogram (ERG).

Stargardt's dystrophy (fundus flavimaculatus), an autosomal recessive disorder, usually becomes symptomatic in the first or second decade, most often around age 10. Again, there is an early loss of the foveal reflex, with more obvious macular changes occurring later. In the fundus flavimaculatus variant, the white flecks become more evident with time. The early lesions may be highlighted by red-free photography, and in early stages the choroid has a characteristically dark appearance on fluorescein angiography. The ERG is normal but the electrooculogram (EOG) is occasionally decreased. The pattern electroretinogram (PERG) is significantly attenuated at a very early stage.

Even when visual loss is minimal, unilateral **optic nerve disease** should be associated with decreased color vision and contrast sensitivity, an afferent pupillary defect, a visual field defect (often a central scotoma), and optic atrophy or retinal nerve fiber layer defects. If these objective signs of monocular optic nerve damage are not present, one should be very suspicious of a functional problem. However, be on the alert for the pituitary tumor, aneurysm, or other parachiasmal mass that compresses the chiasm or both optic nerves, but decreases visual acuity in one eye only; seemingly paradoxically, the apparently unilateral visual loss may not be accompanied by a Marcus Gunn pupil or asymmetry of color vision, optic disc color, or nerve fiber layer density. Nevertheless, in these cases there should be bilateral inextensive pupillary reactions, decreased color vision, optic atrophy, and loss of the nerve fiber layer. Both eyes should show visual field defects.

Rule out *amblyopia* by carefully searching for a history or family history of strabismus, patching, operation, or eye exercises. Check for anisometropia. Test for the crowding phenomenon by testing vision with one letter at a time. Use 4-diopter base-out prisms, neutral-density filter, and stereo tests (see Chapter 2). Evidence is conflicting regarding the affect of amblyopia on pattern electroretinograms (PERGs) and visual evoked potentials (VEPs), so normal test results may not absolutely rule out organic amblyopia.

If a combination of objective and subjective tests has not clearly confirmed the presence of organic monocular visual loss, it is time to pull out your bag of tricks. Most tricks manipulate the testing environment to encourage nonphysiologic responses. Use the simplest tests first. Assemble your own bag of tricks so you are fluid in testing and don't raise the patient's suspicions. Be encouraging. Even malingerers like positive reinforcement.

Vary the testing distance in testing visual acuity and visual fields. The patient reading the 20/40 line at 20 feet should read the 20/20 line at 10 feet; if the visual field subtends 5 degrees (10 inches) at 1 meter with a 1-mm target, it should still subtend the same 5 degrees at 2 meters with a 2-mm target, but should double in size to 20 inches (see below). If the patient is able to read print, a +4 lens should double the near acuity (eg, 20/80 to 20/40, or 20/100 to 20/50).

Put a 4-diopter prism over the "bad" eye while the patient is fixing a distant target less than the patient's claimed acuity for the "bad" eye. If the eye moves, the patient was able to see the target.

Routinely use the screening plates in testing color vision with the **Hardy Rand Ritler (HRR) or other plates.** With any visual acuity greater than 20/500 the patient should be able to resolve the letters. If the patient can't see the screening plates, you have another cause for suspicion—although a large central scotoma rarely may make it impossible to read the plates.

More subtle tests available in ophthalmologists' offices include using the **phoropter** to fog the patient bilaterally and then reducing the fogging in the "bad" eye while appearing to manipulate both eyes. If the bad eye now reads better, your suspicions are confirmed. If a **polarized visual acuity chart** is available, using oppositely polarized lenses in glasses or rotating the polarized lenses in a trial frame can also be useful; the **duochrome test** is similarly employed and can be very effective, as most patients will not have time or knowledge to figure out which eye should be seeing which letters. Use the portable **stereopic test charts,** Titmus or TNO (Fig. 20–1). The visual acuity should correspond with the size of stereopic figure resolved. The patient claiming very poor vision (<20/400) obviously should not briskly

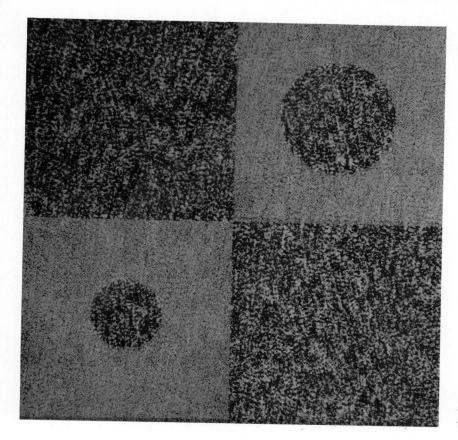

Figure 20–1. TNO Stereo test. When viewed with red-green glasses two of the images are three dimensional.

reach into space for anything smaller than the wings of the stereo fly!

Statements printed in a size smaller than the patient's claimed acuity and flashed before the patient, if insulting, risqué, or otherwise outrageous, may cause an obvious reaction.

If visual acuity is very low (eg, count fingers), you can make use of egocentric human nature by tilting a mirror in front of the bad eye. The image movement of the patient's own face is nearly irresistable and will stimulate the eye to move.

Tests that determine the "retinal acuity," such as the visometer and potential acuity meter (PAM), may be helpful if they yield an acuity better than that the patient describes and unexplained by media opacity.

Optokinetic nystagmus (OKN) tapes or drums can be used similarly. Most patients are unaware of the fact that nystagmus is induced by an OKN stimulus; therefore the use of stripes of appropriate width can, by inducing eye movement, give positive evidence of visual acuity at that level. The sophisticated or experienced functional patient may have learned to blur out or stare through optokinetic targets, and so it is useful to have a selection of tests available and ready for each patient.

Functional Binocular Visual Loss

Obviously, many of the same tests used for the patient with monocular visual loss can be used for patients with binocular visual loss, the major exceptions being those tests that depend on binocular vision: fogging, polaroid, and stereopsis tests.

If you are aware of possible functional binocular visual loss before you begin examining the patient, you have a significant advantage, especially if the visual loss is profound; observation of how the patient navigates from the waiting room to the exam room can be very enlightening. Obviously, a patient with no light perception, hand motion vision, or 5-degree central fields should have difficulty finding the way, especially if you have been conniving enough to place obstacles—chairs, wastebaskets, and so forth—between the door and the patient's chair or bed in the examining room. Additionally, in the ophthalmologist's office the patient who easily puts his or her head into the slit-lamp without first feeling its height by hand usually can see quite well.

Electrophysiologic testing can be helpful to objectively record visual function. Clearly, normal PERGs, VEPs, ERGs, and so forth, effectively rule out all but the most minor of visual problems. Although it is possible for the patient to stare through the stimulus and give spuriously abnormal waveforms, it is unusual to be able to fake delay of a well-developed major positive peak or significant asymmetry between the hemispheres. The latter findings are highly suggestive of an organic lesion, especially multiple sclerosis (MS), and one should go back and look carefully again for a minimal Marcus Gunn pupil in uniocular visual loss or subtle nerve fiber layer changes.

Functional transient visual loss. True transient ischemic attacks (TIAs)—whether due to carotid or vertebrobasilar emboli, inadequate perfusion, migraine, obscurations in association with papilledema, or other causes of transient visual loss (TVL)— usually follow relatively stereotyped patterns and time courses (see Chapter 8). Although there are exceptions to any clinical pattern, TIAs not conforming to the expected criteria should raise suspicion of a functional etiology.

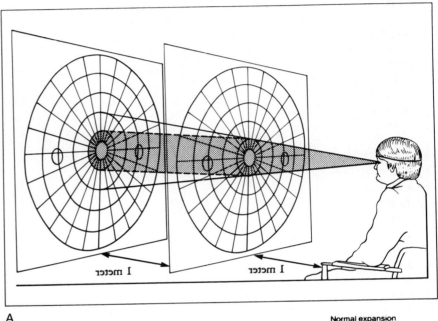

A

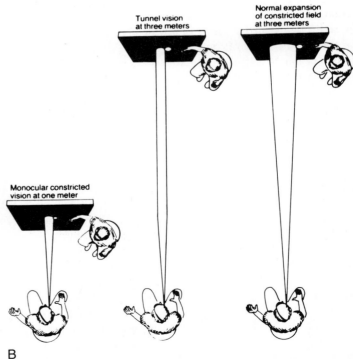

B

Figure 20–2. A. Testing with tangent screen. Testing at 1 and 2 m on a tangent screen to demonstrate nonphysiologic constriction of visual fields. Because light travels in straight lines, the field at 2 m should be twice as large as the field at 1 m for equivalent stimuli (eg, 5-mm disc at 1 m and 10-mm disc at 2 m). When both fields are the same diameter on the screen at two distances, hysteria or malingering should be suspected. **B.** Tunnel vision. The area of a constricted field should expand as the distance from the patient increases. In the functional patient the field will retain the same degree of constriction despite the distance at which it is tested. It is important to remember that when testing at greater distances from the patient, the size of the test object should be increased correspondingly. (**A.** *From Gittinger JW Jr. Neuro-ophthalmology. In: Ophthalmology: A Clinical Introduction. Boston: Little, Brown, 1984, with permission.* **B.** *From Beck RW, Smith CH. Functional diseases in neuro-ophthalmology. In: Symposium on Neuro-ophthalmology. Neurologic Clinics. 1983;1:966, Philadelphia, PA: W.B. Saunders, with permission.*)

Functional visual field loss: The pattern of visual field loss claimed by the patient should be consistent with the other findings. A patient with a central scotoma should also manifest decreased visual acuity, decreased color vision, and if unilateral, an afferent pupillary defect. Field defects due to optic nerve or central nervous system (CNS) lesions should respect the horizontal and vertical meridians, respectively. Unilateral hemianopic visual field defects are not uncommon among patients with functional disorders, but are exceedingly rare in patients with organic disease. Bitemporal defects and binasal defects are also found as functional complaints, but normally have unusual concomitants that can be tested for and that rarely can be simulated by the functional patient. In patients with bitemporal hemianopia there is an area of postfixational blindness where the bitemporal field defects overlap, and in patients with binasal hemianopia (rare even in organic disease) an area of prefixational blindness (see Chapter 2 for more details).

As mentioned above, where there is a question of a functional problem, any visual field defect should be examined at 1 and 2 meters, with test targets of 1 and 2 mm or 5 and 10 mm. Although the angle subtended by the defect remains constant, the area of the defect will be twice as large at the greater test difference (Fig. 20–2). Very gullible patients can be coerced into giving square fields if a large rectangular test object (like an 8½ by 11-inch sheet of paper) is held and the borders of the paper marked obviously on the field screen by the examiner. If then the target is moved along the line, because it is logical that the line should continue linearly, a straight border results. Similar testing extended for the approximate extent of the visual field, turning the paper at the "corners," can yield a square visual field.

When a patient with functional problems is tested on a Goldmann perimeter, three abnormal patterns are likely to result: (1) concentrically constricted visual fields inconsistent with the degree of the patient's visual loss or behavior; (2) fields in which the different isopters overlap; and (3) fields that "spiral," becoming smaller and smaller as testing progresses (Fig. 20–3).

On automated perimetry, responses from the functional patient may be inconsistent, but the patterns of responses or losses of fixation are not sufficiently typical to be considered hard evidence of functional behavior.

A maneuver almost certain to trap the unwary functional patient with bilateral constricted fields is the simple polite gesture of shaking hands either in greeting or goodbye. Clearly, a patient with 10-degree fields should not see the hand that is normally proferred at least 30 degrees into the periphery.

FUNCTIONAL POSITIVE VISUAL PHENOMENA

Positive visual phenomena are rarely described by the functional patient, especially the malingerer, as most of these patients wish to present as normal a facade as possible. Thus, "seeing things" is not likely to be reported. Occasionally the patient with a functional disorder will report an unformed photopsia or hallucination or elaboration of a migraine aura. Again, these phenomena should correspond with those described in organic conditions or raise suspicion.

FUNCTIONAL DISORDERS OF EYE MOVEMENTS

Functional disorders of ocular motility are much less common than claims involving the visual afferent pathways. Perhaps the most common are spasm of accommodation (convergence spasm) and voluntary nystagmus. **Convergence spasm** may present as a complaint of diplopia, an esotropia, or unilateral or bilateral sixth nerve palsies. Usually it is relatively

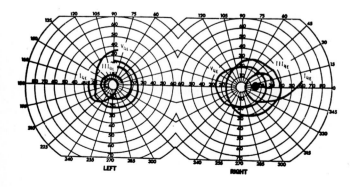

Figure 20–3. Spiral Goldmann field. Goldmann perimetry demonstrating spiraling of the right and left visual fields. Not shown is the inconsistent isopter responses on the binocular Goldmann perimetry examination. *(From Beck RW, Smith CH. Functional diseases in neuro-ophthalmology. In: Symposium on Neuro-ophthalmology. Neurologic Clinics. 1983;1:960, Philadelphia, PA: W.B. Saunders, with permission.)*

easily detected by the accompanying miosis (pupil constriction) and accommodation.

Voluntary nystagmus consists of back-to-back convergent saccades (fast eye movements) at a rapid frequency ($\pm$20/sec). It is difficult to sustain, and just watching while the patient fixes at distance is therefore usually sufficient to observe the abnormal movement fatigue away. It must be differentiated from saccadic intrusions (see Chapter 14), which are of much smaller amplitude; and from ocular flutter, which usually produces only a few beats at a time.

Functional limitation of eye movement can be "caught out" by testing each of the eye movement mechanisms (saccades, pursuit, ocular reflex [vestibular, otolithic, tonic neck], and vergence), as all are affected only in severe brain-stem disorders and patients so affected usually are not able to walk into your office. The oculocephalic maneuver (OCM) (see Chapter 14) may be used to move the eyes into an apparently defective region of gaze, as most patients are unaware that their eyes move relative to the head if they fixate straight ahead while the head is turned. Caloric testing may also be very effective, especially ice water calorics (the latter is sometimes therapeutic for the frustrated examiner).

Functional ptosis can usually be identified by the obvious contraction of the orbicularis oculi and the patient's "inability" to lift the lid above its usual position (which is rarely totally shut) despite an excellent lid fold.

Complaints of *functional diplopia* are assessed by looking for the associated tropia by cover and cross-cover testing. If the degree of diplopia is constant so should be the tropia. If the degree varies with gaze, the underlying muscle palsy should be apparent.

Polyopia and monocular diplopia are most often associated with aberrations of the refractile media, which should be checked with the ophthalmoscope, retinoscope, and slit-lamp for aberrations. True polyopia may also be of CNS origin, occurring rarely in posterior parietal lesions, especially of the right hemisphere. There is often an associated visual field defect and almost always other signs of a "disconnection" syndrome.

OTHER FUNCTIONAL PROBLEMS

Seventh nerve spasm can, on occasion, be simulated by a patient. Usually the best way to detect it is to observe the patient surreptitiously. Few functional patients will continually "spasm."

Instillation of mydriatic drops to affect pupillary function can be detected by appropriate pharmacologic testing; 1% pilocarpine will **not** contract the **pharmacologically dilated pupil** but will constrict the pupil that is large due to a physiologic lesion. The pupil that is small secondary to the use of drops in a functional patient is usually regular and fixed and is uncommon, perhaps because frequent instillation of miotics may be quite uncomfortable.

Although most functional patients are relatively easily diagnosed, be sure not to conclude the patient exhibits functional symptoms only because there is no obvious pathologic diagnosis. The diagnosis of functional disease must be more than just the lack of findings confirming "real" disease. It is incumbent upon us to document *conclusive positive* evidence of nonphysiologic responses before the complaints are considered functional in etiology.

In addition, the most difficult patients of all are those that have some detectable abnormalities; even though abnormal findings are not always manifestations of disease (when looked at with a fine-tooth comb, few patients are *absolutely* normal).

The CRICK (sick crock) is the nearly impossible patient. In this litigious era, a patient who initially impresses us as being functional must be followed. Few progressive diseases, especially the treatable processes most important to diagnose, remain totally quiescent for 3 to 6 months. Most ominous conditions will be progressive and will make themselves known; remitting conditions may resolve and on repeated examinations under stable conditions will show results that are identical within limits of the testing parameters. Three to six months later, few functional patients can perfectly reproduce *all* the results on a battery of tests (especially if you subtly alter the test situation—eg, use a 10-foot lane if a 20-foot lane was used before; use 2- and 4-m fields if 1 and 2 m were used before; or use 2- and +10 mm-targets if 1 and 5 mm were used before, or switch to colored targets). The experienced functional patients will try to *exactly* reproduce results from previous examinations and sometimes trap themselves in doing so.

I find that a frank discussion with some CRICKS can be most illuminating. I tell them that the nonphysiologic responses are masking real damage and that with time some of the confusing parts of the illness may dissipate and the "true" affliction will make itself known. Often on the next visit, the patient is very straightforward, because it is to his or her advantage to have the "real" problem documented. A similar approach emphasizing the "scariness" of the problem is also effective with the preteener (often a girl) with a functional problem. Given a graceful way to give up their symptoms, most will. It is also important to talk frankly with the parents and to caution them against spending the ride home from your office berating their child for all the time and expense suffered "for nothing."

The adult patient may also accept a graceful way out and can sometimes be helped along by intermittent patching of the good eye to strengthen the "bad" eye (nearly everyone knows this is done for children), methylcellulose "tonic" drops to strengthen vision or muscles, or exercises.

In detecting and "treating" these sometimes vexing patients, alertness, guile, persistence, and understanding go a long way.

Section V
Systemic Disorders and the Eye

It is beyond the scope of this book to compile the myriad congenital malformations, systemic disorders, and heritable, neurologic and metabolic diseases implicated in the differential diagnosis of neuro-ophthalmic signs and symptoms. Nevertheless, it is critical to know when the patient with ocular or neurologic disease should be evaluated for associated problems that cause significant morbidity, such as the cardiomyopathies associated with progressive external ophthalmoplegia and Leber's hereditary optic neuropathy. One should also know (1) when genetic counseling is indicated; (2) when prenatal or early diagnosis is possible; (3) when treatable metabolic or medical conditions are associated with neuro-ophthalmic disease; (4) when the neuro-ophthalmic condition itself may respond or be stabilized by treatment, as with Refsum's disease and many lysosomal disorders; and (5) what can be told to the patient or family about the expected course of the disease.

This section approaches the problem in three ways. It tabulates diseases with neuro-ophthalmic manifestations organized (1) by metabolic abnormality or structural problem (Chapter 21), (2) by organ system(s) (Chapter 22), and (3) by ocular signs (Chapter 23). In this way, given a specific neuro-ophthalmic or ocular finding, you can find the systemic problems that might be associated. In a patient with a known systemic disease, disease of an organ system, or hereditary abnormality, you will be able to find the associated ocular and neuro-ophthalmic findings.

Recent advances in diagnostic methods, such as magnetic resonance imaging, prenatal diagnosis, identification of chromosomal abnormalities, and molecular genetics facilitated accurate diagnosis of this bewildering array of syndromes and hereditary disorders. An avalanche of information, methodology, and treatment modalities promises to completely revolutionize the detection, management, and even prevention of many of these disorders. For example, polymerase chain reactions identify products that act as specific probes for portions of DNA associated with infectious, genetic, metabolic, and immune disorders. Abnormal genes, enzymes, and proteins have already been detected in Leber's optic neuropathy and other mitrochondrial diseases, lysosomal storage disorders, multiple sclerosis, myasthenia gravis, ataxia telangectasia, and lymphocytic cancers, to name only a few disorders of neuro-ophthalmic interest (Tables V–1, V–2).

The bibliography for Chapters 21 to 23 appears near the end of Chapter 23. Abbreviations used in Chapters 21 to 23 tables are defined before Chapter 21.

TABLE V–1. PRACTICAL MEDICAL APPLICATIONS OF THE POLYMERASE CHAIN REACTION IN HUMAN GENETICS

Diagnosis

Sickle-cell anemia
Beta-thalassemia and hemoglobin H disease
Phenylketonuria
Diabetes (insulin-gene mutation)
Cystic fibrosis (allele linked)
Hemophilia A (allele linked)
Hemophilia B (gene mutation)
Alpha$_1$-antitrypsin deficiency (allele linked)
Leber's hereditary optic neuropathy (mitochondrial mutation)
Apolipoprotein mutations
Duchenne's muscular dystrophy
Lesch-Nyhan syndrome
Huntington's disease (allele linked)
Residual leukemia (Philadelphia chromosome)
Lymphoma dissemination

Pathogenesis (Allele-linked Disease)

Diabetes mellitus
Pemphigus vulgaris
Myasthenia gravis and multiple sclerosis
Oncogene-linked cancers

From Eisenstein A. The polymerase chain reaction: A new method of using molecular genetics for medical diagnosis. N Engl J Med. 1990;322:181.

TABLE V–2. PRACTICAL MEDICAL APPLICATIONS OF THE POLYMERASE CHAIN REACTION IN INFECTIOUS DISEASE

Diagnosis

HIV
HIV-1 and HIV-2 double infection
HTLV-1 and myelopathy
HTLV-1 and tropic spastic paraparesis
Cytomegalovirus
Hepadnavirus
Papillomavirus in urine
Cutaneous herpes simplex virus
Human parvovirus B$_{19}$
Hepatitis B virus in serum
Slow viruses in brain (BK and JC)
Enterotoxigenic *Escherichia coli*
Legionella pneumophila
Trypanosoma cruzi
Toxoplasma gondii

Viral Associations With Cancer

HTLV-I and leukemia
HTLV-II
Papillomavirus and cervical cancer
Papillomavirus and corneal lesions

HIV-1 and HIV-2 denote human immunodeficiency virus types 1 and 2. HTLV-I and HTLV-II denote human T-cell lymphotropic virus types I and II. *From Eisenstein A. The polymerase chain reaction: A new method of using molecular genetics for medical diagnosis.* N Engl J Med. 1990;322:180.

ABBREVIATIONS FOR CHAPTERS 21–23

Aa uria	Amino acid uria	CVA	Cerebral vascular accident
Abd	Abdomen	Cx	Cortex, cortical
Abn	Abnormal, abnormality, abnormalities	Dcsd	Decreased
AC	Anterior chamber	Defic	Deficit, deficiency
Accel	Accelerated	Degen	Degeneration
AD	Autosomal dominant	Demyelin	Demyelination
AI	Aortic insufficiency	Deter	Deterioration
Anom	Anomaly	Dev	Developmental
Ant	Anterior	Diff dx	Differential diagnosis
Ant seg	Anterior segment	Dis	Disease
AR	Autosomal recessive	Disloc	Dislocated
Art	Artery, arterial	DM	Diabetes mellitus
AVM	Arteriovenous malformation	Dsfxn	Dysfunction
BANF	Bilateral acoustic neurofibromatosis	DT	Delirium tremens
Bilat	Bilateral	DTR	Deep tendon reflex
BMT	Bone marrow transplant	DTS	Delirium tremens
B stem	Brain stem	Dys	Dystrophy
Bx	Biopsy	Dysarth	Dysarthria
C-itis	Conjunctivitis	ED	Early diagnosis via easily accessible material, (eg, blood, urine, tears, skin, conjunctiva)
Ca	Cancer, carcinoma		
Calcif	Calcified, calcification, calcium	EM	Eye movement
Cardiovasc	Cardiovascular	EOM	Extraocular muscle (s)
Car oc	Carotid occlusion	EOG	Electrooculogram
Cat	Cataract	Epithel	Epithelial, epithelium
Cav	Cavernous	ERG	Electroretinogram
CEA	Carcinogenic embryonic antigen	Esp	Especially
Cereb	Cerebral	Exophthal	Exophthalmos
Cerebell	Cerebellar	(f)	frequently
Chrom	Chromosome	FA	Fluorescein angiogram
CME	Cystoid macular edema	FXN	Function
CMV	Cytomegalic inclusion virus	Gen	General
CNS	Central nervous system	GI	Gastrointestinal
Congen	Congenital	GL	Glaucoma
Conj	Conjunctiva (l)	GU	Genitourinary
Contralat	Contralateral	HA	Headache
Cort	Cortex, cortical	HDL	High-density lipoproteins
Cr NN	Cranial Nerve (s)	Hemang	Hemangioma
CR	Chorioretinal	Hematol	Hematologic
CRA	Central retinal artery	Hepatomeg	Hepatomegaly
CRS	Cherry red spot	Hered	Hereditary
CSF	Cerebrospinal fluid	Hmg	Hemorrhage
Cu	Copper	Holopros	Holoprosencephaly
Cut	Cutaneous	HSM	Hepatosplenomegaly

Hydroceph	Hydrocephalus, hydrocephaly
Hyper/Hypopig	Hyper/Hypopigmentation
Hypertel	Hypertelorism
Hypogonad	Hypogonadism
Hypothal	Hypothalamic, hypothalamus
Inc	Including
Incsd	Increased
Inf	Infant, infantile
Inf	Infection, infectious
INO	Internuclear opthelmoplegia
Insuf	Insufficiency
IOP	Intraocular pressure
IQ	Mental capacity
JC	Jacob-Creutzfeldt disease
Juv	Juvenile
K-conus	Keratoconus
KF	Kayser-Fleischer
K-Sicca	Keratoconjunctivitis sicca
LE	Lower extemity, extremities
Leuk	Leukemia
Lymph	Lymphoma, lymphatic
Mac	Macula, maculopathy
Maculopap	Maculopapular
Mal	Malformation
Max	Maxilla, maxillary
Met	Metabolic, metabolism
MG	Myesthenia gravis
MI	Myocardial infarction
Microceph	Microcephaly
Microp	Microphthalmos
Mitochon	Mitochondrion, mitrochondrial
MM	Malignant melanoma
MPS	Mucopolysaccharidosis
MR	Mental retardation
MRI	Magnetic resonance imaging
MS	Multiple sclerosis
MtDNA	Mitochondrial DNA
Musc	Muscular
Myop	Myopia, myopic
N	Normal
Neurol	Neurologic
Neurop	Neuropathy
NLP	No light perception, blindness
NP	Normal pressure
Nys	Nystagmus
O neur	Optic neuritis
OA	Optic atrophy
Occas	Occasional
ON	Optic nerve
ONHD	Optic nervehead drusen
Opac	Opacity
O'plegia	Ophthalmoplegia
Orb	Orbit, orbital
P&T	Pain and temperature
Palp	Palpebral
Pap	Papular
Path	Pathology
PDA	Patent ductus arteriosus

PE	Papilledema
PEO	Progressive external ophthalmoplegia
Periorb	Periorbita (l)
Periph	Peripheral
PHPV	Persistent hyperplastic primary vitreous
Pig	Pigment, pigmentary, pigmented
Pit	Pituitary
PM	Psychomotor
PMR	Psychomotor retardation
PND	Prenatal diagnosis possible
Post	Posterior
Predom	Predominant
Prog	Progressive
Prolif	Proliferative, proliferation
Prom	Prominent
PSC	Posterior subcapsular cataract
Pt	Patient
PTC	Pseudotumor cerebri
Pts	Patients
Pul	Pulmonary, pulmonic
Pyr	Pyramidal
R/O	Rule out
RB	Retinoblastoma
RD	Retinal detachment
Regurg	Regurgitation
Ret	Retina, retinal
Retard	Retardation
RG	Red green
RP	Retinitis pigmentosa
S-W	Sturge-Weber syndrome
Skel	Skeletal
Spor	Sporadic
Strab	Strabismus
Subcut	Subcutaneous
Sublux	Subluxated
Supranuc	Supranuclear
Sx	Symptoms
Syn	Syndrome
T	Tumor
Telang	Telangiectasia
Telangiect	Telangiectasis
TH	Thyroid
Tort	Tortuous, tortuosity
VA	Visual acuity
VAP	Visual afferent path (s)
Vasc	Vascular, vascularity
VEP	Visual evoked potential
Verteb	Vertebral
VFD	Visual field defect
Vit	Vitreous
VLCFA	Very-low-chain fatty acids
VRNF	Von Recklinghausen neurofibromatosis
VSD	Ventriculoseptal defect
WBC	White blood cell
XLR	X-linked recessive
XT	Exotropia
YO	Years old

CHAPTER 21

CORRELATIONS WITH HEREDITARY, METABOLIC, NEUROLOGIC, AND SYSTEMIC DISEASE, AND THE PHAKOMATOSES

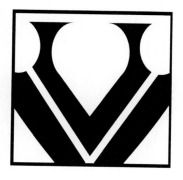

OCULAR-NEURO-CUTANEOUS DISORDERS: THE PHAKOMATOSES

The phakomatoses (Table 21–1) are disorders characterized by tumors and malformations of the eye, neural tissues, and skin. The four classic phakomatoses are (1) neurofibromatosis, (2) tuberous sclerosis (Bourneville's disease), (3) angiomatosis retinae (von Hippel–Lindau disease), and (4) encephalofacial angiomatosis (Sturge-Weber syndrome). I have included in the syndromes discussed below a number of other oculoneurocutaneous syndromes often considered together with the phakomatoses. Most show congenital hamartomas. Some are hereditary and others sporadic. Some are associated with known metabolic abnormalities. Occasionally, patients show stigmata of more than one disease entity.

Neurofibromatosis: Neurofibromatosis is the most frequent phakomatosis. It is autosomal dominant with high penetrance. Recently it has been classified into two primary forms: (1) classic von Recklinghausen's neurofibromatosis (VRNF, NF-1), making up 85% of neurofibromatosis; and (2) bilateral acoustic neurofibromatosis (BANF, NF-2). These appear to be separate genetic entities. The NF-1 gene is on chromosome 17 and the NF-2 gene on chromosome 22. Intermediate forms exist but their genes, if separate, have not been localized.

The most frequent ophthalmic manifestation, present in over 90% of VRNF patients, is the Lisch

nodule (Fig. 21–1), a pigmented iris hamartoma. Von Recklinghausen's neurofibromatosis is associated with optic nerve gliomas but not meningiomas or acoustic neuromas. The most obvious neuro-ocular manifestation usually is a plexiform neuroma involving the lid, filling it with ropey masses. These patients have neurofibromas within the orbit, the superior orbital fissure, and the cavernous sinus. Whether or not an optic glioma is present, the optic canal may be enlarged with or without sphenoid dysplasia, absence of the greater wing of the sphenoid, and pulsating exophthalmos. The sella may be J-shaped with or without an associated chiasmal glioma. Cutaneous neurofibromas and plexiform neuromas of the peripheral nerves occur also; NF-1 seems to be associated with tumors of astrocytes and neurons and NF-2 with tumors of meninges and Schwann cells. Neurofibrosarcoma and other malignant tumors develop with increased frequency, often heralded by pain (frequently referred) and rapid enlargement of a preexisting neurofibroma.

The diagnosis of VRNF (NF-1) is established if two or more of the following criteria are met: (1) six or more café-au-lait spots (> 5 mm in children and 15 mm in adults); (2) two or more neurofibromas or one plexiform neurofibroma; (3) axillary or inguinal freckling; (4) optic glioma; (5) two or more Lisch nodules; (6) a distinctive osseous lesion (eg, sphenoid dysplasia or thinning of long bone cortex; and (7) a first-degree relative with NF-1 (Table 21–2).

TABLE 21–1. OCULAR NEURO-CUTANEOUS DISORDERS[a]

Disorder	Clinical Presentation	
	Ocular	**CNS**
Neurofibromatosis		
VRNF (NF-1)	Iris-Lisch nodules; ON, chiasm glioma; plexiform neuroma of orbit, *Lid*; congenital glaucoma; pulsating exophthalmos; sphenoid bone changes; hypertrophic corneal nerves; MM of iris; choroidal hamartomas	Plexiform neuromas, astrocytomas
BANF (NF-2)	Presenile cats (PSC)	Bilateral acoustic neuromas in teens, meningioma
Tuberous sclerosis	Retinal astrocytic hamartomas (90%)	Calcifications, MR, seizures, subependymal astrocytomas, angiomyolipomas and cardiac rhabdomyosarcomas; skin: Shagreen patches, ungual fibromas, ashleaf spots
Neurocutaneous Angiomatoses		
Von Hippel–Lindau's disease	Retinal hemangioblastomas (50%) bilateral, exudates, RD	Cerebellar hemang. (60%), seizures
Sturge-Weber's syndrome	Choroid hemang. (40%), congenital GL assoc. with lid angioma, homonymous visual field defect	Angioma of meninges, seizures, "train track" calcification, MR, hemiparesis
Klippel-Trenaunay-Weber's syndrome	May have S-W-like ocular and CNS component, conj. telangiect., retinal varicosities, choroidal angioma, GI, buphthalmos	Macrocephaly, angiomas
Wyburn-Mason's syndrome	Retinal/ON AVM	Chiasm, tract AVM, midbrain AVM
Ataxia-telangiectasia (Louis-Bar's syndrome)	Telangiectasia of bulbar conjunctiva (appears age 4–5); nystagmus, supranuc. EM abn, apraxia of saccades	Truncal ataxia, progressive cerebellar degen., choreoathetosis, MR
Hereditary Hemorrhagic Telangiectasia (Osler-Weber-Rendu's syndrome)	Angiomas of lids, conj.	Angiomas of CNS
Fabry's disease	Tort. ret. vessels, telangiectasia of bulbar conj. vessels, cornea verticillata, lens opacities	CVAs Painful polyneuropathy
Familial cerebral cavernous angiomas	No findings	Seizure, stroke, HA, hemangioma
Blue rubber bleb nevus	Hemangioma of conj., iris, ret., and chiasm; blue nevi of lids	Cav. hemang. CNS, cerebellar hemangioblastoma
Epidermal nevus, Sebaceous nevus (linear nevus)	Limbal dermoids; colobomas, ON hypoplasia; linear nevi of lids	Seizures, MR
Multiple endocrine neoplasia (MEN)		
I	VFDs secondary to pit. adenoma	Pituitary adenoma
II	Prominent corneal nerves	—
III	Neuromas of lids, conjunctiva; prominent corneal nerves	—
Ocular spots/myxoma/endocrine excess (Carney's syndrome)	Lid and conj. lentigines, lid myxomas, caruncle lesions	Pituitary adenoma
Cowden's syndrome (multiple hamartoma)	Lid and periorbital tricholemomomas, angioid streaks, retinal glioma	—

[a] Abbreviations used in these tables are defined in the appendix at the end of Chapter 23.

Systemic	Heredity	Other
Cutaneous: axillary freckles, café-au-lait spots; plexiform neuromas, pulmonic stenosis, aortic valve disease, pheochromocytoma, pseudoarthosis	AD	Incsd. nerve growth factor, gene on chromosome 17; 1/4,000
Less prominent cutaneous changes	AD	Separate phenotype, gene on chromosome 22; 1/50,000
Adenoma sebaceum 50% (angiofibromas); dysplasia in most systems, esp. renal	Sporadic, AD	Gene on chromosome 9
Multiple organ hemangioblastomas and cysts, renal cell ca; pheochromocytoma	AD, nearly complete penetrance, highly variable expression	Screen for CNS abn. with MRI, ocular lesions with FA; look for paired feeding vessels of retinal lesion, abn. vasculature on short arm of chromosome 3, genetic linkage analysis may be able to determine which family members are at risk
Port wine stain, esp. V₁; hemihypertrophy; angiomas in many organs	Nonfamilial	Lesions congenital
Extensive dermatomal hemangiomas and hemihypertrophy	Sporadic, (AD)	Spinal variant of S-W?
Facial angioma	Sporadic (AD?)	
Malignancies, esp. leuk/lymph (10%); humoral immune defect; recurrent pulmonary infections; cutaneous telangiectasia; mask-like facies; progeric changes of skin and hair	AR (defect in genetic recombination)	Death in teens; increased alphafeto-protein, CEA onset in infancy; chromosome 11q22–23; abnormal T-cell-receptor antigens
Angiomas of skin, epistaxis, GI/GU bleeds	AD	
Telangiectasia on abd. and LEs, decreased renal function, MIs	XLR	Alpha galactosidase low, PND
	AD, sporadic	Incsd. incidence in Hispanics, study by MRI
Cav. hemang. skin, mucous memb.; GI hmg.; blue nevi	Sporadic, (AD)	
Linear nevi, skin tumors	Sporadic	
Adenomas in multiple organs, lipomas, hypoglycemia; Zollinger-Ellison's syndrome	AD	
Characteristic facies, Thyroid ca., pheochromocytoma, parathyroid adenoma, skeletal anomalies	AD (50%), sporadic (50%)	Chromosome 10; PND?; early thyroidectomy curative for thyroid ca.
Multiple mucosal neuroma, marfanoid habitus, pheochromocytomas, med CA of thyroid, pes cavus		
Myxomas (inc. cardiac), lentigines and blue nevi, endocrine overactivity, endocrine and peripheral nerve tumors	AD	
Facial tricholemomas, keratoses, oral papilloma; ca. of breast and thyroid; multiple other tumors and hamartomas	AD	

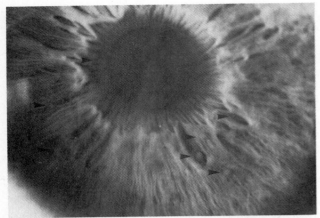

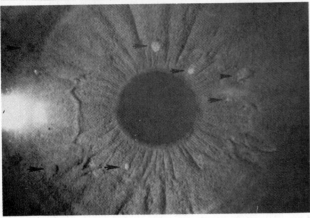

Figure 21–1. Lisch nodules. Photographs of the iris of patients with neurofibromatosis showing varying degrees in number, size, and location of iris nodules. (*From Zehavi C, et al. Lisch Nodules. Clin Genet. 1986;29:51–55, with permission.*)

TABLE 21–2. CRITERIA FOR DIAGNOSIS OF THE NEUROFIBROMATOSES

Neurofibromatosis 1

Neurofibromatosis 1 may be diagnosed when two or more of the following are present:

Six or more café-au-lait macules whose greatest diameter is more than 5 mm in prepubertal patients and more than 15 mm in postpubertal patients

Two or more neurofibromas of any type, or one plexiform neurofibroma

Freckling in the axillary or inguinal region

Optic glioma

Two or more Lisch nodules (iris hamartomas)

A distinctive osseous lesion such as sphenoid dysplasia or thinning of the long-bone cortex, with or without pseudoarthrosis

A parent, sibling, or child with neurofibromatosis 1 according to the above criteria

Neurofibromatosis 2

Neurofibromatosis 2 may be diagnosed when one of the following is present:

Bilateral eighth-nerve masses seen with appropriate imaging techniques (CT or MRI)

A parent, sibling, or child with neurofibromatosis 2 and either unilateral eighth-nerve mass or any two of the following: neurofibroma, meningioma, glioma, schwannoma, or juvenile posterior subcapsular lenticular opacity

From Martuza RL, Eldridge R. Neurofibromatosis 2 (bilateral acoustic neurofibromatosis). N Engl J Med. 1988;318:685.

The bilateral acoustic neuroma BANF (NF-2) form has a more constant expression; all members of the family have the bilateral acoustic tumors. The cutaneous stigmata are more variable and much less frequent. In contrast to patients with the more common unilateral acoustic neuroma, patients with BANF develop symptoms earlier, in their teens. Cataracts (posterior subcapsular) also seem to be a manifestation of this variant of neurofibromatosis. Their appearance in the teens and twenties should suggest this diagnosis. Lisch nodules are rare.

The diagnosis of NF-2 is established in the presence of bilateral acoustic neuromas or a first-degree relative with NF-2 and either a unilateral acoustic neuroma or two of the following: neurofibroma, meningioma, glioma, Schwannoma, or juvenile posterior subcapsular cataract (Table 21–2). The latter may be the first detectable clinical finding in patients at risk for NF-2.

Magnetic resonance imaging (MRI) is extremely valuable in the evaluation and follow-up of these patients with their progressive disease and its predilection for multiple tumors of malignant predisposition (Tables 21–3, 21–4). In fact, MRI studies of asymptomatic patients with NF-1 show gliomatous involvement of the visual afferent pathways in up to 20% of affected individuals, many of whom have normal acuity and fields. Presumed hamartomas are present in the brain of a majority of NF-1 patients who undergo MRI; usually, these are not symptomatic. In NF-2, MRI enhanced with Gadolinium best detects and displays the extent of acoustic tumor penetration.

Tuberous sclerosis. Tuberous sclerosis (TS) also has characteristic cutaneous manifestations. The ash leaf spot is nearly pathognomonic (if more than 3 are present the diagnosis *is* certain). Older patients develop adenoma sebaceum (angiofibromas) and shagreen patches. Tuberous sclerosis patients sometimes have seizures and are retarded as a result of cortical tubers or subependymal glial nodules. Over time, their mental function often declines; death may occur at an early age. Tuberous sclerosis has been assigned to the long arm of chromosome 9.

The primary ocular findings are several forms of retinal astrocytic hamartoma. The most common is a round, gelatinous, light gray, or yellow lesion that is

TABLE 21–3. CRANIAL MRI ABNORMALITIES IN NF-1

Type of Lesion	No. of Patients (n = 53)
Optic glioma	19
"Hamartomas"	32
With optic glioma	17
Without optic glioma (age <20 yr, n = 24)	15
Without optic glioma (age >21 yr, n = 10)	0
Other astrocytomas	8
Cranial nerve tumors	2
Internal auditory canal ectasia	2
Sphenoid dysplasia	2
Extra cranial neurofibromas (plexiform)	18
Few (1–4 lesions)	7
Several (5–9 lesions)	7
Many ≥10 lesions)	4
Aqueductal stenosis	7
Buphthalmos	2

From Aoki S, Bakovich AJ, et al. Neurofibromatosis types 1 and 2: Cranial MR findings. Radiology. 1989;172:528.

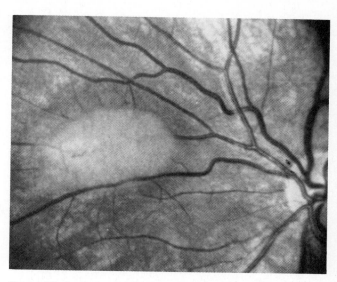

Figure 21–2. Uncalcified retinal hamartoma of tuberous sclerosis. (*From Gomez MR. Tuberous sclerosis. In: Gomez MR, ed. Neurocutaneous Diseases: A Practical Approach. Boston: Butterworths, 1987;30–52, with permission.*)

slightly elevated and usually seen in the posterior pole (Fig. 21–2). Characteristic tapioca-like or mulberry-like tumors may occur at the disc margin or overlying the disc. They grow slowly. Unlike optic nerve head drusen, which small tumors may mimic, they obscure the retinal vessels. Depigmented lesions and retinal pigment epithelial (RPE) hypertrophy have also been described. These lesions rarely produce any effect on vision unless the tumors in the region of the optic disc are large enough to cause a visual field defect.

Hamartomas are also found in the kidneys and lungs; about half of all cardiac rhabdomyosarcomas occurs in patients with tuberous sclerosis. In the central nervous system, subependymal giant-cell astrocytomas of the ventricles are typical. Enamel pits of the teeth are present in 71%.

TABLE 21–4. CRANIAL MRI ABNORMALITIES IN NF-2

Type of Lesion	No. of Patients
Acoustic schwannomas	11
Other cranial nerve tumors (V–XII)	8
Single	3
Multiple	5
Meningiomas	6
Single	2
Multiple	4

From Aoki S, Bakovich AJ, et al. Neurofibromatosis types 1 and 2: Cranial MR findings. Radiology. 1989;172:530.

Neurocutaneous Angiomatoses

Two of the other four major phakomatoses, von Hippel–Lindau disease and Sturge-Weber syndrome, belong to the group of cerebro-neuro-cutaneous angiomatoses, although not all organ systems are involved in each syndrome (eg, von Hippel–Lindau disease does not affect the skin).

Angiomatosis Retinae (Von Hippel–Lindau Disease). This disease is autosomal dominant with nearly complete penetrance and variable expression; its characteristic lesion is the capillary hemangioma. Retinal angiomas are present in more than 50% of the patients and cerebellar hemangiomas in 60%; conversely, 25% of central nervous system (CNS) hemangioblastomas occurs in patients with von Hippel–Lindau disease. Other hemangioblastomas occur in the medulla and spinal cord. Also associated are hypernephromas and pheochromocytomas (Table 21–5). Diagnosis is established in the presence of CNS and retinal hemangioblastomas, or a retinal or CNS tumor with a family history, a hemangioblastoma or cyst in another organ, or a renal cancer.

The retinal hemangioblastomas can be asymptomatic, but may also cause massive exudative changes. Most of the lesions are elevated and peripheral in location, but when peripapillary tend to be flat. Small lesions may be detectable only by fluorescein angiography or angioscopy.

Large hemangioblastomas in the CNS may be associated with substantial erythropoetic activity.

In this disease, the tumors continue to form during the lifetime of the patient, and continued surveil-

TABLE 21–5. MOST COMMON CLINICAL MANIFESTATIONS OF VON HIPPEL–LINDAU DISEASE IN 38 AFFECTED MEMBERS OF A FAMILY IN NEWFOUNDLAND

	Affected (No. and %)		Age at Diagnosis (Range and Median)
Lesion	*Definitely*	*Definitely and Probably*	
Retinal angioma	19(50%)	23(60%)	4–42(19)
Pheochromocytoma	18(47%)	20(53%)	11–58(22)
Hemangioblastoma			
Cerebellar	6(16%)	7(18%)	22–58(—)
Spinal cord	2 (5%)	2 (5%)	39,58(—)
Hypernephroma	1 (3%)	1 (3%)	58(—)

From Green JS, et al. Can Med Assoc J. 1986;134:133–146.

lance by contrast MRI and fluorescein angiography is advisable. Early recognition of the retinal lesions (which may be the earliest sign of the disease) allows them to be treated before they cause symptoms. Thus, these patients should have careful indirect ophthalmoscopy with fluorescein angioscopy annually.

Encephalofacial angiomatosis (Sturge-Weber Syndrome). Unlike the other phakomatoses, the Sturge-Weber syndrome is nonfamilial. The characteristic lesion is the port wine "nevus," which most frequently involves the first and/or second trigeminal dermatomes. There is often an associated ipsilateral leptomeningeal venous abnormality, cortical atrophy, and calcification (the "train track sign"), best seen with computed tomography (CT) scanning. The parieto-occipital changes may be associated with a contralateral hemianopic defect, convulsions, and mental retardation.

Ocular findings include a congenital glaucoma particularly difficult to manage and choroidal hemangiomas, which impart a uniform red "tomato catsup" appearance to the fundus.

Ataxia telangiectasia (Louis-Bar's Syndrome). This autosomal recessive disorder presents in early childhood as a progressive cerebellar ataxia that usually keeps the infant from walking. Telangiectasias of the interpalpebral bulbar conjunctiva also develop during early childhood. They also are prominent over the ears, nose, cheeks, exposed parts of the neck, and extensor surfaces of the forearm. Progressive immunologic deterioration usually occurs in the second decade, leading to death from recurrent infection or neoplasia. Thus, this is one of the clastogenic syndromes (syndromes associated with chromosomal breakage and an increased likelihood of malignancy (Table 21–6).

The Klippel-Trenaunay-Weber's Syndrome. Most cases of this congenital neurocutaneous anomaly are sporadic in occurrence, although some are autosomal dominant. Extensive skin hemangiomas appear in a dermatomal pattern, associated with hemangiomas of the spinal cord and, frequently, tissue hypertrophy in the same dermatomal distribution. It is suggested that this is a spinal variant of the Sturge-Weber syndrome.

Hereditary hemorrhagic telangiectasia (Osler-Weber-Rendu's Syndrome). This syndrome is characterized by angiomas of the skin, mucous membranes, and nervous system. It is autosomal dominant and manifests in childhood with multiple small angiomas. These enlarge and are the cause of recurrent hemorrhages: epistaxis, gastrointestinal (GI), or genito-urinary (GU) hemorrhage. Scattered angiomas occur throughout the CNS and may hemorrhage also.

Wyburn-Mason's Syndrome. This uncommon disorder is characterized by an arteriovenous malformation (AVM) of the midbrain, associated frequently with a unilateral retinal AVM. The retinal AVM may or may not be continuous with the central nervous system AVM. Enlarged vascular channels follow along the optic nerve and through an enlarged optic canal. However, localized AVMs may also occur independent of one another. Mental retardation occurs in this syndrome as well. No hereditary basis has been recognized. The AVMs do not hemorrhage and usually do not cause significant shunting; thus, they

TABLE 21–6. CLASTOGENIC SYNDROMES[a]

Ataxia telangiectasia (Louis-Bar's syndrome)[b]
Bloom's syndrome
Chédiak-Higashi syndrome
Cockayne's syndrome
Fanconi's anemia
Gardner's syndrome
Huntington chorea
Partial trisomy 13
Progeria
Retinoblastoma
Werner's syndrome
Xeroderma pigmentosa[b]

[a] Increased chromosomal breakage, increased propensity for malignancy, and increased sensitivity to ionizing radiation.
[b] Defective repair of DNA.

are symptomatic only by virtue of interfering with neural function. Very large lesions, especially of the retina, can exist despite minimal neural or visual dysfunction.

Fabry's Disease. Fabry's disease has a known biochemical aberration as a basis for the cutaneous and CNS manifestations. It is a lysosomal storage disease with a deficit in alpha galactosidase, leading to alterations in blood vessels that cause multiple small, flat to slightly raised angiokeratomas, predominantly over the lower body and on the bulbar conjunctiva. There is an associated episodic painful polyneuropathy; cerebral thrombo-embolism is not uncommon. This disease is X-linked recessive and thus is seen predominantly in males. When looked for, cornea verticillata, a whorl-like dystrophy of the cornea, is present in 80 to 90% of patients more than 10 years old (as well as female carriers); lens opacities and retinal vessel tortuosity are slightly less frequent.

ABNORMALITIES OF LIPID METABOLISM

This diffuse group of disorders has in common disruption of lipid and lipoprotein metabolism. Lipids form important portions of cell membranes and myelin, the insulating substance of the nervous system, and a major component of the photoreceptors. It is not surprising, therefore, that ocular and neurologic disorders are major portions of these syndromes (Table 21–7).

Hyperlipoproteinemias. The ocular findings depend on which of the lipoproteins are elevated. Those with high triglyceride levels may show lipemia retinalis in which the fat within the bloodstream discolors the retina to a salmon color and the vessels turn milky. Corneal arcus is found if cholesterol is elevated. Xanthelasma and cutaneous and tendinous xanthomas are also present (Fig. 21–3).

Other Disturbances of Lipid and Lipoprotein Metabolism. Disorders of lipid and lipoprotein metabolism associated with neuro-ophthalmic signs and symptoms include lipoprotein deficiency states and diseases that accumulate abnormal fatty acids in the blood.

The lipoprotein deficiency states consist of **abetalipoproteinemia (Bassen-Kornsweig syndrome),** which resembles Freidrich's ataxia in its neuromuscular components: ataxia, spinal cerebellar degeneration, neuropathy, and mental retardation. The ocular findings—similar to those in some other heredofamilial degenerations—consist of retinitis pigmentosa, night blindness, a diminished ERG, and progressive external ophthalmoplegia. The systemic components are characterized by malabsorption, steatorrhea, acanthosis of the red blood cells, and cardiac abnormalities. There is an absence of apolipoprotein B, very-low-density lipoproteins, and low-density lipoproteins in the serum. Heredity is autosomal recessive.

Diagnosis is made by recognition of the typical findings, hopefully in early infancy. Restriction of triglyceride intake is important in obviating the GI manifestations. There is some evidence that high doses of vitamin A and vitamin E forestall the development and/or progression of the ocular and neuromuscular degenerations.

Homozygous familial hypobetalipoproteinemia is even rarer than Bassen-Kornsweig syndrome, to which it is very similar except for milder neuromuscular impairment.

Tangier disease is highlighted clinically by the presence of hyperplastic bright orange tonsils. This is due to storage of cholesterol esters, which also causes corneal deposits and opacity, occasional ptosis, extraocular muscle palsy, and a peripheral neuropathy. There is a deficiency of high-density lipoproteins in the serum. This syndrome is inherited in an autosomal recessive manner.

Familial lecithin/cholesterol acyltransferase (LCAT) deficiency is caused by failure of LCAT to esterify cholesterol in the plasma. Clinically, there are corneal deposits, arcus presenilis, anemia, and renal disease that may progress to life-threatening renal failure. It is a rare autosomal recessive disorder that has been localized to chromosome 16.

Cerebrotendinosis xanthomatosis (CTX) is another rare autosomal recessive disorder of sterol metabolism resulting in massive deposition of lipids. The earliest findings are neurologic with spasticity and ataxia, followed by the development of juvenile cataracts and tendon xanthomas. Enlargement of the xanthomas and neurologic deterioration are progressive, with death resulting from progressive neurologic deterioration and pseudobulbar paralysis between the fourth and sixth decades.

Refsum's disease is yet another autosomal recessive disorder of lipid metabolism associated with phytanic acid accumulation in blood and tissues. The cardinal manifestations are retinal pigmentary degeneration, peripheral neuropathy, cerebellar ataxia, and elevated CSF protein. Treatment with a diet minimizing phytanic acid significantly improves most abnormalities, excepting the cranial nerve dysfunction. Combination of diet with plasmapheresis achieves a faster result. Treatment must be instituted early and continued for life.

LYSOSOMAL ENZYME DISORDERS

This group of maladies is characterized by deficiency of specific lysosomal enzymes, which results in ab-

TABLE 21–7. DEFECTS IN LIPID METABOLISM

	Clinical Presentation		
Defect	*Ocular*	*CNS*	*Systemic*
Hyperlipoproteinemias			
Type I	Lipemia retinalis, lid xanthomas	—	Eruptive xanthomas, abdominal pain, pancreatitis, HSM
Type II	Palpebral xanthelasma, corneal arcus, scleral lipid deposits	—	Tendinous and tuberous xanthomas, polyarthritis, coronary art. disease
Type III	Xanthelasma, corneal arcus, corneal dystrophy	—	Accelerated atherosclerosis, tuberous xanthomas, DM
Type IV	Lipemia retinalis, xanthelasma, corneal arcus	—	Eruptive xanthoma, angina pectoris (40%), HSM (rare), DM, gout
Type V	Xanthelasma, lipemia retinitis, retinal vasc. occlusion	—	Abdominal pain, pancreatitis, hyperuricemia, eruptive xanthoma, DM
Cerebrotendinosis xanthomatosis (cholestanol storage disease)	Cataract	Dementia, cerebellar ataxia, pseudobulbar palsy	Achille's tendon xanthoma, premature atherosclerosis
Lipoprotein Transport Defects			
Abetalipoproteinemia (Bassen-Kornzweig syndrome)	Prog. external o'plegia, ret. pig. degen., night blindness, angioid streaks	Ataxia, spinocerebellar degen., PMR, peripheral neuropathy	Malabsorption (steatorrhea), low serum lipids, acanthocytosis of RBCs, cardiac abn.
Homozygous familial hypobetalipoproteinemia	(Clinically indistinguishable from Bassen-Kornzweig syndrome except for milder neuromuscular impairment)		
Refsum's disease	Ret. pig. degen./OA, night blindness, cat. (50%), nystagmus, pupil chngs.	Cerebellar ataxia, hypertrophic peripheral neuropathy, deafness, hypotonia, high CSF protein without cells	Ichthyosis (50%), bone dysplasia, ECG changes
Tangier disease	Corneal deposits, ptosis, EOM palsy	Periph. neuropathy	Hyperplastic orange tonsils, maculo pap. rash, HSM, anemia, lymphadenopathy
Cerebrotendinous xanthomatosis (cholestanosis)	Juvenile cat., xanthelasma	Prog. dementia, ataxia, spasticity, CNS demyelination	Tendon xanthomas, atherosclerosis, pulmonary insuff.
Peroxisomal Disorders			
XLR adrenoleukodystrophy	OA, cort. NLP, nystagmus	Seizures, demyelin., progressive MR, spasticity, ataxia, deafness	Adrenal insuff., skin pigmentation
Adrenoleukomyeloneuropathy		Spastic paraperesis, polyneurop.	Adrenal dsfxn., hypogonad.
Neonatal adrenoleukodystrophy (Zellweger's syn., hyperpipecolic acidemia)	OA, ret. pig. degen., cataract, GI. nystagmus, speckled iris, cloudy cornea, ret. arteriolar narrowing	Demyelin. hypotonia, seizures	Typical facies, hepatomeg., renal cysts calcif. deposits in patella, adrenal atrophy
Infantile Refsum's disease	Ret. pig. degen.	MR, deafness, ataxia, anosmia	Hepatomegaly, dysmorphic features
Acyl-CoA-oxidase deficiency	Ret. pig. degen.	Hypotonia, neonatal seizures, PMR	Liver dsfxn.
LCAT deficiency	Corneal deposits, arcus in heterozygote	—	Renal disease, anemia

	Clinical Presentation		
Key Diagnostic Finding	**Heredity**	**Treatment**	**Other/Locus**
Hyperlipoproteinemias			
Hyperchylomicronemia, low lipoprotein lipase	Rarely AR	Low-fat diet	Childhood onset
Hypercholesterolemia	AD	Low-fat diet, cholestipol nicotinic acid, probucol	—
Increased low-density lipoproteins	AD?	Low-fat diet, weight loss, clofibrate	—
Very-low-density lipoproteinemia	AD, rarely	Low-fat diet, weight loss, clofibrate	—
Increased chylomicrons and very-low-density lipoproteins	AR?	Low-fat diet, low-carbohydrate diet Clofibrate?	Adult onset
Lipoprotein Transport Defects			
Absent betalipoproteins 0 VLD lipoproteins 0 LDL lipoproteins	AR	Vits. A,E, dietary restriction	PEO, onset 5–10 yr; rare, early death; dcsd. ERG
	AD	—	Normal ERG
High serum phytanic acid, dcsd. phytanic acid alpha hydroxylase	AR	Low phytanic acid diet, plasmapheresis	Dcsd. ERG, PND partially effective, peroxisomal defect?
Dcsd. HDL (anaphalipoproteinemia)	AR	—	
	AR?	Chenodioxycholic acid	
Peroxisomal Disorders			
Elevated VLCFAs MRI changes prior to CNS sxl	XLR	Erucic acid diet	Disorder of long-chain fatty acids
Elevated VLCFAs (test all males with "isolated" Addison's)	XLR	Oleic acid diet	
Cholestanol	AR	—	Prenatal diag., flat ERG
			Milder than ALD
	XLR	—	Extinguished ERG
Lecithin/cholesterol acyltransferase deficiency	AR		Chromosome 16, test pts. with presenile arcus

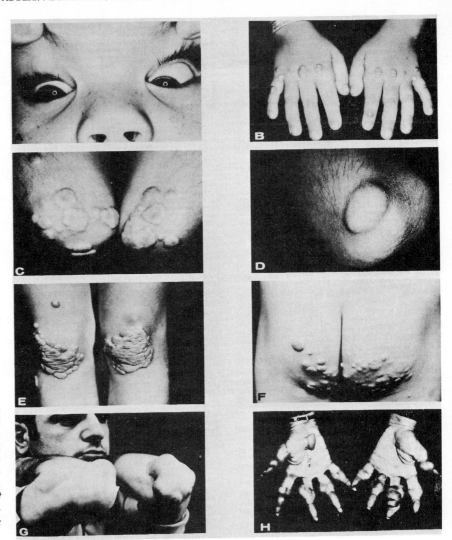

Figure 21–3. Xanthomas. Forms of xanthomas and other lipid deposits frequently seen in FH homozygotes. **A.** Arcucs cornea. **B,C,E,** and **F.** Cutaneous planar xanthomas, usually having a bright orange hue. **C.** and **D.** Tuberous xanthomas on the elbows. **H.** Tendon and tuberous xanthomas. *(From Goldstein JL, Brown MS. Familial hypercholesterolemia. In: Scriver C, et al., eds. The Metabolic Basis of Inherited Disease. 6th ed. New York: McGraw-Hill, 1989;1: 1215–1250, with permission.)*

normal storage of products within the eye, central nervous system, and viscera. A genetic mutation alters enzyme activity critical to cell metabolism. The cells enlarge, degenerate, disappear, and are replaced by gliosis. The ocular tissues most often affected are the retina, conjunctiva, cornea, lens, choroid, and extraocular muscle. One in every 5000 births results in a child with a storage disease.

The nosology of these disorders is extremely confusing. Because of the CNS and ocular manifestations many of them were previously classified as "amaurotic idiocies." In addition, attempts to classify these disorders by enzyme deficiency find many included in several categories. One diagnostic schema is given here (Fig. 21–4).

In general, when the onset of these disorders is in infancy or early childhood, the ocular and CNS involvement is severe. When the onset is later, the involvement is progressively less severe. All lysoso-

mal storage diseases are progressive; they all involve multiple tissues and organs. Most can be diagnosed by conjunctival biopsy (as can cystinosis and type-II glycogenolysis); many if not most can be ameliorated, if not cured, by bone marrow transplantation. However, as bone marrow transplantation may not reverse damage already done, prenatal diagnosis and early diagnosis assume critical roles for managing these patients.

Sphingolipidoses. The ocular changes of the sphingolipidoses (Table 21–8) include cherry-red spots or gray maculas, retinal pigmentary degeneration, and optic atrophy. Demyelination is a common neurologic finding. Visceromegaly is nearly universal. Nearly all are fatal in childhood and inherited in autosomal recessive fashion.

Mucopolysaccharidoses. Corneal opacification, optic atrophy, and retinal pigmentary degeneration are characteristic of these storage syndromes. Cor-

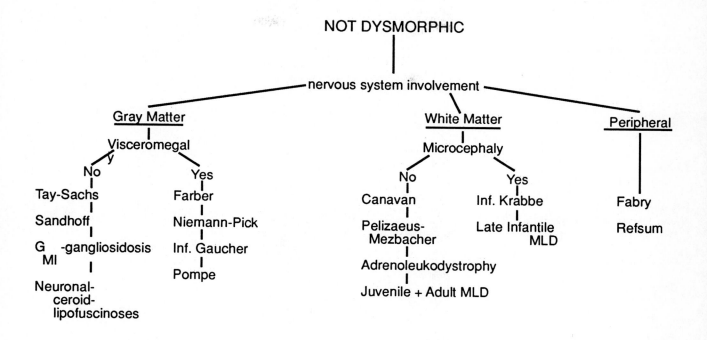

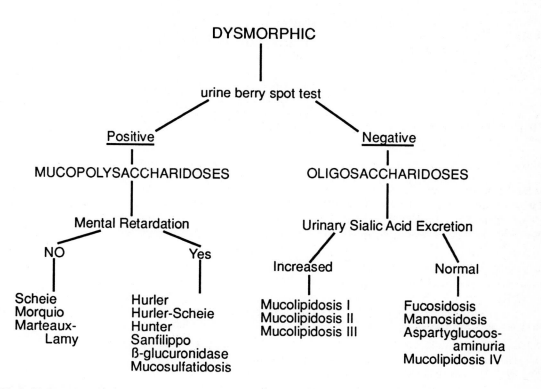

Figure 21-4. Diagnostic schema used by the Lysosomal Lab from the Children's Hospital of Boston.

TABLE 21–8. SPHINGOLIPIDOSES

Name	Clinical Presentation		
	Ocular	*CNS*	*Systemic*
Fabry disease	Cornea vertillata (pigmented whorls), conjunctival and retinal telangiectasia, cataract (PSC), spokes	Paraesthesias, painful crises; CVA	Angiokeratomas, heart disease, renal failure
Farber disease (lipogranulomatosis)	With or without CRS, gray mac., ret. pig. degen., conj. xanthomas		Xanthomas, inflammatory arthropathy, hoarseness
Ganglosidoses[a]			
GM₁-1 infantile (Landing's syndrome)	CRS/OA, conj. and ret. vasc. changes, microaneurysms, tortuosity	Rigidity, seizures, deafness, hypotonia, ataxia	Hurler-like macroglossia, HSM
GM₂-2 juvenile (Derry)	Strabismus		
GM₂-1 (Tay-Sachs disease)	CRS, OA, supranuc. EM abn. (vertical 1st), blindness early	Dementia, ataxia, spasticity, hyperacusis, deafness, hypotonia, macrocephaly, seizures	Doll-like facies
GM₂-2 (Sandhoff disease)	CRS, OA, blindness early	MR, hypotonia, hyperacusis, macrocephaly, seizures	Visceromegaly, doll-like facies
GM₂-3 (juvenile gangliosidosis)	RP, OA, CRS (?), late blindness	Spasticity, ataxia, dysarthria, hyperacousis, seizures, hypotonia	
Gaucher's disease (composite of types)	White spots in fundus, brown pingueculae, strabismus, gray mac.; EM disorder: saccadic defect (horiz. more often than vert.)	Hypertonia, deafness	Anemia, HSM, lytic bone lesions
Krabbe's disease (globoid cell leukodystrophy)	OA, strab./nystagmus, cortical NLP	PM degen., deafness, irritability, long-tract signs, seizures	Rare
Lactosyl ceramidosis	Gray mac., OA	Incsd. CSF pressure	—
Sulfatidelipidoses			
Metachromatic leukodystrophy	CRS, OA, gray mac.	Demyelination, dementia	—
Mucosulfatidosis (multiple sulfatase deficiency)	CRS, OA, lens opacity, corneal clouding, yellowish ret., ret. degen.	Microcephaly, ataxia, PMR	MPS features, ichthyosis, HSM, dyshasia, short stature
Niemann-Pick disease (composite of types)	CRS, gray mac., OA, ret. pig. degen., corneal clouding, cataract, gaze palsies (vertical 1st)	MR, PMR, seizures	Anemia, HSM, pulmonary infiltrates
Cherry red spot myoclonus	CRS, dcsd. VA	Myoclonus	

CRS = cherry red spot, OA = optic atrophy, "RP" = retinal pigmentary degeneration.
Terminology for ganglioside storage disease: G = ganglioside; M,D,T = mono, di, trisialic acid; 1,2,3 = # of hexosides, e.g. tetrahex = 1, tri = 2, di = 3l.

		Clinical Presentation		
Key Diagnostic Finding	Heredity	Treatment	Other/Locus	
Alphagalactosidase A deficiency	XLR	Dilantin, Tegretol for pain, direct enzyme replacement (?) BMT?	PND	
Dcsd. acid ceramidase	AR	— BMT?	Death in childhood, PND	
Dcsd. galactosidase	AR	— BMT?	Death by 2 yr, PND	
	AR	— BMT?	PND	
Dcsd. hexosaminadase A	AR	— BMT?	Detectable by serum assay, PND, chromosome 15, onset 3–6 mo, death 2–5 yr	
Hexosaminadase A,B dcsd.	AR	— BMT?	Detected by serum assay, chromosome 5, onset 3–6 mo, death 2–5 yr, PND	
Hexosaminadase A,B dcsd.	AR	— BMT?	Onset 2–6 yr, death 5–15 yr, PND	
Gaucher cells, dcsd. glucocerebrosidase	AR	Enzyme replacement? BMT?	Most common lysosomal disease, PND	
Dcsd. betagalactosidase, brain bx.	AR	— BMT?	PND, onset 3–6 mo, death by 3 yr	
Dcsd. lactosyl ceramidase	AR	— BMT?	PND	
Dcsd. arylsulfatase	AR	— BMT?	PND, chromosome 22, onset 2 yr, death in 1st decade	
Dcsd. arylsulfatase	AR	— BMT?	PND, chromosome 22	
Dcsd. sphingomyelinase, foam cells in marrow	AR	— BMT?	PND	
Dcsd. alphaneuraminadase (several types)		BMT?	—	

TABLE 21–9. MUCOPOLYSACCHARIDOSES

Name	Clinical Presentation		
	Ocular	*CNS*	*Systemic*
Type I			
Hurler's syndrome	Corneal opac.,[a] ret. pig. degen., photophobia, PE, OA	MR, deafness	Gargoyle facies/HSM, dystosis, dwarfism, coronary art. dis., cardiac valve dis.
Scheie's syndrome	Corneal opac.,[a] ret. pig. degen., OA, GI	N IQ, deafness	Similar to I-H but milder; aortic valve dis., normal stature, hypertrichosis
Type II—Hunter's syndrome	Ret. pig. degen., PE, OA	MR, deafness, hydroceph.	Dystosis, coronary art. dis., cardiac valve dis., nodular skin lesion
Type III—Sanfilippo's syndrome	Ret. pig. degen., OA sometimes	MR,[a] deafness	Behavioral disturbances, dysostosis, HSM
Type IV—Morquio's syndrome	Corneal clouding, OA	Deafness	Skeletal dysplasia,[a]—aortic regurgitation
Type VI—Maroteaux-Lamy syndrome	Corneal clouding,[a] OA	Deafness	Dysostosis,[a] valvular heart dis.
Type VII—Sly's syndrome	Corneal clouding	Deafness	HSM
Winchester's syndrome	Peripheral corneal opacity and furrow	Deafness	—

[a] Ret. pig. degen. manifested only by types that store heparan sulfate (Types I, II, III).

neal changes are prominent in Hurler's, Morquio's, Scheie's, and Maroteaux-Lamy syndromes. Retinal pigmentary degeneration is prominent in Hunter's syndrome and Sanfilippo's syndrome, which do not have corneal clouding (Table 21–9).

The **mucolipidoses** result from a combined disorder of acid mucopolysaccharide and glycosidase metabolism, and thus combine features of the sphingolipidoses and the mucopolysaccharidoses (Table 21–10).

Neuronal Ceroid Lipofuscinoses (Lipopigment Storage Disorders)

This group of diseases—with primarily neurologic and ophthalmologic manifestations, like the sphingolipidoses—was previously termed "amaurotic idiocies." Common to the neuronal ceroid lipofuscinoses is progressive mental and motor neurologic deterioration; the types are distinguished

| | Clinical Presentation | | |
Key Diagnostic Finding	Heredity	Treatment	Other
Alpha-L-iduronidase deficit	AR	BMT?	Death by 10, most common MPS, PND, decreased ERG
Alpha-L-iduronidase deficit	AR	BMT?, corneal transplant	Normal life span (?), decreased ERG, PND?
—	XLR	BMT?	Death by 15, PND, decreased ERG
Decreased heparan sulfatase	AR	BMT?	PND, decreased ERG
—	AR	BMT?	PND?
WBC inclusions	AR	BMT?	Death in 20s, PND, chromosome 5
—	AR	BMT?	Morquio-like, death in 20s, PND, chromosome 7
—	AR	BMT?	PND?

problems are retinal degeneration and optic atrophy mainly by the age of onset. The associated ocular often ending in blindness. Frequently, an abnormal ERG detects retinal degeneration before the diagnosis is otherwise obvious (Table 21–11). Combined, these are the second most common neurodegenerative diseases of childhood. All are autosomal recessive and may be diagnosed by conjunctival biopsy and white blood cell analysis.

OTHER DISORDERS

Disorders of amino acid, metal, and carbohydrate metabolism, which cause a variety of abnormalities, are portrayed in the accompanying tables, as are cytogenic disorders and disorders associated with premature aging and with vitamin deficiency or excess (Tables 21–12 to 21–14, Fig. 21–5, and Tables 21–15 to 21–22). The following sections list disorders by organ system (Chapter 22) and by their significant ocular manifestations (Chapter 22).

TABLE 21–10. MUCOLIPIDOSES

Name	Clinical Presentation				Heredity	Treatment	Other
	Ocular	CNS	Systemic	Key Diagnostic Finding			
Mucolipidosis I	Corneal clouding, CRS	Myoclonus	—	—	AR	BMT?	PND
Mucolipidosis II (I cell disease)	Corneal clouding, gray macula	MR	Hurler's-like gingival hyperplasia	—	AR	— BMT?	PND
Mucolipidosis III (pseudo-Hurler's syndrome)	Some corneal opacity, no retinal changes		Dysostosis, painful joints, aortic regurg.	Dcsd. phosphotransferase activity	AR	— BMT?	PND
Mucolipidosis IV (Goldberg's syndrome)	Corneal clouding, CRS, OA, strab., retinal dystrophy, attenuated ret. vessels	PMR	Hypotonia	Neuramidase defic.		— BMT?	PND
OLIGOSACCHARIDOSES							
Fucosidosis (composite of types)	Tortuous conj. and ret. vessels, cataract, strab., ret. pig. degen., corneal opacities, spider nevi of lid	PMR, dcsd. hearing	Angiokeratomas (like in Fabry's disease), dysostosis, pulmonary infections, coarse facies	Dcsd. alpha fucosidase	AR	— BMT?	Chromosome 1, PND
Mannosidosis (composite of 2 types)	Cataract-spokes in post. cortex, corneal opacities	MR, deafness	Dysostosis, HSM	Dcsd. alpha mannosidase	AR	— BMT?	Chromosome 19, PND
Aspartyl glycososaminuria	Lens opacities	MR		Aspartyl glycosaminidase		— BMT?	PND?
Sialidosis (composite of 2 types)	CRS	MR, myoclonus N IQ	Dysostosis	Dcsd. neuraminosidase	AR	— BMT?	PND?

TABLE 21–11. NEURONAL CEROID LIPOFUSCINOSES (LIPOPIGMENT STORAGE DISORDERS)[a]

| Name | Clinical Presentation | | | Key Diagnostic Finding | Heredity | Treatment | Other |
	Ocular	CNS	Systemic				
Hagberg-Haltia-Santavuori disease (onset 8–18 mo)	RP-hypopig., ret. degen., ret-narrowed arterioles, visual changes early and prom., brown mac., OA	PRM/seizures, ataxia, MR, hypotonia myoclonus	—	a	AR	— BMT?	Death at 5–7 yr, dcsd. ERG
Jansky-Bielschowsky disease (onset 2–5 yr)	Ret. pig. degen, OA, mac. pig. changes +/− bulls eye, narrow ret. art.	PMR/myoclonic, seizures, ataxia, CNS changes	—	a	AR	— BMT?	All 5 forms combined are the 2nd most frequent
Spielmeyer-Vogt-Batten disease (onset 5–10 yr)	Ret. pig. degen., OA, granular mac. changes, bull's eye mac.?, ret.-narrowed art., OA	Dementia/seizures rigidity	a	a	AR	BMT?	Neuro-degen. disease of childhood
Kufs' disease (late onset 2 forms)	Mac. pigment changes, no RP, normal VA	Dementia/seizures, ataxia, myoclonus, facial dyskinesias	—	a	AD/AR	— BMT?	OA on path.
Cherry red spot myoclonus	CRS	Myoclonus	—	a		— BMT?	—

Visual dysfunction worse with earlier onset.
[a] all can be diagnosed by conjunctival biopsy and leucocyte analysis. There are autofluorescent lipopigments in WBCs, neurons, and other tissues.
[b] (Some previously called Batten Mayou).

TABLE 21-12. ABNORMALITIES OF CARBOHYDRATE METABOLISM

Name	Clinical Presentation			Key Diagnostic Findings	Heredity	Treatment	Other
	Ocular	CNS	Systemic				
Diabetes mellitus	Retinopathy, cataract, vit. hmg., RD	Neuropathy	Hyperglycemia, angiopathy	Hyperglycemia	AR?	Insulin, oral hypoglycemics, diet	(see Table 21–10)
G-6-phosphatase deficiency (von Gierke's disease)	Yellow paramacular lesions	Seizures	Hepatomegaly, short stature, renal enlargement, xanthomas, bleeding, hyperglycemia	—			—
Lactic acidemia	OA, o'plegia, RP	MR, ataxia, hypotonia, seizures, Leigh's syndrome, cortical blindness	Hypoglycemia	—	Mitochondrial?	—	PND
Galactosemia (G-1-PUT [GALT] deficiency)	Cataract	MR	Failure to thrive, HSM, renal abn.	—	AR	Diet	40% dies in septicemia if not diagnosed
Galactokinase deficiency (GALK)	Juv. cataract	MR (rare)	No hepatomegaly				—

362

TABLE 21–13. CLASSIFICATION OF DIABETES

A. Primary
   1. Insulin-dependent diabetes mellitus (IDDM, type 1)
   2. Noninsulin-dependent diabetes mellitus (NIDDM, type 2)
      a. Nonobese NIDDM
      b. Obese NIDDM
B. Secondary
   1. Pancreatic disease
   2. Hormonal abnormalities
   3. Drug- or chemical-induced
   4. Insulin receptor abnormalities
   5. Genetic syndromes
   6. Other

From Foster DW. Diabetes mellitus. In: Scriver C, et al, eds. The Metabolic Basis of Inherited Disease. *6th ed. New York: McGraw-Hill, 1989;1:376.*

TABLE 21–14. ABNORMALITIES OF AMINO ACID METABOLISM

Name	Clinical Presentation		
	Ocular	*CNS*	*Systemic*
Cystine			
Cystinosis (composite of all types)	Crystals in cornea, conjunctiva; photophobia; patchy retinal depigmentation	Cerebral atrophy	Renal rickets and failure, dwarfism, hypothyroid
Homocystinuria (composite of forms)	Crystals in cornea, conj.; ectopia lentis; cataract; gl.; myopia; RD; OA; CRA occlusion; (RP in methylmalonic homocystinuria)	MR, dev. delay, seizures	Marfanoid habitus, thromboembolism, osteoporosis, hypopigmentation, pulmonary and aortic dilation, accelerated atherosclorosis
Sulfite oxidase deficiency	Ectopia lentis, OA, spherophakia, strab.	MR, seizures, cerebral atrophy	Renal stones
Cystinuria	RP	Pyr. signs, deafness	Renal lithiasis
Glutamate			
Chinese restaurant syndrome		HA	
Homocarnosinosis	Ret. pig. degen.	Prog. spasticity Mental deterioration Incsd. CSF homocarnisine	
Lysine			
Pipecolicacidemia (variant of Zellweger's syndrome)			
Oxalosis (primary and secondary)	Retinal crystals, black ring maculopathy, orb. myositis, disc pallor	CSF pressure	Nephrolithiasis and calcinosis Renal failure, osteodystrophy
Purine, Pyrimidine			
Xeroderma pigmentosa	Conjunctivitis, blepharitis, keratitis, tumors of lids and periorbita, malignant melanoma, orbital malignancies, photophobia	Microceph., MR, areflexia, choreoathetosis, deafness, seizures	Erythematous, pigmented telangiectatic atrophic and neoplastic skin changes in sun-exposed areas, keratoacanthomas
Tryptophan			
Hooft's disease	RP, gray mac.	PMR, hyperactive	Hypolipidemia; hypoglycemia; abn. hair, nails, teeth
Hartnup disease	Ectropion, nystagmus, scleral ulcers	Cerebellar ataxia, MR	aa uria, pellagra-like rash
Tyrosine			
Albinism (many forms)	Dcsd. VA Mac. dysplasia, nystagmus, strab. (60%), blond fundus, photophobia, no binoc. vision	Chiasmal crossing changes	Light-pigment hair, skin
Chédiak-Higashi disease	Photophobia	Cranial and periph. neuropathy, cereb. atrophy	Immune def., lymphoretic malignancy, early death, cut. ulcers

| | Clinical Presentation | | |
Key Diagnostic Finding	Heredity	Treatment	Other
Crystals, also in bone marrow buffy coat	AR	Symptomatic, renal transplant, cysteamine	PND, diagnose by conjunctival bx, retinal changes may precede sx, lysosomal storage disorder
Dcsd. cystathionine synthetase, urine nitroprusside test	AR	Pyridoxine, low-methionine diet and cystine	Gen. anesth. may cause thromboembolism; PND
	AR		—
	AR		—
	AR		Susceptibility to MSG
			—
	AR		—
	AR (primary), (peroxisomal?)		Reported after methyxyflurane anesthesia; VA good if disc OK
			PND
	AR		Death by 2 yr
			—
	AR (oculocutaneous forms); also AD, XLR		Poor melanin synthesis dcsd. cognitive fnx secondary to misdirected CNS paths ED, PND
Giant granules in blood cells	AR		Defect in melanosomes, not melanin formation; ED, PND

(*Continues*)

TABLE 21–14. ABNORMALITIES OF AMINO ACID METABOLISM (*cont.*)

Name	Clinical Presentation		
	Ocular	*CNS*	*Systemic*
Hermansky-Pudlak syndrome	Albinism		Hemorrhagic diathesis
Phenylketonuria (PKU)	Inf. cat.	MR, seizures	Pale hair and skin, blue eyes, eczema, "mousy" odor
Tyrosinemia II (Richner-Hanhart Syndrome)	Dendritic keratitis, lacrimation, photophobia	MR	Painful keratotic skin lesions on palms and soles
Zellweger syndrome and variants (infantile Refsum's disease, neonatal adrenoleukodystrophy, hyperpipecolic acidemia)	"Leopard spot" RP, cong. cat. and GI, ON hypoplasia	MR, hypotonia	Microcystic kidney, hepatic dysgenesis, aa uria, dysmorphic facies, deformed joints
Parkinsonism	Blepharospasm, EM abnormality	Rigidity, tremor	
Riley-Day syndrome	Dcsd. corneal sensation, alacrima, corneal ulcers, pupil abn. XT, myopia, OA, ret. vasc. tort.	Hypotonia, dcsd. pain and temperature sense, pyr. changes, cerebellar signs, Parkinsonism	Respiratory, feeding difficulties; orthostatic hypotension; episodic pneumonia; aspiration pneumonia; fractures; scoliosis
Urea Cycle			
Hyperornithinemia	Gyrate atrophy (Fig. 21–5) of choroid & retina, high myopia (90%), night blindness, PSC cat. (40%), ret. crystals		Tubular inclusions in type II muscle fibers with or without ECG and EEG abn.
Lowe's syndrome (oculocerebral renal)	Cong. cat. and gl., ret. pig. degen., ON hypoplasia	MR, growth retard.	Early death, met. acidosis, hyperammonemic, aa-uria, renal rickets
Valine, Leucine, Isoleucine			
Maple sugar urine disease	Fluctuating neonatal o'plegia, ptosis	MR, facial diplegia, dystonia	Hypoglycemia
Hypophosphatasia (juvenile Paget's disease)	Band keratopathy, proptosis, PE, spherophakia, blue sclera	Muscle weakness	Fine hair, met. acidosis, hyper Ca^{++}, craniostenosis, fragile bones
Alcaptonuria	Pigment of sclera and cornea		Atherosclerosis, cardiac valvular disease, joint disease, dark urine

Key Diagnostic Finding	Heredity	Treatment	Other
Dcsd. dense bodies, cyclic nucleotides in platelets	AR		Clastogenic (?), ED, PND
Dscd. phenylalanine hydroxylase		Dietary phenylalanine +/− valine, isoleucine, leucine restriction	Test prior to 3 mo of age to prevent MR; ED
Tyrosinaminotransferase	AR		ED
Elevated plasma VLCFA, pipecolic acid, +/− phytanic; elevated bile intermediates	AR		Death usually by 1 yr
			—
	AR	Bethanecol (parasympathomimetic)	Abn. VEPs in 80%
	AR	Some forms are pyridoxine sensitive, low-arginine diet	50% of known cases are Finnish, blind by 40, dcsd. ERG
	AR/XLR?		
Urine odor	AR		ED, PND
	XLR		Anesthesia a risk, PND
	AR		—

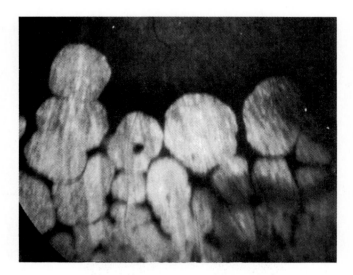

Figure 21–5. Gyrate atrophy. *(From Takki K, Simmell O. Gyrate atrophy of the choroid and retina with hyperornithinemia (HOGA). In: Bergsma D, Bron AJ, Cotlier E, eds.* The Eye and Inborn Errors of Metabolism. *New York: Liss, 1976, with permission. OAS 12(3):373–384.)*

TABLE 21–15. ABNORMALITIES OF METAL METABOLISM

Name	Ocular	CNS	Systemic	Key Diagnostic Finding	Heredity	Treatment	Other
			Clinical Presentation				
Hemochromatosis	Ocular findings are those of the associated diabetes mellitus						Chromosome 6
Menkes' syndrome (steely or kinky hair syndrome)	Retinal degen., iris cysts, OA	Cerebellar signs, seizures	Kinky hair, hypopigmentation, arterial abn., bone changes, hypothermia, hypotonia	Low serum copper; Cu^{++} in gut, mucosa, or liver	XLR	—	PND, mitochon enzyme defect
Wilson's disease	Cornea: Kayser-Fleischer ring[a] (present in 95%, 100% with neurol. symptoms); best seen on gonioscopy; cat. (sunflower)	Ataxia; basal ganglia symptoms—tremor, dysarthria	Cirrhosis, hemolysis, renal dysfxn.	Abn. Cu^{++} deposition, low ceruloplasmin	AR	Penicillamine, zinc rx, 3–6 mo lag to effect; tetramine	Evaluate any undiagnosed liver failure, esp. in children, for Wilson's disease

[a] K-F ring also occurs in copper foreign body and biliary cirrhosis.

TABLE 21–16. DISORDERS OF THE SKULL

Disorder	Clinical Presentation			Heredity	Other
	Ocular	**CNS**	**Systemic**	**Heredity**	**Other**
Fibrous dysplasia of skull (+/− Albright's disease)	Proptosis, strab. OA		Early epiphyseal closure, Albright's syndrome, café-au-lait spots, endocrine malfunction	AD	—
Paget's disease	Angioid streaks,[a] EOM palsies, choroidal sclerosis, OA, RP(?)	Deafness		AD	High alkaline phosphatase
Osteopetrosis (Albers-Schönberg disease)	OA if severe Retinal dystrophy	Deafness	Osteoporosis, macrocephaly, HSM, severe anemia	AR (AD)	PND

[a] May be less common than previously thought.

TABLE 21–17. OCULAR ABNORMALITIES ASSOCIATED WITH SKELETAL DISORDERS

| Abnormality | Clinical Presentation | | | Heredity |
	Ocular	CNS	Systemic	
Conradi syndrome (chrondrodysplasia punctata)	Congen. cat., gl., hypertelorism, heterochromia, OA	MR	Short stature, micromelia, VSD, PDA, skin changes, saddle nose	AD, (AR), XLD
Arthrogryposis multiplex congenita (many forms)	OA, cat., o'plegia, trichiasis, congen. gl.		Rigidity, deformed joints	Spor. AD/AR, XL
Craniometaphyseal dysplasia	OA	Cr nerve palsies, deafness	Facial abn., hyperostosis of skull, abn. of long bones, leonine facies	AD, AR (severe form)

TABLE 21–18. CRANIOFACIAL ABNORMALITIES

Abnormality	Clinical Presentation	
	Ocular	*CNS*
ANOMALIES[A,B]		
Craniostenosis (premature suture closure)	Strab., proptosis, keratoconus, PE, OA in oxycephaly	
Apert's syndrome	OA in 25%, proptosis, iris coloboma	MR
Crouzon's disease	Proptosis, strab., PE, OA (80%)	Hydrocephalus
Mandibulofacial dysostosis (Treacher-Collin's)	Antimongoloid lids, coloboma of lower lid and iris, strab.	Deafness, ear abn.
Hallermann-Streiff-François syndrome (Francheschetti-Klein's syndromes)	Congen. cat., microphthalmos, nystagmus, blue sclera	
Pierre-Robin's syndrome	High myopia, congen. gl., retinal detachment, strab., congen. cat.	MR
Hemifacial microsomia (inc. Goldenhar's syndrome)	Limbal dermoids, orbital lipodermoids, colobomata, Duane's syndrome	Deafness
Meyer-Schwickerath's syndrome	Microp., microcornea, gl.	
Greig's syndrome	OA, hypertelorism, epicanthus, astigmatism	Basilar impression, hearing loss
Craniocleidal dysostosis	Proptosis, upslanting palp. fissures	Brachycephaly
François syndrome (dermato-chrondro-corneal dys.)	Corneal dys.	Seizures
HEMIFACIAL ATROPHY		
Congenital (nonprogressive)	Abn. of cornea, lids	
Progressive (Parry-Romberg's syndrome)	Uveitis; abn. of cornea, pupil, lids, and fundus	Contralat. seizures
Fetal alcohol syndrome	ON hypoplasia, ret. vasc. tort., myopia, strab., corneal opacity, ant. seg. abn., iris defects	Microcephaly, growth retard.

[a] Most associated with strabismus.
[b] Many changes secondary to skull abnormalities.

Systemic	Heredity	Other
	AD	—
Syndactyly, ventricular septal defect	Sporadic (95%), AD	—
PDA, dental abn., syndactyly	AD, sporadic (25%)	—
Maxillary hypoplasia, large mouth, heart defects	AD	—
Mandibular and maxillary hypoplasia, feeding problems, ectodermal dysplasia, hypotrichosis, dwarfism, dental anomalies, characteristic facies	AR?, AD?	Feeding problems
Cleft palate and lip, mandibular hypoplasia, glossoptosis, feeding problems	AR, (AD)	Need to differentiate from Stickler syn.
Preauricular skin tags, fused cervical vertebrae, cardiac and other systemic abnormalities, mandibular hypoplasia, dysplasia of ear	Sporadic, AR	—
Dental anom., syndactyly, typical facies, fine hair		—
Cleft palate, maxillary hypoplasia	AD	—
Short stature, dental anomalies	AD	—
Deformed hands and feet, xanthomatous bodies on dorsal surfaces	AR	—
Systemic abn. rare		—
Linear "Scleroderma" of face	AD?	—
Typical facies		Maternal alcohol abuse

TABLE 21–19. PREMATURE AGING SYNDROMES

Syndrome	Clinical Presentation	
	Ocular	**CNS**
Cockayne's	RP, OA, photophobia, cat., keratopathy, strab., nystagmus, resistant to myriatics	MR, microcephaly, deafness, intracran. Ca^{++}, ataxia, seizures, demyelination
Rothmund-Thomson	Juv. cat., microcornea and other corneal abn., sparse brows and lashes	Microceph. (sometimes)
Progeria	Prominent eyes, ret. vasc. changes	Muscle atrophy, MR
Werner's	PSC cat. (2nd–4th decade), RP, mac. degen., gl. blue sclera	Muscle atrophy
Berardinelli-Siep	Corneal opacities	MR, muscular hypertrophy, hypothalamic harmartomas
De Barsy	Cloudy cornea, cat.	MR, hypotonia, athetosis

See also
Hallerman Streiff (above, craniofacial abn.).

Systemic	Heredity	Other
Dwarfism; sun sensitivity; sparse, gray hair; atherosclerosis	AR	Senile changes at 2–4 YO, dcsd. ERG, PND
Short stature, hypogonad., poikiloderma, skull anomalies, photosensitivity	AR	Cat. at 2–7 YO
Alopecia, thin skin, dcsd. subcutaneous fat, skull hypoplasia, accelerated atherosclerosis, hypogonad. DM, dwarfism	AR? AD?	Death around 14 YO secondary to ASHD
Sparse, gray hair; scleroderma; DM; hypogonadism; cardiomyopathy; birdlike facies; accel. atherosclerosis; neoplasia; growth retardation; skin ulcers	AR	Phenotypic copy of aging; cat. extraction complications, esp. late wound dehiscence and corneal degen.
Lipodystrophy, hyperlipemia, hepatomegaly, acanthosis nigricans, DM	AR	—
Cutis laxa, short stature	Sporadic, AR	—

TABLE 21–20. CHROMOSOMAL DISORDERS[a]

Disorder	Clinical Presentation	
	Ocular	*CNS*
Turner (XO) Syndrome	Epicanthal fold, ptosis, strab., blue sclerae, cat.	
Trisomy 13 (D₁)	Corneal opacity, microphthalmos, colobomata, PHPV, intraocular cartilage, retinal dysplasia, cat., ant. seg. dysgenesis, optic nerve hypoplasia, cyclopia	MR, holoprosencephaly, microceph.
Trisomy 21 (Down's syndrome)	Upslanting palpebral fissures, esotropia (35%), cat. (60%), Brushfield spots (85%), epicanthal folds, high myopia, keratoconus, blepharitis, nystagmus	MR (most common genetic cause)
Trisomy 18 (Edwards's syndrome)	Retinal folds, blepharophimosis, ptosis, corneal opacity, microphthalmos, congenital gl., colobomata, cat., strab., OA, disc anom.	MR, hypertonus deafness
Deletion of long arm of 13	Hypertelorism, ptosis, iris coloboma, cat., gl., RB, strab., orbit abn., epicanthus	Microceph., MR, pineal T
Deletion of short arm of 13	Microphthalmos, hypertelorism, ptosis, post-keratoconus, corneal opacities, cat., ret. degen., OA, deep-set eyes, coloboma, gl.	MR, CNS anom.
Ring D 13	Microphthalmos, hypertelorism, strab., ptosis, retrocorneal membrane, iris coloboma, optic nerve hypoplasia	
Cri-du-chat syndrome (5p−)	Strab., ptosis, dcsd. tearing, hypertelorism, absence of brows, iris/choroid colobomas, cat., ret. vasc. tort., OA, epicanthal folds	Microceph., hypotonia
Schmid-Fraccaro (cat eye syndrome)	Microphthalmos, strab., coloboma iris/ret., hypertelorism Cataract, epicanthal folds, telecanthus, dry eye syn.	
4p (Wolf-Hirschhorn syndrome)	Ptosis, nystagmus, cat., hypertelorism, exotropia, epicanthal folds, coloboma	Seizures, MR (profound)
Deletion of short arm of 11p−	Aniridia, epicanthal folds	PMR
Deletion of long arm of 15 (present in 50% of Praeder-Willi cases)	Strab., epicanthal folds	MR
Partial trisomy 10g	Abn. discs, yellow post pole deposits, hypertelorism, antimongoloid lids, microphthalmia, ptosis, cat., sclerocornea	PMR, microceph.

[a] Chromosomal abnormalities are detected by PND.

Systemic	Other/Prevalence
Short stature, webbed neck, facial and skull anom., hypogonad	1/1,500 births, women, incidence of X-linked disorders equal to males
Cardiac defects, GU abn., cleft palate, polydactyly, hematol. abn., hemangiomas	Death in 1st mo, 1/15,000 births
Short stature, characteristic facies, cardiac abn., broad hands and feet, leukemia, Alzheimer's	Sensitivity to atropine, 1/600 births (most common chromosomal abn.) extra chromosome 95% of maternal origin
Cardiac anomalies, micrognathia, microstomia, low-set ears, clenched fists, rocker-bottom feet	Death in 1st yr, 1/5000 births
Micrognathia, dysplastic thumbs, congen. heart dis., malignancies, short stature	Chromosome 13q/14, deletion in 10% of RB patients
Short stature	—
	—
Micrognathia, short stature	—
Anal atresia, cardiac anom., preauricular skin tags or pits	—
Midfacial anomalies, characteristic facies, congenital heart disease, skeletal defects	—
Wilm's tumor, characteristic facies, hemihypertrophy	—
Short stature, hypogonad., obesity, small hands and feet	—
Heart defects, micrognathia, cleft palate, abn. hands and feet	—

TABLE 21–21. OTHER MULTIPLE DEVELOPMENTAL ANOMALIES

Syndrome	Clinical Presentation			Heredity
	Ocular	*CNS*	*Systemic*	
De Lange's	Synophorys (confluent eyebrows), long lashes, ptosis, corneal opacity, OA, strab., post-coloboma	MR	Short neck, micrognathia, limb defects, cardiac defects, GU defects	
Fraser's	Cryptophthalmos, microphthalmos	CNS defects, encephalocele	GU anom., skeletal anom., esp. syndactyly; renal anom.; ear abn.	AR
Rieger's	Gl., cat., ectopia lentis, colobomata, cornea anom., OA, iris and angle anom.	Occas. MR, muscular dystrophy	Dental anom., limb anom., typical facies	AD
Peter's anomaly	Corneal clouding, iridolenticulo-corneal adhesions	CNS abn., hydroceph., MR	Skeletal anom., GI anom.	
Rubenstein-Taybi's syndrome	Antimongoloid palpebral fissures, epicanthus, strab., cat., long lashes	PMR	PDA, pul. stenosis, broad toes and thumbs	Cardiac arrhythmia with succinylcholine

TABLE 21–22. DISORDERS OF VITAMIN METABOLISM

Disorder	Clinical Presentation			Key Diagnostic Finding	Heredity	Treatment	Other
	Ocular	CNS	Systemic				
Vitamin A deficiency	Xerophthalmia, Bitot's spot, night blindness, yellow ret. spots, keratomalacia, ret. vasculitis						Dcsd. ERG
Vitamin A excess	PE, VI nerve palsy	Pseudotumor cerebri					—
Thiamine deficiency	Gaze palsies	DTs	Beriberi	Dcsd. thiamine		Thiamine	—
Wernicke's syndrome (vitamin B₁ deficiency)	Nystagmus, corneal epithel. damage	Wernicke's encephelopathy					—
Leigh's syndrome	Visual loss, supranuc. EM disorder	Weakness, dcsd. hearing, MR, seizures	Tachypnea, tachycardia	Dcsd. thiamine	Mitochondrial(?)	Thiamine	—
Vitamin B₂ deficiency (riboflavin)	Corneal vasc.						—
Vitamin B₆ deficiency (pyridoxine)	Optic neuropathy					Pyroxidine in pts. taking isoniazid hydralizine penicillamine	—
Vitamin B₁₂ deficiency	OA	Tropical neuropathy	Pernicious anemia				—
Vitamin C deficiency	Subconjunctival hemorrhage; lid, conj,. AC retinal hemorrhage		Scurvy, bleeding				—
Vitamin D excess	Conj. crystals, band keratopathy, zonular cat.	Tetany	Renal damage				—
Vitamin E deficiency	Ret. pig. degen. nyctalopia ptosis o'plegia						—
Vitamin K	Ret. hemorrhage in neonates?		Bleeding				—
Nicotinic acid			Pellagra				—

CHAPTER 22

SYSTEMIC DISORDERS OF NEURO-OPHTHALMIC INTEREST BY ORGAN SYSTEM

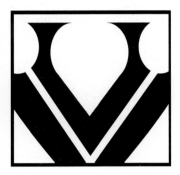

NERVOUS SYSTEM DISORDERS

Disorders of neuro-ophthalmic interest include many of the metabolic and hereditary neurodegenerative diseases that have already been briefly discussed and outlined. Several categories of neurologic disease associated with tapetoretinal degenerations, optic atrophy, or both, will be outlined below. These diseases may affect many other organ systems and present a panoply of signs and symptoms that occur together sufficiently often to constitute named syndromes. However, the nosology of many of these disorders is very difficult and confusing. For example, retinitis pigmentosa, optic atrophy, and a progressive external ophthalmoplegia all occur singly and in concert with spinocerebellar degenerations, muscular disorders, and disorders of other organ systems, especially deafness, diabetes mellitus, and cutaneous manifestations.

The classification that follows is modified from *Nelson's Textbook of Pediatrics* (Table 22–1). Some disorders are listed in multiple sections of this chapter, as their etiology and manifestations logically place them into several categories. As the precise metabolic defects, gene location, and pathophysiology of the disorders are elucidated, it becomes increasingly difficult to define some of these diseases narrowly. For example, metachromatic leukodystrophy is a disorder with the controlling gene on the long arm of chromosome 22 (22q); it might also be classified as a lysosomal storage disease (one of the sulfatidelipidoses) and/or a leukodystrophy.

In addition, as our understanding of the metabolic abnormalities in these diseases increases, there emerge new categories of disorders with common mechanisms, such as mitochondrial disorders and peroxisomal disorders. Among the mitochondrial diseases are included Freiderich's ataxia, Leigh's disease, Leber's optic neuropathy, Zellweger's syndrome, and the Kearns-Sayre syndrome. In some of these disorders, specific defects in mitochondrial DNA, metabolism, or both have been defined; in others they are suspected; in others the inheritance of the disorder itself is thought to be via the mitochondria; in still others, only a structural abnormality of the mitochondria is identified.

Mitochondria have their own genetic material as well as their own translation and transcription processes. For each zygote, almost all the mitochondria are contributed by the ovum, making possible maternal inheritance of defective mitochondrial metabolism (as for Leber's optic neuropathy). Variable genetic expression in disorders of mitochondrial metabolism may relate to the relative proportions of mitochondria contributed by the maternal and paternal lines or the stage of development at which a DNA deletion occurs. It is also of interest that the receptor elements (the rods and cones) contain particularly dense aggregations of mitochondria in their cytoplasm, as many mitochondrial disorders are associated with retinal pigmentary degeneration.

TABLE 22–1. CLASSIFICATION OF CNS DISEASES OF NEURO-OPHTHALMIC INTEREST

I. Degeneration of gray matter
  A. Neuronal storage diseases
    1. Lysosomal storage diseases—sphingolipidoses, mucopolysaccaridoses, mucolipidoses, neuronal ceroid lipofuscinoses
    2. Glycogen storage disease—von Gierke's disease
  B. Other: Alper's, Leigh's, and Menkes' diseases, subacute sclerosing panencephalitis (SSPE)
II. Degeneration of white matter
  A. Leukodystrophies
    1. Lysosomal storage disorders—Metachromatic leukodystrophy (MLD), Krabbe's disease (globoid)
    2. Sudanophilic storage diseases—Adrenoleukodystrophy, Pelizaeus-Merzbacher disease
    3. Canavan's disease, Alexander's disease
  B. Demyelinating (nongenetic?)
  C. Other—Cockayne's syndrome
III. System degenerations
  A. Spinocerebellar and cerebellar—Freidreich's ataxia, ataxia-telangiectasia, Bassen-Kornzweig syndrome, Refsum's disease
  B. Basal ganglia disorders—Wilson's disease, dystonia musculorum deformans, Huntington's disease, Parkinson's disease

From Vaughan VC, Nelson WE, eds. Textbook of Pediatrics. 13th ed. Philadelphia: Saunders, 1987:1311.

TABLE 22–2. PEROXISOMAL DISORDERS

Group I	Zellweger's syndrome[a] Neonatal adrenoleukodystrophy (ALD)[a] Infantile Refsum's disease[a] Hyperpipecolic acidemia	Decreased peroxisomes, VLCFAs
Group II	Rhizomelic chrondrodysplasia punctata	Deficiency of peroxisome enzymes
Group III	X-linked adrenoleukodystrophy CoA-thiolase deficiency (pseudo-Zellweger's syndrome) Acyl-CoA oxidase deficiency[a] Adult Refsum's disease[a] Adrenomyeloneuropathy (AMN) Hyperoxaluria Acatalasemia	Genetic lack of single peroxisomal enzyme (?)

[a] Ocular findings.
Modified from Singh I, et al. Peroxisomal disorders and clinical diagnostic considerations. Am J Dis Child. 1988;142:1299.

Peroxisomal deficiency is associated with a wide range of phenotypic defects that involve virtually every tissue. Peroxisomes are abundantly present during active myelination (eg, in the early postnatal nervous system and in the processes that form the myelin sheath). They are required to synthesize plasmalogens, essential myelin constituents. Thus, their disorder presumably contributes to the characteristic defects of neuronal migration in peroxisomal deficiency disorders. Peroxisomes are rare in the mature central nervous system (CNS).

Peroxisomal disorders (Table 22–2) commonly present with neonatal seizures, hypotonia, dysmorphic features, psychomotor retardation, optic atrophy, retinal pigmentary degeneration and a decreased electroretinogram (ERG) amplitude, hearing defects, hepatomegaly and dysfunction, and chrondrodysplasia punctata. If several of these signs are present, consider a peroxisomal disorder. Diagnostic measures include measurement of plasma very-long-chain fatty acids (VLCFA), plasmalogen and plasmalogen enzymes, pipecolic acid, bile acid intermediates, and phytanic acid. All are amenable to prenatal diagnosis and ameliorated by a dietary regimen. Bone marrow transplantation potentially benefits these patients.

With respect to **neurodegenerative processes,** recall that **disorders of gray matter** usually initially present with dementia and seizures; on the other hand, **white matter disorders** tend to affect motor function early, frequently presenting with spasticity and ataxia. With progression, distinctions between the involvement of white and gray matter become blurred and many neural structures are involved (Tables 22–3 to 23–9).

The paraneoplastic syndromes are nonmetastatic complications of cancer, especially small-cell carcinoma of the lung, breast carcinoma, and gynecologic cancer. More readily recognized syndromes include subacute cerebellar degeneration, opsoclonus–myoclonus, carcinoma-associated retinopathy, and the Lambert-Eaton syndrome. The cerebellar degeneration appears to result from an immune response (an "anti-onconeural immune response") to neural antigens expressed by the tumor. These entities often present prior to recognition of the neoplasm and necessitate careful evaluation for an occult malignancy.

INFECTIOUS DISORDERS

Nearly any infectious agent, congenital or acquired, may cause neuro-ophthalmic signs and symptoms by involving either the eye or the CNS. Both tissues have in common a barrier to blood-borne infection. Thus, it is unusual for blood-borne agents to cause infection in healthy individuals with intact ocular and CNS tissues. When this happens—especially with opportunistic infections such as cytomegalovirus (CMV), *Candida*, or toxoplasmosis—consider immune deficient states—lymphoma, transplant patients, or HIV infection.

The neuro-ocular apparatus is also affected by diseases such as tuberculosis, brucellosis, and tularemia, which cause chronic and/or granulomatous infections. These affect the eye and CNS, but with the exception of tuberculosis are relatively rare. Some viruses that are neurotropic show a similar predilection and not infrequently present with optic neuritis, papillitis, and/or chorioretinitis as their ocular manifestations; there may be associated anterior segment inflammation, vitritis, or orbital involvement.

The neuro-ophthalmic manifestations are dependent upon the part of the brain, orbit, or eye involved. Meningeal involvement may be heralded by cranial nerve palsies, photophobia, and nuchal rigidity. Both the orbit and CNS may be secondarily involved by infections of the sinus and nasopharynx. In patients with immune compromise and/or diabetes mellitus, a fungal etiology should be suspected. Also be alert to potential neuro-ophthalmic complications (eg, optic atrophy) of antibiotic agents used to treat the infections, vascular occlusion with antimalarial agents, and optic atrophy and eighth nerve involvement with antituberculous medications. Don't forget the parasitic protozoal infestations such as *Cryptococcus* and *Toxocara*; and if the patient has traveled in endemic areasa, even more exotic species should be considered.

Additionally, unusual neurologic complications of ocular diseases may occur—for example, the neurologic complications (cranial nerve paralysis, poliolike syndrome) of acute hemorrhagic conjunctivitis (EV 70 infection).

Other reactions related to infection and vaccination include autoimmune responses such as the Guillain-Barré and Miller-Fisher syndromes.

Still other agents such as herpes virus remain latent in the CNS. The exact mechanisms of involvement by other viruses remain obscure; for example, the Epstein-Barr virus appears to have multiple neuro-ophthalmic manifestations.

Treponemal infections again appear to be on the rise. Still most frequent is the "great mimick," syphilis. More than 50% of patients presenting in an oculoplastics clinic (Table 22–10) had positive FTA-Abs tests, but only one quarter of those was VDRL positive. The majority had significant ocular findings (Table 22–11). Another treponemal disease, Lyme disease, is being recognized with increasing frequency. It has three stages and numerous manifestations, as does syphilis; it may also yield a false-positive FTA or HATTS test. Bell's palsy is a frequent manifestation. Guillain-Barré type neuritis also occurs (Tables 22–12, 22–13).

The protean manifestations, low sensitivity of diagnostic testing during the early stages of the disease, cross-reactivity with syphilis, and interlaboratory variability make diagnosis problematic. Clinical suspicion is paramount. However, a new assay using the polymerase chain reaction (PCR) promises more secure diagnosis. The current recommended therapy is parenteral antibiotics (Table 22–14) comparable to those used in treating CNS syphilis. Ceftriaxone has the lowest minimal inhibitory concentration, best penetration of the blood–brain barrier, and widest clinical margin between tissue level and curative dose. As with *T. pallidum*, a Herxheimer reaction should be anticipated and appropriate steroid coverage given.

Congenital infections with frequent neuro-ophthalmic manifestations include rubella (cataract, deafness, cardiac anomalies, salt-and-pepper fundi, microphthalmus, glaucoma, and mental retardation; Tables 22–14, 22–15); CMV infection (fetal malformation in 50% of maternal infections—chorioretinitis, optic atrophy, optic nerve hypoplasia, cataract, deafness, microcephaly); toxoplasma infection (chorioretinal scarring, especially in the macula, CNS calcification, hydrocephalus, seizures); and congenital syphilis (Hutchinson's triad—interstitial keratitis, deafness, and notched incisors—and other ocular inflammations).

Outside of the Western hemisphere and Europe, one may encounter leprosy, which frequently causes blindness, usually from corneal complications of seventh-nerve palsy combined with anesthetic corneas. Lumpy or prominent corneal nerves are very characteristic of this disease (they are also found in multiple endocrine neoplasia and neurofibromatosis). Onchocerciasis (river blindness) is a filarial disease that is a frequent cause of blindness worldwide. Loa Loa is another frequent cause of visual loss in third-world countries.

Diseases of organ systems are listed in the accompanying tables (Tables 22–1 to 22–21) followed by tables of diseases listed by the affected part of the eye.

TABLE 22–3. WHITE MATTER DISEASES (LEUKODYSTROPHIES)

Disorder	Clinical Presentation		
	Ocular	*CNS*	*Systemic*
PEROXISOMAL DISORDERS			
Adrenoleukodystrophy (ALD), typical	Vision defect, eventually very low VA, OA, cortical NLP	Demyelin., seizures, dementia, spasticity, ataxia, deafness	Adrenal atrophy (Addison's disease)
Adrenomyeloneuropathy (AMN)		Spastic paraperesis, polyneuropathy	Addison's disease, hypogonadism
Infantile Refsum's disease	Ret. pig. degen.	MR, deafness, ataxia, anosmia	Hepatomegaly, dysmorphic features
Congenital neonatal leukodystrophy	OA, ret. pig. degen.	Hypotonia, seizure, PMR	Adrenal atrophy
Zellweger's syndrome	OA, ret. pig. degen., speckled iris, cloudy cornea, cat., gl, nystagmus	PMR, hypotonia, seizures	Dysmorphic facies, hepatomegaly, renal cysts, calcific deposits in patella
Lysosomal Storage Disorders			
Multiple sulfatase deficiency	CRS, OA, corneal clouding		MPS-like, ichythyosis, HSM
Metachromatic leukodystrophy (many forms)	OA, RP, CRS?, gray mac.	Gait abn., dementia, spasticity, psychiatric presentation, dystonia, seizures	Nonfilling gallbladder
Krabbe's disease (globoid)	OA, strab., nystagmus, cortical NLP	Myoclonic seizures, spasticity, high CSF protein, periph. neurop., PMR	Swallowing problems
Other leukodystrophies			
Pelizaeus-Merzbacher's disease	Roving EMs, nystagmus, mild OA, RP	Head trembling, ataxia, tremor, MR, spasticity, choreoathetosis	Pes cavus, scoliosis, short stature, autonomic disturbance in adult form
Infantile neuroaxonal dystrophy	OA, NLP	MR, seizures, myoclonus, motor signs	
DEMYELINATING DISEASES			
Canavan's disease	OA, ret. pig. degen., retinal vacuoles?	Hypotonia, seizures, spasticity, poor head control, macroceph.	Failure to thrive
Cockayne's syndrome	OA, RP, cat., corneal clouding, pupil changes, strab., nystagmus, photophobia	MR (severe), microceph., deafness, ataxia, seizures, NP hydrocephalus	Dwarfism, premature aging, sparse gray hair, atherosclerosis, skin sensitivity, hypertension
Smith-Lemli-Optiz syndrome	Congen. cat., strab., ptosis, OA, choroidal hemangioma	Microceph., MR, midline anom., hypotonia	Ambiguous genitalia, typical facies, failure to thrive, heart defects, syndactyly
Multiple sclerosis	O neur.; EM disorders: INO, skew; sheathing of retinal veins	Ataxia, dysarthria, spasticity	
Schilder's disease	O neur., OA, cx NLP, EM abn., nystagmus	Spasticity, cortical deafness, seizures, dementia	
Devic (neuromyelitis optica)	O neur., EM abn.	Myelitis	

Clinical Presentation			
Key Diagnostic Findings	*Heredity*	*Treatment*	*Other*
Elev. VLCFAs, MRI changes prior to CNS sx!	XLR	Erucic acid, diet, BMT	Boys 4–8, death in early to late teens, PND; on Xq28 (same locus as R-G color gene!)
Elevated VLCFAs (test *all* males with "isolated" Addison's disease)	XLR	Oleic acid, diet?	Variant adult-onset form of ADL; involves spinal cord and peripheral nerves predom; PND; milder than ALD
			—
Elevated VLCFAs	AR		Defect in multiple peroxisomal functions; defect in peroxisomal biogenesis
Elevated VLCFAs, pipecolic acid, phytanic acid, bile intermediates	AR		Defect of peroxisomal biosynthesis, death in childhood, PND
			—
Arylsulfatase A	AR	BMT	See also sphingolipidoses
Globoid cells in CNS, dcsd. galactocerebrosidase	AR		Onset 4–6 mo, PND
	XLR, AD (adult onset)		Males only, onset 1st mos, elliptical pendular, upbeat nystagmus combination may be diagnostic death in early childhood
	AR		Onset and death in first decade, form of severe Hallervorden-Spatz syndrome(?)
	AR		Death by age 6, N ERG, dcsd. VEP
	AR		PND, dcsd. ERG, senile at 2–4 YO
	AR		Death in childhood, mitochondrial disorder?
			Only 1% <15 YO, relapsing
			—

TABLE 22–4. GRAY MATTER DEGENERATIONS

Disorder	Clinical Presentation		
	Ocular	CNS	Systemic
Subacute sclerosing panencephalitis (SSPE)	Mac. changes	Mental deter., myoclonus seizures	
Menke's disease (kinky or steely hair)	Ret. degen., iris cysts	PMR, cerebellar signs	Kinky, steely hair; arterial changes; bone changes; hypothermia; hypopig.
Lysosomal storage diseases	(See Chapter 1 Tables 8–11)		
Leigh's disease (subacute necrotizing encephalopathy), familial/infantile, juv/adult	OA, nystagmus, supranuc. EM dis.	Ataxia, seizures, b stem sx., periph. neurop.	
Alper's disease	Visual disturbances	PMR, seizures, spasticity, ataxia	Lactic acidosis, cirrhosis
Acetyl-CoA oxidase deficiency	Ret. pig. degen.	Hypotonia, neonatal seizures, PMR	Liver dsfxn
Adrenoleukomyeloneuropathy		Spastic paraperesis, polyneurop.	Adrenal dsfxn, hypogonadism

Key Diagnostic Finding	Heredity	Treatment	Other
			Slow virus; after measles, most frequent cause of infant hospitalization for neurologic degenerative disease; onset late 1st decade; death in infancy; mitochondrial enzyme def.
AbN Cu^{++} metab, dcsd. ceruloplasm	XLR		Death in infancy, mitochondrial enzyme def.
Pyruvate, carboxylase	AR, spor. (XLR), mitochondrial?	Thiamine	Onset 2 mo to 6 yr; defect in electron transport chain
	AR, mitochondrial defect?		—
	XLR		Extinguished ERG
	XLR, peroxisomal		—

TABLE 22–5. HEREDITARY NEURODEGENERATIVE DISEASES

| | Clinical Presentation | | |
Disorder	Ocular	CNS	Systemic
SPINOCEREBELLAR ATAXIAS			
Friedreich's disease	OA, strab., nystagmus	Spinocerebellar degen. Ataxia, dysarth.	Pes cavus, DM, cardiac myop.
Pierre-Marie's syndrome	OA, o'plegia, nystagmus, pig. retinopathy	Ataxia, hypotonia	
Behr's disease	OA, nystagmus	Ataxia, pyr. signs, MR	
Cerebellar degen, with slow eye movements	Absent saccades, slow pursuit	Ataxia, MR	
Olivopontocerebellar ataxia (OPCA), composite of 5 forms	RP (starts central, spreads to periph.); abn. EMs; o'plegia; OA, nystagmus, cat., bull's-eye maculopathy	Ataxia, dysarth., rigidity, dementia, tremor	
Marinesco-Sjögren's syndrome	Congen. cat., nystagmus, strab., epicanthus	MR, spinocereb. ataxia, PMR	Skeletal anom.
Sjögren-Larson's syndrome	Mac. degen., ret. pig. degen.	MR, spastic ataxia	Ichthyosis
Hallgren's disease	RP, OA; cat. only occurs in midlife	Ataxia, MR, deafness	
Refsum's disease	RP, abn. pupils, OA, cat., night blindness, nystagmus	Ataxia, polyneuritis, deafness, anosmia (?), high CSF protein without cells	Ichthyosis, cardiac arrhythmias, bone dysplasia
Bassen-Kornzweig syndrome	Ret. pig. degen., PEO, night blindness	Ataxia, spinocerebellar degen., PMR, neuropathy	Malabsorption, stearorrhea, cardiac abn.
Neuronal intranuclear hyaline inclusion disease (NIHID)	OA, pupil change, abn. EMs, oculogyric crises ptosis, blepharospasm	Extrapyr. and pyr. signs, mental deter.	
Ataxia-telangiectasia (Louis-Barr syndrome)	Nystagmus, conj. telang., supranuc. EM abn.	Ataxia, dysarth., choreo-athetosis	Skin telang., immune def., incsd. incidence of malignancy, recurrent pul. infection, progeric changes of skin, hair
Cerebello trigeminal dermal dysplasia	Corneal anesthesia and scarring	Trigeminal hypesthesia	Alopecia
Joubert's syndrome	Abn. EMs	Ataxia, MR	Episodic hyperpnea
Misc. ataxic syndromes of neuro-ophthalmic interest	Aniridia, retinal coloboma cat., mac. dys., mac. pig.	MR, ataxia, spastic diplegia, MR MR or Marinesco/Sjögren syndrome MR, pyramidal degen. signs	Congen. skin pig.

Key Diagnostic Findings	Heredity	Treatment	Other
	AR		Can be phenotypically similar to Bassen-Kornzweig's syndrome, childhood Refsum's diseases, with DM; death 3rd–4th decade
	AD, (AR)		Onset after 20, probably heterogenous
	AR		Onset in childhood
	AD		—
	AD, OPCA II AR		Dcsd. ERG Peroxisomal (?), lysosomal (?) storage; similar to neuronal ceroid lipofucsinosis
	AD		—
	AR		—
	AR		Related (?) to Laurence-Moon/Bardet-Biedel syndromes with DM and obesity
High serum phytanic acid	AR (peroxisomal dexase?)	Low phytanic acid diet, plasma pheresis	ERG, PND, peroxisomal disease (?)
Absent beta-lipoproteins, very low serum cholesterol, acanthocytosis of RBCs	AR	Vitamins A and E, low-fat diet	—
Intranuclear eosinophilic inclusions in neurons			Depressed ERG
	AR		Onset in infancy
			—
	AR		—
	Familial		—

(Continues)

TABLE 22–5. HEREDITARY NEURODEGENERATIVE DISEASES (cont.)

Disorder	Clinical Presentation		
	Ocular	*CNS*	*Systemic*
MITOCHONDRIAL MYOPATHY/ ENCEPHALOPATHY/ CYTOPATHY[a]			
Kearns-Sayre's syndrome (KSS)	O'plegia, ptosis, ret. pig. degen.	Cerebellar ataxia, deafness, myopathy, seizures, increased CSF protein	Heart block, short stature
Myoclonic epilepsy with ragged red fibers (MERRF)	OA	Ataxia, seizures, sensory loss, dementia, hearing loss	Short stature
MELAS (mitochondrial myopathy, encephalopathy, lactic acidosis, stroke)	Hemianopia, cx NLP	Seizures, stroke-like episodes, dementia, hearing loss	Growth retardation, episodic vomiting
Leber optic neuropathy	OA	Occas. CNS symptoms	Cardiac preexcitation syndrome
Facioscapulohumeral dystrophy	Orbicularis weakness, ret. telang.	Facial, shoulder weakness	
Alper's disease (progressive infantile poliodystrophy)	Visual disturbances	PMR, spastic paresis, ataxia, myoclonic jerks	Lactic acidosis cirrhosis
Leigh's disease (subacute necrotizing encephalo-myelopathy)	Supranuc. EM disorder, nystagmus, OA	Pyramidal, cerebellar, extrapyramidal signs; seizures	
OTHER NEUROLOGIC DISORDERS			
Familial dysautonomia (Riley-Day syndrome)	Dcsd. corneal sensation, alacrima, corneal ulcers, pupil abn., XT, myopia, OA, ret. vasc. tort.	Hypotonia, dcsd. P+T sense, pyr. changes., cerebellar, signs, Parkinsonism	Respiratory, feeding difficulties; orthostatic hypotension; episodic hypertension; aspiration pneumonia; fractures; scoliosis
Hallervorden-Spatz disease	Ret. pig. degen., OA, yellow flecks, bull's-eye maculop.	Dementia, spasticity, athetosis, dysarthr., ataxia	
Dystonia, blepharospasm pigmentary retinopathy	Bull's-eye maculop. ret. pig. degen. blepharospasm	Dystonia	
Aicardi's syndrome	Pigmented and depig. lacunes, OA—gray disc, disc colob., scleral ectasia, microphthalmos, coloboma	Infantile spasms, CNS anom., absent corpus callosum, MR—profound	Skeletal anom.
Norrie's disease	RD, retrolental mass	MR, deafness, seizures	
Usher's syndrome	RP	Deafness (congenital)	
MISC. SYNDROMES			
Laurence-Moon's syndrome	Ret. pig. degen.	Spastic paraplegia	Hypogonadism
Bardet-Biedl's syndrome	Ret. pig. degen.; rarely oplegia, cat, OA	Paraplegia, MR, misrouted VAP	Polydactyly, obesity, hypogenitalism, cardiac anom., renal anom.
Prader-Willi's syndrome	Albinotic, strab., nystagmus	Hypotonia, misrouted VAP, MR	Hypogonadism, obesity, short stature, poor feeding
Rud's syndrome	RP, strab., ptosis, nystagmus, blepharospasm	MR, seizures, polyneurop., deafness	Ichthyosis; hypogonadism; DM; dwarfism; abn. hair, teeth, nails
Biemond's syndrome	Iris coloboma	MR	Hypogonadism, obesity, polydactyly
MUSCULAR DISORDERS			
Charcot-Marie-Tooth's disease (composite of types)	OA, RP, PEO, nystagmus	Prog. musc. dyst., dcsd. DTRs	Bilat. foot drop, pes cavus
Ocular pharyngeal muscular dystrophy	O'plegia, ptosis at 45–55 yr	VII weakness	Pharyngeal weakness, dysphagia
Fascioscapulo humeral dystrophy	Ret. telang., orbic. weakness	Facial, shoulder weakness	
Myotonic dystrophy	X-mas tree cats., ptosis, RP, low IOP	MR, myotonia	DM, testicular atrophy, baldness, heart block

[a] Some mitochondrial encephalopathies/myopathies are differentiated by immunohistochemistry.

Key Diagnostic Findings	Heredity	Treatment	Other
	Sporadic AD?, mtDNA deletion with mitotic segregation		Onset by 15 yr
	Mitochondrial?		onset before <20 yr
	Mitochondrial?		First years
	Maternal mitochondrial		—
	AD		—
	AR		—
Pyruvate carboxylase	AR, sporadic, (XLR)	Thiamine	Onset 2 mo–6 yr
	AR	Bethanecal (parasympathomimetic)	Abn. VEPs in 80%
Radiographic densities in basal ganglia (iron deposition)?	AR		Onset 7–10 YO
			Dcsd ERG
Females only	Possibly new mutation for X-linked dominant gene that is lethal in males		—
	XLR		—
	AR (at least 2 separate genes)		—
	AR		—
	AR		ERG dcsd.
	AD		Abn. chrom 15 (50%), abn VEP
	AR		—
			—
	AD, XLR, AR		—
	AD		Many are French Canadian
	AD		Mitochondrial?
	AD		Chromosome 19(?), do serial ECGs

TABLE 22–6. SENSORY NEUROPATHIES

| Neur-opathy | Clinical Presentation | | | Heredity |
	Ocular	CNS	Systemic	
Congenital sensory neuropathy	Ret. pig. degen.	Lack of pain sense, MR, deafness	Ulceration, loss of digits, anhidrosis	AR
Cerebello-trigemino-dermal dysplasia	Hypertension, absent corneal reflexes, cloudy cornea	Facial analgesia, cerebellar hypoplasia, MR, hypotonia	Patchy alopecia	

TABLE 22–7. OTHER CENTRAL NERVOUS SYSTEM DISORDERS

| Disorder | Clinical Presentation | | | | Heredity | Treatment | Other |
	Ocular	CNS	Systemic	Key Diagnostic Findings			
BASAL GANGLIA **Wilson's disease**	KF ring	Tremor, dysarth., bulbar signs, dementia	Hepatic failure	Low ceruloplasm	AR	Liver transplant	
AUTONOMIC **Familial dysautonomia (Riley-Day syndrome)**	Dcsd. corneal sensation, alacrima, corneal ulcers, pupil abn., XT, myopia, OA, ret. vasc. tort.	Hypotonia, dcsd. P+T sense, pyr. changes, cerebellar signs, Parkinsonism	Respiratory, feeding difficulties; orthostatic hypotension; episodic hypertension; aspiration pneumonia; fractures; scoliosis; blotchy skin; absence of fungiform papillae on tongue;		AR	Bethanecal (parasympa-thomimetic)	Abn. VEPs in 80%
Shy-Drager's syndrome	Iris atrophy, pupil changes, K-sicca, nystagmus	Extrapyr. cerebellar, pyr. signs	autonomic abn., esp. orthostatic hypotension		AD		

TABLE 22–8. CENTRAL NERVOUS SYSTEM DISORDERS ASSOCIATED WITH DEAFNESS

Disorder	Clinical Presentation			
	Ocular	CNS	Systemic	Heredity
Usher's syndrome	RP	Congen. deafness		AR (2 genes)
Halgren's syndrome	RP, OA, cat. in midlife	Ataxia, MR		
Alström's syndrome	RP	Deafness	Obesity, DM, nephropathy, hypogonadism	
Alport's syndrome	Cat. (10%), myop., ant. lenticonus, perimacular granularity, K-conus, nystagmus		Nephritis	
Norrie's disease	RD, retrolental mass	MR, deafness, seizures		XLR
Craniostenosis, esp. oxycephaly	OA			
LEUKODYSTROPHIES				
Metachromatic leukodystrophy (MLD)	OA, CRS, gray mac.	Cerebellar signs, dementia, gait abn.	Nonfilling gallbladder	
Lysosomal storage disorders	(see Section I)			
TOXIC DRUG REACTIONS				
Streptomycin	OA			
Isoniazid	Optic neuritis			
Sulfonamides				
Chloramphenicol				
Charge syndrome	Colobomas, blocked tear ducts	MR	Choanal atresia, heart anomaly, renal malfunction	AR
Morgagni's syndrome	Cat., OA		Hyperostosis frontalis, obesity, hypertension	
Mitochondrial Cytopathies:				
KSS, MERFF, MELAS	(see above Hered. Neuro. Dys. Disease, Ch 22 Table 3)			
also Refsum, Hallgren	(see above Hered. Neuro. Dys. Disease, Ch 22 Table 3)			

See also MPS—Ch 21 Table 9 (Fucosidosis, Mannosidosis)
MLS—Ch 21 Table 10 (nearly all)
CT dis.—Ch 21 Tables 16 & 17 (Paget's, osteopetrosis, osteogenesis imperfecta)
Aminoacidopathies—Ch 21 Table 14 (Cystinuria)
Demyelination—Ch 22 Table 3 (Cockayne's, Schilder's)
Mitochondrial—Ch 22 Table 5 (Refsum's)
Other Neurodegenerative Diseases—Ch 22 (Bardet Biedel, Congenital Sensory Neurodystrophy)
Trisomy 18—Ch 21 Table 20
Treacher Collins—Ch 21 Table 18

TABLE 22–9. PARANEOPLASTIC SYNDROMES[a]

Disorder	Clinical Presentation			Treatment	Other
	Ocular	CNS	Systemic		
Encephalomyelitis	Dependent on part of CNS affected	Forms: cerebral, cerebellar, bstem, limbic, myelitis; incsd. CSF pressure			Esp. with bronchogenic ca. (70%); lymphoma; adenoca of breast, ovary
Opsoclonus/ myoclonus	Opsoclonus	Ataxia myoclonus			In child, R/O neuro-blastoma. In adult, R/O breast and other ca.
Lambert-Eaton syndrome	Muscle palsies	MG-like		Guanedine, plasmapheresis	EMG facilitation
Cancer-associated retinopathy (CAR)	Ret. pig. degen. Initially N, then narrow arteries; OA				Dcsd. ERG; esp. with oat cell ca, temporary response to steroids serum antibodies to photoreceptors;
Optic neuritis	OA				Serum antibodies to ON
Leukoencepha-lopathies	OA	MS-like but may be progressive			
Autoimmune neuropathy	Tonic pupils				

[a] All are probably "antionconeural immune responses." Occur in 7–15% of cancer patients.

TABLE 22–10. FTA-ABS REACTIVITY IN UNSELECTED PATIENTS (n = 227)

Patients	Age (yr)	No. Patients	Reactive to FTA-Abs	
			No.	Percentage
Urban	68.5	146	76	52
Suburban	53.5	81	44	54.3
Total		227	120	52.8

From Spoor TC, et al. Ocular syphilis 1986: Prevalence of FTS-Abs reactivity and CSF fluid findings. J Clin Neuro-Ophthalmol. 1987;7:191–195.

TABLE 22–11. OCULAR FINDINGS IN PATIENTS WITH REACTIVE SERUM FTA-ABS TESTS (n = 50)

Ocular Finding	Percentage of Patients
Optic atrophy	40
Chorioretinitis	28
Iritis	12
Interstitial keratitis	4
Papillitis	4
Hemianopia/ dementia	4
Abnormal pupils	2
Sixth-nerve paresis	2
Periscleritis	2
Ocular trauma	2

From Spoor TC, et al. Ocular syphilis 1986: Prevalence of FTS-Abs reactivity and CSF fluid findings. J Clin Neuro-Ophthalmol. 1987;7:191–195.

TABLE 22–12. NEUROLOGIC SIGNS AND SYMPTOMS OF LYME DISEASE

Amyotrophy
Anorexia-nervosa-like illness
Carpal tunnel syndrome (often bilateral)
Chorea
Cranial neuropathies
Dementia
Headache
Hearing impairment
Impaired concentration
Motor neuropathy
Multiple-sclerosis-like illness
Paralysis (transverse myelitis)
Personality changes
Psychosis
Seizures
Sensory neuritis
Short-term memory problems
Stiff neck
Vertigo

From MacDonald AB. Lyme disease: A neuro-ophthalmologic view. J Clin Neuro-Ophthalmol. 1987;7:185–190.

TABLE 22–14. MINIMAL BACTERIOCIDAL CONCENTRATIONS (*BORRELIA BURGDORFERI*)

Antibiotic	Concentration	CD_{50}[a] (mg/kg)
Penicillin G	6.5 μg/mL	1975
Ceftriaxone	0.04 μg/mL	240
Tetracycline	0.80 μg/mL	287
Erythromycin	0.05 μg/mL	2352

[a] CD_{50} curative dose 50% for hamsters experimentally infected with *Borrelia burgdorferi.*
Data from Johnson, et al.

TABLE 22–15. INCIDENCE OF ASSOCIATED OCULAR DISORDERS IN 328 CASES OF CONGENITAL RUBELLA

Disorder	No. Patients	Percentage
Retinopathy	78	23.8
Strabismus	38	17.7
Esotropia	41	12.5
Exotropia	17	3.2
Cataracts	34	16.5
Nystagmus	44	13.4
Microphthalmia and micro-cornea	31	9.5
Optic atrophy and abnormalities of the disc	29	8.8
Corneal haze and leukomas	25	7.6
Glaucoma	13	4.6
Buphthalmos	11	3.4
Lid defects, colobomas, ptosis, blepharophimosis	10	3.0
Persistent hyaloid artery	9	2.7
Retinal disorders	7	2.1
Phthisis bulbi	7	2.1
Iris atrophy	7	2.1
Lacrimal stenosis	5	1.5
Miscellaneous[a]	1	0.3

[a] One patient each had the following disorders: Brown's syndrome, dermoid cyst, cortical.
Wolff.

TABLE 22–13. OPHTHALMOLOGIC SIGNS AND SYMPTOMS OF LYME DISEASE

Blurred vision
Conjunctivitis
Cortical blindness
Diplopia
Exposure keratitis
Horner's syndrome (reversible)
Optic neuritis
Orbital myositis
Panophthalmitis
Papilledema
Photophobia
Symptoms of eye pressure

From MacDonald AB. Lyme disease: A neuro-ophthalmologic view. J Clin Neuro-Ophthalmol. 1987;7:185–190.

TABLE 22–16. ASSOCIATED SYSTEMIC FINDINGS OF THE POSTRUBELLA SYNDROME IN PATIENTS WITH OCULAR DISEASE (24 CASES)

Systemic Findings	No.	%
Heart	23	96
Patent ductus arteriosus	16	67
Peripheral pulmonary stenosis	6	25
Ventricular septal defect	4	17
Pulmonary artery stenosis	2	8
Atrial septal defect	2	8
Wolff-Parkinson-White syndrome	1	4
Transposition	1	4
Endocardial cushion defect	1	4
Premature (wt < 5.5 lb)	10	42
Hearing loss	12	50
Mental retardation	9	38
Thrombocytopenic purpura	3	13
X-ray evidence of bony changes	3	13
Pancytopenia	1	4
Porencephaly	1	4
Pyloric stenosis	1	4
Biliary atresia	1	4
Kidney deformity	1	4

TABLE 22–17. SLOW VIRUS CENTRAL NERVOUS SYSTEM DISEASES

Disease	Clinical Presentation				
	Ocular	CNS	Systemic	Treatment	Other
Progressive multifocal leuko-encephalopathy (PML)	Visual field defects	Progressive spasticity, dementia, dysarthria	Immune def., lymphoma, AIDS		Papovavirus
Creuzfeldt-Jakob's syndrome	Supranuc. gaze paresis	Ataxia, dementia			A few cases may be AD
Subacute sclerosing panencephalitis (SSPE)	Mac. pig. changes	Mental changes, high CSF gamma glob., myoclonus, seizures		Inosiplex?	Onset age 7–8 after measles, age 2–3 in persistent measles inf. of CNS
Myoclonic encephalopathy	Opsoclonus, nystagmus	Ataxia, myoclonus		Steroids?	Also with occult neuroblastoma

TABLE 22–18. CONNECTIVE TISSUE/COLLAGEN DISORDERS

Disorder	Clinical Presentation			Heredity	Other
	Ocular	CNS	Systemic		
Pseudoxanthoma elasticum (PXE) (composite of 4 types)	Angioid streaks, peau d'orange of retina, blue sclera, keratoconus, ret. detachment		Skin, vascular dis.; joint laxity; yellow rash; arterial rupture	AR, (AD)	
Marfan's syndrome	Dislocated lens (79%), gl., retinal detachment, strab. (20%), myopia		Tall stature, arachnodactyly, cardiac defects, hi arched palate	AD 15% sporadic	Chromosome 15
Ehlers-Danlos syndrome (composite of types)	Sublux. lens, hi myop, blue sclera, RD, angioid streaks		Cutis laxa, hypermobility of joints, hemorrhagic death, arterial dilation	AD, (AR), (XLR)	
Osteogenesis imperfecta (composite of types)	Blue sclera, hyperopia, gl., keratoconus, megalocornea, easy rupture of cornea	Deafness	Brittle bones, AI	AD/AR	
Menke's syndrome	Ret. degen., iris cysts, OA	Cerebellar signs, seizures	Steely, kinky hair; hypopigmentation; bone changes; arterial abn.; hypothermia; hypotonia	XLR	PND, mitochon. enzyme defect
Homocystinuria (several different genetic defects)	Subluxated lens, myopia, OA, cat., ret. pig. degen. in 1 type	MR, dev. delay	Marfanoid, accelerated arteriothromboembolism, osteoporosis, hypopigmentation, pulmonary and aortic stenosis	AR	Gen. anesth. may cause thromboembolism
Alcaptonuria	Pig. sclera and cornea		Degen. joint dis., atherosclerosis, cardiac valve dis., dark urine		
Pseudohyperparathyroidism	Lentic opac., strab., OA	MR, seizures, basal ganglia calcifications	Short stature and extremities		

TABLE 22–19. ABNORMALITIES OF ENDOCRINE METABOLISM

Disorder	Clinical Presentation		
	Ocular	CNS	Systemic
Pseudohyperparathyroidism	OA, nystagmus, cat.	MR, seizures, basal ganglia Ca^{++}	Calcifications, short stature and extremities
Thyroid disorders			
Thyroid orbitopathy	(See Chapter 18)		
Hypothyroidism	Ptosis, cat., K-sicca, EOM myotonia	Hearing dcs., myotonia	Lethargy, skin changes, hypothermia
Pituitary disorders	(See Chapter 6)		
Parathyroid disorders			
Hyperparathyroidism	Conj. Ca^{++}, band keratop.		
Hypoparathyroidism	K-conjunctivitis, blepharospasm, cat., PE	PTC	
Pancreatic disorder			
Diabetes mellitus	(See Chapter 21, Table 21–12)		

TABLE 22–20. RENAL DISORDERS

	Clinical Presentation	
Disorder	**Ocular**	**CNS**
Alport's syndrome	Cat., myopia, lenticonus, keratoconus, nystagmus, microspherophakia, drusen-like mac. changes	Deafness
Lowe's syndrome	Congen. cat., congen. gl., ret. pig. degen ON hypoplasia	MR
Marinesco-Sjögren syndrome	Congen. cat., nystagmus, strab., epicanth.	Ataxia, MR
Alström's syndrome	Ret. pig. degen, nystagmus	MR, deafness
Jeune's syndrome (asphyxiating thoracic dystrophy)	Retinal dystrophy	
Senior-Loken's syndrome	Ret. pig. degen.	Ataxia
Renal retinal dysplasia	Retinal dysplasia	Ataxia in some
Pseudohyperparathyroidism	Cat., nystagmus, OA	MR, seizures, basal ganglia Ca^{++}
Cystinuria	Ret. pig. degen.	Pyr. signs, deafness
Cystinosis (composite of types)	Crystals in cornea and conj., photophobia, patchy ret. depig., crystals in ret.	Cerebral atrophy
Oxalosis	Retinal crystals, orb. myositis	
Tyrosinemia II (Richner-Hanhart's syndrome)	Dendritic keratitis, lacrimation, photophobia	MR
Laurence-Moon's syndrome	RP	Spastic paraplegia
Bardet-Biedl's syndrome	RP, cat., OA; rare: oplegia	MR, paraplegia, misrouted VAP
Zellweger's syndrome and variants (infantile Refsum's disease, neonatal adrenoleukodystrophy, hyperpipecolic acidemia)	"Leopard-spot" RP, congen. cat., gl., ON hypoplasia	MR, hypotonia
Nail patella syndrome	Keratoconus	
Trisomy 13	Corneal opac., microp., colobomata, PHPV, cat., ON hypoplasia, ret. dysplasia, ant. seg., abn., intraocular cartilage	MR, holoprosenceph., microcep. dysgenesis
Sulfite oxidase Def.	Ectopia lentis, OA, spherophakia, strab.	MR, seizures, cerebral atrophy, spastic quadraparesis
Fabry's disease	Cornea verticillata (pigmented whorls), conjunctival and retinal telangiectasia, cataract (PSC), spokes	Paresthesias, painful crises, CVAs

Systemic	Heredity	Treatment	Other
Hemorrhagic nephritis	AD, (XLR)	Dialysis, transplant	
Aa uria, renal rickets, dwarfism, early death	XLR		
Skel anom.	AR		
Hypogonadism, obesity	AR		
Malformed rib cage; skeletal dysplasia; polydactyly; cystic kidney, liver, pancreas	AR		
Renal dysplasia, amino aciduria, hepatic fibrosis, skeletal anomalies	AR		Dcsd. ERG
Renal dysplasia	AR		Heterogenous
Short stature, alopecia, hypocalcemia, brachydactyly, calcifications			
Renal lithiasis	AR		
Renal rickets and failure, dwarfism, hypothyroidism	AR		
Nephrolithiasis and calcinosis, renal insufficiency	AR		
Painful keratotic skin lesions on palms and soles	AR		
Hypogonadism	AR		
Polydactyly, obesity, hypogenitalism, cardiac anom., renal anom.	AR		
Microcystic kidney, hepatic dysgenesis, aa uria, dysmorphic facies, deformed joints	AR		
Nephropathy	AD		
Cardiac defects, cleft palate, polydactyly, GU abn., hematol. abn., hemangiomas			
Renal stones	AR		
Angiokeratomas, heart disease, renal failure	XLR	Dilantin, Tegretol for pain, direct enzyme replacement?	PND

TABLE 22–21. DERMATOLOGIC ABNORMALITIES

Disorder	Clinical Presentation		
	Ocular	*CNS*	*Systemic*
Incontinentia pigmenti (Bloch-Sulzberger syndrome)	Uveitis, myopia, blue sclera, ret. vasc. changes, retrolental mass, RD, corneal opacities, OA, nystagmus, strab., pig. ret. degen., microp.	MR, seizures, spasticity, hydrocephalus, microcephaly	Blisters progress to hyperpig. skin lesions, abn. dentition, cardiac anomalies
ICHTHYOSIS			
Sjögren-Larsen syndrome	Mac. lesion, RP, "glistening spots," myopia	MR, spastic paresis, seizures	Ichthyosis, short stature, abn. of hair and teeth, skeletal dysplasia
Rud's syndrome Ichthyosis and crystalline maculopathy	RP, crystalline maculopathy strab., nystagmus, blepharospasm	MR, seizures, polyneurop., deafness	Ichthyosis, ichthyosis hypogonadism, dwarfism, abn. hair, teeth, nails
Refsum's disease	RP/OA, night blindness, cat. (50%), nystagmus, pupil changes	Hypertrophic polyneur., ataxia, deafness, anosmia, incsd. CSF protein	Ichthyosis, bone changes, ECG changes
Conradi's syndrome	Congen. cat., OA, heterochromia iridis	PMR	Ichthyosis, short stature, slipped epiphyses, heart defects
Ichthyosis and neutral lipid storage	Cat.	Deafness, myopathy, devel. delay, ataxia	
Tay's disease	Cat.	Microceph., ataxia, spasticity, Ca^{++} in basal ganglion	Hypogonadism, progeria, abn. hair
KID (keratitis, ichthyosis, deafness) syndrome	Keratitis, photophobia	Deafness	Ichthyosis, squamous cell Ca. of tongue, scanty hair, skin infections
Migratory ichthyosis neuro-ocular defects	Retinal colobomas	Seizures, cerebral atrophy, dcsd. hearing, MR	Abn. dermatoglyphics, typical facies
Anosmia, ichthyosis, hypogonadism	Congen. nystagmus, dcsd. VA, strab., hypopig. of iris, hypoplastic optic disc	Anosmia, mirror movements	Congen. ichthyosis, hypogonadism
FAIR SKIN AND HAIR			
Albinism (composite of forms)	Mac. dysplasia, nystagmus, strab., photophobia, no binoc. vision	Chiasmal crossing changes, cerebral atrophy	Light hair, skin
Cystinosis	Corneal and ret. crystals, ret. pig. degen.		Renal dysfxn, dwarfism

Key Diagnostic Finding	Hereditary	Treatment	Other
	Females, XLD?, lethal in males	Cryotherapy for retinal vascular tufts	Skin lesions present at birth
	AR		
	AR		
Incsd. serum phytanic acid	AR	Low phytanic acid diet	Dcsd. ERG
	AR, AD, XLR	—	—
Lipid granules in eosinophiles	AR	—	—
	AR		
Lysosomal enzyme def.?	AD	—	—
	AR	—	—
Dcsd. steroid sulfatase and arylsulfatase C	XLR	—	—
	XLR	—	—

(*Continues*)

TABLE 22–21. DERMATOLOGIC ABNORMALITIES (*cont.*)

	Clinical Presentation	
Disorder	*Ocular*	*CNS*
Lowe's syndrome (oculocerebral renal)	Congen. cat., gl.	MR
Tyrosinemia type II (Richner-Hanhart syndrome)	Dendritic keratitis	MR
PREMATURE AGING		
Rothmund-Thomson syndrome	Juv. cat. (75%), photophobia, microcornea and other corneal abn., spare brows and lashes	
Werner's syndrome	PSC cat (2nd–4th decades), RP, blue sclera, mac. degen., gl.	Muscle atrophy
Progeria	Prominent eyes, ret. vascular changes	MR, muscle atrophy
Cockayne's syndrome	RP, OA, cat., keratopathy, strab., nystagmus, resistant to mydriatics, photophobia	MR (severe), ataxia, deafness, seizures, microcephaly, intracranial Ca^{++}, normal pressure hydrocephalus, demyelination
Short syndrome	Rieger's anom.	Retarded speech
De Barsy's syndrome	Cloudy cornea, cat.	MR, hypotonia, athetosis
Atopic dermatitis	Ant. sub. cap. cat., keratoconus, RD	
Focal dermal hypoplasia (Goltz's syndrome)	Nystagmus, strab., microp., colobomata, sublux. lens	PMR
An(hypo)hidrotic ectodermal dysplasia	Keratopathy, photophobia, cat., spare lashes and brows, uveitis, strab., CR atrophy	
Epidermal nevus, Sebaceous nevus (linear nevus) (Jadassohn's anetoderma)	Dermoids	CNS anom.

Systemic	Hereditary	Other
Renal rickets, aa uria, hypotonia, dwarfism		
Painful keratotic skin lesions on palms and soles	AR	ED
Poikiloderma, hypogonadism, short stature, skeletal anomalies	AR	
Scleroderma, accelerated atherosclerosis, sparse gray hair, short stature, DM, hypogonadism, skin ulcers, neoplasia, birdlike facies, cardiomyopathy	AR	Cat. surg. causes corneal degen. and wound dehiscence; phenotypic copy of aging
Sparse hair, accelerated atherosclerosis, hypogonadism, DM, thin skin or subcut. fat, skull hypoplasia		
Dwarfism, sparse gray hair, atherosclerosis, sun sensitivity	AR	PND, dcsd. ERG, senile cat. at 2–4 YO
Short stature, micrognathia	AR	
Cutix laxa, short stature	Sporadic AR	
Linear hyperpig.; skel., nail, and hair abn.	XLD?	Cat. surg. often complicated
Sweating absent, heat intolerance, abn. hair and teeth	XLR	
Linear nevi, skull deform.	Nonhered.	(See Chapter 21, Table 1)

(*Continues*)

TABLE 22–21. DERMATOLOGIC ABNORMALITIES (*cont.*)

Disorder	Clinical Presentation		
	Ocular	**CNS**	**Systemic**
Basal cell nevus (Gorlin's syndrome)	Cat., OA, colobomata, strab., lid and periorb. tumors, gl., hypertel.	MR, absent corp. callosum, Ca++ falx, medulloblastoma	Basal cell Ca., other neoplasms, broad face, odontogenic cysts, palmer and plantar pits
Juvenile xanthogranuloma (JXG)	JXG in orbit or iris, hyphema, heterochromia		
Xeroderma pigmentosa	Photophobia; c-itis; blepharitis; keratitis; tumors of lids, conj., cornea, and periorb.; MM; orb. malig.; loss of lashes; ectropion	Microceph., choreoath., MR, deafness, seizures, areflexic	Erythematous, pigmented, telangiectalic, and neoplastic skin changes; light sensitivity; keratoacanthomas
Bloom's syndrome	C-itis, conj. telang., p. pole drusen		Photosensitivity, dwarfism, malignancy, resp. and GI infection, immune defect
Multiple hamartoma neoplasia (Cowden's disease)	Cat., gl., ret. hamartomas, ret. drusen, angioid streaks		Malign. papules, keratoses
Malignant atrophic papulosis (Dego's disease)	Conj. papules, telangiectasia, retinal, CR lesions; OA, VFDs	CNS infarcts	Skin papules, peritonitis (fatal)
Urbach-Wiethe's disease	Lid papules (string of beads), conj.-yellow nodules, mac. degen., drusen		Chronic infections, hoarseness
Hypomelanosis of Ito	Strab., OA, microp., nystagmus, hypertel., corneal opacity, choroidal atrophy	MR, seizures	Linear hypopigmentation of skin, musculoskeletal deformities
Hallermann-Streiff's syndrome	Congen. cat., microp., nystagmus, strab., colobomata, blue sclera, ret. pig. degen.	PMR	Craniofacial, dental abn.; hypotrichosis; bird's-head dyscephaly; dwarfism
Fabry's disease	Tort. conj. and ret. vessels, cornea verticillata cat. (PSC)	Painful crises, CVAs	Angiokeratomas, cardiovasc. dis., renal failure
Fucosidosis type III	Corneal opacities, cat., tort. conj. and ret. vessels	MR, deafness	Angiokeratomas (Fabry-like), dysostosis, pulmonary infections, coarse facies
Hyperlipoproteinemias	Xanthelasma, corneal arcus, lipemia ret.		Xanthomas
Farber's disease	CRS, gray mac., RP, conj. xanthomas		Xanthomas, inflammatory arthro-hoarseness
Ataxia telangiectasia (Loùis-Bar's syndrome)	Cong. telang., nystagmus, strab., supranuc. EM disorder	Ataxia, dystonia	Telangiectasis, immune def., reticuloendothelial neoplasia
Waardenburg's syndrome	Heterochromia iridis, poliosis, dystropia canthorum, albinotic fundi	Cochlear deafness	White forelock, leukoderma, premature graying
Pseudoxanthoma	Angioid streaks		Skin, vascular dis.
Elasticum (PXE) (composite of 4 types)	Angioid streaks, peau d'orange of retina, blue sclera, keratoconus, ret. detachment		Joint laxity, yellow rash, arterial rupture
Ehlers-Danlos syndrome (composite of types)	Sublux. lens, hi myop, blue sclera, RD, angioid streaks		Cutis lava, hypermobility of joints, hemorrhagic death, arterial dilation
Familial dysautonomia (Riley-Day's syndrome)	Dcsd. corneal sensation, alacrima, corneal ulcers, pupil abn., XT, myopia, OA, ret. vasc. tort.	Hypotonia, P+T sense decreased, pyr. changes, cerebellar signs, Parkinsonism	Respiratory, feeding difficulties; blotchy skin, orthostatic hypotension, episodic hypertension, aspiration pneumonia, fractures, scoliosis, absence of fungi form papillae on tongue

Key Diagnostic Finding	Hereditary	Treatment	Other
	AD		
	AR		Defective DNA repair (clastogenic)
	AR		Clastogenic
	AD		
	Nonhered.		
	(AD?)		
Decreased alpha-galactosidase A	XLR	Dilantin, Tegretol for pain, direct enzyme replacement	PND
	AR		Chromosome 1, PND
(See Chapter 21 Table 7 for details) Dcsd. acid ceramidase	AR		Death in childhood, PND
	AR		
	AD		
	AR (AD)		
	AD, (AR), (XLR)		
	AR	Bethanecal (parasympathomimetic)	Abn. VEPs in 80%

CHAPTER 23

SYSTEMIC DISORDERS OF NEURO-OPHTHALMIC INTEREST BY PART OF EYE INVOLVED

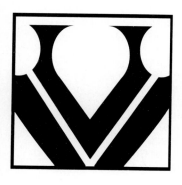

TABLE 23–1. DISORDERS AFFECTING SKIN/LIDS

Type of Lesion Involved	Clinical Presentation				
	Disorder	**Other Ocular Signs**	**CNS**	**Systemic**	**Other**
ICHTHYOSIS					
	Refsum's disease	RP, OA, night blindness, cat., nystagmus, pupil changes	Ataxia, hypertrophic polyneurop., deafness, incsd. CSF protein, MR	Cardiac arrythmia, bone changes	See Chapter 21 Table 7
	Rud's syndrome	RP, strab., ptosis, nystagmus, blepharospasm	MR, seizures, deafness, polyneurop.	Hypogonad; DM; dwarfism; abn. hair, teeth, nails	—
	Sjögren-Larsson's syndrome	Mac. degen., glistening dots, ret. pig. degen., myopia	MR, spastic diplegia, seizures	Short stature; abn. hair, teeth, nails; hypogonadism	—
	Conradi's syndrome	Congen. cat., OA	PMR	Slipped epiphyses, other bone abn., heart defects	—
	KID (Keratitis, ichthyosis, deafness) syndrome	Keratitis, photophobia	Deafness	Squamous cell Ca. of tongue, scanty hair, skin infections	—
	Ichthyosis and neutral lipid storage	Cat.	Deafness, myopathy, devel. delay, ataxia		—
	Tay's disease	Cat.	Microceph., ataxia, spasticity, Ca^{++} in basal ganglion		—
	PREMATURE AGING				
	Progeria	Prominent eyes, ret. vasc. changes	Muscle atrophy, MR	DM, short stature, micrognathia, alopecia, resorption of phalanges and clavicles, accelerated atherosclerosis	See Chapter 21 Table 19
	Cockayne's syndrome	OA, RP, cat., cor. clouding, resistance to mydriatics, strab., photophobia	MR (severe), microceph., deafness, ataxia, seizures, intracranial Ca^{++}, demyelination, N pressure hydroceph.	Dwarfism, sun sensitivity, sparse gray hair, atherosclerosis	
	Rothmund-Thomson syndrome	Juv. cat., corneal abn.—microcornea; strab.; photophobia; spare brows and lashes		Short stature, hypogonadism, bone and skin abn., poikiloderma	
	Werner's syndrome	Cat., blue sclerae, ret. pig. degen.		Short stature, skin changes, ulcers	Sx. in 2nd decade; cat. surg. leads to complications

Type of Lesion Involved	Clinical Presentation				
	Disorder	*Other Ocular Signs*	*CNS*	*Systemic*	*Other*
DEPOSITS					
Xanthelasma	Hyperlipidemias	Arcus, lipemia ret.		Xanthomas, atherosclerosis	See Chapter 21 Table 7
PIGMENT CHANGES					
Vitiligo	Vogt-Koyanagi-Harada syndrome	Uveitis, RD, ret. pig. changes	Deafness, tinnitus, meningoenceph., incsd. CSF cells	Poliosis, alopecia	—
Hypopigmentation	Albinism	Foveal dysplasia, nystagmus	Abn. VAPs, abn. CNS paths		See Chapter 21 Table 14
TUMORS					
	VRNF (NF-1)	Lisch nodules; glioma of ON, chiasm; plexiform neuroma of lid, orbit; gl.; pulsating exophthalmos; sphenoid bone changes; hypertrophic corneal nerves; MM of iris	Plexiform neuromas, acoustic neuromas, meningiomas	Axillary freckles, café-au-lait spots, plexiform neuromas, neuromas, pulmonic stenosis, aortic coarctation, pheochromocytoma	—
	BANF (NF-2)	Cat.	Bilat. acoustic neuromas in teens	Less prominent skin changes, other tumors	—
	Multiple mucosal neuromas				—
Adenoma sebaceum (angiofibromas)	Tuberous sclerosis	Ret. astrocytic hamartomas	Ca^{++}, MR, seizures, subependymal hamartomas	Ashleaf spots, ungual fibromas, dysplasia in most organ systems, Shagreen patches	—
Hemangiomas	Von Hippel–Lindau's disease	Ret. hemangiomas (50%), exudates, RD	Cerebellar hemangioma (60%)	Other hemangiomas, cysts, hypernephroma, pheochromocytoma	—
	Disseminated hemangiomatosis	Lid, ret. hemangiomatosis	Cavernous skin, hemangiomas	Visceral hemangiomas	—
Angiomas	Sturge-Weber's syndrome	Choroid hemangioma (40%) Congen. gl. assoc. with lid angioma	Angioma of meninges, seizures, "train track" Ca^{++}, MR	Port wine stain, esp. V_1; hemihypertrophy; angiomas in many organs	—
	Klippel-Trenaunay-Weber's syndrome	May have Sturge-Weber-like ocular and CNS component		Extensive hemangiomas and hypertrophy	—
	Hereditary hemorrhagic telangiectasia (Osler's, Weber's, Rendu's syndromes)	Angiomas of lids, conj.	Angiomas of CNS	Angiomas of skin, epistaxis, GI/GU bleeds	—
Blue nevus	Blue rubber bleb nevus	Hemangiomas of conj., iris, retina, chiasm; blue nevi of lids	Cav. hemang., CNS	Cav. hemang. skin, mucous membranes; GI hemorrhage, blue nevi	—

(Continues)

TABLE 23–1. DISORDERS AFFECTING SKIN/LIDS (*cont.*)

Type of Lesion Involved	Clinical Presentation				
	Disorder	*Other Ocular Signs*	*CNS*	*Systemic*	*Other*
Linear nevus	Epidermal nevus (Sebaceous nevus of Jadassohn)	Linear nevi of lids, colobomas, limbal dermoids, ON hypoplasia	Seizures, MR	Linear nevi, tumors	—
Lentigenes	Ocular spots/myxoma/ endocrine excess	Lid lentigenes, lid myxomas, caruncle lesions	Pit. ad.	Myxomas, inc. cardiac; lentigenes; endocrine overactivity	—
MALIGNANT TUMORS	Xeroderma pigmentosa	Conjunctivitis, photophobia, keratitis	Microcephaly, MR, areflexia	Blistering, carcinomas	—
	Basal cell nevus syndrome	Basal cell. ca., corneal dystrophy, cat., glaucoma, strab., colobomata	Ca^{++}	Basal cell ca., other tumors, broad face, abn. teeth, verteb. abn., genital infantilism	—
	Incontinentia pigmenti (Bloch-Sulzberger syndrome) retrolental mass, uveitis, OA, RD, ret. pig. degen., strab.		MR, seizures, spasticity	Skin lesions, hyperpig., growths; hypoplasia of hair; dental abn.	—
	Juvenile xanthogranu-lomatosis	Lid/iris nodules, hyphema		Xanthogranulomas of skin	—
	Multiple hamartoma-Neoplasia (Cowden's disease)	Cat., gl. ret. glioma, ret. drusen		Mucosal papil-lomas, facial papules, malig-nancies of breast and thyroid	—
	Epidermal nevus (Sebaceous nevus of Jadassohn)	Limbal dermoids, colobomas, ON hypoplasia(?), linear nevi of lids	Seizures, MR	Linear nevi, tumors	—
GRANULOMAS, PAPULES	Urbach-Weithe's disease	Yellow conj. nodules (gray/white string of beads), posterior pole drusen, ret. pig. degen., mac. degen.	CNS abn.	Skin and muc. membrane lesions, hoarseness	—
MALFORMATIONS COLOBOMAS	Epidermal nevus syndrome (Sebaceous nevus of Jadassohn)'s syndrome	Limbal dermoids, ON hypoplasia, linear nevi of lids	Seizures, MR	Linear nevi, tumors	—
	Goldenhar/ hemifacial microsomia	Limbal dermoids, orbital lipodermoids, Duane's syndrome (?)	Deafness	Ear dysplasia, preauricular skin tags, fused cervi-cal vertebrae, cardiac and other systemic abnormalties, maxillary hypoplasia	—

Type of Lesion Involved	Clinical Presentation				
	Disorder	*Other Ocular Signs*	*CNS*	*Systemic*	*Other*
	Treacher-Collins'-Fransheschetti syndrome	Antimongoloid lids, strabismus	Deafness	Maxillary hypoplasia, hypoplasia, large mouth, ear and heart defects	—
	Hallerman-Streiff's syndrome	Cat., microp., nystagmus, strab., blue sclera	PMR	Dwarfism, skull and face mal., dental anom., hypoptrichosis, ectodermal dysplasia	—
	Chromosomal abn.	(Colobomas very frequent in dysgenetic syndromes)			See Chapter 21 Table 20
Other	Familial amyloidosis	Vitreous opacity	CNS, cr. nn. abn.		—
Xanthelasma	Hyperlipoproteinemia types III and IV				See Chapter 21 Table 8
Xanthoma	Farber's disease	CRS, gray ma., ret. pig. degen., conjunc. xanthomas	Xanthomas, inflammatory arthropathy, hoarseness		Death in childhood, PND

TABLE 23–2. DISORDERS AFFECTING CONJUNCTIVA

Type of Lesion Involved	Clinical Presentation				
	Disorder	*Other Ocular Signs*	*CNS*	*Systemic*	*Other*
VASCULAR ALTERATIONS					
Conjunctival telangiectasis	Ataxia-telangiectasia (Louis-Bar's syndrome)	Nystagmus, supranuc. EM disorders, apraxia of saccades	Truncal ataxia, progressive cerebellar degen., choreoathelosis	Malignancies, esp. leuk/lymphoma (10%); humoral immune defect; recurrent pulmonary infections	Death in teens, incsd. alpha-fetal protein, CEA, PND
	Fabry's disease	Corneal verticillata, ret. telangiectasia	Parasthesias, painful crises, CVAs	Angiokeratomas, heart disease, renal failure	—
Tortuous conjunctival vessels	Fucosidosis	Tor. ret. vessels, cat., corneal opacity	MR, deafness	Angiokeratomas (Fabry-like), dysostosis	—
Arterialized conjunctival veins	Carotid cavernous fistula	Red eye, gl., engorged ret. veins	Bruit, CNS sx.		—
	Farber's disease	Conjunctival xanthoma, CRS, gray mac.		Xanthoma, inflammatory arthropathy, hoarseness	—
Hemangioma of lid and face	Klippel-Trenaunay-Weber's syndrome	May have Sturge-Weber-like ocular and CNS component		Extensive hemangiomas and hypertrophy	—
Lid angioma	Sturge-Weber's syndrome	Choroidal hemangioma (40%), congen. gl. with lid angioma	Angioma of meninges, seizures, "train track" Ca^{++}, MR		—
	Osler-Weber-Rendu's disease	Angioma of lids, conj.	CNS, angioma	Angioma of skin, epistaxis, Gi/Gu bleeds	—
Sludging	Hemoglobinopathies				
	Sickle cell disease	Ret. vasc. changes	Cerebrovasc. occ.	Sickle crisis infarcts	See Chapter 3
	Waldenström's disease	Conj. crystals, ret. vasc. abn.	Neurol. signs	Proliferation of B-lymphocytes/ plasma cells, bone pain, renal failure, parapro-teinemia, incsd. blood viscosity	—
	Multiple myeloma	Orbital tumor, ret. vasc. abn.		Bone lesions, hyperviscosity	—
CONJUNCTIVITIS	Reiter's syndrome	Keratitis, uveitis, episcleritis, secondary corneal changes, iridocyclitis		Urethritis, arthritis, "psoriatric" skin lesions	—
	Behçet's disease	Hypotony or iritis, ret. vascular changes		Venous occlusion, necrotizing folliculitis, aphthous ulcers of mouth and genitalia	—
	Xeroderma pigmentosa	Photophobia, keratitis	Microcephaly, MR, areflexia	Blistering carcinomas	—

Type of Lesion Involved	Clinical Presentation				
	Disorder	*Other Ocular Signs*	*CNS*	*Systemic*	*Other*
	Acrodermatitis enteropathia			Diarrhea, dermatitis, alopecia	Rx—iodoquin
	Lysosomal storage disorders	(diagnosed by conjunctival biopsy)			See Chapter 21 Tables 8–11
Abnormal Deposits					
	Wiskott-Aldrich's syndrome	Periorbit and conj. bleeding, ret. hemorrhage		Purpura, immune deficiency	—
Nodules	Urbach-Wiethe's disease	Yellow nodules, post. pole drusen, mac. degen.	CNS abn.	Skin and muc. membrane lesions, hoarseness	—
Crystals					
	Cystinosis	Crystals in conj., cornea, retina; photophobia; ret. pig. degen.	Cerebral atrophy	Renal rickets and failure, dwarfism	—
	Hypophosphatasia	Calcium deposits			See Table 23–4
Pigmentation	Gaucher's disease				See Chapter 21 Table 8
White Conjunctiva	Tyrosinemia type II	Dendritic keratitis, lacrimation, photophobia	MR	Painful keratotic skin lesions on palms and soles	ED
	Waldenström's disease	Conj. crystals, ret. vasc. abn.		Proliferation of B-lymphocytes/ plasma cells, bone pain, renal failure, paraproteinemia, incsd. blood viscosity, vascular occlusion	—

TABLE 23–3. DISORDERS AFFECTING THE CORNEA

Type of Lesion Involved	Clinical Presentation				
	Disorder	*Other Ocular Signs*	*CNS*	*Systemic*	*Other*
Clouding	Lysosomal storage diseases (gangliosidoses, sphingolipidoses, mucolipidoses, mucopolysaccharidoses, neuronal ceroid lipofucsinoses)	Mac. changes, OA, ret. pig. degen.			See Chapter 21 Tables 8–11
	Gyrate atrophy (hyperornithinemia)	Gyrate atrophy of choroid, myopia (90%), night blindness, PSC cat. (40%)			See Chapter 21 Table 11
	LCAT insufficiency	Corneal deposits, arcus in heterozygote		Renal disease, anemia, atherosclerosis	Test pts. with presenile arcus
	Congenital rubella	Salt-and-pepper ret. pig. changes, cat., gl., microphthalmos	MR, deafness	Cardiac anom.	See Chapter 22 Tables 10–16
	Tangier disease	Ptosis, EOM palsy	Peripheral neuropathy	Hyperplastic orange tonsils	See Chapter 21
	Niemann-Pick's disease	CRS, OA, corneal clouding, cat.	MR, PMR, seizures, gaze palsies	Anemia, HSM, pulmonary infiltrates, foam cells in marrow	PND; see Chapter 21
Keratoconus	Down's syndrome	Upslanting palp. fissures, esotropia (35%), cataract (60%), Brushfield spots (85%), myopia	MR	Short stature, cardiac abn., broad hands and feet, leukemia	Sensitivity to atropine
	Marfan's syndrome	Retinal detachment, strab. (20%), myopia, dislocated lens (79%), gl.		Tall stature, arachnodactyly, cardiac defects, hi arched palate	—
	Rieger's syndrome	Ant. chamber dysgen., microcornea with opacity, iris hypoplasia, ant. synechia, gl.		Dental abn., anal stenosis	Linkage with myotonic dystrophy
	Focal dermal hypoplasia (Gorlin-Goltz syndrome)	Nystagmus, strab., microp., colobomata, sublux. lens	PMR	Linear hyperpig.; skin, nail, and hair abn.	—
	Apert's syndrome	OA (25%) proptosis	PMR	Syndactyly, heat intolerance, abn. hair and teeth	—
	Crouzon's disease	Proptosis, strab., PE, OA (80%)	Hydrocephalus	PDA, coarctation	—
	Ostegenesis imperfecta	Blue sclera, hyperopia, gl., megalocornea, easy rupture	Deafness	Brittle bones, AI	—

Type of Lesion Involved	Clinical Presentation				
	Disorder	*Other Ocular Signs*	*CNS*	*Systemic*	*Other*
Megalocornea	Lowe's syndrome	Congen. cat., RP, ON hypoplasia	MR	Aa uria, renal rickets, dwarfism, early death	—
	Marfan's syndrome	Ret. detachment, strab. (20%), myopia, dislocated lens (79%)		Tall stature, arachnodactyly, cardiac defects	—
	Pierre-Robin's syndrome	High myopia, gl., ret. detachment, strab., congen. cat.		Cleft palate, mandibular hypoplasia, glossoptosis, feeding problems	—
	Congenital rubella	Cat., "salt-and-pepper" ret. pig. changes, microphthalmos, gl.	Deafness, MR	Cardiac anom.	—
	Sturge-Weber syndrome	Choroid hemang. (40%), Congen. gl. assoc. with lid angioma	Angioma of leptomeninges, seizures, "train track" Ca^{++}, MR	Port wine stain, esp. V_1; hemihypertrophy	Lesions congenital
	Trisomy 13	Ret. dysplasia, cat., ant. segment dysgenesis, ON hypoplasia	MR, microcephaly, corneal opacity, micropthalmos, colobomata, PHPV, intracular cartilage	Cardiac defects, GU abn., cleft palate, polydactyly, hematol. abn., hemangiomas	Death in 1st months, 1/15,000
Microcornea	Chromosome 18 deletion	Microcornea, nystagmus, DA, colobomata, ret. pig. degen.	Microceph., MR	Short stature	—
	Ehlers-Danlos syndrome	Sublux. lens, hi myop., blue sclera, RD, angioid streaks		Cutis laxa, hypermobility of joints, hemorrhagic death, arterial dilation	—
	Hallermann-Streiff-François syndrome	Congen. cat., microp., nystagmus, blue sclera		Mandibular and maxillary hypoplasia ectodermal dysplasia, hypotrichosis, dwarfism, dental anomalies, characteristic facies	Feeding problems
	Laurence-Moon syndrome	Ret. pig. degen.	Spastic paraplegia	Hypogonadism	—
	Bardet-Biedl syndrome	Ret. pig. degen.; rarely: o'plegia, cataract, OA	Paraplegia, MR, misrouted VAP	Polydactyly, obesity, hypogenitalism, cardiac anom., renal anom.	ERG dcsd.
	Congenital rubella	Cat., gl., microphthalmos, "salt-and-pepper" ret. pigmentary changes	Deafness, MR	Cardiac defects	—

(Continues)

TABLE 23–3. DISORDERS AFFECTING THE CORNEA (cont.)

Type of Lesion Involved	Clinical Presentation				
	Disorder	*Other Ocular Signs*	*CNS*	*Systemic*	*Other*
Hyperplastic Corneal Nerves	VRNF (NF-1)	Iris—Lisch nodules; ON, chiasm glioma; plexiform neuroma of orb., lid; glaucoma; pulsating exophthal.; sphenoid bone changes; MM of iris	Plexiform neuromas, meningiomas	Cut: axillary freckles, café-au-lait spots (>5mm); plexiform neuromas	Incsd. nerve growth factor
	Multiple endocrine neoplasia II (MEN)		Pit. adenoma	Characteristic facies, thyroid Ca., pheochromocytoma, parathyroid adenoma, skeletal anom.	—
	Leprosy	Corneal opac. and ulcer, loss of lashes	Cr. nn; periph. neurop.	Lionine facies, anesthesia, skin changes	—
Decreased Sensation/Scarring (Frequent in diseases that disturb lid function, tear function)	Familial dysautonomia (Riley-Day's syndrome)	Dcsd. corneal sensation, ulcers, alacrima, XT, myopia, pupil abn., OA, ret. vasc. tort.	Hypotonia, dcsd. P+T sensation, pyr. changes, cerebellar signs, Parkinsonism	Resp. and feeding difficulties, orthostatic hypotension, episodic hypertension	—
	(An)hypoectodermal dysplasia	Keratopathy, photophobia, cat., spare lashes and brows, uveitis, strab., CR atrophy		Hypohydrosis, hypotrichiasis, defective teeth, absent sweating, heat intolerance	—
Dermoids	Duane's syndrome	Strab., limbal dermoids, orbital lipodermoids, colobomata	Deafness	Dysplasia of ear, preauricular skin tags, fused cervical vertebrae, cardiac and other systemic abnormalities, mandibular hypoplasia	—
	Hemifacial microsomia	Limbal dermoids	Dysplasia of ear		
	Goldenhar's syndrome	Orbital lipodermoids, colobomata, Duane's syndrome (?)		Preauricular skin tags, fused cervical vertebrae, cardiac and other systemic abnormalities, mandibular hypoplasia	—
	Epidermal nevus, (Sebaceous nevus of Jadassohn)	Limbal dermoids, colobomas, ON hypoplasia, linear nevi of lids	Seizures, MR	Linear nevi, tumors	—

Type of Lesion Involved	Clinical Presentation				
	Disorder	*Other Ocular Signs*	*CNS*	*Systemic*	*Other*
DRUG TOXICITY	Amiodarone				—
	Amantadine				—
	Chloroquine				—
Opacities	Berardinelli-Siep disease		MR, muscular hypertrophy, hypothalamic hamartomas	Lipodystrophy, hyperlipemia, hepatomegaly, acanthosis nigricans, DM	—
Arcus	Hyperlipopro- teinemias				
	Type III	Xanthelasma, corneal dystrophy		Accelerated atherosclerosis, tuberous xanthomas, DM	See Tables 21–7
	Type IV	Lipemia ret., xanthelasma		Eruptive xanthoma, angina pectoris (40%), HSM (rare), DM, gout	See Table 21–7
	LCAT insuf.	Corneal deposits, arcus in heterozygote		Renal disease, anemia	Test pts. with presenile arcus
	Hyperlipoproteinemia type III				
	Fucosidoses	Tort. conj. and ret. vessels, cat.	MR, deafness	Angiokeratomas (Fabry-like), dysostosis	—
Herpetiform Lesion	Tyrosinemia (Richner-Hanhart disease)	Cat.	MR, PMR	Hyperkeratotic skin lesions	Chapter 21 Table 14
Interstitial Keratitis	Congenital syphilis	Pig. retinopathy	Deafness	Notched incisors, bone changes, saddle nose	See Chapter 22 Tables 10–16
Cornea Verticillata (Wheel-like epithelial dystrophy)	Fabry's disease	Conj. and ret. telangiectasia, cat.	Paraesthesias, painful crises	Angiokeratomas, heart disease, renal failure	Similar changes in amiodarone, amantidine, and chloroquine toxicity
Crystals	Cystinosis	Photophobia, crystals in cornea and conj., patchy retinal depigmentation	Cerebral atrophy	Renal rickets and failure, dwarfism	PND by conjunctival bx., retinal change may precede symptoms
	Multiple myeloma	Orbital tumor, ret. vasc. abn.		Bone lesions, hyperviscosity	—
	Osteogenesis imperfecta	Blue sclera, hyperopia, gl., keratoconus, megalocornea, easy rupture	Deafness	Brittle bones, AI	—
Pigment	Alcaptonuria	Scleral pig.		Arthritis, dark urine, joint disease	—
Kayser-Fleischer Ring	Wilson's disease	Sunflower cat. (20%), EM abn.	Ataxia, basal ganglia symptoms	Liver failure, hemolytic crisis	—

(*Continues*)

TABLE 23–3. DISORDERS AFFECTING THE CORNEA (*cont.*)

Type of Lesion Involved	Clinical Presentation				
	Disorder	*Other Ocular Signs*	*CNS*	*Systemic*	*Other*
Deformity	Ehlers-Danlos syndrome	Sublux. lens, hi myop., blue sclera, RD		Cutis laxa, arterial dilation, hyper-mobile joints, hemorrhagic diathesis	—
Anterior Segment Dysgenesis	Rieger's syndrome	GI.			—
	Alagille	Post. embryotoxon., ectopic pupils, subcap. cat., band keratop-athy, kerato-conus, myopia, strab., ret. pig. degen. (mild)		Neonatal jaundice, cholestasis, HSM, typical facies, congen. heart disease	—
	Short syndrome	Rieger's anomalies	Retarded speech	Short stature, premature aging, micrognathia	—
Sclerocornea	Partial trisomy 10$_q$	Abn. disks, yellow post. pole deposits, hyper-telorism, anti-monogoloid lids, microcephthalmia, ptosis, cat., sclerocornea	PMR, microceph.	Heart defects, mictognathia, cleft palate, abn. hands and feet	—
Nonspecific Corneal Changes	An(hypo)-hidrotic ectodermal dysplasia (Goltz)	Photophobia, cat., strab., spare lashes and brows, uveitis, CR atrophy		Hypohydrosis, hypotrichosis, defective dentition	—

TABLE 23–4. DISORDERS AFFECTING THE SCLERA

Type of Lesion Involved	Clinical Presentation				
	Disorder	*Other Ocular Signs*	*CNS*	*Systemic*	*Other*
Blue Sclera	Osteogenesis imperfecta	Hyperopia, gl., k-conus, megalocornea, easy rupture	Deafness	Brittle bones, AI	See Chapter 22 Table 18
	Ehlers-Danlos syndrome	Sublux. lens, high myop., RD		Hemorrhage	See Chapter 22 Table 18
	Hallerman-Streiff-François syndrome	Cat., microp., strab.	PMR	Dwarfism, skull and face mal., dental anom., hypotrichosis, ectodermal dysplasia	—
	Turner's syndrome	Epicanthal folds, ptosis, strab., cat., PE, proptosis		Short stature, webbed neck, facial and skull anom., hypogonadism	—
	Hyperphosphatasia (juvenile Paget's disease)	OA, pig, ret., angioid streaks		Large head, dwarfism, fragile bones, deformities	—
	Hypophosphatasia	Band keratopathy, conj. Ca^{++}, cataract, papilledema	Complications of craniostenosis, muscle weakness	Fine hair, met. acidosis, hyper Ca^{++}, craniostenosis, rarefication of bones	See Chapter 21 Table 14
	Werner's syndrome	Cat., ret. pig. degen.		Short stature, skin changes, ulcers	See Chapter 21 Table 19 cat. extraction complications,
	Alcaptonuria	Brown/black pig. between limbus and muscle insertion		Atherosclerosis, cardiac valve, joint dis.	Diff. diagnosis: MM; use of antimalarial meds.
Ulcers	Hartnup's disease	Ectropion, nystagmus	Cerebellar ataxia, MR	Aa uria, pellagra-like rash	—

TABLE 23–5. GLAUCOMA

Type of Lesion Involved	Clinical Presentation				
	Disorder	Other Ocular Signs	CNS	Systemic	Other
Glaucoma	Lysosomal Storage Defects				
	MPS				
	Hunter's syndrome (MPS II)	RP, OA	MR, deafness, hydroceph.	Dysostosis, coronary art. dis., cardiac valve dis.	—
	Hurler's syndrome (MPS I)	Corneal opac., RP, OA	MR	Gargoyle facies, dysostosis, dwarfism, cardiovasc. abn., coronary art. dis., cardiac valve dis.	—
	PHAKOMATOSES				
	Neurofibromatosis (VRNF, VF-1)	Iris—Lisch nodules; ON, chiasm glioma; plexiform neuroma of orbit, lid; pulsating exophthal.; sphenoid bone changes; hypertrophic corneal nerves; MM of iris	Plexiform neuromas, meningiomas	Cut: axillary freckles, café-au-lait spots (>5mm); plexiform neuromas, pulmonic stenosis, AO, pheochromo-cytoma	Incsd. nerve growth factor
	Sturge-Weber's syndrome	Choroid hemang. (40%), congen. gl. assoc. with lid angioma	"Train track" angioma of leptomeninges, seizures, Ca⁺⁺, MR	Port wine stain, esp. V_1; hemihypertrophy; angiomas in many organs	Nonfamilial lesion
	Klippel-Trenaunay-Weber's syndrome			Extensive hemangiomas and hemihypertrophy	Sprinal variant of Sturge-Weber syndrome (?), may have S-W-like ocular and CNS findings
	MEN			Thyroid Ca., adrenal Ca., pheochromo-cytoma, parathyroid adenoma, Cushing's disease	Detect on chromosome 10, PND, early thyroidectomy curative for T_4 ca.
	Other				
	Homocystinuria (composite of forms)	Ectopia lentis, myopia, RP, (in methyl melanic acidemia form), OA	MR, developmental delay	Marfanoid habitus, thromboembolism, hypopigmentation, accelerated atherosclerosis, pulmonary and aortic dilation	Gen. anesth. dangerous
	Marfan's syndrome	Dislocated lens (79%), RD, strab. (20%), myopia		Tall stature, arachnodactyly, cardiac defects	—
	Marchesani's syndrome	Dislocated lens, spherophakia		Short stature	—

Type of Lesion Involved	Clinical Presentation				
	Disorder	*Other Ocular Signs*	*CNS*	*Systemic*	*Other*
FACIAL DYSGENESIS					
	Pierre-Robin's syndrome	High myopia, congen. cat., strab., RD	MR	Cleft palate, mandibular hypoplasia, glossoptosis, feeding problems	—
	Hallerman-Strieff-François syndrome	Cat., microp., nystagmus		Mandibular hypoplasia, ectodermal dysplasia, hypotrichosis, feeding problems	
CHROMOSOMAL DISORDERS					
	Trisomy 18	Corneal opacity, microp., coloboma, cat., blepharophomosis, ant. seg. dys., ret. folds, PHPH, intraocular cartilage, ret. dysplasia, ON hypoplasia	MR	Cardiac defects, GU abn., cleft palate, polydactyly, hemat. abn., hemangiomas, holoprosencephaly, microcephaly	—
	Chromosome 18—del. of long arm	Microcornea, nystagmus, OA, colobomata, ret. pig. degen.	Microceph., MR	Short stature	—
	Trisomy 13	Microp., coloboma	MR, holoprosencephaly	Cleft lip/palate, polydactyly, congen. heart disease	—
	Trisomy 21	Mongoloid lids, esotropia (35%), cat. (60%), Brushfield spots (85%), keratoconus, myopia	MR	Short stature, characteristic facies, cardiac abn., broad hands and feet, leukemia	*Sensitivity to Atropine, extra chromosome 95% maternal
	Chrom 18 deletion	Microphthalmos, hypertelorism, ptosis, post. keratoconus, corneal opacities, cat., ret. pig. degn., OA, deep-set eyes, coloboma	MR, CNS anom.	Short stature	—
Disorders of Lipid Metabolism					
	Zellweger's syndrome, neonatal leukodys. inf. Refsum's disease, hyperpipecolic acidemia	"Leopard spot" ret. pig. degen., congen. cat., ON hypoplasia, OA, nystagmus	MR	Microcystic kidney, hepatic dysgenesis, aa uria, typical facies	—

(Continues)

TABLE 23–5. GLAUCOMA (*cont.*)

Type of Lesion Involved	Clinical Presentation				
	Disorder	*Other Ocular Signs*	*CNS*	*Systemic*	*Other*
	Homocystinuria	Ectopia lentis, gl., ret. pig. degen., myopia, RD, OA	MR	Thromboembolism, osteoporosis, hypopigmentation	Gen. anesthesia
	Lowe's syndrome	Congen. cat., RP, ON hypoplasia	MR	Aa uria, congen. renal rickets, dwarfism, early death	—
	Carotid cavernous fistula (CCF)	Conj. arterialized veins	Bruits		—
	Focal dermal hypoplasia (Goltz Gorlin's syndrome)	Nystagmus, strab., microphthalmos, colobomata, subluxed lens	PMR	Linear hyperpig.; skeletal, nail, and hair abn.	—
	Juvenile xanthogranuloma (JXG)	Iris lesions, hyphema, lid papules			Yellow papules regress spontaneously
	Hurler's syndrome	Corneal opac., RP, OA	MR	Gargoyle facies, deafness, HSM, dysostosis/CV abn., dwarfism	Death by 10, most common MPS
	Hunter's syndrome	RP, OA	MR, deafness, hydroceph.	Dystosis	Death by 15
	Thyroid orbitopathy and other restrictive myopathies	Forced ductions abnormal, pseudoglaucoma secondary to restriction			—
	Congenital rubella	Cat., ret. pig. degen., microphthalmos	Deafness, MR	Cardiac anom.	—
	Vogt-Koyanegi-Harada's syndrome	Exudative RD, uveitis, poliosis	Meningoencephalitis, tinnitus	Vitiligo	—
	ANTERIOR SEGMENT DYSGENESIS				
	Rieger's syndrome		MR	Anal stenosis, renal mal., heart mal.	—
	Alagille's syndrome	Post. embryotoxin, ectopic pupils, subcap. cat., band keratopathy, keratoconus, myopia, strab, mild ret. pig. degen.		Neonatal jaundice, cholestasis, HSM, typical facies, congen. heart dis.	—
	Short's syndrome	Rieger's anomalies	Retarded speech	Short stature, micrognathia, premature aging	—
Congenital Glaucoma (Buphthalmos)					
	Zellweger's syndrome	"Leopard spot" ret. pig. degen., cong. cat., ON hypoplasia	MR	Microcystic kidney, hepatic dysgenesis, aa uria, typical facies	See Chapter 21 Table 14

Type of Lesion Involved	Clinical Presentation				
	Disorder	*Other Ocular Signs*	*CNS*	*Systemic*	*Other*
	Conradi's syndrome	Congen. cat., OA, hypertel., heterochromia	MR	Stippled epiphyses, short stature, micromelia, VSD, PDA	—
	Hurler's syndrome	Corneal clouding, nystagmus, strab.	MR, deafness	Infection, coarse facies, dysostosis, macroglossia, dwarfism, cardiac sx.	See Chapter 21 Table 9
	Lowe's syndrome (oculo-cerebral-renal)	Congen. cat., ret. pig. degen., ON hypoplasia	MR	Aa uria, congen., renal rickets, dwarfism	XLR
	Congenital rubella	Cat., RP, microp.	Deafness, MR	Cardiac anom.	See Chapter 22 Tables 9–16, Neurol. infections most frequent cause of congen. cat.
	Krabbe's disease (globoid cell leukodystrophy)	OA, strab., nystagmus, cortical blindness	PMR, myoclonic seizures, spastic, hi CSF prot., deafness	Swallowing problems (rare)	See Chapter 21 Table 11, Onset 3–6 mo., death by 3 yr

TABLE 23—6. DISORDERS AFFECTING THE IRIS

	Clinical Presentation				
Ocular Finding	*Disorder*	*Other Ocular Signs*	*CNS*	*Systemic*	*Other*
Brushfield Spots	Trisomy 21	Mongoloid lids, esotropia (35%), cat. (60%), myopia, keratoconus	MR	Short stature, characteristic facies, cardiac abn., broad hands and feet, leukemia	1/600 births
Lisch Nodules	Neurofibromatosis (VRNF) (NF-1)	MM of iris, ON, chiasm glioma, plexiform neuroma of orb. and *lid*, gl., pulsating exophthal., sphenoid bone changes, hypertrophic corneal nerves	Cut: axillary freckles, café-au-lait spots (>5mm); plexiform neuromas	Plexiform neuromas, meningiomas	Incsd. nerve growth factor
Koeppe Nodules	Sarcoidosis	Uveitis, ret. phlebitis, ON infiltration	Hypothal., meningeal involvement	Hilar nodes, skin changes	—
Depigmentation	Albinism (many types)	Dcsd. VA, mac. dysplasia, nystagmus, strab. (60%), blond fundus, photophobia, no binoc. vision	Chiasmal crossing changes	Light pigment hair and skin	Poor melanin synthesis, dcsd. cognitive function secondary to misdirected CNS paths, ED, PND
Heterchromia	Congen. Horner's syndrome	Ptosis, miosis	Ipsilateral sympathetic lesion	Dcsd. sweating in affected area	—
	Juvenile xanthogranuloma	Iris lesions, hyphema, lid papules		Yellow papules—regress spont.	Infants and small children
	Progressive hemifacial atrophy (Parry-Romberg syndrome)	Uveitis; abn. of cornea, pupil, lid		Linear "scleroderma" of face and scalp	—
Iridicyclitis	Beçhet's syndrome	Hypopyon. uveitis, ret. vasculitis		Secondary venous occlusion, urethritis, ulcers, vaso-occlusion	—
Coloboma	Maternal phenylketonuria				—
	Many chromosomal abnormalities		See Chapter 21, Table 2		
	Rieger's syndrome (cat's eye)	Anterior chamber dysgenesis, gl.	MR	Anal. stenosis, renal mal., heart mal.	—

Ocular Finding	Clinical Presentation				
	Disorder	*Other Ocular Signs*	*CNS*	*Systemic*	*Other*
Coloboma (*cont.*)	Alagille's (arteriohepatic dysplasia)	Post. embryotoxon, ectopic pupils, subcap. cat., band keratopathy, keratoconus, myopia, ret. pig. degen. deepset eyes hypertelorism strab., mild ret. pig. degen.	PMR	Neonatal jaundice, cholestasis, HSM, typical facies, congen. heart disease, vertebral anomalies	AD early treatment with fat soluble vitamins A and E by injection may abort pigmentary retinopathy
Aniridia	WAGR syndrome	sl.	MR	Wilm's tumor gtl malf.	deletion of chromosome II

ªSensitive to atropine.

TABLE 23–7. DISORDERS AFFECTING THE LENS

Ocular Finding	Clinical Presentation				
	Disorder	*Other Ocular Signs*	*CNS*	*Systemic*	*Other*
Cataract	Neurofibromatosis (BANF) (NF-2)	Presenile PSC	Bilat. acoustic neuromas in teens	Cutaneous changes	—
	Cockayne's syndrome	RP, OA, photophobia	MR, microcephaly, deafness, intracranial Ca^{++}, ataxia, seizures	Dwarfism, dermatitis, sparse gray hair, atherosclerosis	—
	Marinesco-Sjögren's syndrome	Congen. cat., nystagmus, strab., epicanthus	Spinocereb. ataxia, MR	Skeletal anom.	—
	Conradi's syndrome	Heretochromia, iritis, OA and ON hypoplasia		Stipped epiphyses	—
	Marfan's syndrome	Dislocated lens, megalocornea, myopia, RD, gl., iris changes, strab.		Tall stature, arachnodactyly, cardiovasc. dis.	—
	Pseudohyperpara-thyroidism	OA, nystagmus		Calcifications, short stature, malabsorption	—
	Abetalipopro-teinemia (Bassen-Kornzweig's syndrome)	PEO, true RP-like retinop., night blindness	Ataxia, spinocerebellar degen., PMR, neurop.	Steatorrhea, low serum lipids, acanthosis of RBCs, cardiac abn.	—
	Refsum's disease	True RP-like retinop., night blindness, nystagmus, pupil changes	Cerebellar ataxia, hypertrophic periph. neuropathy, deafness, hypotonia, MR	Ichthyosis, bone disease, ECG changes	—
	Zellweger's syndrome (inc. neonatal adrenoleukodys.)	OA, RP, nystagmus, congen. gl., speckled iris, cloudy cornea, ret. arteriolar narrowing	Demyelin. hypotonia, seizures, psychomotor retardation	Typical facies deformations, hepatomeg., renal cysts, calcif. deposits in patella, adrenal atrophy	PND, flat ERG
	Incontinenta pigmenti (Bloch-Sulzberger's syndrome)	Retrolental mass, corneal opacities, OA, pig. ret., nystagmus strab., ret. dysplasia	MR, seizures	Hyperpig. skin lesions, blisters progress to growths, abn. dentition, alopecia	—
	Congenital rubella	Pig. ret., gl. microphthalmos	Deafness, MR	Cardiac anom.	—
	Hypocalcemia				—
	Galactosemia		MR	Failure to thrive, HSM, renal abn.	—
	Galactokinase def.	Juv. cat.	No hepatomegaly		—
	Hyperornithinemia (gyrate atrophy)	Gyrate atrophy of choroid, myopia, night blindness, PSC			—

Ocular Finding	Clinical Presentation				
	Disorder	*Other Ocular Signs*	*CNS*	*Systemic*	*Other*
	Mannosidoses (composite of 2 types)	Nystagmus, post. cortical spokes, dendritic keratitis	MR, deafness	Dysostosis, HSM, painful keratotic skin lesions on palms and soles	—
	Tyrosinemia II (Richner-Hanhart's syndrome)	Lacrimation, photophobia, mac. dysplasia, nystagmus, strab. (60%), blond fundus	Chiasmal crossing changes	Light pigmented hair and skin, skin neoplasia	—
	Trisomy 21	Upslanting lids, esotropia (35%), keratoconus, Brushfield spots (85%)	MR	Short stature, characteristic facies, cardiac abn., broad hands and feet, leukemia	Extra chromosomes 95% of maternal origin
Christmas tree cataract	Myotonic dystrophy	Ptosis, pig. retinopathy, low IOP	MR	DM, testicular atrophy, baldness	—
Propeller cataract	Fabry's disease	Corneal verticillata, conj. and ret. telang.	Parathesias, painful crises, CVAs	Angiokeratoma, heart disease, renal failure	—
"Sunflower" cataract	Wilson's disease	Cornea: Kayser-Fleischer ring best seen on gonioscopy (present in 95%), 100% of those with neurol. symptoms	Ataxia, basal ganglia symptoms, tremor, dysarthria	Cirrhosis, hemolysis	Evaluate any undiagnosed liver failure, esp. in children, for Wilson's disease
Posterior cortical spokes	Fabry's disease	Cornea verticillata (pigmented whorls), conjunctival and retinal telangiectasia	Paraesthesias, painful crises, CVAs	Angiokeratomas, heart disease, renal failure	PND
Congenital Cataract	Trisomy 13 (Patau's syndrome)	Corneal opacity, microphthalmos, colobomata, PHPV, intraocular cartilage, ret. dysplasia, ant. seg. dysgenesis, ON hypoplasia	MR, holoprosencephaly, microcephaly	Cardiac defects, GU abn. cleft palate, polydactyly, hematol. abn., hemangiomas	Death in 2nd mo., 1/15,000
	Trisomy 21	Upslanting lids, esotropia (35%), Brushfield spots (85%)	MR	Short stature, characteristic facies, cardiac abn., broads hands and feet, leukemia	Sensitivity to atropine, 1/600, extra chromosome 95% of maternal origin
	Trisomy 18 (Edward's syndrome)	Ret. folds blepharophimosis, ptosis, corneal opacity, microphthalmos, congenital gl., colobomata, strab., OA, disc. anom.	MR, hypertonus, deafness	Cardiac anom., micrognatha, microstomia, low-set ears, clenched fists, rocker-bottom feet	Death in 1st year

(Continues)

TABLE 23–7. DISORDERS AFFECTING THE LENS (*cont.*)

Ocular Finding	Clinical Presentation				
	Disorder	*Other Ocular Signs*	*CNS*	*Systemic*	*Other*
Congenital Cataract (*cont.*)	Turner's syndrome	Epicanthal fold, ptosis, strab., blue sclerae		Short stature, webbed neck, facial and skull anom., hypogonadism	1/1500 births, women, incidence of X-linked disorders equal to males
	Mandibular facial dysostosis (Treacher-Collin's syndrome) (Franceschetti-Klein's syndrome)	Antimongoloid lids, coloboma of lower lid and iris, strab., nystagmus, microp.	Deafness, ear abnormalities	Max. hypoplasia, large mouth, heart defects, cardiac abn., microglioma, mandibular hypoplasia, ectodermal dysplasia, hypotrichosis	—
	Hallerman-François-Streiff's syndrome	Microphthalmos		Bird's-head dyscephaly, dental anom., dwarfism, hypotrichosis	—
	Pierre-Robin's syndrome	High myop., strab., congen. gl. ret. detachment		Feeding problems, cleft palate, mandibular hypoplasia, glossoptosis	—
	Laurence-Moon's syndrome	Ret. pig. degen.	Spastic paraplegia	Hypogonadism	—
	Bardet-Biedl's syndrome	Ret. pig. degen., OA, rare: o'plegia	MR, paraplegia, misrouted VAP	Polydactyly, obesity, hypogenitalism, cardiac anom., renal anom.	—
	Stickler-Wagner's syndrome	Myopia, strab., vitreous degen., ret. degen. (lattice)	Deafness	Facial hypoplasia, bone and joint changes	—
	Hand-Schüller-Christian's syndrome	Exopth., PE, OA, swelling lids, orbit	Cranial neuropathies, complications of tumors	Histiocytic prolif., skin, skull lesions	—
	Hyperphosphatasia (juvenile Paget's disease)	Blue sclera	Premature synostosis	Fragile bones, shortness, large head	—
	Hypoparathyroidism	K-conjunctivitis, blepharospasm, PE	PTC		
	Diabetes mellitus	Retinopathy, vit. hemorrhage	Neuropathies, coma	Hyperglycemia, immune deficiency	—
	Norrie's syndrome	Ret. dysplasia, retrolental mass, corneal opac., phthisis	MR, deafness		—
	Lowe's syndrome (oculo-cerebral-renal)	Congen. gl., ON hypoplasia, ret. pig. degen.	MR, hypotonia	Renal dis., renal rickets, atrophic skin with pig. and depigmented patches	—

Ocular Finding	Clinical Presentation				
	Disorder	**Other Ocular Signs**	**CNS**	**Systemic**	**Other**
	Rothmund-Thomson's syndrome	Sparse brows and lashes, microcornea, corneal abn.	Demyelination, microceph.	Short stature, hypogonadism, poikiloderma, skull anom., photosensitivity	—
	An(hypo)hidrotic ectodermal dys.	Microphthalmos., PHPV		Anhydrosis, hypotrichosis, adontia	—
	Smith-Lemli-Optizes syndrome		Microceph., MR		—
	Rubinstein-Taybi's syndrome	Photophobia	MR	Peculiar facies, broad thumbs and toes	—
	Intrauterine infections: rubella, influenza, syphilis, toxoplasmosis, CMV		Deafness	Heart defects	—
Dislocated Lens	Syphilis				
	Congenital	Interstitial keratitis, ret. pig. degen., lens dislocation	Deafness, gumma, meningitis	Notched incisors	—
	Acquired	O neur., perineuritis; uveitis, pig. retinopathy			—
	Marfan's syndrome	Megalocornea, myopia, gl., RD, strab.		Tall stature, arachnodactyly, CV dis.	—
	Homocystinuria	Ectopia lentis, gl., pig. retinopathy, myopia, RD, OA	MR	Thromboembolism, osteoporosis, hypopigmentation, cardiovasc. abn.	Gen. anesth. may cause thromboembolism
	Sulfite oxidase deficiency	OA, strab.	MR, seizures, hemiplegia	Renal stones	—
	Hyperlysinemia	Spherophakia	MR, seizures	Anemia	—
	Ehlers-Danlos syndrome	High myop., blue sclera, RD, angioid streaks		Cutis laxa, hypermobile joints, hemorrhagic death, arterial dilation	—
	Rieger's syndrome	Ant. seg. dysgenesis, microcornea, corneal opacity, gl.		Anal stenosis, typical facies	—
	Alport's syndrome	Nystagmus myopia, lenticonus, keratoconus, drusen-like macular changes, microspherophakia	Deafness	Hemorrhagic nephritis	—
Spherophakia	Hyperlysinemia	Disloc. lens	MR, hypotonia, spastic diplegia		—
	Sulfite oxidase deficiency	Ectopia lentis, OA, strab.	MR, seizures, cerebral atrophy	Renal stones	—

(Continues)

TABLE 23–7. DISORDERS AFFECTING THE LENS (*cont.*)

Ocular Finding	Clinical Presentation				
	Disorder	*Other Ocular Signs*	*CNS*	*Systemic*	*Other*
Spherophakla (*cont.*)	Marfan's disease	Dislocated lens (79%), gl., ret. detachment, strab. (20%), myopia		Tall stature, arachnodactyly, cardiac defects, hi arched palate	—
	Alport's syndrome	Cat., myopia, lenticonus, keratoconus, nystagmus, microspherophakia, drusen-like macular changes	Deafness	Hemorrhagic, nephritis	—
	Weill-Marchesani syndrome	Microspherophakia		Short stature, short digits	—
	Galactosemia	Cat.	MR	HSM, failure to thrive, renal abn., jaundice	40% dies in septicemia if not diagnosed

TABLE 23–8. DISORDERS AFFECTING THE RETINA

Ocular Finding	Clinical Presentation				
	Disorder	*Other Ocular Signs*	*CNS*	*Systemic*	*Other*
Retinitis Pigmentosa					
	True RP (many forms)	Waxy pallor of optic disc, ONHD, NFBDs, telang., cat.			Dcsd ERG, type I AD form on chromosome 3; in at least 20% by a mutation in the rhodopsin gene
	Leber's congenital amaurosis	Pendular nystagmus, very low VA from birth, refractive errors	Misc. malformations, occasional seizures, MR		Dcsd. ERG
	Leber's with marbelized fundus			Renal disease	—
Retinal Pigmentary Degeneration in Disorders of Lipid Metabolism (Pigmentary Retinopathy)					
	Abetalipopro-teinemia Bassen-Kornzweig's syndrome)	Prog. external o'plegia, night blindness, nystagmus ptosis	Ataxia, spinocerebellar degen., PMR, neurop.	Malabsorption (steatorrhea), low serum lipids, acanthocytosis of RBCs, cardiac abn.	—
	Familial hypobetalipopro-teinemia	(Bassen-Kornzweig-like, but CNS symptoms less)			—
	Refsum's disease	OA, night blindness, cat. (50%), nystagmus, pupil changes	Hypertrophic periph. neurop., cerebellar ataxia, deafness, hypotonia, MR, anosmia, increased CSF protein	Ichthyosis, bone dis., ECG changes	—
	Zellweger's syndrome	OA, ret. pig. degen. cat., gl., nystagmus, speckled iris, cloudy cornea, ret. arteriolar narrowing, ON hypoplasia	Demyelin., hypotonia, seizures, MR	Typical facies, hepatomegaly, renal cysts, calcif. deposits in patella, adrenal atrophy	PND, flat ERG

Mucopolysaccharidoses (types I, II, III), Neuronal ceroid lipofuscinoses, mucolipidoses, sphingolipidoses, spinocerebellar degens.: see Chapter 21 Tables 8–11

	Lysosomal Storage Diseases				
	Menke's syndrome	Cat., ret. vasc. tort., iris cysts	MR	Kinky, steely hair; hypopigmentation; arterial abn.; bone changes; hypothermia	—

(Continues)

TABLE 23–8. DISORDERS AFFECTING THE RETINA (cont.)

Ocular Finding	Clinical Presentation				
	Disorder	**Other Ocular Signs**	**CNS**	**Systemic**	**Other**
PIGMENTARY RETINOPATHY AND CNS DISORDERS					
	Marinesco-Sjögren's syndrome	Congen. cat.	MR, spinocerebellar ataxil amyotrophy		
	Cockayne's syndrome	OA, cat., corneal clouding, pupil changes	MR, microceph., deafness, ataxia, seizures	Dwarfism, premature aging	—
	Kjellin's syndrome	Perifoveal specks	Spastic paraplegia, dementia		—
	Sjögren-Larson syndrome	Mac. degen.	MR, spastic ataxia	Ichthyosis	—
	Abetalipoproteinemia (Bassen-Kornzweig syndrome)	PEO, night NLP ptosis nystagmus	Ataxia, spinocerebellar degen., PMR, neuropathy	Malabsorption (steatorrhea), acanthosis of RBCs, low serum lipids, cardiac anom.	—
	Hallervorden-Spatzes syndrome	Ret. flecks, RP-like, mac. bull's-eye, blepharospasm, ERG, apraxia of lid opening	Basal ganglia disorder, dementia	Early death	—
	Dystonia, blepharospasm, pigmentary retinopathy	ret. pig. degen. bull's eye mac. blepharospasm	dystonia		ERG
	Pelizaeus-Merzbacher's disease	"Wandering eyes"	Spasticity, cerebellar ataxia, dementia, head trembling	Pes cavus, scoliosis, short stature	—
	Neuronal ceroid lipofuscinoses	Dcsd. VA	MR, seizures	See Chapter 21 Table 11	—
	Friedreich's ataxia	Nystagmus, OA, strab.	Ataxia, post. column disease, dysarthria	Pes cavus, DM (10%), cardiac myopathy	—
	Pigmentary retinopathy and pallidal degen. (Saldino's syndrome)		Extrapyr. ridigity, dysarthria, cerebellar ataxia	Nephropathy, skeletal anom.	—
	Olivopontocerebellar degeneration (composite of forms)	Nystagmus, o'plegia, ptosis, OA	Cerebellar, pyramidal, extrapyramidal, bstem dysfxn.	Esophageal, bladder, bowel dysfunction	—
	Myotonic dystrophy	X-mas tree cat., ptosis, low IOP	Myotonia, MR	testicular atrophy, baldness	—
	Muscular dystrophy RP with spastic diplegia	Cat.	Proximal dystrophy, spastic diplegia		—

Ocular Finding	Clinical Presentation				
	Disorder	*Other Ocular Signs*	*CNS*	*Systemic*	*Other*
	Flynn-Aird's syndrome	Cat., myopia	Ataxia, dementia, seizures, muscle wasting, deafness, peripheral neurop., elevated CSF protein	Cutaneous changes, cystic bone changes, baldness, caries, stiff joints	
	Bardet-Biedl's syndrome	Rarely: o'plegia, cat., OA	Paraplegia, MR, misrouted VAP	Polydactyly, obesity, hypogenitalism, cardiac anom., renal anom.	—
	Laurence-Moon's syndrome		Spastic paraplegia	Hypogonadism, obesity, hypogenitalism, polydactyly	—
	Biemond's II syndrome	Iris coloboma	MR		
	Infantile Refsum's disease	Mac. degen.	Hypotonia, deafness, MR	HM	Peroxisomal
	Canavan's disease	OA, retinal vacuoles?	Hypotonia, seizures, failure to thrive, spasticity, poor head control, macrocephaly	Renal cysts	—
PEROXISOMAL DISEASES					
	Zellweger's syndrome	OA, nystagmus, hypertelorism, cat., gl., corneal clouding	Developmental retardation, PMR, hypotonia, seizures	Hepatomegaly, high forehead, dysmorphic facies, renal cysts	Dscd. ERG
	Hyperpipecolic acidemia variant	Speckled iris, cloudy cornea, OA, cat. nystagmus	PMR	Dysmorphic facies, hepatomegaly	—
	Juvenile adreno-leuko-dystrophy	Vision defect, eventually very low VA, OA, cortical NLP	Demyelination, seizures, dementia, spasticity, ataxia, deafness	Adrenal atrophy (Addison's)	Boys 4–8 yr, death in early to late teens, PND; on Xq28 (same locus as R-G color gene!)
	Refsum's disease	Cat., nystagmus, OA, night NLP, pupil changes	Cerebellar ataxia, periph. neuropathy, deafness, hypotonia	Ichthyosis, bone disease, ECG changes, diabetes	—
	Congenital/neonatal adrenoleukodystrophy	OA, cat.	Hypotonia, seizures, PMR	Adrenal atrophy	Defect in multiple peroxisomal functions, defect in peroxisomal biogenesis
	Infantile phytanic acid storage disease (Refsum's disease)		MR, deafness, ataxia, anosmia	Hepatomegaly, dysmorphic features	Milder than ALD
SUDANOPHILIC LEUKODYSTROPHIES					
	Adrenoleukodystrophy	Low VA, OA	Dwarfism, seizures, dementia, spasticity, ataxia	Adrenal atrophy (Addison's disease)	—
	Multiple sulfatase deficiency	CRS, OA, corneal clouding		MPS-like ichthyosis, HSM	—

(Continues)

TABLE 23–8. DISORDERS AFFECTING THE RETINA (cont.)

Ocular Finding	Clinical Presentation				
	Disorder	**Other Ocular Signs**	**CNS**	**Systemic**	**Other**
	SUDANOPHILIC LEUKODYSTROPHIES (cont.)				
	Metachromatic leukodystrophy	OA, CRS, gray mac.	Gait abn., dementia, spasticity	Nonfilling gallbladder	—
	Zellweger's syndrome (hyperpipecolic acid variant)	OA, speckled iris, cloudy cornea, cat.	PMR	Dysmorphic facies, hepatomeg.	—
	MITOCHONDRIAL DISEASES				
	Kearn-Sayre's syndrome	PEO, ptosis	Cerebellar ataxia, deafness, myopathy, seizures, ncsd CSF protein	Heart block, short stature	—
	Myoclonic epilepsy	OA, supranue o'plegia	Ataxia, seizures, sensory loss, dementia, hearing loss	Short stature	—
	Cystinosis (composite of types)	Crystals in cornea, conj., photophobia, patchy ret. pig.	Cerebral atrophy	Renal rickets and failure, dwarfism	—
	DERMATOLOGIC DISORDERS				
	Rud's syndrome	Strab., ptosis, nystagmus, blepharospasm	MR, seizures	Ichthyosis, hypogonadism, DM	—
	Sjögren-Larson syndrome	Mac. lesion	MR, spastic paresis, seizures	Ichthyosis, short stature, abn. of hair and teeth, skeletal dysplasia	—
	Hallgren's disease		Ataxia, MR, deafness		—
	Werner's syndrome	PSC 2nd-4th decade, mac. degen., gl., blue sclera	Gray hair, scleroderma, ASCHD, DM, hypogonadism, increased neoplasia		Phenotypic copy of aging cat. extraction complications, esp. late wound dehiscince
	Psoriasis	Lesions on lids, corneal vasc. and opacities, PSC cat.		Red skin plaques	—
	An(hypo)hidrotic ectodermal dysplasia	Keratopathy, photophobia, cat., spare lashes and brows, uveitis, strab.		Absent sweating, heat intolerance, abn. hair and teeth	—
	Alström's syndrome	Iris coloboma, ret. vascular attenuation, nystagmus, cat.	N IQ, deafness	Hypogonadism, obesity, acanthosis nigricans, DM, renal failure, polydactyly, hypertriglyceridemia	—

Ocular Finding	Clinical Presentation				
	Disorder	Other Ocular Signs	CNS	Systemic	Other
	Cockayne's syndrome	RP, OA, photophobia, cat., keratopathy, strab., nystagmus, resistant to mydriatics	MR, microcephaly, deafness, intracran. Ca⁺⁺, ataxia, seizures	Dwarfism, sun sensitivity, sparse gray hair, atherosclerosis	Senile changes at 2–4 YO, dcsd. ERG, PND
	Incontinentia pigmenti	Pseudogliomas, persistent hyaloid art., corneal opac., cat., OA, nystagmus, strab., Coats-like perih. ret. vasc. changes	MR, seizures	Skin lesions, blisters, dental anom., alopecia	—
	Focal dermal hypoplasia (Goltz-Gorlin syndrome)	OA, colobomata, EM abn. nystagmus, microp., sublux. lens		Focal dermal hypoplasia	—
	Atopic dermatitis	Cat.—ASC, keratoconus, RD			Cat. surg. often complicated
	Urbach-Wiethe's disease	mac. degen., post. pole drusen, gray/white papules on lid, yellow conj. nodules		Hyperkeratoses	—
	Flynn-Aird disease	Cat., myopia	Prog. hearing loss, ataxia, periph. neuritis, seizures, dementia, peripheral neuropathy, elevated CSF protein, muscle wasting	Skin atrophy and ulceration, baldness, caries, cystic bone changes, stiff joints	—
DISORDERS OF AMINO ACID METABOLISM					
	Homocarnosinosis		Prog. spasticity, mental deterior. ncsd. CSF homocarnosine		—
	Homocystinuria	Ectopia lentis, gl., myopia, RD, OA	MR	Marfanoid habitus, thromboembolism, osteoporosis, hypopigmentation, arterial dilatation	Gen. anesthesia may cause thromboembolism
	Cystinosis (composite of types)	Crystals in cornea, conj.; photophobia; patchy ret. depigmentation	Cerebral atrophy	Renal rickets and failure, dwarfism	—
	Cystinuria		Pyr. signs, deafness	Renal lithiasis	—
	Hyperornithinemia (gyrate atrophy)	Myopia (80%), night blindness, PSC (40%)			—
	Oxalosis	Ret. crystals, orbital myositis, pigmented rings		Nephrolithiasis and calcinosis, renal insufficiency	Reported in methoxyflurane anesthesia

(Continues)

TABLE 23–8. DISORDERS AFFECTING THE RETINA (*cont.*)

		Clinical Presentation			
Ocular Finding	**Disorder**	**Other Ocular Signs**	**CNS**	**Systemic**	**Other**
	DISORDERS OF AMINO ACID METABOLISM (*cont.*)				
	Hooft's disease	gray macula	PMR, hyperactive	hypolipidemia, hypoglycemia, abn. hair, nails, teeth	
	Senior-Loken syndrome		PMR	Renal dysplasia early death, met. acidosis, hyperamonemia, aa urla	Dcsd. ERG
	Lowe's syndrome	Congen. cat. and gl., ON hypoplasia	Ataxia, MR, growth retard.	Renal dysplasia early death, met. acidosis, hyperammonemia, aa uria	Dcsd. ERG
	Imidazone amino acid uria				—
	OTHER METABOLIC ABNORMALITIES				
	Metal Metabolism: Menkes' syndrome	Iris cysts	Cerebellar signs	Steely, kinky hair; hypopigmentation; bone changes; arterial abn.; hypothermia	—
	Alagille's syndrome (arteriohepatic dysplasia)	Axenfeld anomaly, corectopia, strab.	Absent DTRs	Neonatal jaundice, pulmonic stenosis, periph. arterial stenosis, abn. vertebrae, typical facies	Dcsd. ERG, EOG
	Vitamin E deficiency	ret. pig. deg. ptosis o'plegia nyctalopia blepharospasm			Dcsd. ERG
	Jeune's syndrome	retinal dystrophy, decreased VA, nystagmus, strab.		Malformed rib cage; skeletal dysplasia; polydactyly; cystic kidney, liver, pancreas; dwarfism; resp. insuff., renal failure	Abn. ERG
	Megacolon	Polar cat., strab., nystagmus			—
	RETINITIS PIGMEN-TOSA AND DEAFNESS				
	Alport's syndrome	Cat. (10%), myop., ant. lenticonus, perimacular granularity, K-conus, nystagmus		Nephritis	—
	Refsum's disease (phytanic acid storage disease)	Pupil changes, OA, night blindness, cat. (50%), nystagmus	Cerebellar ataxia, hypertrophic periph. neuropathy, deafness, hypotonia, MR	Ichthyosis (50%), bone dis., ECG changes	AR, incsd. phytanic acid

Ocular Finding	Clinical Presentation				
	Disorder	*Other Ocular Signs*	*CNS*	*Systemic*	*Other*
	Usher's disease		Congen. deafness, cerebellar atrophy		AR, dcsd. ERG
	Cockayne's syndrome	Cat., OA, corneal dys., nystagmus	PMR, MR, macroceph., extrapyr. signs, leucodystrophy	Dwarfism, premat. aging, derm. changes, photosensitivity, skeletal dyslasia, birdlike facies	AR
	Alström's syndrome	OA, nystagmus	IQN	Obesity, nephritis, DM	—
	Bardet-Biedl's syndrome	O'plegia (rare), cat., OA, macular atrophy	MR, spastic diplegia, misrouted VAP, deafness	Polydactyly, diabetes mellitus, hypogonadism, cardiac anom., renal disease	—
	McGovern's syndrome	Low VA	Deafness		—
	Kearn-Sayre syndrome	PEO, ptosis	Deafness, ataxia	Heart block, short stature	—
	Norrie's disease	Microp., retrolental mass	Severe MR		—
	Familial hypogonadism	OA, cat.		Obesity, short stature, hypogonadism	—
	Flynn-Aird syndrome	Cat.	Ataxia, dementia, seizures, muscle wasting, deafness, peripheral neurop.	Cutaneous changes, cystic bone changes	—
	Hallgren's syndrome	RP, OA, cat. in midlife	Ataxia, MR, deafness		AR, related to LM/BB (?), with DM and obesity
	Osteopetrosis (Albers-Schönberg disease)	OA if severe, retinal dystrophy	Deafness	Osteoporosis, macrocephaly, HSM, severe anemia	AR, (AD), PND
	Waardenburg's syndrome	Hypertelorism, heterochromia iridis		White forelock	—
Leber's type "RP"	Familial juvenile nephrophthisis (Senior-Loken syndrome)			Renal disease, hematol. abn., chrondoectodermal dysplasia polydactyly	—
	Cystinosis/uria	Corneal/conj. crystals			—
	Saldino-Mainzer syndrome	Senior-Loken syndrome		Cone-shaped epiphyses of hand	—
	Osteopetrosis (Albers-Schönberg disease)	OA if severe, retinal dystrophy	Deafness	Osteoporosis, macrocephaly, HSM, severe anemia	PND

(Continues)

TABLE 23–8. DISORDERS AFFECTING THE RETINA (*cont.*)

Ocular Finding	Disorder	Other Ocular Signs	CNS	Systemic	Other
				Clinical Presentation	
Atypical Retinal Pigmentary Retinopathy					
	Cystinosis	Crystals in cornea and conj., photophobia, patchy retinal depigmentation	Cerebral atrophy	Renal rickets and failure	—
	Homocystinuria	Ectopia lentis, gl., ret. pig. degen., myopia, RD, OA	MR	Thromboembolism, osteoporosis, hypopigmentation, pulmonary and aortic dilatation	—
	Hyperomithinemia (gyrate atrophy)	Gyrate atrophy, myopia (50%), night blindness, PSC (40%)			—
Other					
	Infection/inflammation				

Most infections and inflammatory processes involving the outer retinal layers and RPE will produce pigment alterations, including Behçet's disease, Vogt-Koyanagi-Harada syndrome, congenital rubella, subacute sclerosing panencephalitis, and congenital and acquired syphilis among others.

Ocular Finding	Disorder	Other Ocular Signs	CNS	Systemic	Other
	Vascular occlusion				—
	Trauma				—
	Toxic reactions	Chloroquine, metalloses, phenothiazine, tamoxifen			—
Retinal Depigmentation	Albinism (10 forms)	Mac. dysplasia, nystagmus, strab., blond fundus, photophobia, no binoc. vision	Chiasmal crossing changes	Light pigmented hair and skin	—
	Laurence-Moon syndrome		Spastic paraplegia	Hypogonadism	—
	Bardet-Biedl syndrome	Rarely: o'plegia, cat., OA	Paraplegia, MR, misrouted VAP	Polydactyly, obesity, hypogenitalism, cardiac anom., renal anom.	—
	Prader Willi's syndrome	albinotic strab., nystagmus	Hypotonia, MR, misrouted VAP	Hypogonadism, obesity, short stature	—

Ocular Finding	Clinical Presentation				
	Disorder	*Other Ocular Signs*	*CNS*	*Systemic*	*Other*
Retinal Spots, Flecks and Crystals	PRIMARY RETINAL DISORDERS				
	Bietti crystalline corneal and retinal dystrophy, gyrate atrophy, calcified drusen, tamoxifen toxicity, canthaxanthine, flurane (secondary oxalosis)				—
	Emboli	TIA, ret. VFD, ret. vasc. sheathing	CNS sx.	Cardiac valve dis. ?, atrial thrombus, car. oc. dis.	—
	Vitamin A retinopathy				—
	Primary hyperoxaluria	Mac. crystals (also in ciliary body and choroid)		Renal stones	—
	Retinal punctata albescens				—
	Fundus albipunctatus				PERG
	Fundus flavimaculatus	NFBDs			—
	Flecked retina of Kandori				—
	Familial drusen				—
	Hallervorden-Spatz syndrome	OA, bull's-eye maculopathy	Neurol. deterioration, spasticity, athetosis, dysarthria, ataxia		—
Crystals	DISORDERS OF AMINO ACID METABOLISM				
	Cystinosis	Crystals in conj. and cornea, photophobia	Cerebral atrophy	Renal rickets and failure, dwarfism	Retinal changes may precede sx.
	Homocystinuria	Ectopia lentis, gl., myopia, RD, OA	MR	Thromboembolism, hypopigmentation, pulmonary and aortic stenosis	Gen. anesthesia may cause thromboembolism
	Oxalosis	Orbital myositis, pigmented rings		Nephrolithiasis and calcinosis, renal insufficiency	—
	Hyperornithinemia (gyrate atrophy)	Gyrate atrophy of choroid, myopia (90%), night blindness, PSC (40%)			—
	Other Disorders Bietti crystalline corneal and retinal dystrophy				—

(*Continues*)

TABLE 23–8. DISORDERS AFFECTING THE RETINA (*cont.*)

Ocular Finding	Clinical Presentation				
	Disorder	**Other Ocular Signs**	**CNS**	**Systemic**	**Other**
Crystals (*cont.*)	Sjögren-Larson syndrome	Mac. degen.	MR, spastic ataxia, spastic paresis, seizures	Ichthyosis, short stature, abn. of hair and teeth, skeletal dysplasia	
	Ichthyosis			Ichthyosis	—
	Juxtafoveal telangiectasia	Mac. lesions			—
	Talc, canthaxanthine, or tamoxifen toxicity				—
	Alport's syndrome	Cat., myopia, lenticonus, keratoconus, nystagmus, microspherophakia, drusen-like macular changes	Deafness	Hemorrhagic nephritis	—
Retinal Detachment: Rhegmentogenous					
	Incontinentia pigmenti	Retrolental mass, corneal opac., cat., strab., microp., OA anomalies	MR, seizures	Hyperpig. skin lesions, blisters, growths, abn. dentition	—
	Pierre-Robin syndrome	High myop., congen. gl., strab., congen. cat.	MR	Cleft palate, mandibular hypoplasia, glossoptosis	—
	Ehler-Danlos syndrome	Sublux. lens, high myop., angioid streaks, vit. hemorrhage, blue sclerae		Elastic skin, lax joints, vascular dilatation hemorrhage	—
	Homocystinuria	Sublux. lens, ret. pig. degen., myopia, OA	MR	Marfanoid habitus, accelerated atherosclerosis, thromboembolic osteoporosis, hypopigmentation, pulmonary and aortic stenosis	Gen. anesth. may cause embolism
	Marfan's syndrome	Disloc. lens, gl., strab., myopia		Tall stature, arachnodactyly, cardiovasc. defects	—
	Vogt-Koyanagi-Harada syndrome	Exudative RD, uveitis, poliosis	Meningo-encephalitis, deafness, tinnitus	Vitiligo	—
	Wildervark-Duane's syndrome	Strab., limbal dermoid colobomata	Deafness	Fused cervical vertebrae	—
	Norrie's disease	Ret. dysplasia	MR (20%)	Boney abn.	—

Ocular Finding	Clinical Presentation				
	Disorder	*Other Ocular Signs*	*CNS*	*Systemic*	*Other*
	Wagner-Stickler disease	Progressive myopia, RD, cat., strab., vasc. sheathing, OA, vitreous degen. ("empty vit."), choroidal atrophy	Dcsd. hearing	Orofacial abn. similar to Pierre-Robin syndrome	Dcsd. ERG
	Median clefting-skeletal and joint abn-(esp. if associated with Pierre-Robin, Wagner-Stickler syndromes)				
	Zellweger's + other peroxisomal disorders	cataracts	hypotonia		
		optic nerve hypoplasia	MR		
			dysmorphic features		
Angioid Streaks	A-betalipoproteinemia (see appropriate tables in Chapter 21 for details)				
	Hypobetalipoproteinemia				
	Acromegaly				
	Drusen				
	Dwarfism with retinal atrophy and deafness				
	Ehlers-Danlos syndrome				
	François diencephalic syndrome				
	Hemoglobinopathies				
	High myopia				
	Hyperphosphatasia				
	Hypertension				
	Idiopathic (50%)				
	Lead poisoning				
	Marfan's syndrome				
	Osteitis deformans				
	Paget's disease; recent studies suggest association is less than previously reported				
	Pseudoxanthoma elasticum (PXE)				
	Acanthocytosis				
	Thrombocytopenia				
	Trauma				

(Continues)

TABLE 23–8. DISORDERS AFFECTING THE RETINA (*cont.*)

| Ocular Finding | Clinical Presentation | | | | |
	Disorder	Other Ocular Signs	CNS	Systemic	Other
Exudative Retinal Detachment Secondary to peripheral retinal vascular changes					
	Periarteritis nodosa and other vascular inflammatory diseases	See Chapter 3			
	Vogt-Koyanagi-Harada syndrome	Poliosis, uveitis	Meningo-encephalitis, deafness, tinnitus	Vitiligo	—
	Coats' disease Eales' disease von Hippel–Lindau disease Hemoglobinopathies Uveitis Retinopathy of prematurity	See Chapter 3			

TABLE 23–9. DISORDERS AFFECTING THE MACULA

Ocular Finding	Clinical Presentation				
	Disorder	*Other Ocular Signs*	*CNS*	*Systemic*	*Other*
Gray Macula					
	Farber's disease	CRS, RD, conj. xanthomas	Hypotonia, seizures	Xanthomas, inflammatory arthritis, hoarseness	—
	Lysosomal Storage Diseases Gangliosidoses Mucopolysaccharid- oses Mucolipidoses Neuronal ceroid- lipofuscinoses Renal glycosuria				
	Senior-Loken's syndrome (familial juvenile nephronophthisis)	Ret. pig. degen.	Ataxia, deafness	Renal dysplasia, amino aciduria, hepatic fibrosis, skeletal anomalies	See Chapter 21 Dcsd. ERG
	Spinocerebellar degeneration				
	Myotonic dystrophy	Christmas tree cat., ptosis, RP, low IOP	MR, myotonia	DM, testicular atrophy, baldness	—
	Congenital rubella	Pig. ret. gl., microphthalmos	Deafness, MR	Cardiac anom.	—
	Subacute sclerosing panencephalitis (SSPE)		Mental deter., myoclonus, seizures		Slow virus; after measles, most frequent cause of infant hospitali- zation for neuro- logic degenera- tive dis.; onset late 1st decade; death in infancy; mitochondrial enzyme def.
Macular Degeneration: Primary	Stargardt's Cone Dystrophy				—
	Associated With Systemic Disease				
	Cockayne's syndrome	Cat., OA, corneal dys., nystagmus, ret. pig. degen.	PMR, macrocephaly, extrapyr. signs, leucodystrophy	Dwarfism, premature aging, derm. changes, photosensitivity, skeletal dysplasia	—
	Alström's syndrome	OA, nystagmus	Leucodystrophy	Obesity, nephritis, DM	—
	Laurence-Moon syndrome	Ret. pig. degen.	Spastic paraplegia	Hypogonadism	—
	Bardet-Biedl syndrome	Ret. pig. degen., o'plegia (rarely), cat., OA	Paraplegia, MR, misrouted VAP	Polydactyly, obesity, hypogenitalism, cardiac anomalies, renal anomalies	—

TABLE 23–9. DISORDERS AFFECTING THE MACULA (*cont.*)

Ocular Finding	Clinical Presentation				
	Disorder	*Other Ocular Signs*	*CNS*	*Systemic*	*Other*
Macular Degeneration: Primary (*cont.*)	Hallgren's syndrome	OA, cat. in midlife	MR, ataxia, deafness		—
	Refsum's disease	Ret. pig. degen., OA, night blindness, cat. (50%), nystagmus, pupil changes	Cerebellar ataxia, hypertrophic peripheral neuropathy, deafness, hypotonia, MR	Ichthyosis (50%), bone disease, ECG changes	—
	Bassen-Kornzweig syndrome	Prog. external o'plegia, ret. pig. degen., night blindness, angioid streaks	Ataxia, spinocerebellar degen., PMR, peripheral neuropathy	Malabsorption (steatorrhea), low serum lipids, acanthocytosis of RBCs, cardiac abn	PEO onset 5–10 yr; rare, early death; dcsd. ERG
	Sjögren-Larson syndrome	Mac. lessons, RP	MR, spastic paresis, seizures	Ichthyosis, short stature, abn. of hair and teeth, skeletal dysplasia	—
Bull's-Eye Maculopathy	SYSTEMIC DISEASES, NEURAL DISORDERS				
	Olivoponto- cerebellar atrophy (OPCA)	RP, OA, abn. Ems, o'plegia, cat.	Ataxia, dysarthria, rigidity, dementia, tremor		—
	Hallervorden- Spatz's syndrome	Ret. pig. degen., OA, yellow flecks	Dementia, spasticity, athetosis, dysarthr., ataxia		Onset 7–10 YO
	Dystonia blepharospasm pigmentary retinopathy	Ret. pig. degen. blepharospasm	dystonia		Dcsd. ERG
	LYSOSOMAL STORAGE DISORDERS				
	Fucosidosis (composite of types)	Tort. conj. and ret. vessels, cat., strab., corneal opacities, spider nevi of lid	PMR, dcsd. hearing	Angiokeratomas (like Fabry's), dysostosis, pulmonary infections, coarse facies	Chromosome 1, PND
	Neuronal ceroid lipofuscinoses	RP	Neuronal degeneration		See Chapter 21 Table 11
	Niemann-Pick's disease (composite of types)	CRS, OA, corneal clouding, cat., gaze palsies (vertical)	MR, PMR, seizures	Anemia, HSM, pulmonary infiltrates foam cells in marrow	PND
	IN DERMATOLOGIC DISORDERS				
	Sjörgren-Larsen's syndrome	Mac. lesions, RP, "glistening spots," myopia	MR, spastic paresis, seizures	Ichthyosis, short stature, abn. of hair and teeth skeletal dysplasia	—
	Ichthyosis	Crystalline retinopathy			
	TOXIC				
	Canthaxanthine	Crystalline retinop.			—
	Chloroquine				—

Ocular Finding	Clinical Presentation				
	Disorder	Other Ocular Signs	CNS	Systemic	Other
	Indomethacine				—
	PRIMARY OCULAR DISEASES				
	Congenital cone dystrophy				
	Bull's-eye macular dystrophy				
	RP (inverse, central)				
	Benign concentric maculopathy				
	Annular macular dystrophy				
	Stargardt's/fundus flavimaculatus				
	Central areolar macular dystrophy				
	Fenestrated sheen macular dystrophy				
Cherry Red Spot					
	Lysosomal storage diseases	See Chapter 21, Tables 8–11			
	CRAO				
	Macular hole (true, pseudo)				
	Trauma with posterior pole edema				
	Solar retinopathy				
	Macular hemorrhage				
Yellow Paramacular Flecks	Von Gierke's disease			HSM, short stature, xanthomas, bleeding diathesis	—

TABLE 23–10. DISORDERS AFFECTING THE OPTIC NERVE

Ocular Tissue Involved	Clinical Presentation				
	Disorder	**Other Ocular Signs**	**CNS**	**Systemic**	**Other**
Optic Atrophy[a]					
	HEREDOFAMILIAL				
	Autosomal dominant				
	Autosomal recessive		See Chapter 5		
	Leber optic neuropathy				
	Behr optic neuropathy				
	Lysosomal storage disease		See Chapter 21, Tables 8–11		
	MPS (all exc. Maroteaux-Lamy syndrome), MLS, sphingo-lipidosis; NCL				
	Hallervorden-Spatz syndrome	RP (25%), maculopap. flecks, bull's-eye		Neurol. deterior spasticity, athetosis, dyarthr., ataxia	—
	Dejerine-Sottas	EM, pupil abn.		Hypertrophic neuropathy	—
	Lipid metab. disorders: Refsum's disease	See Chapter 21, Table 7			
	DEAFNESS				
	Prog. OA and congen. deafness	Vis. loss progressive, later onset	Deafness—severe	AD	—
	OA, DM, and deafness	OA by 17 YO		AR	—
	OA, ataxia, and deafness (Sylvester's syndrome)		Ataxia, muscle wasting	AD	Onset 2 ½ YO
	Opticocochlear dentate degeneration	Vis. loss, infancy	MR, prog. spas. quadriplegia	AR	Death in childhood
	OA, polyneurop., deafness (Rosenberg-Chutorian syndrome)	VA dcsd. by 20 YO	Deafness, polyneurop., prog. hearing loss, ataxia, spasticity, MR	XLR/AR	—
	OA, diabetes insipidus, DM, deafness (DIDMOAD)		Deafness, DI, DM		—
	PHAKOMATOSES				
	Neurofibromatosis	Iris-Lisch nodules, ON, chiasm glioma, plexiform neuroma of orb. and lid, gl., pulsating exophthal., sphenoid bone changes, hypertrophic corneal nerves, MM of iris	Plexiform neuromas, meningiomas	Cut: axillary freckles café-au-lait spots (>5mm), plexiform neuromas	AD Incsd. nerve growth factor, R/O ON glioma

TABLE 23–10. DISORDERS AFFECTING THE OPTIC NERVE (*cont.*)

Ocular Tissue Involved	Clinical Presentation				
	Disorder	*Other Ocular Signs*	*CNS*	*Systemic*	*Other*
	Tuberous sclerosis	Ret. astrocytic hamartomas (90%)	Ca^{++}, MR, seizures, subependymal astrocytomas	adenoma, sebaceum 90% (angiofibromas)	Gene on chromosome 9
	Rubenstein-Taybi's syndrome				
	Laurence-Moon's syndrome	Ret. pig. degen.	Spastic paraplegia	Hypogonadism, polydactyly, obesity, hypogenitalism, cardiac anomalies, renal anom.	—
	Bardet-Biedl's syndrome	Ret. pig. degen., o'plegia (rarely)	Paraplegia, MR, misrouted VAP		
	Cockayne's syndrome	Cat., corneal dys., nystagmus, ret. pig. degen.	PMR, macroceph., extrapyr. signs, leucodystrophy	Dwarfism, premat. aging, derm. changes, photosensitivity, skeletal dysplasia	—
	DERMATOLOGIC DISORDERS				
	Incontinentia pigmenti	Retrolental mass, corneal opac., cat., strab., microp.	MR, seizures	Hyperpig. skin lesion, progress to blisters, growths; abn. dentition	—
	METABOLIC ABNORMALITIES				
	Homocystinuria	Ectopia lentis, gl., ret. pig. degen., myopia, RD	MR	Thromboembolism, osteoporosis, hypopigmentation, pulmonary and aortic stenosis	—
	Hypophosphatasia (juvenile Paget's disease)	Band keratopathy, proptosis, PE, spherophakia, blue sclera	Muscle weakness	Fine hair, met. acidosis, hyper Ca^{++}, craniostenosis, fragile bones	—
	Menke's syndrome	Ret. degen., iris cysts	Cerebellar signs	Steely, kinky hair; hypopigmentation; bone changes; arterial abn.; hypothermia	—

(*Continues*)

TABLE 23–10. DISORDERS AFFECTING THE OPTIC NERVE (*cont.*)

Ocular Tissue Involved	Clinical Presentation				
	Disorder	*Other Ocular Signs*	*CNS*	*Systemic*	*Other*
	SKULL AND BONE DISORDERS				
	Osteopetrosis (Albers-Schönberg disease)			Osteopetrosis	—
	Paget's disease	Angioid streaks, EOM palsies, choroidal sclerosis	Deafness		—
	Fibrous dysplasia	Proptosis, strab.		Albright's:café-au-lait spots, early epiphyseal closure	—
	Craniostenosis Craniodystosis Facial anomalies				
	Hypophosphatasia (juvenile Paget's disease)	Band keratopathy, proptosis, PE, spherophakia, blue sclera	Muscle weakness	Fine hair, met. acidosis, hyper Ca^{++}, craniostenosis, fragile bones	—
	Bassen-Kornzweig syndrome	Prog. external, o'plegia, ret. pig. degen. night blindness	Ataxia, spinocerebellar degen. PMR	Malabsorption (steatorrhea), low serum lipids, acanthocytosis of RBCs, cardiac abn.	—
	LCAT (lecithin/cholesterol acyltransferase deficiency)	Corneal deposits, arcus in heterozygote	Renal disease, anemia	Typical facies	—
	Zellweger's syndrome	Nystagmus, ret. pig. degen., cat.	Demyelin., hypotonia, seizures		—
	Behr's disease	Gaze abn., nystagmus, strab., supranuc.	PMR, chorea, spastic paresis, ataxia, movement disorder		—

*a*Optic atrophy is a common feature of paraneoplastic leucodystrophy, ret. dystrophies (primary and secondary), cranial stenosis, and other dysostoses.

TABLE 23–11. DISORDERS AFFECTING THE CHOROID

Type of Lesion Involved	Clinical Presentation				
	Disorder	*Other Ocular Signs*	*CNS*	*Systemic*	*Other*
Choroidal Atrophy:					
	PRIMARY OCULAR DISEASE				
	Malignant Myopia				
	Central choroidal Atrophy				
	Choroderemia				
	Other				
	Hyperomithinemia (gyrate atrophy of choroid)	myopia (90%) night blindness			
	Aicardi's syndrome	PSC cataracts (40%) gray disc lacunes scleral ectasia	inf. spasms severe MR absent corpus callosum other CNS anom.		
Chorioretinal Changes					
	Scars in: Toxoplasmosis; Epstein-Barr virus (EBV); histoplasmosis; toxocara, cytomegalovirus (CMV); Candida; Roth spots;				
	Syphilis—primary, secondary, congenital; Congen. rubella, subacute sclerosing panencephalitis (SSPE); Leprosy; onchocerosis; Loa Loa				
	Vitamin A deficiency				
	Vascular occlusions trauma high myopia toxic reactions				

BIBLIOGRAPHY

General

Aita JA. *Congenital Facial Anomalies With Neurologic Defects: A Clinical Atlas.* Springfield, IL: Thomas, 1969.

Behrman R, Vaughan VC III, Nelson WE, eds. *Textbook of Pediatrics.* 13th ed. Philadelphia: Saunders, 1987.

Geeraets WJ. *Ocular Syndromes.* Philadelphia: Lea & Febiger, 1969.

Gomez MR. *Neurocutaneous Diseases: A Practical Approach.* Boston: Butterworths, 1987.

Mausolf FA, ed. *The Eye and Systemic Disease.* 2nd ed. St. Louis: Mosby, 1980.

McKusick VA. *Mendelian Inheritance in Man: Catalog of Autosomal Dominant, Autosomal Recessive, and X-Linked Phenotypes.* 8th ed. Baltimore: Johns Hopkins, 1988.

Nyhan WL, Sakati NA. *Diagnostic Recognition of Genetic Disease.* Philadelphia: Lea & Febiger, 1987.

Renie WA. *Goldberg's Genetic and Metabolic Eye Disease.* 2nd ed. Boston: Little, Brown, 1986.

Rosa PA, Schwan TG. A specific and sensitive assay for the Lyme disease spirochete *Borrelia burgdorferi* using the polymerase chain reaction. *J. Infect. Dis.* 1989; 160: 1018–1029.

Scriver C, et al., eds. *The Metabolic Basis of Inherited Disease.* 6th ed. New York: McGraw-Hill, 1989.

Vinken PJ, Bruyn GW. Neuroretinal degeneration. In: *Handbook of Clinical Neurology.* New York: American Elsevier, 1972; 13.

Ocular Spots and Myxomas

Kennedy RH, Waller RR, Carney JA. Ocular pigmented spots and eyelid myxomas. *Am J Ophthalmol.* 1987; 104: 533–538.

Ataxia Telangiectasia

Schindler D, et al. Screening test for ataxia telangiectasia. *Lancet.* 1988; 2:1398–1399. Letter.

Neurofibromatosis

Barker D, Wright E, Nguyen K. Gene for VRNF is in the pericentromeric region of chromosome 17. *Science.* 1987; 236:1100–1102.

National Institutes of Health consensus development conference. Neurofibromatosis: Conference statement. *Arch Neurol.* 1988; 45:575–578.

Neuronal Ceroid Lipofuscinosis

Berkovic SF, et al. Kuf's Disease: A clinical reappraisal. *Brain.* 1988; 111:27–62.

Brod RD, Packer AJ, Van Dyck HJL. Diagnosis of neuronal ceroid lipofuscinosis by ultrastructural examination of peripheral blood lymphocytes. *Arch Ophthalmol.* 1987; 105:1388–1393.

François J. Metabolic tapetoretinal degeneration. *Surv Ophthalmol.* 1982;26: 293–333.

Metal Metabolism

Hoogenbaad TH, Van Hattum J. Zinc therapy as the initial treatment for Wilson's disease. *Arch Neurol.* 1988; 45: 378–488. Letter.

Naidu S, et al. Mitochondrial enzyme defects in kinky hair disease. *Neuropaed.* 1988; 19:46–48.

Amino Acid Metabolism

Cole GF, et al. Cognitive functioning in albino children. *Dev Med Child Neurol.* 1987; 29:659–665.

Infections

Macdonald AB. Lyme disease: A neuro-ophthalmic/neurologic view. *J Clin Neuro-ophthalmol.* 1987; 7:185–190.

Macdonald AB. Lyme Disease and its neurological complications. *Arch Neurol.* 1988; 45: 99–104.

Spoor TC, et al. Ocular syphilis 1986: Prevalance of FTA-Abs Reactivity and CSF fluid findings. *J Clin Neuro-ophthalmol.* 1987; 7; 191–195.

Mitochondrial Inheritance Disorders

Zeviani M, et al. Deletions of mitochondrial DNA in Kearns-Sayre syndrome. *Neurology.* 1988;38: 1339–1346.

Peroxisomal Disorders

Moser HW. The peroxisome: Nervous system role of a previously underrated organelle. *Neurology.* 1988; 38: 1617–1627.

Paraneoplastic Disorders

Furneaux HM, Rosenblum MC, et al. Selective expression of Purkinje-cell antigens in tumor tissue from patients with paraneoplastic cerebellar degeneration. *N Engl J Med.* 1990; 322:1844–1851.

INDEX

Abducens nerve. *See also* Sixth
  nerve disorders
  anatomy of, 205, 207*f*
  in cavernous sinus, 201*f*, 206
  congenital absence, 206
  fasciculus, 193
  nuclei of, 175–9, 189, 193, 197,
    205, 219
  in orbit, 269
  palsies of, 205–208
    benign, 206
    vs. divergence palsy, 206
    in Duane's retraction syndrome,
      205
    etiology of, 207*t*, 208*t*
    evaluation associated with, 208
    following lumbar puncture, 205
    Horner's syndrome in, 251
    in nasopharyngeal carcinoma,
      145
    prognosis of, 206–207
    pseudo 192, 241
      in esotropia, 228
      in spasm of near reflex, 228
      in temporal bone fracture, 209
    treatment of, 207–208
  in superior orbital fissure, 265, 269
Abducting nystagmus. *See also* Medial longitudinal fasciculus,
  internuclear ophthalmoplegia,
  182, 217, 220
Aberrant regeneration. *See also* Synkinesis, misdirection
  oculomotor nerve, 199
  fascial nerve, 256
Abetalipoproteinemia, 351, 352*t*–

Page numbers followed by *t* or *f* indicate
tables or figures, respectively

363*t*, 388–389. *See also*
  Bassen-Kornzweig syndrome
  pigmentary retinopathy in, 432*t*
Abscess, pituitary, 143
AC/A ratio, in accommodative es-
  otropia, 233–234. *See also* Cy-
  loplegia
Accessory optic tract, 9
Accommodation, 197, 239, 248, 249
  in diphtheria, 209, 210, 250
  increased in Horner's Syndrome,
    250
  and vergence, 177
Accommodative esotropia, 228–229
  AC/A ratio in, 233–234
Acetyl-CoA oxidase deficiency,
  386*t*–387*t*
Acoustic nerve. *See* Eighth nerve
Acoustic neurinoma, 263, 348
Acoustic neurofibromatosis, bilateral,
  345–348
Acquired immunodeficiency syn-
  drome (AIDS), 73, 80, 94. *See
  also* Human Immunodefi-
  ciency Virus
Acrodermatitis enteropathia, 413*t*
Acromegaly, 138, 140. *See also* Pituitary adenoma
ACTH secretion by pituitary tumors,
  140
Acute hemorrhage conjunctivitis, 382
Acute posterior multifocal placoid
  pigment epitheliopathy, 95
Acyl-CoA oxidase deficiency, 352*t*–
  353*t*
Adduction lag, 185. *See also* intranuclear ophthalmoplegia, MLF
  syndrome.
Adenoid cystic carcinoma of lacrimal gland, 289

Adenoma pituitary, 138–142, 140*t*.
    See also Pituitary Adenoma
  hemorrhage into, and pituitary ap-
    oplexy, 143
  management of, 141–142
Adenoma sebaceum, 348, 409*t*
Adenomatous polyposis, 95
Adie's pupil, 241, 243, 249–250,
    270
  acute, 250
  evaluation of, 245*t*, 249
  pharmacologic test for, 250
Adie's syndrome, 250
Adrenoleukodystrophy, 122, 384*t*–
    385*t*
  neonatal, 398*t*–399*t*
    cataract in, 426*t*
    retina in, 433*t*
  X-linked recessive, 352*t*–353*t*
Adrenoleukomyeloneuropathy, 352*t*–
    353*t*, 386*t*–387*t*
Adrenomyeloneuropathy, 122, 384*t*–
    385*t*
Afferent papillary defect. *See also*
  Marcus Gunn pupil, 34, 242
Afferent visual pathway, system,
    1–25. *See also* Visual afferent
    pathway
Aging, premature, 374*t*–375*t*, 402*t*–
    403*t*, 408*t*
Agnosia, 149
Agraphia, 148, 149
Aicardi's syndrome, 96*t*, 390*t*–391*t*
  choroidal atrophy in, 449*t*
AIDS, retinal vascular changes in, 80
Air embolus, 75. *See also* emboli
Alagille's syndrome
  coloboma in, 425*t*
  glaucoma in, 414*t*, 422*t*
  retina in, 436*t*

451

Page numbers followed by t or f indicate tables or figures, respectively

Antidepressants
  affecting eye movements, 195t
  affecting prolactin levels or lactation, 142t
  affecting pupil, 241t
  hallucinations from, 167t
  in migraine prophylaxis, 315t
Antihistamines, affecting pupil, 241t
Antiinflammatory drugs in migraine prophylaxis, 315t
Antimalarial agents, hallucinations from, 167t
Antimony, optic neuropathy from, 131t
Antiphospholipid antibodies in retinal vascular occlusion, 80
Anton's syndrome, 149
AO-HRR color plates, 34, 332
Apert's syndrome, 327t–373t, 415t
Apoplexy
  occipital, 150, 313, 326
  pituitary, 143
    painful ophthalmoplegia in, 323t
Apraxia, oculomotor, 189–190, 190f
  acquired, 190
  congenital, 189–190
Aqueduct of Sylvius, 197, 247
  block, 202
Arcus, corneal, in hyperlipoproteinemia, 351, 413t
Arachnoid cyst sellar, 142
Areflexia, 209, 250
Argyll Robertson pupil, 243, 247–248, 249f
  evaluation of, 245t
Arnold Chiari malformation, 224, 250
  and downbeat nystagmus, 220
Arsenic, optic neuropathy from, 131t
Artane, affecting pupil, 241t
Arterial occlusion, retinal, 75–76
Arterial spasm, retinal, 81
Arteriohepatic syndrome. See Alagille's syndrome
Arteriolar spasm, retinal, 81, 81t
Arteriovenous malformation, 20
  bleeding, 326
  differential diagnosis vs. migraine, 150, 313
  occipital, 150
  in Wyburn-Mason syndrome, 350
Arteritis, temporal, 317–320. See also Temporal arteritis
  arterior ischemic optic neuropathy in, 113–116
  and the orbit, 285
Arthrogryposis multiplex congenita, 371t
Ash leaf spot, 348
Aspartyl glycosoaminuria, 360t

Aspergillosis, 287. See also Mycosis
Asphyxiating thoracic dystrophy, 398t–399t
Aspidium, optic neuropathy from, 131t
Aspirin in migraine prophylaxis, 315t
Assymetric convergence, 194, 220
Astereoagnosia in parietal lobe lesions, 148
Astigmatism, 3
Astrocytic hamartomas, retinal and subependymal, in tuberous sclerosis, 348–349, 349f
Ataxia, 121, 209, 223, 313
Ataxias. See also individual disorder
  olivopontocerebellar, 388t–389t
  spinocerebellar, 388t–389t
Ataxia-telangiectasia (Louis-Bar's syndrome), 346t, 350, 388t–389t
  conjunctiva in, 412t
  skin in, 404t–405t
Atenolol in migraine prophylaxis, 315t
Atrophy
  choroidal, 96t, 449t
  gyrate, 96t
    in hyperornithinemia, 366t, 368f, 415t, 426t, 435t, 438t, 439t, 449t
  hemifacial, 372t–373t
    progressive, 424t
  olivopontocerebellar, bull's eye maculopathy in, 444t
  optic nerve, 54, 125–126, 446t
  in retinal nerve fiber layer, 89–94, 91f
Atropine sulfate, cycloplegia from, 242t
Atypical facial pain, 310
Auditory artery occlusion, vertigo in, 262t
Aura, 311. See also migraine seizures
Autoimmune neuropathy in cancer patients, 394t
  optic, 122
Automated perimetry, 51. See also visual field testing
Autonomic dysfunction, 329
  familial dysantonomia (Riley Day syndrome) 390–392
Autonomic nervous system. See parasympathic nervous system, sympathetic nervous system
Axoplasmic flow, 6, 9
  and optic disc swelling, 105
  retinal, 6
  stasis, 6, 7, 73
    and retinal opacity, 76, 94

Baclofen
  in blepharospasm, 260t
  hallucinations from, 167t
  In trigeminal neuralgia, 307t
Balint's syndrome, 149
Barbiturates
  affecting eye movements, 195t
  nystagmus from, 219
  optic neuropathy from, 130t
Bardet-Biedl syndrome, 390t–391t
  cataract in, 428t
  macular degeneration in, 443t
  microcornea in, 416t
  optic nerve in, 447t
  pigmentary retinopathy in, 433t
  renal disease in, 398t–399t
  retinal depigmentation in, 438t
  retinitis pigmentosa and deafness in, 437t
Basal cell nevus syndrome, 404t–405t, 410t
Basilar artery aneurysm, 144, 199
Basilar migraine, 312–313
Bassen-Kornzweig syndrome, 351, 352t–353t, 388t–389t
  cataract in, 426t
  macular degeneration in, 444t
  ophthalmoplegia in, 212
  optic nerve in, 448t
  pigmentary retinopathy in, 431t, 432t
Bear tracks sign in retinal pigment epithelium hypertrophy, 95, 95t
Behçet's syndrome
  conjunctivitis in, 412t
  iridocyclitis in, 424t
  retinal vascular changes in, 80
Behr's disease, 388t–389t, 448t
Behr's pupil, 147, 246
Bell's palsy, 256. See also Facial nerve palsies
Bell's phenomenon, 185–186, 192, 255
Benadryl, affecting pupil, 241t
Benedikt's syndrome, 198–199
Benign mixed tumor of lacrimal gland, 289
Benign paroxysmal positional vertigo, 261
Berardinelli-Siep syndrome, 374t–375t, 413t
Bergmeister's papilla, remnants of, 99
Beta blockers in migraine prophylaxis, 315t
Bielschowsky head-tilt test, 202, 231
Biemond's syndrome, 390t–391t
  pigmentary retinopathy in, 433t
Bietti crystalline corneal and retinal dystrophy, 439t

Page numbers followed by t or f indicate tables or figures, respectively

---

Page numbers followed by *t* or *f* indicate
tables or figures, respectively

Page numbers followed by *t* or *f* indicate
tables or figures, respectively